THE
PHYSICIANS'
AND
PHARMACISTS'
GUIDE
TO YOUR
MEDICINES

THE
PHYSICIANS'
AND
PHARMACISTS'
GUIDE
TO YOUR
MEDICINES

United States Pharmacopeial Convention

Ballantine Books • New York

Library of Congress Cataloging in Publication Data

United States Pharmacopeial Convention.
  The physicians' and pharmacists' guide to your medicines.

  Abstracted from the 1981 USP dispensing information.
  Includes index.
  1. Drugs—Side effects. 2. Drugs—Safety measures. 3. Drug utilization. I. Title. [DNLM: 1. Drugs—Popular works. 2. Pharmacology—Popular works. QV 55 U66p]
  RM302.5.U54 1981   615.5′8   80-70522
  ISBN 0-345-29724-5
  ISBN 0-345-29635-4 (pbk.)

Manufactured in the United States of America

Contents

The Physicians' and Pharmacists' Guide to Your Medicines

To The Reader

When purchasing a medicine, whether over-the-counter (nonprescription) or with a doctor's prescription, you may have questions about its usefulness to you, the best way to take it, possible side effects, and advisable precautions. For instance, some medicines should be taken with meals, others between meals. Some may make you drowsy while others may tend to keep you awake. Alcoholic or other beverages, other medicines, certain foods, or smoking may affect the way your medicine works. As for side effects, some are merely bothersome and may go away while others may require medical attention.

The Physicians' and Pharmacists' Guide to Your Medicines contains information which may provide general answers to some of your questions as well as suggestions for the correct use of your medicine. *It is important to remember, however, that medicines are complex and may act differently on different people. If you feel that you need additional information about your medicine or its possible side effects, ask your doctor, nurse, or pharmacist. They are there to help you.*

ORGANIZATION OF INFORMATION: *The Physicians' and Pharmacists' Guide to Your Medicines* contains a section of general information about the correct use of any medicine, as well as individual discussions of a wide variety of commonly and not so commonly used medicines. *You should read both the general information and the information specific to the medicine you are taking.* See page viii for this general information.

Each medicine appears under its generic rather than brand name. If you already know the generic name of your medicine, you can find it listed in alphabetic order beginning on page 1. If not, look in the index starting on page 503. Common brand names are given in the index also. It is a good idea for you to learn both the generic and brand names of your medicine and even to write them down and keep them for future use.

Information for each medicine is divided according to the area of the body which is affected. For example, some common divisions used are:

SYSTEMIC—For general effects throughout the body; applies to most medicines when taken by mouth or given by injection.

TOPICAL—For local effects when applied directly to the skin.

NASAL—For local effects when used in the nose.

OPHTHALMIC—For local effects when applied directly to the eyes.

OTIC—For local effects when used in the ear.

RECTAL—For local effects when used in the rectum.

VAGINAL—For local effects when used in the vagina.

As a general rule, information for one type of use will not be the same as for other types of use. Thus, if you take tetracycline capsules by mouth for their systemic effect in treating an infection, the information will not be the same as for tetracycline ointment which is applied directly to the skin for its topical effects.

NOTICE: The information about the drugs contained herein is general in nature and is not intended to replace specific instructions or directions or warnings given to you by your physician or other prescriber or accompanying a particular product. The information is selective and it is not claimed that it includes all known precautions, contraindications, effects, or interactions possibly related to the use of a drug. The information may differ from that contained in official product labeling required by law. The information is not sufficient to make an evaluation as to the risks and benefits of taking a particular drug in a particular case or to provide medical advice for individual problems and should not alone be relied upon for these purposes. Since the inclusion or exclusion of particular information about a drug is judgmental in nature and since opinion as to drug usage may differ, you may wish to consult additional sources. Should you desire additional information or if you have any questions as to how this information may relate to you in particular, ask your doctor, pharmacist, or other health care provider.

Since previously unreported side effects, newly recognized precautions, or other new information for any given drug may come to light at any time, continuously updated drug information sources should be consulted as necessary. Please be advised that USPC makes available on subscription a newsletter providing substantive corrections and selected updates on the information contained in this volume (see page 522 for subscribing information).

There are many brands of drugs on the market. The listing of selected brand names is intended only for ease of reference. The inclusion of a brand name does not mean the USPC has any particular knowledge that the brand listed has properties different from other brands of the same drug, nor should it be interpreted as an endorsement by the USPC. Similarly, the fact that a particular brand has not been included does not indicate that the product has been judged to be unsatisfactory or unacceptable.

If any of the information in this book causes you special concern, do not decide against taking any medicine prescribed for you without first checking with your doctor.

ABOUT USP: The information in this volume is prepared by the United States Pharmacopeial Convention, Inc. (USPC). This is the same body that sets the official standards of strength, quality, purity, packaging, and labeling for medical products used in the United States.

The United States Pharmacopeial Convention is an independent, non-profit corporation composed of representatives from accredited colleges of medicine and pharmacy in the U.S.; state medical and pharmaceutical associations; many national associations concerned with medicines, such as the American Medical Association, the American Nurses Association, the American Dental Association, and the American Pharmaceutical Association; and various departments of the federal government, including the Food and Drug Administration. It was established over 150 years ago, and is the only national body that represents the professions of both pharmacy and medicine.

The first convention came into being on January 1, 1820, and within the year published the first national drug formulary of the United States. The U.S. Pharmacopeia of 1820 contained 217 drug names, divided into two groups according to the level of general acceptance and usage.

When Congress passed the first major drug safety law in 1906, the standards recognized by that statute were those set forth in the United States Pharmacopeia and in the National Formulary. Today, the USP and NF continue to be the official U.S. compendia for standards for drugs and for the inactive ingredients in drug dosage forms. The United States Pharmacopeia is now the world's oldest regularly revised pharmacopeia and is generally accepted as being the best.

The work of the USPC is carried out by the Committee of Revision. This committee of experts is elected by the Convention and currently consists of 83 outstanding physicians, pharmacists, dentists, nurses, chemists, and other individuals particularly qualified to judge the merits of drugs and the standards and information that should apply to them. Committee members serve without pay and are assisted by numerous advisory panels, other outside reviewers, and USPC staff.

USP DISPENSING INFORMATION: The information contained in *The Physicians' and Pharmacists' Guide to Your Medicines* is extracted from *USP Dispensing Information* (USP DI).

Three years in the making, USP DI was first published in 1980. It is a continuously reviewed and revised base of drug information intended for use by prescribers, dispensers, and consumers of medications. The information is developed by the consensus of the USP Committee of Revision and its Advisory Panels and anyone, including ordinary citizens, may contribute through review and comment on drafts of the monographs published in *USP DI Review*.

For further information about USP DI or if you have any comments as to how the information published in this volume might better meet your information needs, please contact:
    USP Drug Information Division
    12601 Twinbrook Parkway
    Rockville, Maryland   20852
    (301)881-0666

For your own safety, health, and well-being, it is important that you learn about your medicines. The information that follows is general in nature and applies to the use of any medicine. This information must be supplemented with the drug-specific information which is found in the individual listings of this book.

● *Tell your doctor and pharmacist about any medical problems you may have and all medicines you are now taking or have taken in the past few weeks.* Don't forget over-the-counter (nonprescription) medicines such as aspirin, laxatives, and antacids.

● Before having any kind of surgery (including dental surgery) or emergency treatment, tell the doctor or dentist in charge about any medicine you are taking.

● Tell your doctor and pharmacist if you have ever had an allergic or unusual reaction to any medicine.

● Most medicines contain more than their active ingredient. If you are on a low-salt, low-sugar, or any other special diet, or if you are allergic to any substance, such as yellow dye, before taking any medicine check with your doctor or pharmacist about what is contained in it.

● *If you are pregnant or if you plan to become pregnant, check with your doctor before taking any medicine.* Certain medicines may cause birth defects or other problems in the unborn child. For other medicines, safe use during pregnancy has not been established. *The use of any medicine during pregnancy must be carefully considered.*

● *If you are breast-feeding a baby, check with your doctor before taking any medicine.* Some medicines may pass into the breast milk and cause unwanted effects in the infant.

● Take medicine exactly as directed, at the right time, and for the full length of time prescribed by your doctor. If you are using an over-the-counter (nonprescription) medicine, follow the directions on the label, unless otherwise directed by your doctor. If you feel that your medicine is not working for you, check with your doctor.

● *Keep all medicines out of the reach of children.*

● Child-proof caps on most prescription medicines for oral use are required by law. However, if there are no children in your home, and you find it hard to open such caps, you may ask your pharmacist for a regular, easier-to-open cap. He or she is authorized by law to furnish you with a regular cap if you request it.

● *How to store your medicine:* Store medicine away from bright light in a cool, dry place such as a kitchen cabinet or the bedroom, out of the reach of children. Do not store medicine in the bathroom, where it is too warm and humid, or in the refrigerator unless you are told to do so.

● Different medicines should never be mixed in one container. Always store your medicine in its original container, kept tightly capped when not in use. Do not remove the label since directions for use and other special information appear there.

● To avoid mistakes, do not take medicine in the dark. Always read the label before taking, noting especially the expiration date, if any, of the contents.

● *If you think you have taken an overdose of any medicine or if a child has taken a medicine by accident:* Call your poison control center or your doctor or pharmacist, at once. Keep those telephone numbers handy. Also, keep a bottle of Ipecac Syrup safely stored in your home in case you are told to cause vomiting. Read the directions on the label of Ipecac Syrup before using.

● If you notice unusual reactions or side effects while taking any medicine, check with your doctor or pharmacist.

● After your doctor has told you to stop taking a medicine, ask if you should save it for future use. If not, discard by flushing it down the toilet. *Never give your medicine to anyone else.* It has been prescribed for your personal medical problem and may not be the correct treatment for another person.

● It is a good idea for you to learn both the generic and brand names of your medicine and even to write them down and keep them for future use.

● Do not be embarrassed to ask questions about any medicine you are taking. To help you remember, it may be helpful to write down any questions you have and bring these questions with you on your next visit to your doctor or pharmacist. Also, if you want more information about your medicines, ask your doctor, nurse, or pharmacist.

● Remember that with many prescription refills, your pharmacist will have to first check with your doctor before he or she can refill it. Therefore, do not wait until you are completely out of your medicine before you have it refilled. This is especially important if you must take your medicine every day. Also, give your pharmacist enough advance notice so that you will not have to wait.

Members of the Subcommittee who served as Chairman or Co-Chairmen are listed first

Panel on Allergy, Immunology, and Connective Tissue Disease—ALBERT L. SHEFFER, M.D., Boston, Mass.; RONALD ANDERSON, M.D., Boston, Mass.; DOMINGO M. AVIADO, M.D., Morristown, N.J.; ELLIOTT ELLIS, M.D., Buffalo, N.Y.; DAVID P. JACOBUS, M.D., Princeton, N.J.; STEPHEN R. KAPLAN, M.D., Providence, R.I.; JAMES R. KLINENBERG, M.D., Los Angeles, Calif.; DANIEL J. STECHSCHULTE, M.D., Kansas City, Kans.; MARTIN D. VALENTINE, M.D., Baltimore, Md.

Panel on Analgesics, Sedatives, and Anti-inflammatory Agents—WILLIAM T. BEAVER, M.D., Washington, D.C.; JOHN BAUM, M.D., Rochester, N.Y.; J. WELDON BELLVILLE, M.D., Los Angeles, Calif.; THOMAS G. KANTOR, M.D., New York, N.Y.; WILLIAM R. MARTIN, M.D., Lexington, Ky.; WILLIAM M. O'BRIEN, M.D., Charlottesville, Va.; ANTHONY S. RIDOLFO, M.D., PH.D., Indianapolis, Ind.; NAOMI ROTHFIELD, M.D., Farmington, Conn.; WALTER L. WAY, M.D., San Francisco, Calif.; MURRAY WEINER, M.D., Cincinnati, Ohio.

Panel on Anesthesiology—ARTHUR S. KEATS, M.D., Houston, Texas; J. WELDON BELLVILLE, M.D., Los Angeles, Calif.; BURNELL R. BROWN, JR., M.D., Tucson, Ariz.; WALTER L. WAY, M.D., San Francisco, Calif.

Panel on Cardiovascular Drugs—DANIEL L. AZARNOFF, M.D., Chicago, Ill.; KARL ENGELMAN, M.D., Philadelphia, Pa.; EDWARD D. FROHLICH, M.D., New Orleans, La.; KEITH L. MacCANNELL, M.D., PH.D., Calgary, Alberta, Canada; ALBERT J. WASSERMAN, M.D., Richmond, Va.; STEVEN WOLFSON, M.D., New Haven, Conn.

Panel on Dentistry—SAMUEL V. HOLROYD, D.D.S., St. Louis, Mo.; SEBASTIAN G. CIANCIO, D.D.S., Buffalo, N.Y.; ALFRED E. CIARLONE, D.D.S., Augusta, Ga.; TOMMY W. GAGE, D.D.S., Dallas, Texas; JOHN J. LYTLE, D.D.S., Glendale, Calif.; H.D. MILLARD, D.D.S., Ann Arbor, Mich.

Panel on Dermatology—JOHN J. VOORHEES, M.D., Ann Arbor, Mich.; DAVID R. BICKERS, M.D., Cleveland, Ohio; HOWARD DUBIN, M.D., Ann Arbor, Mich.; THOMAS B. FITZPATRICK, M.D., PH.D., Boston, Mass.; JOHN HANIFIN, M.D., Portland, Ore.; HENRY JOLLY, M.D., New Orleans, La.; JOHN A. KENNEY, M.D., Washington, D.C.; EDMUND KLEIN, M.D., Buffalo, N.Y.; JOHN MAIZE, M.D., Buffalo, N.Y.; MILTON ORKIN, M.D., Minneapolis, Minn.; ANDREW H. RUDOLPH, M.D., Houston, Texas; ALAN SHALITA, M.D., Brooklyn, N.Y.; MAREK STAWISKI, M.D., Ann Arbor, Mich.; RICHARD STOUGHTON, M.D., San Diego, Calif.; WILLIAM B. TAYLOR, M.D., Ann Arbor, Mich.; EUGENE VAN SCOTT, M.D., Philadelphia, Pa.

Panel on Diagnostic Agents (Non-radioactive) and Radiological Contrast Media—HARRY W. FISCHER, M.D., Rochester, N.Y.; FRANCIS BURGENER, M.D., Rochester, N.Y.; STEVEN H. CORNELL, M.D., Iowa City, Iowa; DANIEL KIMBERG, M.D., New York, N.Y.; P. RUBEN KOEHLER, M.D., Salt Lake City, Utah; ELLIOTT C. LASSER, M.D., San Diego, Calif.; ROSCOE MILLER, M.D., Indianapolis, Ind.; MANUEL VIAMONTE, M.D., Miami, Fla.

Panel on Electrolytes, Large-volume Parenterals, and Renal Drugs—ROBERT D. LINDEMAN, M.D., Louisville, Ky.; JACK W. COBURN, M.D., Los Angeles, Calif.; LAURENCE FINBERG, M.D., Bronx, N.Y.; STUART A. KLEIT, M.D., Indianapolis, Ind.; JOHN F. MAHER, M.D., Farmington, Conn.; CARLOS A. VAAMONDE, M.D., Miami, Fla.; DONALD G. VIDT, M.D., Cleveland, Ohio.

Panel on Endocrinology—EDWIN D. BRANSOME, JR., M.D., Augusta, Ga.; LOUIS V. AVIOLI, M.D., St. Louis, Mo.; SALVADOR CASTELLS, M.D., Brooklyn, N.Y.; LESLIE J. DEGROOT, M.D., Chicago, Ill.; KARL ENGELMAN, M.D., Philadelphia, Pa.; ARTHUR L. HERBST, M.D., Chicago, Ill.; OLOF H. PEARSON, M.D., Cleveland, Ohio; GERALD M. REAVEN, M.D., Palo Alto, Calif.

Panel on Gastroenterology and Nutrition—DAVID H. LAW, M.D., Albuquerque, N.M.; LLOYD BRANDBORG, M.D., San Francisco, Calif.; COLONEL JOHN E. CANHAM, M.D., Presidio of San Francisco, Calif.; MURRAY DAVIDSON, M.D.,

xiii

ALASKA

Alaska Pharmaceutical Association: Jacqueline L. Warren,*
10902 Howland Drive, Reston, VA 22091.

ARIZONA

University of Arizona, College of Medicine: Thomas F. Burks,
Ph.D., Professor & Head, Dept. of Pharmacology, Univ. of
Arizona, College of Medicine, Tucson, AZ 85724.
Arizona Medical Association: Gerald C. Moczynsk, M.D.,
6036 N. 19th Ave., Suite 206, Phoenix, AZ 85015.

ARKANSAS

University of Arkansas College of Medicine: William Y.
Au, M.D., Dept. of Pharmacology, Univ. of Arkansas College
of Medicine, 4301 West Markham, Little Rock, AR 72205.
University of Arkansas Medical Sciences Campus, College of Pharmacy: James R. McCowan, Ph.D.,* College of Pharmacy,
University of Arkansas Medical Sciences Campus, 4301 West
Markham, Little Rock, AR 72205.
Arkansas Pharmacists Association: Marcus Jordin, R.Ph.,
Ph.D.,* Prof. of Pharmacology, Univ. of Arkansas, School of
Pharmacy, 4301 West Markham, Little Rock, AR 72205.

CALIFORNIA

University of California, Davis School of Medicine: Larry G.
Stark, Ph.D.,* Dept. of Pharmacology, 4453 M.S.I-A, School
of Medicine, University of Calif., Davis, CA 95616.
University of California, Los Angeles, School of Medicine:
Matthew E. Conolly, M.D.,* Dept. of Pharmacology, UCLA
School of Medicine, Center for Health Science, Room 23-150,
Los Angeles, CA 90024.
University of California, San Diego, School of Medicine: Philip
O. Anderson, Pharm.D.,* Director, Drug Information Service, University of California, Medical Center, 225 Dickinson
St., (H-765), San Diego, CA 92103.
University of California, San Francisco, School of Medicine:
Walter L. Way, M.D.,* Dept. of Anesthesia, UCSF School of
Medicine, 513 Parnassus Ave., Rm. 436, San Francisco,
CA 94143.
University of California, School of Pharmacy: Robert L. Day,
Pharm.D.,* School of Pharmacy, University of California,
San Francisco, CA 94143.
University of the Pacific, School of Pharmacy: Charles W.
Roscoe, Ph.D.,* 2444 River Dr., Stockton, CA 95211.
California Pharmacists Association: Max Stollman,* 8314
Wilshire Blvd., Beverly Hills, CA 90211.

COLORADO

University of Colorado, School of Pharmacy: Robert W.
Piepho, Ph.D., Box C238, UCHSC, 4200 East 9th Ave.,
Denver, CO 80262.
Colorado Pharmacal Association: Thomas G. Arthur, R.Ph.,
R.R. 2, Box 403, Conifer, CO 80433.

CONNECTICUT

University of Connecticut Health Center, School of Medicine:
Anthony J. Kubica, Pharm.D.,* Director of Pharmacy, Univ.
of Connecticut Health Center, Farmington, CT 06032.
Yale University, School of Medicine: Thomas R. Tritton,* Yale
University School of Medicine, 333 Cedar Street, New Haven,
CT 06510.
University of Connecticut, School of Pharmacy: Arthur E.
Schwarting, Ph.D.,* University of Connecticut, School of
Pharmacy, Storrs, CT 06268.
Connecticut State Medical Society: James E. O'Brien, M.D., 31
Surrey Drive, Wethersfield, CT 06109.
Connecticut Pharmaceutical Association: Henry A. Palmer,
Ph.D.,* 26 Timber Drive, Storrs, CT 06268.

DELAWARE

Medical Society of Delaware: Vincent DelDuca, Jr., M.D.,*
Suite 5, Professional Building, Wilmington, DE 19803.
Delaware Pharmaceutical Society: Charles H. Newman,* 736
Taunton Road, Wilmington, DE 19803.

DISTRICT OF COLUMBIA

Georgetown University, School of Medicine: Frank G.
Standaert, M.D., Professor & Chairman, Pharmacology,
Georgetown University School of Medicine, Washington,
DC 20007.
Howard University, College of Medicine: H. Lloyd Garvey,
Ph.D., Howard University, College of Medicine, 520 W St.,
N.W., Washington, DC 20059.
Howard University College of Pharmacy and Pharmacal Sciences:
Wendell T. Hill, Jr., Pharm.D.,* Howard University College
of Pharmacy & Pharmacal Sciences, 2300 - 4th Street, N.W.,
Washington, DC 20059.

FLORIDA

University of Florida, College of Medicine: Thomas F. Muther,
Ph.D.,* Box J-267 JHMHC, Gainesville, FL 32610.
University of Miami School of Medicine: Earl Brill, Dept. of
Pharmacology, University of Miami School of Medicine, P. O.
Box 016960, Miami, FL 33101.
University of South Florida, College of Medicine: Donn L.
Smith, M.D., Ph.D., Univ. of South Florida, Tampa,
FL 33612.
Florida A&M University, School of Pharmacy: Henry Lewis
III, Pharm.D.,* Florida A&M University, School of Pharmacy, Tallahassee, FL 32307.
University of Florida, College of Pharmacy: Michael A.
Schwartz, Ph.D.,* University of Florida, College of Pharmacy, Box J-4, JHMHC, Gainesville, FL 32610.
Florida Pharmacy Association: J. B. Powers, Florida Pharmacy Association, P. O. Box 960, Tallahassee, FL 32302.

GEORGIA

Medical College of Georgia, School of Medicine: Raymond R.
Ahlquist, Ph.D.,* Medical College of Georgia, 1120 15th
Street, Augusta, GA 30912.
Mercer University, Southern School of Pharmacy: Oliver M.
Littlejohn, Ph.D.,* Dean, Mercer Univ., Southern School of
Pharmacy, 345 Blvd., N.E., Atlanta, GA 30312.
University of Georgia, School of Pharmacy: Howard C. Ansel,
Ph.D.,* Dean, University of Georgia, School of Pharmacy,
Athens, GA 30602.
Medical Association of Georgia: Stanley P. Aldridge, M.D.,*
755 Columbia Dr., Decatur, GA 30030.
Georgia Pharmaceutical Association: Norman H. Franke,
Ph.D.,* 345 Boulevard, N.E., Atlanta, GA 30312.

HAWAII

University of Hawaii, John A. Burns School of Medicine: Bert
K. B. Lum, M.D., Ph.D., University of Hawaii, 1960 East
West Road, Honolulu, HI 96822.

IDAHO

Idaho State University, College of Pharmacy: Eugene I.
Isaacson, Ph.D.,* 1619 East Terry, Pocatello, ID 83201.
Idaho State Pharmaceutical Association: Rosemary S. Wells,*
1365 No. Orchard, Room 103, Boise, ID 83706.

ILLINOIS

The Chicago Medical School/University of Health Sciences:
Vel Nair, Ph.D., D.Sc.,* The Chicago Medical School, 2020
West Ogden Ave., Chicago, IL 60612.
Loyola University of Chicago, Stritch School of Medicine: Nae
J. Dun, Ph.D., Dept. of Pharmacology, Stritch School of
Medicine, 2160 S. First Ave., Maywood, IL 60153.
Northwestern University Medical School: George T. Okita,
Ph.D.,* Northwestern University Medical School, 303 E.
Chicago Ave., Chicago, IL 60611.
Pritzker School of Medicine, University of Chicago: David
Kornhauser, M.D., Chairman, Comm. on Pharmacy & Therapeutics, University of Chicago Hosp. & Clinics, 950 E. 59th
St., Chicago, IL 60637.
Rush Medical College of Rush University: Donald S.
Ebersman, Ph.D.,* Rush Medical College of Rush University,
1753 West Congress Parkway, Chicago, IL 60612.

Southern Illinois University, School of Medicine: Ronald A. Browning, Ph.D.,* Southern Illinois University School of Medicine, Carbondale, IL 62901.

University of Illinois, College of Medicine: Marten M. Kernis, Ph.D., Univ. of Illinois, College of Medicine, 1853 West Polk St., Room 131, Chicago, IL 60612.

University of Illinois, College of Pharmacy: Martin I. Blake, Ph.D.,* University of Illinois College of Pharmacy, 833 S. Wood St., Chicago, IL 60612.

Illinois State Medical Society: Joseph H. Skom, M.D.,* 55 East Monroe Street, Suite 3510, Chicago, IL 60603.

Illinois Pharmacists Association: Hillory Still,* 9750 Holy Cross Road, Fairview Heights, IL 62208.

INDIANA

Indiana University, School of Medicine: Lynn Roger Willis, Ph.D., Indiana University School of Medicine, 1100 West Michigan St., Indianapolis, IN 46223.

Butler University College of Pharmacy: Edward J. Rowe, Ph.D.,* Butler University College of Pharmacy, 4600 Sunset Ave., Indianapolis, IN 46208.

Purdue University, School of Pharmacy and Pharmacal Sciences: Adelbert M. Knevel, Ph.D.,* 62 Thise Court, Lafayette, IN 47905.

Indiana State Medical Association: Anthony S. Ridolfo, M.D.,* R.R. 1, Box 121, Zionsville, IN 46077.

Indiana Pharmacists Association: Dale W. Doerr, Ph.D.,* Butler University College of Pharmacy, 4600 Sunset Ave., Indianapolis, IN 46208.

IOWA

Drake University, College of Pharmacy: Wendell H. Southard, Ph.D.,* Drake University College of Pharmacy, 25th & University, Des Moines, IA 50311.

University of Iowa, College of Pharmacy: Dale E. Wurster, Ph.D.,* Dean, College of Pharmacy, The University of Iowa, Iowa City, IA 52242.

Iowa Pharmacists Association: Gale W. Stapp,* 606 North 10th Street, Oskaloosa, IA 52577.

KANSAS

University of Kansas, School of Medicine: Edward J. Walaszek, Ph.D.,* Dept. of Pharmacology, University of Kansas School of Medicine, 39th and Rainbow, Kansas City, KS 66103.

University of Kansas, School of Pharmacy: Larry A. Sternson, Ph.D., School of Pharmacy, The University of Kansas, Lawrence, KS 66045.

Kansas Medical Society: Wayne O. Wallace, Jr., M.D., 1301 North 3rd, Atchison, KS 66002.

Kansas Pharmacists Association: Roger Miller,* 503 Coronado, Bonner Springs, KS 66012.

KENTUCKY

University of Louisville, School of Medicine: Peter R. Rowell, Ph.D.,* Associate Professor, Dept. of Pharmacology, Univ. of Louisville, 500 South Preston St., Louisville, KY 40292.

University of Kentucky, College of Pharmacy: Howard Hopkins, Ph.D.,* 1020 Celia Lane, Lexington, KY 40504.

Kentucky Medical Association: E. C. Seeley, M.D.,* University of Kentucky, Dept. of Family Practice, 915 South Limestone, Lexington, KY 40536.

Kentucky Pharmacists Association: George W. Grider,* 230 West Lexington Ave., Danville, KY 40422.

LOUISIANA

Louisiana State University, School of Medicine in New Orleans: Paul L. Kirkendol, Ph.D., Pharmacology Dept., LSU Medical Center, 1100 Florida Ave., New Orleans, LA 70119.

Louisiana State University Medical Center: John W. Dailey, Ph.D.,* 9908 Village Green Dr., Shreveport, LA 71115.

Northeast Louisiana University, School of Pharmacy: Kenneth R. Shrader, Ph.D.,* School of Pharmacy, Northeast Louisiana University, Monroe, LA 71209.

Xavier University of Louisiana, College of Pharmacy: Ludmila Stass, Ph.D.,* Xavier University of Louisiana College of Pharmacy, 7325 Palmetto Street, New Orleans, LA 70125.

Louisiana State Medical Society: John Adriani, M.D.,* 67 N. Park Place, New Orleans, LA 70124.

Louisiana Pharmacists Association: Thomas Cerullo, J.D.,* 3701 Severn Ave., New Orleans, LA 70002.

MAINE

Maine Medical Association: Stephen A. Ross, M.D.,* Penobscot Bay Physicians Building, Glen Cove, Rockland, ME 04841.

MARYLAND

Johns Hopkins University, School of Medicine: David A. Blake, Ph.D.,* Director of Research Admin., The Johns Hopkins University S/M, 720 Rutland Ave., Baltimore, MD 21205.

Uniformed Services University of the Health Sciences, School of Medicine: Carl Peck, M.D., Dept. of Pharmacology, Uniformed Services Univ. of the Health Sciences School of Medicine, 4301 Jones Bridge Rd., Bethesda, MD 20014.

University of Maryland at Baltimore, School of Pharmacy: Ralph F. Shangraw, Ph.D.,* University of Maryland, School of Pharmacy, 636 W. Lombard St., Baltimore, MD 21201.

Medical & Chirurgical Faculty of the State of Maryland: Frederick H. Wilhelm, M.D., 5807 Annapolis Rd., Hyattsville, MD 20784.

Maryland Pharmaceutical Association: Paul Freiman,* 7504 Monita Rd., Baltimore, MD 21208.

MASSACHUSETTS

Harvard Medical School: Peter Goldman, M.D.,* Beth Israel Hospital, 330 Brookline Ave., Boston, MA 02215.

Tufts University, School of Medicine: Edward L. Decker, Pharm.D., 171 Harrison Ave., Box 420, Boston, MA 02111.

University of Massachusetts Medical Center: Brian Johnson, M.D., University of Massachusetts Medical Center, 55 Lake Avenue North, Worcester, MA 01605.

Massachusetts College of Pharmacy and Allied Health Sciences: Sumner M. Robinson, Ph.D.,* Massachusetts College of Pharmacy & Allied Health Sciences, 179 Longwood Ave., Boston, MA 02115.

Northeastern University College of Pharmacy and Allied Health Professions: John L. Neumeyer, Ph.D.,* Northeastern University, College of Pharmacy & Allied Health Professions, 360 Huntington Ave., 211 Mugar, Boston, MA 02115.

Massachusetts State Pharmaceutical Association: George Narinian, R.Ph.,* 43 Avon Circle, Needham, MA 02194.

MICHIGAN

Michigan State University, College of Human Medicine: Theodore M. Brody, Ph.D., Chairman, Dept. of Pharmacology, College of Human Medicine, Michigan State University, East Lansing, MI 48824.

Wayne State University School of Medicine: Ralph Kauffman, M.D.,* 3901 Beaubien Blvd., Detroit, MI 48201.

Ferris State College, School of Pharmacy: Gerald W. A. Slywka, Ph.D.,* 7630 Crestview Dr., Reed City, MI 49677.

University of Michigan, College of Pharmacy: Ara G. Paul, Ph.D.,* Dean, College of Pharmacy, University of Michigan, Ann Arbor, MI 48109.

Wayne State University, College of Pharmacy and Allied Health Professions: Bhupendra Hajratwala, Ph.D.,* College of Pharmacy and Allied Health Professions, 515 HSB, Wayne State University, Detroit, MI 48202.

Michigan Pharmacists Association: Louis M. Sesti, Michigan Pharmacists Association, 815 N. Washington Ave., Lansing, MI 48906.

MINNESOTA

University of Minnesota Medical School: Frederick E. Shideman, M.D., Ph.D.,* 105 Millard Hall, University of Minnesota, Minneapolis, MN 55455.

University of Minnesota College of Pharmacy: Edward G. Rippie, Ph.D.,* College of Pharmacy, University of Minnesota, 128 Pleasant Street, S.E., Minneapolis, MN 54455.

Minnesota State Pharmaceutical Association: Arnold D. Delger,* 1533 Grantham Street, St. Paul, MN 55108.

MISSISSIPPI

University of Mississippi, School of Medicine: Fred W. McEwen, Jr., Ph.D.,* University of Mississippi School of Medicine, 2500 North State St., Jackson, MS 39216.
University of Mississippi, School of Pharmacy: Robert W. Cleary, Ph.D.,* School of Pharmacy, University of Mississippi, University, MS 38677.

MISSOURI

St. Louis University, School of Medicine: Andrew J. Lonigro, M.D.,* St. Louis VA Hospitals (J.C.), St. Louis, MO 63125.
University of Missouri-Kansas City, School of Medicine: David R. Rush, Pharm.D.,* Truman Medical Center-East, Little Blue & Lee's Summit Road, Kansas City, MO 64139.
Washington University, School of Medicine: H. Mitchell Perry, 1983 Karlin Drive, St. Louis, MO 63110.
University of Missouri-Kansas City, School of Pharmacy: Wayne M. Brown, Ph.D.,* School of Pharmacy, University of Missouri-Kansas City, Kansas City, MO 64110.
Missouri Pharmaceutical Association: Lawrence E. Schreiber, Jr., 2805 Newbridge Court, St. Louis, MO 63129.

MONTANA

University of Montana, School of Pharmacy and Allied Health Sciences: Donald H. Canham, Ph.D., School of Pharmacy, University of Montana, Missoula, MT 59812.
Montana State Pharmaceutical Association: Frank J. Davis,* 613 Beth Drive, Great Falls, MT 59405.

NEBRASKA

Creighton University, School of Medicine: John T. Elder, Jr., Ph.D.,* Professor and Acting Chairman of Pharmacology, Creighton University School of Medicine, 2500 California St., Omaha, NB 68178.
University of Nebraska, College of Medicine: Manuchair Ebadi, Ph.D., Chairman, Dept. of Pharmacology, University of Nebraska College of Medicine, 42nd & Dewey Ave., Omaha, NB 68105.
Creighton University, School of Pharmacy: James M. Crampton, Ph.D.,* 1512 N. 75 Ave., Omaha, NB 68114.
University of Nebraska, College of Pharmacy: David Newton, Ph.D., University of Nebraska College of Pharmacy, 42nd and Dewey Ave., Omaha, NB 68105.
Nebraska Pharmacists Association: Rex Higley, R.P.,* 3110 South 42nd St., Lincoln, NB 68506.

NEVADA

University of Nevada-Reno, School of Medicine: Emile C. VanRemoortere, M.D., Department of Pharmacology, Anderson Bldg., Reno, NV 89557.
Nevada State Medical Association: Richard G. Pugh, CAE, Executive Director, Nevada State Medical Association, 3660 Baker Lane, Reno, NV 89509.

NEW HAMPSHIRE

New Hampshire Pharmaceutical Association: William J. Lancaster,* Mary Hitchcock Hospital, Hanover, NH 03755.

NEW JERSEY

New Jersey Medical School - CMDNJ: George A. Condouris, Ph.D., New Jersey Medical School - CMDNJ, 100 Bergen St., Newark, NJ 07103.
Rutgers University, College of Pharmacy: Thomas Medwick, Ph.D.,* Rutgers University, College of Pharmacy, P. O. Box 789, Piscataway, NJ 08854.
Medical Society of New Jersey: Frank J. Malta, M.D., 7 Hospital Drive, Toms River, NJ 08753.
New Jersey Pharmaceutical Association: Jacob Eisen,* 1155 Corrinne Terrace, Mountainside, NJ 07092.

NEW MEXICO

University of New Mexico, College of Pharmacy: Carman A. Bliss, Ph.D.,* University of New Mexico, College of Pharmacy, Albuquerque, NM 87131.

NEW YORK

Albany Medical College of Union University: David B. Ludlum, M.D., Dept. of Medicine, Albany Medical College of Union University, 47 New Scotland Ave., Albany, NY 12208.
Albert Einstein College of Medicine of Yeshiva University: George C. Escher, M.D.,* Dept. of Surgery, Box 126, Hospital of the Albert Einstein College of Medicine, 1825 Eastchester Rd., Bronx, NY 10461.
Columbia University College of Physicians and Surgeons: Joseph H. Graziano, Ph.D., Babies Hospital, 3959 Broadway BHA-B-19, New York, NY 10032.
Cornell University Medical College: Marcus M. Reidenberg, M.D., Cornell University Medical College, 1300 York Avenue, New York, NY 10021.
State University of New York at Buffalo, School of Medicine: Robert J. McIsaac, Ph.D.,* 127 Farber Hall, State Univ. of NY at Buffalo, School of Medicine, Buffalo, NY 14214.
State University of New York Downstate Medical Center: Julius Belford, Ph.D.,* SUNY Downstate Medical Center, 450 Clarkson Ave., Brooklyn, NY 11203.
State University of New York at Stony Brook, School of Medicine: Arthur P. Grollman, M.D.,* Dept. of Pharmacology, HSC, SUNY at Stony Brook, Stony Brook, NY 11794.
University of Rochester Medical Center: Michael Weintraub, M.D.,* University of Rochester Medical Center, 601 Elmwood Avenue, Rochester, NY 14642.
Albany College of Pharmacy: Walter Singer, Ph.D.,* 5 Barry Court, Loudonville, NY 12211.
Arnold & Marie Schwartz College of Pharmacy and Health Sciences: John J. Sciarra, Ph.D.,* Executive Dean, Arnold and Marie Schwartz College of Pharmacy and Health Sciences of Long Island University, 75 DeKalb Avenue at University Plaza, Brooklyn, NY 11201.
St. John's University, College of Pharmacy and Allied Health Professions: Andrew J. Bartilucci, Ph.D.,* Dean, St. John's University College of Pharmacy and Allied Health Professions, Jamaica, NY 11439.
Medical Society of the State of New York: Alfred A. Angrist, M.D., Medical Society of the State of New York, 420 Lakeville Road, Lake Success, NY 11042.

NORTH CAROLINA

Bowman Gray School of Medicine of Wake Forest University: James Maxwell Little, Ph.D.,* Bowman Gray School of Medicine, 300 S. Hawthorne Road, Winston-Salem, NC 27103.
University of North Carolina, School of Medicine: Svein U. Toverud, D.M.D., Dr. Odont.,* University of North Carolina, Dept. of Pharmacology, Dental Research Center 210H, Chapel Hill, NC 27514.
University of North Carolina at Chapel Hill, School of Pharmacy: Raymond Jang, Ph.D.,* School of Pharmacy, The University of North Carolina at Chapel Hill, Beard Hall 200 H, Chapel Hill, NC 27514.
North Carolina Medical Association: T. Reginald Harris, M.D.,* 808 Schenck Street, Shelby, NC 27611.

NORTH DAKOTA

North Dakota State University, College of Pharmacy: William B. Henderson, Ph.D.,* College of Pharmacy, North Dakota State University, Fargo, ND 58105.
North Dakota Pharmaceutical Association: William H. Shelver, Ph.D.,* 2948 Edgemont Street, Fargo, ND 58102.

OHIO

University of Cincinnati College of Medicine: Leonard T. Sigell, Ph.D.,* University of Cincinnati, College of Medicine, 231 Bethesda Ave., Room 7701 Bridge, Cincinnati, OH 45267.
Medical College of Ohio at Toledo: Robert D. Wilkerson, Ph.D., Dept. of Pharmacology & Therapeutics, Medical College of Ohio, C.S. #10008, Toledo, OH 43699.
Northeastern Ohio Universities, College of Medicine: J. Mark Braughler, Ph.D.,* Asst. Prof. of Pharmacology, Northeastern Ohio Universities College of Medicine, Rootstown, OH 44272.

The Ohio State University, College of Medicine: Joseph R. Bianchine, Ph.D., M.D.,* 333 West Tenth Ave., Columbus, OH 43210.

Wright State University, School of Medicine: John O. Lindower, M.D., Ph.D.,* 3301 Stonebridge, Kettering, OH 45419.

Ohio Northern University, College of Pharmacy and Allied Health Sciences: LeRoy D. Beltz, Ph.D.,* Dean, College of Pharmacy and Allied Health Sciences, Ohio Northern University, Ada, OH 45810.

Ohio State University, College of Pharmacy: Louis Malspeis, Ph.D.,* College of Pharmacy, Ohio State University, 500 West 12th Avenue, Columbus, OH 43210.

University of Cincinnati, College of Pharmacy: Latif S. Shenouda, Ph.D.,* University of Cincinnati, College of Pharmacy, Mail Location 4, Cincinnati, OH 45267.

University of Toledo, College of Pharmacy: Norman F. Billups, Ph.D.,* Dean, College of Pharmacy, University of Toledo, 2801 West Bancroft Street, Toledo, OH 43606.

Ohio State Pharmaceutical Association: J. Richard Wuest, Pharm.D.,* 2720 Topichills Drive, Cincinnati, OH 45211.

OKLAHOMA

Oral Roberts University, School of Medicine: Clinton N. Corder, M.D., Ph.D.,* Oral Roberts University School of Medicine, 7777 S. Lewis Ave., Tulsa, OK 74171.

Southwestern Oklahoma State University, School of Pharmacy: William G. Waggoner, Ph.D., School of Pharmacy, Southwestern Oklahoma State Univ., Weatherford, OK 73096.

University of Oklahoma, College of Pharmacy: Loyd V. Allen, Jr., Ph.D.,* Rt. 12, Box 160, Midwest City, OK 73115.

Oklahoma Pharmaceutical Association: Bernard G. Keller, Jr., Ph.D., P. O. Box 60304, Oklahoma City, OK 73146.

OREGON

University of Oregon Health Sciences Center, School of Medicine: Elton L. McCawley, M.S., Ph.D.,* Dept. of Pharmacology, School of Medicine of the University of Oregon Health Sciences Center, 3181 S.W. Sam Jackson Park Road, Portland, OR 97201.

Oregon Medical Association: Richard E. Lahti, M.D., P.C.,* 2350 S.W. Multnomah Blvd., Portland, OR 97219.

Oregon State Pharmaceutical Association: Mrs. Hallie L. Lahti,* 1601 S.E. Oak Shore Lane, Milwaukie, OR 97222.

PENNSYLVANIA

Hahnemann Medical College and Hospital of Philadelphia: Benjamin Calesnick, M.D.,* Hahnemann Medical College and Hospital of Philadelphia, 230 North Broad Street, Philadelphia, PA 19102.

The Medical College of Pennsylvania: Claire M. Lathers, Ph.D., Medical College of Pennsylvania, 3300 Henry Ave., Philadelphia, PA 19129.

Pennsylvania State University College of Medicine: John D. Connor, Ph.D., The Milton S. Hershey Medical Center, Hershey, PA 17033.

Temple University, School of Medicine: Charles A. Papacostas, Ph.D.,* Temple University School of Medicine, Dept. of Pharmacology, 3400 North Broad Street, Philadelphia, PA 19140.

University of Pennsylvania, School of Medicine: Winifred Angenent Koelle, M.D.,* Dept. of Pharmacology, Medical School/G3, University of Pennsylvania, Philadelphia, PA 19104.

The University of Pittsburgh, School of Medicine: Robert H. McDonald, Jr., M.D., Univ. of Pittsburgh School of Medicine, 448 Scaife Hall, Pittsburgh, PA 15261.

Duquesne University, School of Pharmacy: Joseph A. Feldman, Ph.D.,* Duquesne University School of Pharmacy, Pittsburgh, PA 15219.

Philadelphia College of Pharmacy and Science: Alfonso R. Gennaro, Ph.D.,* Philadelphia College of Pharmacy and Science, 43rd St., Woodland Ave., & Kingsessing Mall, Philadelphia, PA 19104.

Temple University, School of Pharmacy: Murray M. Tuckerman, Ph.D.,* The Philadelphian, 14A-11, 2401 Pennsylvania Ave., Philadelphia, PA 19130.

University of Pittsburgh, School of Pharmacy: Lewis W. Dittert, Ph.D.,* Dean, University of Pittsburgh School of Pharmacy, 1103 Salk Hall, Pittsburgh, PA 15261.

Pennsylvania Medical Society: Arthur Hull Hayes, Jr., M.D.,* The Milton S. Hershey Medical Center, Hershey, PA 17033.

Pennsylvania Pharmaceutical Association: Joseph A. Mosso, R.Ph.,* 319 Carolyn Avenue, Latrobe, PA 15650.

PUERTO RICO

University of Puerto Rico, College of Pharmacy: José A. Aponte, M.S., College of Pharmacy, University of Puerto Rico, G.P.O. Box 5067, San Juan, PR 00936.

RHODE ISLAND

University of Rhode Island, College of Pharmacy: Heber W. Youngken, Ph.D.,* College of Pharmacy, University of Rhode Island, Kingston, RI 02881.

Rhode Island Medical Society: Peter L. Mathieu, Jr., M.D., 255 Waterman Street, Providence, RI 02906.

Rhode Island Pharmaceutical Association: Leonard R. Worthen, Ph.D.,* College of Pharmacy, University of Rhode Island, Kingston, RI 02881.

SOUTH CAROLINA

Medical University of South Carolina, College of Medicine: James A. Richardson, Ph.D.,* Dept. of Pharmacology, M.U.S.C., 171 Ashley Avenue, Charleston, SC 29403.

University of South Carolina, School of Medicine: Thomas D. Derby, Ph.D., University of South Carolina, School of Medicine, T-28, VA, Columbia, SC 29208.

Medical University of South Carolina, College of Pharmacy: James F. Cooper, M.S., Pharm.D.,* Medical Univ. of South Carolina, College of Pharmacy, 171 Ashley Ave., Charleston, SC 29403.

University of South Carolina, College of Pharmacy: Robert L. Beamer, Ph.D.,* College of Pharmacy, University of South Carolina, Columbia, SC 29208.

SOUTH DAKOTA

South Dakota State University, College of Pharmacy: Gary S. Chappell, Ph.D.,* College of Pharmacy, South Dakota State University, Brookings, SD 57007.

TENNESSEE

East Tennessee State University College of Medicine: Ernest A. Daigneault, Ph.D.,* Chairman, Dept. of Pharmacology, P. O. Box 19, 810A, East Tennessee State University, Johnson City, TN 37601.

University of Tennessee, College of Pharmacy: Ramachander Gollamudi, Ph.D.,* Room 406, S.D. Feurt Building, College of Pharmacy, The University of Tennessee Center for the Health Sciences, Memphis, TN 38163.

TEXAS

University of Texas Health Science Center at Dallas: D. Craig Brater, M.D.,* 6650 Lakeshore, Dallas, TX 75214.

University of Texas Health Science Center at San Antonio: Arthur H. Briggs, M.D.,* The University of Texas Health Science Center at San Antonio, 7703 Floyd Curl Dr., San Antonio, TX 78284.

University of Texas Medical Branch: Sydney Ellis, Ph.D.,* 1223 Marine, Galveston, TX 77550.

Texas Southern University, School of Pharmacy: Mary Ann Williams, Pharm.D.,* 3805 Gertin Street, Houston, TX 77004.

University of Houston, College of Pharmacy: Joseph P. Buckley, Ph.D.,* 13714 Pebblebrook, Houston, TX 77079.

University of Texas at Austin, College of Pharmacy: Jaime N. Delgado, Ph.D.,* College of Pharmacy, University of Texas at Austin, Austin, TX 78712.

Texas Medical Association: August J. A. Watzlavick, P. O. Box 458, Schulenburg, TX 78956.

Texas Pharmaceutical Association: Bob Gude, R.Ph.,* 5654 Meadowbrook Drive, Fort Worth, TX 76112.

UTAH

University of Utah, College of Medicine: Stewart C. Harvey, Ph.D., Dept. of Pharmacology, Univ. of Utah, College of Medicine, 50 North Medical Dr., Salt Lake City, UT 84132.

University of Utah, College of Pharmacy: Arthur G. Lipman, Pharm.D.,* College of Pharmacy, University of Utah, Salt Lake City, UT 84112.

VERMONT

University of Vermont, College of Medicine: Geoffry Redmond, M.D.,* Dept. of Pharmacology, University of Vermont, College of Medicine, Given Building, Burlington, VT 05405.

Vermont Pharmaceutical Association: Thomas R. Reif, R.Ph.,* Route 1-A, Box 30, Shaftsbury, VT 05262.

VIRGINIA

Eastern Virginia Medical School: Desmond R.H. Gourley, Ph.D.,* Dept. of Pharmacology, Eastern Virginia Medical School, P. O. Box 1980, Norfolk, VA 23501.

Medical College of Virginia/Virginia Commonwealth University, School of Medicine: Louis S. Harris, Ph.D., P. O. Box 27 MCV Station, Richmond, VA 23298.

University of Virginia, School of Medicine: Peyton E. Weary, M.D.,* Chairman, Dept. of Dermatology, University of Virginia School of Medicine, Box 134, Charlottesville, VA 22908.

Medical College of Virginia/Virginia Commonwealth University, School of Pharmacy: William H. Barr, Pharm.D., Ph.D.,* Box 581 MCV Station, Richmond, VA 23298.

The Medical Society of Virginia: William J. Hagood, Jr., M.D.,* Little Retreat Clinic, Clover, VA 24534.

Virginia Pharmaceutical Association: Elmer R. Deffenbaugh, R.Ph.,* 1407 Sherwood Ave., Richmond, VA 23220.

WASHINGTON

University of Washington, School of Pharmacy: Lynn R. Brady, Ph.D.,* Dept. of Pharmaceutical Sciences, BG-20, University of Washington, Seattle, WA 98195.

Washington State University College of Pharmacy: Melvin R. Gibson, Ph.D.,* College of Pharmacy, Washington State University, Pullman, WA 99164.

Washington State Pharmaceutical Association: Gertrude M. Reavis, P. O. Box 397, Pullman, WA 99163.

WEST VIRGINIA

Marshall University, School of Medicine: Donald S. Robinson, M.D., Dept. of Pharmacology, Marshall University School of Medicine, Huntington, WV 25701.

West Virginia University, School of Medicine: Robert E. Stitzel,* Dept. of Pharm. and Tox., West Virginia University Medical Center, Morgantown, WV 26505.

West Virginia University, School of Pharmacy: Louis A. Luzzi, Ph.D.,* Dean, West Virginia University, School of Pharmacy, Morgantown, WV 26506.

West Virginia Pharmacists Association: J. Frank McClendon, 272 Barton Drive, Barboursville, WV 25504.

WISCONSIN

Medical College of Wisconsin: Richard I. H. Wang, M.D., Ph.D., Veterans Administration Hospital, Wood, WI 53193.

University of Wisconsin Medical School: Joseph M. Benforado, M.D.,* 730 Seneca Place, Madison, WI 53711.

University of Wisconsin-School of Pharmacy: Glenn Sonnedecker, Ph.D.,* Prof., School of Pharmacy, University of Wisconsin, 425 N. Charter Street, Madison, WI 53706.

Wisconsin Pharmaceutical Association: Louis W. Busse, Ph.D.,* 6967 Applewood Drive, Madison, WI 53711.

WYOMING

University of Wyoming, School of Pharmacy: Jack N. Bone, Ph.D., School of Pharmacy, University of Wyoming, Box 3375, Univ. Station, Laramie, WY 82071.

Members-At-Large

J. Weldon Bellville, M.D.,* Prof. of Anesthesia, Univ. of Calif. at Los Angeles, Medical Center, Los Angeles, CA 90024.

John V. Bergen, Ph.D.,* Wright State Univ., Office of Health Affairs, Box 1064, Dayton, OH 45401.

Edwin D. Bransome, Jr., M.D.,* Div. of Metabolic & Endocrine Disease, Medical College of Georgia, Augusta, GA 30902.

Lester Chafetz, Ph.D.,* Warner-Lambert Research Institute, 170 Tabor Road, Morris Plains, NJ 07950.

Durward F. Dodgen,* Food Chemicals Codex, National Academy of Sciences, 2101 Constitution Ave., N.W., Washington, DC 20037.

Klaus G. Florey, Ph.D.,* Squibb Institute for Medical Research, New Brunswick, NJ 08903.

Felix B. Gorrell, 5035 35th Rd. N., Arlington, VA 22207.

Joseph B. Jerome, Secy.* United States Adopted Names Council, 535 North Dearborn Street, Chicago, IL 60610.

Irwin Lerner, President & Chief Executive Officer, Hoffmann-LaRoche, Inc., Nutley, NJ 07110.

James Long, M.D.,* National Science Foundation, 1800 G Street, N.W., Washington, DC 20006.

Fred A. Morecombe,* Head, Corporate Compendial Liaison/Senior Corporate Q.A. Consultant, Abbott Laboratories, North Chicago, IL 60064.

Mark Novitch, M.D.,* Deputy Associate Commissioner for Medical Affairs, HFM 1, 5600 Fishers Lane, Rockville, MD 20857.

Jane C. Sheridan, Ph.D.,* Hoffman-LaRoche, Inc., Nutley, NJ 07110.

Vernon Trygstad, D.Sc.,* National Pharmaceutical Council, Suite 468, 1030 Fifteenth Street, N.W., Washington, DC 20005.

Henry Verhulst,* 5917 Walton Road, Bethesda, MD 20034.

Joseph D. Williams, President, Warner-Lambert Company, 201 Tabor Road, Morris Plains, NJ 07950.

Ex-Officio Members

Clifford E. Barnett, J.D.,* 1809 Suncrest Drive, Boise, ID 82705.

Louis W. Busse, Ph.D.,* University of Wisconsin-Madison, School of Pharmacy, 425 North Charter Street, Madison, WI 53706.

Jan Koch-Weser, M.D.,* 16, rue d'Ankara, 67000 Strasbourg, FRANCE

Margaret McCarron, M.D., Los Angeles County/USC Medical Center, 1200 North State Street, Room 1102, Los Angeles, CA 90027.

Fred T. Mahaffey, Pharm.D., Secretary, National Association of Boards of Pharmacy, One East Wacker Drive, Room 2210 Chicago, IL 60601.

John H. Moyer, M.D., D.Sc.,* Director of Prof. Affairs, Conemaugh Valley Memorial Hospital, 1986 Franklin Street, Johnstown, PA 15905.

Committee Chairmen

USP Credentials Committee: Joseph M. Benforado, M.D.,* Clinical Pharmacology Section, Dept. of Medicine, Univ. of Wisconsin, 600 Highland Ave., Madison, WI 53792.

USP Constitution & Bylaws Committee: Paul L. McLain, M.D.,* 33 McKelvey Avenue, Pittsburgh, PA 15218.

USP Nominating Committee for the Committee of Revision: John M. Woodside,* 909 E. 82nd St., Indianapolis, IN 46240.

USP Nominating Committee for Officers & Trustees: Joseph M. Pisani, M.D.,* The Proprietary Association, 1700 Pennsylvania Avenue, N.W., Washington, DC 20006.

USP Resolutions Committee: John T. Fay,* Jr., Ph.D., National Wholesale Druggists Association, 1511 K Street, N.W., Suite 800, Washington, DC 20005.

Honorary Members

George F. Archambault, Pharm.D., J.D.,* 5916 Melvern Drive, Bethesda, MD 20014.

Lloyd C. Miller, Ph.D.,* 1625 Skyhawk Road, Escondido, CA 92025.

Justin L. Powers, Ph.D., Cathedral Terrace, Apt. 304, 701 North Ocean St., Jacksonville, FL 32202.

Keeping Current

You can stay informed about the medicines described in this book and the drug-use issues in the news through a subscription to the ABOUT YOUR MEDICINES NEWSLETTER.

Published every other month, each issue will bring you timely articles and updated drug information from the same experts who produced this book and the authoritative United States Pharmacopeia (USP)—National Formulary (NF) and the USP Dispensing Information used by physicians, dentists, pharmacists, and nurses in their professional work.

Even if you only take an occasional aspirin or vitamin, you owe it to yourself to know more about these and all the medicines available to you over-the-counter or on prescription by staying informed ABOUT YOUR MEDICINES.

For further information about the newsletter, please see page 522.

DRUG MONOGRAPHS

ACETAMINOPHEN (Systemic)

Some commonly used brand names are:

Algophen*	Exdol*	Tempra
Atasol*	Liquiprin	Tivrin*
Atasol Forte*	Phenaphen	Tylenol
Campain*	Robigesic*	Tylenol Extra
Datril	Rounox*	Strength
Empracet*	SK-APAP	Valadol

*Not available in the United States.

Acetaminophen (a-seat-a-MEE-noe-fen) is a medicine used to relieve pain and reduce fever. Unlike aspirin, it does not relieve the redness or swelling caused by arthritis. Acetaminophen can be taken by mouth in the form of capsules, elixir, oral suspension, syrup, tablets, or chewable tablets. It can also be used rectally in the form of suppositories. This medicine is available without a prescription; however, your doctor may have special instructions on the proper dose of acetaminophen for your medical condition.

Before Using This Medicine

In order to decide on the best treatment for your medical problem, your doctor should be told:

—if you have ever had any unusual reaction to acetaminophen in the past. This medicine should not be taken if you are allergic to it.

—if you are pregnant, if you intend to become pregnant, or if you are breast-feeding an infant. Although acetaminophen has not been shown to cause problems, the chance always exists.

—if you have any of the following medical problems:

Kidney disease (severe)	Virus infection of the liver
Liver disease	

Proper Use of This Medicine

Unless otherwise directed by your doctor:

• *Do not take more of this medicine than is recommended on the package label.* If too much is taken, liver damage may occur.

• Children up to 12 years of age should not take this medicine for more than 5 days in a row.

• Adults should not take this medicine for more than 10 days in a row.

If you have been directed to take this medicine for a longer period of time, it is important that your doctor check your progress at regular visits.

This medicine will not relieve the redness or swelling that may occur with arthritic or rheumatic conditions. If you plan to take this medicine for these conditions, check with your doctor first.

Keep this medicine out of the reach of children since overdose is very dangerous in young children.

For patients using the suppository dosage form of this medicine:

• How to insert suppository: First remove the foil wrapper and moisten the suppository with water. Lie down on side and push the suppository well up into rectum with finger.

Precautions While Using This Medicine

Check with your doctor:

—if your symptoms do not improve or if they get worse.

—if you are taking this medicine to bring down a fever, and the fever lasts for more than 3 days or returns.

Check the labels of all over-the-counter (OTC), nonprescription, and prescription medicines you now take. If any contain acetaminophen be especially careful, since taking them while taking this medicine may lead to overdose. If you have any questions about this, check with your doctor or pharmacist.

There may be a greater risk of liver damage if you use large amounts of alcoholic beverages while taking this medicine.

Side Effects of This Medicine

Along with its needed effects, a medicine may cause some unwanted effects. Although not all of these side effects appear very often, when they do occur they may require medical attention. When this medicine is used for short periods of time at low doses, side effects usually are rare. However, check with your doctor or pharmacist if any of the following occur:

Rare

Itching or skin rash	Unusual tiredness or
Unexplained sore	weakness
throat and	Yellowing of eyes or
fever	skin
Unusual bleeding or	
bruising	

Possible signs of overdose

Diarrhea	Stomach cramps or
Nausea or vomiting	pain

Other side effects may occur which usually do not require medical attention. These side effects may go away during treatment as your body adjusts to the medicine. However, check with your doctor or pharmacist if any of the following side effects continue or are bothersome:

> *Rare*
> Dizziness
> Drowsiness

Other side effects not listed above may also occur in some patients. If you notice any other effects, check with your doctor.

ACETAMINOPHEN AND CODEINE
(Systemic)

Some commonly used brand names are:

Aceta with Codeine	Phenaphen with
Capital with	Codeine
Codeine	Proval
Empracet with	SK-APAP with
Codeine	Codeine
Papa-Deine	Tylenol with
Pavadon	Codeine

Acetaminophen and codeine (a-seat-a-MEE-noe-fen and KOE-deen) is a combination of pain relievers. It is available only with your doctor's prescription.

Before Using This Medicine

In order to decide on the best treatment for your medical problem, your doctor should be told:

—if you have ever had any unusual reaction to acetaminophen or codeine in the past. This medicine should not be taken if you are allergic to it.

—if you are pregnant, if you intend to become pregnant, or if you are breast-feeding an infant. Although this medicine has not been shown to cause problems, the chance always exists.

—if you have any of the following medical problems:

Brain disease or	Enlarged prostate or
injury	problems with
Colitis	urination
Emphysema,	Gallbladder disease
asthma, or	or gallstones
chronic lung	
disease	

Kidney disease	Underactive thyroid
Liver disease or	Unusually slow or
cirrhosis of the	irregular
liver	heartbeat
Underactive adrenal	Virus infection of
gland (Addison's	the liver
disease)	

—if you are now taking other central nervous system (CNS) depressants such as:

Antihistamines or	Sedatives, tran-
medicine for hay	quilizers, or
fever, other	sleeping
allergies	medicine
or colds	Seizure medicine
Barbiturates	Tricyclic
Other narcotics	antidepressants
Other prescription	(medicine for
pain medicine	depression)

—if you are now taking prescription medicine for stomach cramps or spasms.

—if you are now taking or have taken within the past 2 weeks monoamine oxidase (MAO) inhibitors such as:

Isocarboxazid	Phenelzine
Pargyline	Tranylcypromine

Proper Use of This Medicine

Take this medicine only as directed by your doctor. Do not take more of it, do not take it more often, and do not take it for a longer period of time than your doctor ordered. If too much is taken, it may become habit-forming or cause liver damage.

Keep this medicine out of the reach of children since overdose is very dangerous in young children.

Precautions While Using This Medicine

Check the labels of all over-the-counter (OTC), nonprescription, and prescription medicines you now take. If any contain acetaminophen, codeine, or other narcotics, be especially careful, since taking them while taking this medicine may lead to overdose. If you have any questions about this, check with your doctor or pharmacist.

If you will be taking this medicine for a long period of time (for example, for several months at a time), your doctor should check your progress at regular visits.

This medicine will add to the effects of alcohol and other medicines (CNS depressants) that slow down the nervous system. Some examples of

CNS depressants are antihistamines or medicine for hay fever, other allergies, or colds; sedatives, tranquilizers, or narcotics; barbiturates; medicine for seizures; tricyclic antidepressants (medicine for depression); or anesthetics, including dental anesthetics. Also, there may be a greater risk of liver damage if you use large amounts of alcoholic beverages while taking this medicine. *Check with your doctor before taking any of the above while you are taking this medicine.*

This medicine may cause some people to become drowsy or less alert than they are normally. *Make sure you know how you react to this medicine before you drive, use machines, or do other jobs that require you to be alert.*

Dizziness, lightheadedness, or fainting may occur, especially when you get up from a lying or sitting position. Getting up slowly may help lessen this problem.

Nausea may occur, especially after the first couple of doses. This effect usually goes away if you lie down for awhile.

Side Effects of This Medicine

Along with its needed effects, a medicine may cause some unwanted effects. Although not all of these side effects appear very often, when they do occur they may require medical attention. Check with your doctor or pharmacist if any of the following side effects occur:

Less common

Shortness of breath	Unusual excitement
Troubled breathing	(especially in children)
	Unusually slow heartbeat

Rare

Itching or skin rash	Unusual tiredness or
Unexplained sore throat and fever	weakness
Unusual bleeding or bruising	Yellowing of eyes or skin

Possible signs of overdose

Diarrhea	Stomach cramps
Nausea or vomiting	or pain

Other side effects may occur which usually do not require medical attention. These side effects may go away during treatment as your body adjusts to the medicine. However, check with your doctor if any of the following side effects continue or are bothersome:

More common

Constipation
Drowsiness

Less common

Difficult urination	Nausea or vomiting
Dizziness	Redness or flushing
Feeling faint	of face
Frequent urge to urinate	Unusual increase in sweating
Lightheadedness	Unusual tiredness or
Loss of appetite	weakness

Other side effects not listed above may also occur in some patients. If you notice any other effects, check with your doctor.

ACRISORCIN (Topical)

A commonly used brand name is Akrinol.

Acrisorcin (ak-ri-SOR-sin) belongs to the group of medicines called antifungals. It is applied to the skin to treat some types of fungal infections. This medicine is available only with your doctor's prescription.

Before Using This Medicine

In order to decide on the best treatment for your medical problem, your doctor should be told:

—if you have ever had any unusual reaction to acrisorcin in the past. This medicine should not be used if you are allergic to it.

—if you are pregnant, if you intend to become pregnant, or if you are breast-feeding an infant, although acrisorcin has not been shown to cause problems.

Proper Use of This Medicine

To help clear up your infection completely, *keep using this medicine for the full time of treatment* even though your condition may have improved.

Apply enough acrisorcin to cover the affected area. Before applying this medicine at night, wash with warm soapy water the area to be treated. Rinse thoroughly to remove all the soap and then dry thoroughly with a towel.

Keep this medicine away from the eyes.

If you miss a dose of this medicine, apply it as soon as possible. Then go back to your regular dosing schedule. If you have any questions about this, check with your doctor.

Precautions While Using This Medicine

To help cure the infection and to help prevent

reinfection, good health habits are required. These include the following:

• Wash all towels and bedding after use.

• Use only freshly laundered clothes each time clothing is changed.

If you have any questions about this, check with your doctor, nurse, or pharmacist.

This medicine may cause itching of the area to which it is applied if the area is exposed to ultraviolet light. When you first begin using this medicine, avoid too much sun or use of a sunlamp until you see how you react. If you have any questions about this, check with your doctor.

Side Effects of This Medicine

Along with its needed effects, a medicine may cause some unwanted effects. Although not all of these side effects appear very often, when they do occur they may require medical attention. Check with your doctor if any of the following side effects occur:

> Skin rash or hives, blistering, burning, itching, or other sign of irritation not present before using this medicine

Other side effects not listed above may also occur in some patients. If you notice any other effects, check with your doctor.

ADRENOCORTICOIDS (Dental)

This information applies to the following medicines:
Hydrocortisone (hye-droe-KOR-ti-sone)
Triamcinolone (trye-am-SIN-oh-lone)

Some commonly used brand names are:	Generic names:
Orabase HCA	Hydrocortisone
Kenalog in Orabase	Triamcinolone

This medicine is an adrenocorticoid (cortisone-like medicine). It belongs to the general family of medicines called steroids. These cortisone-like medicines are used in the mouth to relieve the discomfort and redness of some mouth and gum problems. Dental adrenocorticoids are available only with your physician's or dentist's prescription.

Before Using This Medicine

In order to decide on the best treatment for your medical problem, your physician or dentist should be told:

—if you have had any unusual reaction to dental adrenocorticoids in the past. This medicine should not be used if you are allergic to it.

—if you have an infection of the mouth or throat.

Proper Use of This Medicine

Press (do not rub) a small amount of paste onto the area to be treated until the paste sticks and a smooth, slippery film forms. Apply the paste at bedtime so the medicine can work overnight. The other applications of the paste should be made following meals.

Do not use this medicine more often or for a longer period of time than your physician or dentist ordered. To do so may increase the chance of absorption through the lining of the mouth and the chance of side effects.

Do not use any left-over medicine for future mouth problems without first checking with your physician or dentist. The medicine should not be used on many kinds of bacterial, viral, or fungal infections.

If you miss a dose of this medicine, apply it as soon as possible. Then continue with your regular dosing schedule. But if it is almost time for your next dose, do not apply the missed dose at all. Instead, continue with your regular dosing schedule. If you have any questions about this, check with your physician or dentist.

Precautions While Using This Medicine

Check with your physician or dentist:

—if signs of a throat or mouth infection occur.

—if your symptoms do not improve within 1 week.

—if your condition gets worse.

Side Effects of This Medicine

Along with its needed effects, a medicine may cause some unwanted effects. Although not all of these side effects appear very often, when they do occur they may require medical attention. Check with your physician or dentist if the following side effects occur:

> Signs of infection or irritation such as burning, itching, blistering, or peeling not present before therapy

Other side effects not listed above may also occur in some patients. If you notice any other effects, check with your doctor.

ADRENOCORTICOIDS (Ophthalmic)

This information applies to the following medicines:

Cortisone (KOR-ti-sone)
Dexamethasone (dex-a-METH-a-sone)
Fluorometholone (flure-oh-METH-oh-lone)
Hydrocortisone (hye-droe-KOR-ti-sone)
Medrysone (ME-dri-sone)
Prednisolone (pred-NISS-oh-lone)

Some commonly used brand names and other names are:	Generic names:
Decadron Maxidex Novadex*	Dexamethasone
FML Liquifilm	Fluorometholone
Cortamed* Cortisol Hydrocortone Optef	Hydrocortisone
HMS Liquifilm	Medrysone
AK-Pred AK-Tate Econopred Hydeltrasol Inflamase Metreton Pred Forte Pred Mild Predulose	Prednisolone

*Not available in the United States.

This medicine is an adrenocorticoid (cortisone-like medicine). It belongs to the general family of medicines called steroids. Ophthalmic adrenocorticoids are used in the eye in the form of drops or ointment to prevent permanent damage to the eye which may occur with certain eye problems. They also provide relief from redness, irritation, and other discomfort. Adrenocorticoids for use in the eye are available only with your doctor's prescription.

Before Using This Medicine

In order to decide on the best treatment for your medical problem, your doctor should be told:

—if you have ever had any unusual reaction to adrenocorticoids in the past. This medicine should not be used if you are allergic to it.

—if you have any other eye infection, glaucoma, or cataracts, or if you have ever had herpes of the eye.

Proper Use of This Medicine

Do not use any leftover medicine for future eye problems without first checking with your doctor. The medicine should not be used on many kinds of bacterial, viral, or fungal infections. To do so may make the problem worse and possibly lead to eye damage.

If you miss a dose of this medicine, apply it as soon as possible. Then go back to your regular dosing schedule. But if it is almost time for your next dose, do not apply the missed dose at all. Instead, go back to your regular dosing schedule. If you have any questions about this, check with your doctor.

For patients using the eye drop form of this medicine:

• How to apply this medicine: First, wash hands. Tilt head back and pull lower eyelid away from eye to form a pouch. Drop the medicine into the pouch and gently close eyes. Do not blink. Keep your eyes closed for 1 or 2 minutes to allow the medicine to be absorbed. If you think you did not get the drop of medicine into your eye properly, use another drop.

• To prevent contamination of the eye drops, do not touch the applicator tip to any surface (including the eye), and keep the container tightly closed.

For patients using the ointment form of this medicine:

• How to apply this medicine: First, wash hands. Pull the lower eyelid away from the eye to form a pouch. Squeeze a thin strip of ointment into the pouch. A 1-cm (approximately 1/3 inch) strip of ointment is usually enough unless otherwise directed by your doctor. Gently close your eyes and keep them closed for 1 or 2 minutes to allow the medicine to spread over the surface of the eye and be absorbed.

• To prevent contamination of the eye ointment, do not touch the applicator tip to any surface (including the eye). After using, wipe the tip of the ointment tube with a clean tissue and keep the tube tightly closed.

• After application, eye ointments may be expected to cause your vision to blur for a few minutes.

Precautions While Using This Medicine

If you will be using this medicine for more than several weeks, your doctor should examine your eyes at regular visits.

If your symptoms have not improved after 5 to 7 days, or if your eye condition becomes worse, check with your doctor.

Side Effects of This Medicine

Along with its needed effects, a medicine may cause some unwanted effects. Although not all of these side effects appear very often, when they do occur they may require medical attention. Check with your doctor if any of the following side effects occur:

Less common or rare

Blurred vision	Seeing halos around
Drooping of the	lights
eyelids	Unusually large
Eye pain	pupils
Headache	

Other side effects may occur which usually do not require medical attention. These side effects may go away during treatment as your body adjusts to the medicine. However, check with your doctor if any of the following side effects continue or are bothersome:

Less common

Burning, stinging, or watering of the eyes

ADRENOCORTICOIDS (Otic)

This information applies to the following medicines:

Dexamethasone (dex-a-METH-a-sone)
Prednisolone (pred-NISS-oh-lone)

Some commonly used brand names are:	Generic names:
Decadron	
Maxidex	Dexamethasone

Hydeltrasol	
Metreton	Prednisolone

This medicine is an adrenocorticoid (cortisone-like medicine). It belongs to the general family of medicines called steroids. Otic adrenocorticoids are used in the ear in the form of drops or ointment to relieve the redness, itching, and swelling caused by certain ear problems. Adrenocorticoids for use in the ear are available only with your doctor's prescription.

Before Using This Medicine

In order to decide on the best treatment for your medical problem, your doctor should be told:

—if you have ever had any unusual reaction to adrenocorticoids in the past. This medicine should not be used if you are allergic to it.

—if you have any of the following medical problems:

Any other ear	Punctured ear drum
infection or	
condition	

Proper Use of This Medicine

Do not use any leftover medicine for future ear problems without first checking with your doctor. The medicine should not be used on many kinds of bacterial, viral, or fungal infections.

Before applying this medicine, wash the area to be treated (including the ear canal) with soap and water, and dry thoroughly. The ear canal should be dried with a sterile cotton applicator.

If you miss a dose of this medicine, apply it as soon as possible. Then go back to your regular dosing schedule. But if it is almost time for your next dose, do not apply the missed dose at all. Instead, go back to your regular dosing schedule. If you have any questions about this, check with your doctor.

For patients using the liquid form of this medicine:

• How to apply this medicine: Lie down or tilt the head so that the infected ear faces up. For adults, gently pull the ear lobe up and back to straighten the ear canal. (For children, gently pull the ear lobe down and back to straighten the ear canal.) Drop medicine into the ear canal. Keep ear facing up for several minutes to allow medicine to run to the bottom of the ear canal. A clean, soft cotton plug may be gently inserted into the ear opening to prevent the medicine from leaking out.

• To prevent contamination of the drops, do not touch the applicator tip to any surface (including the ear), and keep the container tightly closed.

For patients using the ointment form of this medicine:

• How to apply this medicine: Squeeze a small amount of ointment onto a sterile cotton-tipped applicator and gently apply to the ear canal.

• To prevent contamination of the ointment, do not touch the applicator tip of the ointment tube to any surface (including the ear). After using, wipe the tip of the ointment tube with a clean tissue and keep the tube tightly closed.

Precautions While Using This Medicine

If your symptoms have not improved after 5 to 7 days, or if your ear problem becomes worse, check with your doctor.

Side Effects of This Medicine

After application of this medicine to the ear, occasional stinging or burning may be expected.

There have not been any other common or important side effects reported with this medicine. However, if you notice any unusual effects, check with your doctor.

ADRENOCORTICOIDS (Topical)

Applies to:

Amcinonide (am-SIN-oh-nide)
Betamethasone (bay-ta-METH-a-sone)
Desonide (DESS-oh-nide)
Desoximetasone (des-ox-i-MET-a-sone)
Dexamethasone (dex-a-METH-a-sone)
Diflorasone (dye-FLOR-a-sone)
Flumethasone (floo-METH-a-sone)
Fluocinolone (floo-oh-SIN-oh-lone)
Fluocinonide (floo-oh-SIN-oh-nide)
Fluorometholone (flure-oh-METH-oh-lone)
Flurandrenolide (flure-an-DREN-oh-lide)
Halcinonide (hal-SIN-oh-nide)
Hydrocortisone (hye-droe-KOR-ti-sone)
Methylprednisolone (meth-ill-pred-NISS-oh-lone)
Prednisolone (pred-NISS-oh-lone)
Triamcinolone (trye-am-SIN-oh-lone)

Some commonly used brand names and other names are:	Generic names:
Cyclocort	Amcinonide
Benisone Betacort* Betaderm* Betnovate* Celestoderm* Celestone Valisone	Betamethasone
Tridesilon	Desonide
Topicort	Desoximetasone
Aeroseb-Dex Decaderm Decadron Decaspray Hexadrol	Dexamethasone
Florone	Diflorasone
Locacorten* Locorten	Flumethasone
Dermalar* Fluoderm* Fluonid Flurosyn Synalar	Fluocinolone
Lidemol* Lidex Topsyn	Fluocinonide
Oxylone	Fluorometholone
Cordran Drenison*	Flurandrenolide
Halciderm Halog	Halcinonide
Cortaid Cort-Dome Cortef Corticreme* Cortisol Cortril Dermacort Hyderm* Hydrocortone Hytone Texacort	Hydrocortisone
Medrol	Methylprednisolone
Meti-Derm	Prednisolone
Aristocort Aristogel Kenalog Kenalog-E* Spencort Triacet Triaderm* Triamalone* Trimacort*	Triamcinolone

*Not available in the United States.

This medicine is an adrenocorticoid (cortisone-like medicine). It belongs to the general family of medicines called steroids. Topical cortisone-like medicines are applied to the skin to help relieve redness, swelling, itching, and discomfort of many skin problems. Most adrenocorticoids are available only with your doctor's prescription. Some strengths of hydrocortisone are available without a prescription; however, your doctor may have special instructions on its proper use for your medical condition.

Before Using This Medicine

In order to decide on the best treatment for your medical problem, your doctor should be told:

—if you have ever had any unusual reaction to adrenocorticoids in the past. This medicine should not be used if you are allergic to it.

—if you are pregnant or if you intend to become pregnant while using this medicine. Although topical adrenocorticoids have not been shown to cause birth defects or other problems in humans, the chance always exists. In addition, use in large amounts or for prolonged periods of time is not recommended since the medicine may be absorbed through the skin.

—if you are breast-feeding an infant. Although topical adrenocorticoids have not been shown to cause problems, the chance always exists.

—if you think you may have an infection at the site of treatment.

Proper Use of This Medicine

Do not use this medicine more often or for a longer period of time than your doctor ordered. To do so may increase the chance of absorption through the skin and the chance of side effects. In addition, too much use, especially on thin skin areas (for example, face, armpits, groin), may result in thinning of the skin and stretch marks.

Do not bandage or otherwise wrap the area of the skin being treated unless directed to do so by your doctor.

If your doctor has ordered an occlusive dressing (for example, kitchen plastic wrap) to be applied over this medicine, make sure you know how to apply it. Since occlusive dressings increase the amount of medicine absorbed through your skin and the possibility of side effects, use them only as directed. If you have any questions about this, check with your doctor.

This medicine was prescribed for a specific skin problem. *Do not use it on other skin problems without first checking with your doctor* since the medicine should not be used on many kinds of bacterial, viral, or fungal skin infections.

If you miss a dose of this medicine, apply it as soon as possible. Then go back to your regular dosing schedule. But if it is almost time for your next dose, do not apply the missed dose at all. Instead, go back to your regular dosing schedule. If you have any questions about this, check with your doctor.

For patients using the topical aerosol form of this medicine:

• This medicine usually comes with patient directions. Read them carefully before using this medicine.

• It is important to avoid breathing in the vapors from the spray.

• Do not use near heat, near open flame, or while smoking.

• Store away from heat and direct sunlight. Do not puncture, break, or burn the container.

For patients using flurandrenolide tape:

• This medicine usually comes with patient directions. Read them carefully before using this medicine.

Precautions While Using This Medicine

This medicine may be absorbed through the skin and can affect growth. *Children who must use this medicine should be followed closely by their doctor.*

If this medicine is to be used on the diaper area, avoid using tight-fitting diapers or plastic pants on the child. Wearing these may increase the chance of absorption of the medicine through the skin and the chance of side effects.

Side Effects of This Medicine

Along with its needed effects, a medicine may cause some unwanted effects. Although not all of these side effects appear very often, when they do occur they may require medical attention. Check with your doctor if any of the following side effects occur:

Signs of irritation or infection such as burning, itching, blistering, or peeling not present before using this medicine

When the gel, solution, lotion, or aerosol form of this medicine is applied, a mild, temporary stinging may be expected.

Other side effects not listed above may also occur in some patients. If you notice any other effects, check with your doctor.

ADRENOCORTICOIDS (Systemic)
Combined Glucocorticoid and
Mineralocorticoid Effects

This information applies to the following medicines:

Betamethasone (bay-ta-METH-a-sone)
Cortisone (KOR-ti-sone)
Dexamethasone (dex-a-METH-a-sone)
Fluprednisolone (floo-pred-NISS-oh-lone)
Hydrocortisone (hye-droe-KOR-ti-sone)
Meprednisone (me-PRED-ni-sone)
Methylprednisolone (meth-ill-pred-NISS-oh-lone)
Paramethasone (par-a-METH-a-sone)
Prednisolone (pred-NISS-oh-lone)
Prednisolone, Buffered
Prednisone (PRED-ni-sone)
Triamcinolone (trye-am-SIN-oh-lone)

The following information does *not* apply to desoxycorticosterone or fludrocortisone.

Some commonly used brand names are:	Generic names:
Betnelan* Betnesol* Celestone	Betamethasone
Cortone	Cortisone
Decadron Dexasone Hexadrol	Dexamethasone
Alphadrol	Fluprednisolone
A-Hydrocort Cortef Cortenema Hydrocortone Solu-Cortef	Hydrocortisone
Betapar	Meprednisone
A-MethaPred Duralone Medralone Medrol Methylone	Methylprednisolone
Haldrone	Paramethasone
Delta-Cortef Hydeltrasol Meticortelone Sterone	Prednisolone
Predoxine	Prednisolone, Buffered
Colisone* Deltasone Meticorten Orasone Sterapred Winpred*	Prednisone
Aristocort Aristospan Cinonide Kenacort Kenalog Tramacort	Triamcinolone

*Not available in the United States.

This medicine is an adrenocorticoid (cortisone-like medicine). It belongs to the general family of medicines called steroids. Your body naturally produces certain cortisones which are necessary to maintain good health. If your body does not pro-

duce enough, your doctor may have prescribed this medicine to help make up the difference.

Cortisone-like medicines are used also to provide relief for inflamed areas of the body. They lessen swelling, redness, itching, and allergic reactions. They are often used as part of treatment for a number of different diseases such as severe allergies or skin problems, asthma, or arthritis.

Adrenocorticoids are taken by mouth or by injection, used rectally, or inhaled into the lungs. They are available only with your doctor's prescription.

Before Using This Medicine

In order to decide on the best treatment for your medical problem, your doctor should be told:

—if you have ever had any unusual reaction to adrenocorticoids in the past. This medicine should not be taken if you are allergic to it.

—if you are using the inhalation aerosol and have ever had an unusual reaction to aerosol spray inhalation medicines.

—if you are pregnant or if you intend to become pregnant while taking this medicine. Too much use of adrenocorticoids during pregnancy may cause the baby to have problems after birth. Be sure you have discussed this with your doctor before taking this medicine. In addition, although adrenocorticoids have not been shown to cause birth defects in humans, the chance always exists.

—if you are breast-feeding an infant. Adrenocorticoids pass into breast milk and may cause problems with growth or other unwanted effects in infants of mothers taking this medicine. Be sure you have discussed this with your doctor before taking this medicine.

—if you have an infection at the place of treatment.

—if you have any of the following medical problems:

Bone disease	Kidney disease or
Colitis	kidney stones
Diabetes	Liver disease
Diverticulitis	Myasthenia gravis
Glaucoma	Stomach ulcer or
Heart disease	other stomach
Herpes simplex of	problems
the eye	Tuberculosis
High blood pressure	(positive
High cholesterol	skin test, latent
levels	TB, or past
Infections (fungal)	history of)
	Underactive thyroid

—if you are now taking any of the following medicines or types of medicine:

Amphotericin B
Anticoagulants
(blood thinners)
Aspirin or other
salicylates
Diabetes medicine
you take by
mouth
Digitalis (heart
medicine)

Diuretics (water
pills) or antihy-
pertensives (high
blood pressure
medicine)
Inflammation
medicine
(for example,
arthritis medicine)
Insulin
Phenobarbital
Phenytoin
Rifampin
Somatropin

Proper Use of This Medicine

Use this medicine only as directed by your doctor.
Do not use more or less of it, do not use it more
often, and do not use it for a longer period of
time than your doctor ordered.

*Do not stop using this medicine without first
checking with your doctor.* Your doctor may
want you to reduce gradually the amount you
are using before stopping completely.

If you miss a dose of this medicine and your dosing
schedule is one dose to be taken:
Every other day—
Take the missed dose as soon as possible
if you remember it the same morning,
then go back to your regular dosing
schedule. If you do not remember the
missed doses until that afternoon, wait
and take it the following morning. Then
skip a day and start your dosing
schedule again.
Once a day—
Take the missed dose as soon as possible, then go back to your regular dosing
schedule. If you do not remember until
the next day, do not take the missed
dose at all and do not double the next
one. Instead, go back to your regular
dosing schedule.
Several times a day—
Take the missed dose as soon as possible, then go back to your regular dosing
schedule. If you do not remember until
your next dose is due, double the next
dose. Then, go back to your regular
dosing schedule.

If you have any questions about this, check
with your doctor.

For patients taking this medicine by mouth:
• This medicine may upset your stomach.
Eating something may help. If stomach upset,

burning, or pain continues, check with your
doctor.

• Stomach problems may be more likely to occur if you drink alcoholic beverages while being
treated with this medicine. You should not
drink alcoholic beverages while taking this
medicine, unless you have first checked with
your doctor.

• If you are taking buffered prednisolone and
you are also taking a tetracycline antibiotic, do
not take these two medicines within 1 or 2
hours of each other. Taking them together may
prevent the tetracycline from being absorbed
by your body.

For patients using dexamethasone sodium
phosphate inhalaion aerosol:
• This medicine usually comes with patient
directions. Read them carefully before using
this medicine.

• This medicine is used with a special inhaler.
Save your inhaler. Refill units of the medicine
may be available at lower cost.

• Container provides about 170 measured
sprays. Store away from heat and direct
sunlight. Do not puncture, break, or burn.

• This medicine may be absorbed through the
lungs and can affect growth. Therefore,
children using it should be followed closely by
their doctor.

• If signs of a mouth, throat, or lung infection
occur, if your condition gets worse, or if your
symptoms do not improve, check with your
doctor.

• Cough, hoarseness, or throat irritation may
occur. Gargling and rinsing your mouth after
each dose may help prevent the hoarseness and
irritation; however, check with your doctor if
these or any other side effects continue or are
bothersome.

If you are using hydrocortisone enema:
• For best results, use this medicine right after
a bowel movement (BM). Lie on your left side
and stay there for at least 30 minutes after the
enema is given so the medicine can work. If
you can, keep the enema inside all night.

• Gently insert the rectal tip of the enema to
prevent damage to the rectal wall.

• Each bottle contains a single dose. Use it all,
unless otherwise directed by your doctor.

If you are using hydrocortisone acetate rectal foam
aerosol:
• This medicine is used with a special applicator. Do not insert any part of the aerosol
container into the rectum.

• Container provides about 14 applications of foam. Store away from heat and direct sunlight. Do not puncture, break, or burn.

If you are using methylprednisolone acetate for enema:

• Gently insert the rectal tip of the enema to prevent damage to the rectal wall.

• Shake the bottle every half-hour while you are giving the enema.

• Each bottle contains a single dose. Use it all, unless otherwise directed by your doctor.

• Save your applicator. Refill units of this medicine may be available at lower cost.

Precautions While Using This Medicine

Your doctor should check your progress at regular visits. Your progress may have to be checked after you have stopped using this medicine also, since some of the effects may linger.

If you will be using this medicine for a long time:
• *Your doctor may want you to follow a low-salt diet and/or a potassium-rich diet.*

• Your doctor may want you to have your eyes examined by an ophthalmologist before and also sometime later during treatment.

• Your doctor may want you to carry a medical identification card stating that you are using this medicine.

• Your doctor may want you to watch your calories to prevent weight gain.

Tell the doctor in charge that you are using this medicine:
—*before having a vaccination, other immunizations, or skin tests.*

—*before having any kind of surgery (including dental surgery) or emergency treatment.*

—*if you get a serious infection or injury.*

Caution: Diabetics—This medicine may cause your blood sugar levels to rise. If you notice a change in the results of your urine or blood sugar test or if you have any questions, check with your doctor.

For patients having this medicine injected into their joints:
• If this medicine is injected into one of your joints, you should be careful not to put too much stress or strain on it. Make sure your doctor has told you how much you are allowed to move this joint while it is healing.

• If redness or swelling occurs at the place of injection, and continues or gets worse, check with your doctor.

For patients using this medicine rectally:
• This medicine usually comes with patient directions. Read them carefully before using this medicine.

• This medicine may be absorbed through the lining of the rectum and can affect growth. Therefore, children using it should be followed closely by their doctor.

• Check with your doctor if you notice rectal bleeding, pain, burning, itching, blistering, or other sign of irritation not present before you started using this medicine, or if signs of infection occur.

Side Effects of This Medicine

Along with its needed effects, a medicine may cause some unwanted effects. Although not all of these side effects appear very often, when they do occur they may require medical attention. When this medicine is used for short periods of time, side effects usually are rare. However, check with your doctor if any of the following side effects occur:

Less common

Decreased or blurred vision	Frequent urination Increased thirst

Rare

Skin rash

Additional side effects may occur if you take this medicine for a long period of time. Check with your doctor if any of the following side effects occur:

Acne or other skin problems	Irregular heartbeats
Back or rib pain	Menstrual problems
Bloody or black tarry stools	Mood or mental changes
Continuing stomach pain or burning	Muscle cramps or pains
Depression	Muscle weakness
Fever or sore throat	Nausea or vomiting
Filling or rounding out of the face	Seeing halos around lights
Infections that will not heal	Swelling of feet or lower legs
	Unusual tiredness or weakness

Other side effects may occur which usually do not require medical attention. These side effects may go away during treatment as your body adjusts to the medicine. However, check with your doctor if any of the following side effects continue or are bothersome:

More common

Indigestion

Less common

False sense of well-being	Restlessness
	Trouble in sleeping
Increase in appetite	Weight gain
Nervousness	

After you stop using this medicine, your body may need time to adjust. The length of time this takes depends on the amount of medicine you were using and how long you used it. During this period of time check with your doctor if you notice any of the following side effects:

Abdominal or back pain	Prolonged loss of appetite
Dizziness or fainting	Shortness of breath
Fever	Unusual tiredness or weakness
Muscle or joint pain	
Nausea or vomiting	Unusual weight loss

Other side effects not listed above may also occur in some patients. If you notice any other effects, check with your doctor.

ADRENOCORTICOIDS (Systemic)
Mineralocorticoid Effects

This information applies to the following medicines:

Desoxycorticosterone
(des-ox-i-kor-ti-koe-STER-one)
Fludrocortisone (floo-droe-KOR-ti-sone)

Some commonly used brand names are:	Generic names:
Doca	
Percorten	Desoxycorticosterone

Florinef	Fludrocortisone

This medicine is an adrenocorticoid (cortisone-like medicine). It belongs to the general family of medicines called steroids. Your body naturally produces certain cortisones which are necessary in order to maintain good health. If your body does not produce enough, your doctor may have prescribed this medicine to help make up the difference.

These adrenocorticoids are taken by mouth, used by injection, or placed under the skin in pellet form, and are available only with your doctor's prescription.

Before Using This Medicine

In order to decide on the best treatment for your medical problem, your doctor should be told:

—if you have ever had any unusual reaction to adrenocorticoids in the past. This medicine should not be taken if you are allergic to it.

—if you are allergic to sesame seeds or sesame oil (for desoxycorticosterone injection only).

—if you are pregnant, if you intend to become pregnant, or if you are breast-feeding an infant. Although these adrenocorticoids have not been shown to cause problems, the chance always exists.

—if you have any of the following medical problems:

Heart disease	Kidney disease
High blood pressure	Liver disease

—if you are now taking any of the following medicines or types of medicine:

Amphotericin B	Phenobarbital
Digitalis (heart medicine)	Phenytoin
	Rifampin
Diuretics (water pills) or antihypertensives (high blood pressure medicine)	

Proper Use of This Medicine

Use this medicine only as directed by your doctor. Do not use more or less of it, do not use it more often, and do not use it for a longer period of time than your doctor ordered.

If you miss a dose of this medicine, take it as soon as possible. If it is almost time for your next dose, do not take the missed dose at all and do not double the next one. Instead, go back to your regular dosing schedule. If you have any questions about this, check with your doctor.

Precautions While Using This Medicine

Your doctor should check your progress at regular visits.

If you will be using this medicine for a long time, your doctor may want you to carry a medical identification card stating that you are using this medicine.

If you are using desoxycorticosterone acetate pellets:
• If a pellet comes out from under your skin, see your doctor as soon as possible for replacement.

Side Effects of This Medicine

Along with its needed effects, a medicine may cause some unwanted effects. Although not all of these side effects appear very often, when

they do occur they may require medical attention. Check with your doctor if any of the following side effects occur:

Less common or rare

Dizziness	Swelling of feet
Increase in blood	or lower legs
pressure	Unusual weight gain
Severe or continuing	
headaches	

Other side effects not listed above may also occur in some patients. If you notice any other effects, check with your doctor.

ALCOHOL AND ACETONE (Topical)
Some commonly used brand names are Seba-Nil, Sebasum, and Tyrosum.

Alcohol and acetone (AL-koe-hol and A-se-tone) combination is used to cleanse oily or greasy skin associated with acne or other oily skin conditions. This medicine is available without a prescription; however, your doctor may have special instructions on the proper use of this medicine for your medical condition.

Before Using This Medicine
In order to decide on the best treatment for your medical problem, your doctor should be told:

—if you have ever had any unusual reaction to alcohol or acetone in the past. This medicine should not be used if you are allergic to it.

—if you are pregnant, if you intend to become pregnant, or if you are breast-feeding an infant, although alcohol and acetone combination has not been shown to cause problems.

—if you are now using any topical acne preparation or preparation containing a peeling agent such as benzoyl peroxide, resorcinol, salicylic acid, sulfur, or tretinoin.

Proper Use of This Medicine
Apply this medicine by wiping gently over the face and other affected areas to remove dirt and oily secretions.

Keep this medicine away from the eyes.

This medicine is flammable. Do not use near heat, near open flame, or while smoking.

If you miss a dose of this medicine, apply it as soon as possible. Then go back to your regular dosing schedule. But if it is almost time for your next dose, do not apply the missed dose at all. Instead, go back to your regular dosing schedule. If you have any questions about this, check with your doctor or pharmacist.

Precautions While Using This Medicine
Do not use any acne preparation or preparation containing a peeling agent (for example, benzoyl peroxide, resorcinol, salicylic acid, sulfur, or tretinoin) *on the same affected area as this medicine,* unless otherwise directed by your doctor. To do so may cause severe irritation of the skin.

Side Effects of This Medicine
When you apply this medicine, a mild temporary stinging may be expected.

Other side effects may also occur in some patients. If you notice any other effects, check with your doctor or pharmacist.

ALCOHOL AND SULFUR (Topical)
Some commonly used brand names are:

Acne Aid	Postacne
Acnomead	Transact
Epi-Clear	Xerac
Liquimat	

Alcohol and sulfur (AL-koe-hol and SUL-fur) combination is used in the treatment of acne and oily skin. This medicine is available without a doctor's prescription; however, your doctor may have special instructions on the proper use of this medicine for your medical condition.

Before Using This Medicine
In order to decide on the best treatment for your medical problem, your doctor should be told:

—if you have ever had any unusual reaction to alcohol or sulfur in the past. This medicine should not be used if you are allergic to it.

—if you are pregnant, if you intend to become pregnant, or if you are breast-feeding an infant, although alcohol and sulfur combination has not been shown to cause problems.

—if you are now using any topical acne preparation or preparation containing a peeling agent such as benzoyl peroxide, resorcinol, salicylic acid, or tretinoin.

—if you are now using any topical medicine containing mercury, such as ammoniated mercury ointment.

Proper Use of This Medicine

Use this medicine only as directed. Do not use it more often than recommended on the label, unless otherwise directed by your doctor.

Before using this medicine, wash the affected areas thoroughly and gently pat dry. Then apply a small amount to the affected areas and rub in gently.

Keep this medicine away from eyes. If you should accidentally get some in your eyes, flush them thoroughly with water.

This medicine is flammable. Do not use near heat, near open flame, or while smoking.

If you miss a dose of this medicine, apply it as soon as possible. Then go back to your regular dosing schedule. But if it is almost time for your next dose, do not apply the missed dose at all. Instead, go back to your regular dosing schedule. If you have any questions about this, check with your doctor or pharmacist.

Precautions While Using This Medicine

Do not use any acne preparation or preparation containing a peeling agent (for example, benzoyl peroxide, resorcinol, salicylic acid, or tretinoin) *on the same affected area as this medicine,* unless otherwise directed by your doctor. To do so may cause severe irritation of the skin.

Do not use any topical mercury-containing preparation such as ammoniated mercury ointment on the same affected area as this medicine. To do so may cause a foul odor, be irritating to the skin, and stain the skin black. If you have any questions about this, check with your doctor or pharmacist.

Side Effects of This Medicine

Along with its needed effects, a medicine may cause some unwanted effects. Although not all of these side effects appear very often, when they do occur they may require medical attention. Check with your doctor or pharmacist if the following side effect occurs:

Irritation of skin not present before using this medicine

After you apply this medicine, a stinging or tingling sensation may be expected.

After you use this medicine for a few days, you may have some drying and peeling of the skin.

Other side effects not listed above may also occur in some patients. If you notice any other effects, check with your doctor or pharmacist.

ALLOPURINOL (Systemic)

Some commonly used brand names are Lopurin, Purinol*, and Zyloprim.

---

*Not available in the United States.

Allopurinol (al-oh-PURE-i-nole) is taken by mouth to treat chronic gout. It is also used to prevent the body from producing too much uric acid that may cause other medical problems. This medicine is available only with your doctor's prescription.

Before Using This Medicine

In order to decide on the best treatment for your medical problem, your doctor should be told:

—if you have ever had any unusual reaction to allopurinol in the past. This medicine should not be taken if you are allergic to it.

—if you are pregnant, if you intend to become pregnant, or if you are breast-feeding an infant. Although allopurinol has not been shown to cause problems, the chance always exists.

—if you have kidney disease.

—if you have or any member of your immediate family has idiopathic hemochromatosis.

—if you are now taking any of the following medicines or types of medicine:

Ampicillin	Diuretics (water
Anticoagulants	pills)
(blood thinners)	Medicine to make
Azathioprine	the urine more
Cyclophosphamide	acid
	Mercaptopurine
	Pyrazinamide

Proper Use of This Medicine

In order for this medicine to help you, it must be taken regularly as ordered by your doctor. Up to 1 or more weeks may pass before you feel the full effects of this medicine.

Allopurinol is used to help prevent gout attacks. It will not relieve an attack that has already started. *Even if you take another medicine for gout attacks, continue to take this medicine also.* If you have any questions about this, check with your doctor.

If this medicine upsets your stomach, it may be taken after meals. If stomach upset (nausea, vomiting, diarrhea, or stomach pain) continues, check with your doctor.

To help prevent kidney stones while taking allopurinol, *adults should drink at least 10 to 12 full glasses (8 ounces each) of fluids each day* unless otherwise directed by their doctor. The doctor should be asked about the amount of fluids to be taken each day by children being treated with this medicine.

If you miss a dose of this medicine and your dosing schedule is one dose to be taken:

Once a day —
Take the missed dose as soon as possible. Then go back to your regular dosing schedule. But if you do not remember the missed dose until the next day, do not take it at all and do not double the next one. Instead, go back to your regular dosing schedule.

More than once a day —
Take the missed dose as soon as possible. Then go back to your regular dosing schedule. But if you do not remember the missed dose until it is almost time for your next dose, do not take the missed dose at all and do not double the next one. Instead, go back to your regular dosing schedule.

If you have any questions about this, check with your doctor.

Precautions While Using This Medicine

Your doctor should check your progress at regular visits in order to make sure that this medicine does not cause unwanted effects.

Drinking too much alcohol may lessen the effects of allopurinol. Therefore, *do not drink alcoholic beverages while taking this medicine,* unless you have first checked with your doctor.

Taking too much vitamin C may make the urine more acidic and increase the possibility of kidney stones forming while you are taking allopurinol. Therefore, *do not take vitamin C while taking this medicine,* unless you have first checked with your doctor.

This medicine may cause some people to become drowsy or less alert than they are normally. *Make sure you know how you react to this medicine before you drive, use machines, or do other jobs that require you to be alert.*

Side Effects of This Medicine

Along with its needed effects, a medicine may cause some unwanted effects. Although not all of these side effects appear very often, when they do occur they may require medical attention. Check with your doctor if any of the following side effects occur:

More common
Skin rash, hives, or itching
Rare

Numbness, tingling, pain, or weakness in hands or feet	Unusual bleeding or bruising
Unexplained sore throat and fever	Unusual tiredness or weakness
	Yellowing of eyes or skin

Other side effects may occur which usually do not require medical attention. These side effects may go away during treatment as your body adjusts to the medicine. However, check with your doctor if any of the following side effects continue or are bothersome:

Less common

Diarrhea	Nausea
Drowsiness	Stomach pain
	Vomiting

Other side effects not listed above may also occur in some patients. If you notice any other effects, check with your doctor.

AMANTADINE (Systemic)
A commonly used brand name is Symmetrel.

Amantadine (a-MAN-ta-deen) is used in the treatment of Parkinson's disease (sometimes called paralysis agitans or shaking palsy) either alone or with other medicines. It is also used in the prevention and treatment of virus infections caused by influenza type A. Amantadine is available only with your doctor's prescription.

Before Using This Medicine

In order to decide on the best treatment for your medical problem, your doctor should be told:

—if you have ever had any unusual reaction to amantadine in the past. This medicine should not be taken if you are allergic to it.

—if you are pregnant, if you intend to become pregnant, or if you are breast-feeding an infant. Although amantadine has not been shown to cause problems in humans, the chance always exists.

—if you have any of the following medical problems:

Eczema (recurring)	Mental or emotional illness
Epilepsy	
Heart disease	Stomach ulcer
Kidney disease	Swelling of feet and ankles or other circulation problems
Liver disease	

—if you are now taking any of the following medicines or types of medicine:

Amphetamines	Phenothiazines
Appetite	(medicine
suppressants	for mental or
(diet pills)	emotional illness)
Medicine for	Tricyclic an-
Parkinson's	tidepressants
disease	(medicine for
Medicine for	depression)
stomach cramps,	
intestinal spasms,	
or ulcers	

Proper Use of This Medicine

Take this medicine exactly as directed by your doctor. Do not miss taking any doses and do not take more medicine than your doctor ordered.

If you are taking this medicine for Parkinson's disease, improvement usually occurs in about 2 days. However, for a few patients amantadine must be taken for up to 2 weeks   before satisfactory improvement occurs.

If you do miss a dose of this medicine, take it as soon as possible. If your next scheduled dose is within 4 hours, do not take the missed dose at all and do not double the next one. Instead, go back to your regular dosing schedule.

Precautions While Using This Medicine

It is important that your doctor check your progress at regular visits, especially if you are taking amantadine regularly for longer than 3 months.

This medicine will gradually lose its effect in a few parkinsonism patients after it has been used regularly for 3 months to 1 year. An adjustment of the dosage by the doctor often restores the effectiveness.

Avoid alcoholic beverages while taking this medicine until you have discussed their use with your doctor, because alcohol may cause increased side effects such as circulation problems, dizziness, fainting, or mental confusion.

This medicine may cause some people to become dizzy, faint, or less alert than they are normally and also may cause blurred vision. *Make sure you know how you react to this medicine before you drive, use machines, or do other jobs that require you to be alert.*

Dizziness, lightheadedness, or fainting may occur, especially when you get up from a lying or sitting position. Getting up slowly may help. If the problem continues or gets worse, check with your doctor.

Your mouth and throat may feel very dry while you are taking this medicine. To relieve mouth dryness chew sugarless gum or dissolve bits of ice in your mouth.

Parkinsonism patients must be careful not to overdo physical activities as their condition improves and body movements become easier, since injuries resulting from falls may occur. Such activities must be gradually increased to allow your body to adjust to changing balance, circulation, and coordination.

A side effect of amantadine therapy that may unnecessarily alarm some patients is the appearance on the skin of purplish red, net-like, blotchy areas with the medical name of livedo reticularis. This effect occurs more often in female patients and is usually noticed on the legs and/or feet after continuous treatment for 1 month or longer. This effect may remain during the period of amantadine treatment, but then gradually disappears (usually within 2 to 12 weeks after the medicine is discontinued) with no bad effects to the patient.

If you are taking amantadine for Parkinson's disease, do not suddenly stop taking the doses as scheduled, because your condition may become worse very quickly. Follow your doctor's instructions when this medicine is to be stopped.

Side Effects of This Medicine

Along with its needed effects, a medicine may cause some unwanted effects. Although not all of these side effects appear very often, when they do occur they may require medical attention. Check with your doctor if any of the following side effects occur:

Less common

Difficult urination	Mental confusion
Fainting	Mental depression

Usually only with long-term therapy

Swelling of ankles and feet	Weight gain, rapid
Unexplained shortness of breath	

Rare

Convulsions	Uncontrolled
Slurred speech	rolling of eyes
	Unexplained sore throat and fever

Other side effects may occur which usually do not require medical attention. These side effects may go away during treatment as your body adjusts to the medicine. However, check with your doctor if any of the following side effects continue or are bothersome:

More common

Dizziness or light-headedness	Nervousness
Irritability	Purplish, blotchy spots on skin
Loss of appetite	Sleeping difficulty
Nausea	Tiredness and weakness

Less common

Blurred vision	Hallucinations (seeing, hearing, or feeling things that are not there)
Constipation	
Dry mouth	
	Headache

Rare

Skin rash

Other side effects not listed above may also occur in some patients. If you notice any other effects, check with your doctor.

AMINOCAPROIC ACID (Systemic)
A commonly used brand name is Amicar.

Aminocaproic (a-mee-noe-ka-PROE-ik) acid belongs to the group of medicines called hemostatics. It is taken by mouth or given by injection to treat excessive bleeding caused by certain conditions. This medicine is available only with your doctor's prescription.

Before Using This Medicine

In order to decide on the best treatment for your medical problem, your doctor should be told:

—if you have ever had any unusual reaction to aminocaproic acid in the past. This medicine should not be taken if you are allergic to it.

—if you are pregnant, if you intend to become pregnant, or if you are breast-feeding an infant. Although aminocaproic acid has not been shown to cause problems in humans, the chance always exists.

—if you have any of the following medical problems:

Heart disease	Liver disease
Kidney disease	

—if you are now taking any of the following medicines or types of medicine:

Estrogens	Oral contraceptives (birth control pills)

Proper Use of This Medicine

Take this medicine only as directed by your doctor. Do not take more of it, do not take it more often, and do not take it for a longer period of time than your doctor ordered.

Precautions While Using This Medicine

Your doctor should check your progress at regular visits in order to make sure that the medicine does not cause unwanted effects.

Side Effects of This Medicine

Along with its needed effects, a medicine may cause some unwanted effects. The following side effects may go away during treatment as your body adjusts to this medicine; however, check with your doctor if any of the following side effects continue or are bothersome:

Headache or dizziness	Ringing or buzzing in ears
Nausea, stomach pain, or diarrhea	Skin rash
Red or bloodshot eyes	Stuffy nose

Other side effects not listed above may also occur in some patients. If you notice any other effects, check with your doctor.

AMINOGLYCOSIDES (Systemic)
This information applies to the following medicines:

Amikacin (am-i-KAY-sin)
Gentamicin (jen-ta-MYE-sin)
Kanamycin (kan-a-MYE-sin)
Neomycin (nee-oh-MYE-sin)
Streptomycin (strep-toe-MYE-sin)
Tobramycin (toe-bra-MYE-sin)

Some commonly used brand names are:	Generic names:
Amikin	Amikacin
Apogen Bristagen Cidomycin* Garamycin U-Gencin	Gentamicin
Kantrex Klebcil	Kanamycin
Mycifradin	Neomycin
	Streptomycin
Nebcin	Tobramycin

*Not available in the United States.

Aminoglycosides (a-mee-noe-GLYE-coe-sides) belong to the general family of medicines called antibiotics. They are given by injection to help the body overcome infections. Some of them may also be given with one or more other medicines for tuberculosis (TB). Aminoglycosides are available only with your doctor's prescription.

Before Using This Medicine

In order to decide on the best treatment for your medical problem, your doctor should be told:

—if you have had allergic reactions to any of the aminoglycosides.

—if you are pregnant or if you intend to become pregnant. Prolonged use of aminoglycosides may damage the infant's hearing and sense of balance.

—if you are breast-feeding an infant, although aminoglycosides have not been shown to cause problems.

—if you have any of the following medical problems:

Eighth-cranial-nerve disease (loss of hearing and/or balance)	Kidney disease Myasthenia gravis Parkinson's disease

—if you are now receiving any of the following medicines or types of medicine:

Aminoglycosides (more than one at a time) Capreomycin Cephaloridine Cephalothin Cisplatin Colistimethate	Colistin Ethacrynic acid Furosemide Mercaptomerin Polymyxin B Vancomycin

Side Effects of This Medicine

Along with its needed effects, a medicine may cause some unwanted effects. Although not all of these side effects appear very often, when they do occur they may require medical attention. Check with your doctor if any of the following side effects occur:

More common

Blood in urine Clumsiness or unsteadiness Dizziness Excessive thirst Greatly decreased frequency of urination or amount of urine Loss of appetite Loss of hearing	Nausea Numbness, tingling, or burning of face or mouth (streptomycin only) Rash (neomycin only) Ringing or buzzing sound or a feeling of fullness in the ears Vomiting

Less common

Any loss of vision (streptomycin only)

Rare

Difficulty in breathing Drowsiness	Weakness

Other side effects may occur which usually do not require medical attention. These side effects may go away during treatment as your body adjusts to the medicine. However, check with your doctor if any of the following side effects continue or are bothersome:

Less common

Itching, rash, redness, or swelling (streptomycin only)

Other side effects not listed above may also occur in some patients. If you notice any other effects, check with your doctor.

4-AMINOQUINOLONES (Systemic)

This information applies to the following medicines:

Amodiaquine (am-oh-DYE-a-kwin)
Chloroquine (KLOR-oh-kwin)
Hydroxychloroquine (hye-drox-ee-KLOR-oh-kwin)

Some commonly used brand names are:	Generic names:
Camoquin	Amodiaquine
Aralen	Chloroquine
Plaquenil	Hydroxychloroquine

The 4-aminoquinolones belong to the group of medicines called antiprotozoals. Although sometimes used for other medical problems, they are used most often in the prevention and treatment of malaria. Also, hydroxychloroquine may be used in the treatment of arthritis. These medicines are available only with your doctor's prescription.

Before Using This Medicine

In order to decide on the best treatment for your medical problem, your doctor should be told:

—if you have ever had any unusual reaction to amodiaquine, chloroquine, or hydroxychloroquine.

—if you are pregnant or if you intend to become pregnant while using this medicine. Amodiaquine, chloroquine, or hydroxychloroquine may cause birth defects if taken during pregnancy.

—if you are breast-feeding an infant. Although these medicines have not been shown to cause problems, the chance always exists.

—if you have any of the following medical problems:

Alcoholism	Intestinal disease
Blood disease	Liver disease
Eye or vision prob-	Nerve or brain
lems	disease
Glucose-6-phosphate	including seizures
dehydrogenase	Porphyria
(G6PD) deficiency	Psoriasis

—if you are now taking any of the following medicines or types of medicine:

Gold salt injections	Oxyphenbutazone
for arthritis	Phenylbutazone

Proper Use of This Medicine

If you are taking this medicine for malaria, *keep taking it for the full time of treatment* to help prevent or clear up your infection completely.

It is very important that you *take this medicine only as directed.* Do not take more of it, do not take it more often, and do not take it for a longer period of time than your doctor ordered. To do so may increase the chance of serious side effects.

Take this medicine with meals or milk to lessen possible stomach upset, unless otherwise directed by your doctor.

Keep this medicine out of the reach of children since overdose is especially dangerous in children.

If you miss a dose of this medicine and your dosing schedule is one dose to be taken:

Every seven days—
Take the missed dose as soon as possible. Then go back to your regular dosing schedule.

Once a day—
Take the missed dose as soon as possible. Then go back to your regular dosing schedule. But if you do not remember the missed dose until the next day, do not take it at all and do not double the next one. Instead, go back to your regular dosing schedule.

More than once a day—
Take it right away if you remember within an hour or so of the missed dose. Then go back to your regular dosing schedule. But if you do not remember until later, do not take the missed dose at all and do not

double the next one. Instead, go back to your regular dosing schedule.

If you have any questions about this, check with your doctor.

If you are taking hydroxychloroquine for arthritis:

• This medicine must be taken regularly as ordered by your doctor in order for it to help you. Several months may pass before you feel its full effects.

Precautions While Using This Medicine

If you will be taking this medicine for a long period of time:

• Your doctor should check your progress at regular visits.

• Your doctor may want you to have your eyes examined by an ophthalmologist before, during, and after treatment.

Side Effects of This Medicine

Along with its needed effects, a medicine may cause some unwanted effects. Although not all of these side effects appear very often, when they do occur they may require medical attention. When this medicine is used for short periods of time, side effects usually are rare. However, when it is used for long periods of time and/or in high doses, side effects are more likely to occur and may be serious. Check with your doctor if any of the following side effects occur:

With short- or long-term use

Unexplained sore
throat and fever

With long-term use

Mood or mental	Unusual bleeding or
changes	bruising
Numbness, tingling,	Unusual muscle
pain, or weakness	weakness
in hands or feet	Yellowing of eyes or
Seizures	skin

With long-term use and/or high doses

Blurred vision or	Ringing or buzzing
any change in	in ears or any
vision	loss of hearing

Other side effects may occur which usually do not require medical attention. These side effects may go away during treatment as your body adjusts to the medicine. However, check with your doctor if any of the following side effects continue or are bothersome:

More common

Diarrhea	Nausea or vomiting
Headache	Stomach cramps or
Loss of appetite	pain

Less common

Bleaching of hair or unusual hair loss (with long-term use)	Dizziness or light-headedness
Blue-black coloration of skin, fingernails, or inside of mouth (with long-term use)	Nervousness or restlessness
	Skin rash or itching (with long-term use)
	Unusual tiredness

After you stop using this medicine, it may still cause some side effects that need attention. During this period of time check with your doctor if you notice the following:

Blurred vision or any change in vision

Although not all of the side effects listed above have been reported for all three of these medicines, they have been reported for at least one of them. However, since amodiaquine, chloroquine, and hydroxychloroquine are very similar, any of the above side effects may occur with any of these medicines.

Other side effects not listed above may also occur in some patients. If you notice any other effects, check with your doctor.

AMINOSALICYLATES (Systemic)
Some commonly used brand names are:

Nemasol*	Parasal
P.A.S.	Teebacin

*Not available in the United States.

Aminosalicylates (a-mee-noe-sal-i-SILL-ates) belong to the general family of medicines called anti-infectives. They are used to help the body overcome tuberculosis (TB). They are given by mouth with one or more other medicines for TB. Aminosalicylates are available only with your doctor's prescription.

Before Using This Medicine

In order to decide on the best treatment for your medical problem, your doctor should be told:

—if you have had allergic reactions to aspirin or other salicylates including methyl salicylate (oil of wintergreen) or to other related medicines such as sulfonamides (sulfas) or dyes.

—if you are pregnant, if you intend to become pregnant, or if you are breast-feeding an infant, although aminosalicylates have not been shown to cause problems.

—if you are taking aminosalicylate calcium and have any of the following medical problems:

Cancer	Overactive para-thyroid glands
Glucose-6-phosphate dehydrogenase (G6PD) deficiency	Overactive thyroid gland
	Sarcoidosis
Kidney stones or other kidney disease	Stomach ulcer
	Underactive adrenal glands
Liver disease	

—if you are taking aminosalicylate potassium and have any of the following medical problems:

Glucose-6-phosphate dehydrogenase (G6PD) deficiency	Liver disease
	Stomach ulcer
	Underactive adrenal glands
Kidney disease	

—if you are taking aminosalicylate sodium and have any of the following medical problems:

Glucose-6-phosphate dehydrogenase (G6PD) deficiency	Heart disease
	Kidney disease
	Liver disease
	Stomach ulcer

—if you are now taking any of the following medicines or types of medicine:

Aminobenzoic acid (PABA)	Probenecid
	Rifampin
Oral anticoagulants (blood thinners you take by mouth)	Sulfinpyrazone

—if you are now taking aminosalicylate calcium and are also taking any of the following medicines (tetracyclines):

Demeclocycline	Minocycline
Doxycycline	Oxytetracycline
Methacycline	Tetracycline

—if you are now taking aminosalicylate potassium and are also taking any of the following medicines or types of medicine:

Diuretics, potassium-sparing (water pills, such as spironolac-tone, triamterene)	Potassium-containing medicines
	Potassium supplements

—if you are now taking aminosalicylate potassium and are also using salt substitutes or drinking low-salt milk.

Proper Use of This Medicine

Aminosalicylates may be taken with or after meals or with an antacid if they upset your stomach.

If you are taking the dry powder form of this medicine:
• Dissolve the contents of each packet in water immediately before taking. Stir well. Be sure to drink all the liquid in order to get the full dose of medicine.

If you are taking the enteric-coated tablet form of this medicine:
• Swallow tablets whole to keep this medicine from upsetting your stomach. Do not break or crush.

To help clear up your tuberculosis (TB) completely, *it is important that you keep taking this medicine for the full time of treatment* even if you begin to feel better after a few weeks. You may have to take it every day for as long as 1 to 2 years or more. *It is important that you do not miss any doses.*

If you do miss a dose of this medicine, take it as soon as possible. However, if it is almost time for your next dose, do not take the missed dose or double your next dose. Instead, go back to your regular dosing schedule.

Precautions While Using This Medicine

Do not take aminosalicylates within 6 hours of the time you take rifampin since this may keep rifampin from working as well.

Do not take aminosalicylate calcium within 1 to 3 hours of the time you take tetracyclines by mouth since this may keep tetracyclines from working as well.

If your symptoms do not improve within 2 to 3 weeks or if they become worse, check with your doctor.

Caution: Diabetics—This medicine may cause false test results with some urine sugar tests. Check with your doctor before changing your diet or the dosage of your diabetes medicine.

Side Effects of This Medicine

Along with its needed effects, a medicine may cause some unwanted effects. Although not all of these side effects appear very often, when they do occur they may require medical attention. Stop taking this medicine and check with your doctor if any of the following side effects occur:

More common

Chills	Rash
Itching	Unexplained sore
Lower-back pain	throat or fever
Pain or burning	Unusual tiredness or
while urinating	weakness

Less common

Blood in urine	Increased sensitivity
Changes in	of eyes to light
menstrual periods	Swelling of front
Coldness	part of neck
Decreased sexual	Unusual weight gain
ability (males)	Yellowing of eyes or
Dry, puffy skin	skin
Headache	

Signs of too much calcium

Constipation	Loss of appetite
Drowsiness	Mental confusion
Greatly increased	and depression
frequency of	Nausea
urination or	Unusual thirst
amount of urine	Vomiting

Signs of too much potassium

Irregular heartbeat	Weakness or
Mental confusion	heaviness of
Numbness, tingling	legs
pain, or weakness	
in hands or feet	

Other side effects may occur which usually do not require medical attention. These side effects may go away during treatment as your body adjusts to the medicine. However, check with your doctor if any of the following side effects continue or are bothersome:

More common

Diarrhea	Stomach pain
Red discoloration of	
urine on contact	
with certain	
chlorine bleaches	

This medicine may cause the urine to turn red when it comes into contact with certain chlorine bleaches (such as those used to clean toilet bowls). This side effect does not require medical attention.

Other side effects not listed above may also occur in some patients. If you notice any other effects, check with your doctor.

AMPHETAMINES (Systemic)

This information applies to the following medicines:

Amphetamine (am-FET-a-meen)
Dextroamphetamine (dex-troe-am-FET-a-meen)
Methamphetamine (meth-am-FET-a-meen)

Some commonly used brand names are:	Generic names:
Benzedrine	Amphetamine
Dexampex Dexedrine Diphylets Ferndex Obotan Oxydess Spancap	Dextroamphetamine
Desoxyn Methampex	Methamphetamine

Amphetamines (am-FET-a-meens) belong to the group of medicines called central nervous system (CNS) stimulants. They are used in the treatment of narcolepsy (uncontrolled desire for sleep or sudden attacks of sleep at irregular intervals). They are also used to treat behavior problems in children.

Amphetamines should not be used for weight loss or for control of weight. When used for this purpose, they are not considered to be effective and may be dangerous to your health.

These medicines are available only with your doctor's prescription. Prescriptions cannot be refilled. A new prescription must be obtained from your doctor each time you need this medicine.

Before Using This Medicine

In order to decide on the best treatment for your medical problem, your doctor should be told:

—if you have ever had any unusual reaction to amphetamine, dextroamphetamine, ephedrine, epinephrine, isoproterenol, metaproterenol, methamphetamine, norepinephrine (levarterenol), phenylephrine, phenylpropanolamine, pseudoephedrine, or terbutaline.

—if you are pregnant or if you intend to become pregnant while using this medicine. Amphetamines may increase the chance of birth defects if taken during the early months of pregnancy.

—if you are breast-feeding an infant. Although amphetamines have not been shown to cause problems, the chance always exists.

—if you have any of the following medical problems:

Glaucoma	Severe anxiety or
Heart or blood	tension
vessel disease	Severe mental
High blood pressure	illness (especially
Overactive thyroid	in children)

—if you are now taking any of the following medicines or types of medicine:

Acetazolamide	Sodium bicarbonate
Guanethidine	Tricyclic an-
Medicine to make	tidepressants
the urine less acid	(medicine for
Phenothiazines	depression)

—if you are now taking or have taken within the past 2 weeks monoamine oxidase (MAO) inhibitors such as:

Isocarboxazid	Phenelzine
Pargyline	Tranylcypromine

Proper Use of This Medicine

Take this medicine only as directed by your doctor. Do not take more of it, do not take it more often, and do not take it for a longer period of time than your doctor ordered. If too much is taken, it may become habit-forming.

If you are taking the short-acting form of this medicine:

• Take the last dose for each day at least 6 hours before bedtime to help prevent trouble in sleeping.

If you are taking the long-acting form of this medicine:

• Take the daily dose about 10 to 14 hours before bedtime to help prevent trouble in sleeping.

• These capsules or tablets are to be swallowed whole. Do not break, crush, or chew before swallowing.

If you miss a dose of this medicine and your dosing schedule is one dose to be taken:

Once a day—
Take the missed dose as soon as possible, but not later than stated above. Then go back to your regular dosing schedule. But if you do not remember the missed dose until the next day, do not take it at all and do not double the next one. Instead, go back to your regular dosing schedule.

Two or three times a day—
If you remember within an hour or so of the missed dose, take it right away. Then go back to your regular dosing schedule. But if you do not remember

until later, do not take the missed dose at all and do not double the next one. Instead, go back to your regular dosing schedule.

If you have any questions about this, check with your doctor.

Precautions While Using This Medicine

Your doctor should check your progress at regular visits in order to make sure that this medicine does not cause unwanted effects.

If you will be taking this medicine in large doses for a long period of time, do not stop taking it without first checking with your doctor. Your doctor may want you to reduce gradually the amount you are taking before stopping completely.

Dryness of the mouth may occur while you are taking this medicine. Sucking on hard sugarless candy or ice chips or chewing sugarless gum may help relieve the dry mouth.

This medicine may cause some people to feel a false sense of well-being or to become dizzy, lightheaded, or less alert than they are normally. *Make sure you know how you react to this medicine before you drive, use machines, or do other jobs that require you to be alert.*

Side Effects of This Medicine

Along with its needed effects, a medicine may cause some unwanted effects. Although not all of these side effects appear very often, when they do occur they may require medical attention. Check with your doctor if any of the following side effects occur:

Rare

Chest pain or irregular heartbeat	Unusual and uncontrolled movements of head, neck, arms, and legs
Skin rash or hives	

With long-term use or high doses

Mood or mental changes

Other side effects may occur which usually do not require medical attention. These side effects may go away during treatment as your body adjusts to the medicine. However, check with your doctor if any of the following side effects continue or are bothersome:

More common

False sense of well-being	Nervousness
Irritability	Restlessness
	Trouble in sleeping

Note: After such stimulant effects have worn off, drowsiness, trembling, unusual tiredness or weakness, or mental depression may occur.

Less common

Blurred vision	Headache
Changes in sexual desire or decreased sexual ability	Loss of appetite
	Nausea or vomiting
Constipation	Stomach cramps or pain
Diarrhea	Unusual sweating
Dizziness or lightheadedness	Unusual weight loss
Dryness of mouth or unpleasant taste	Unusually fast or pounding heartbeat

After you stop using this medicine, your body may need time to adjust. The length of time this takes depends on the amount of medicine you were using and how long you used it. During this period of time check with your doctor if you notice any of the following side effects:

Mental depression	Trembling
Nausea or vomiting	Unusual tiredness or weakness
Stomach cramps or pain	

Other side effects not listed above may also occur in some patients. If you notice any other effects check with your doctor.

AMPHOTERICIN B (Systemic)
A commonly used brand name is Fungizone.

Amphotericin (am-foe-TER-i-sin) B belongs to the group of medicines called antifungals. It is given by injection to treat certain fungal infections. This medicine is available only with your doctor's prescription.

Before Using This Medicine

In order to decide on the best treatment for your medical problem, your doctor should be told:

—if you have ever had any unusual reaction to amphotericin B in the past. This medicine should not be taken if you are allergic to it.

—if you are pregnant, if you intend to become pregnant, or if you are breast-feeding an infant. Although amphotericin B has not been shown to cause problems, the chance always exists.

—if you have kidney disease.

—if you are now taking any of the following medicines or types of medicine:

Aminoglycoside antibiotics (such as amikacin, gentamicin, kanamycin, streptomycin, or tobramycin)
Capreomycin
Cephaloridine
Cephalothin
Cisplatin
Corticosteroids (cortisone-like medicines)
Digitalis glycosides (heart medicine)
Ethacrynic acid
Flucytosine
Furosemide
Medicine to make the urine less acid
Mithramycin
Polymyxin B
Vancomycin

Side Effects of This Medicine

Along with its needed effects, a medicine may cause some unwanted effects. Although not all of these side effects appear very often, when they do occur they may require medical attention. Check with your doctor if any of the following side effects occur:

With intravenous injection
More common

Fever and chills
Irregular heartbeat
Muscle cramps or pain
Redness, swelling, or pain at place of injection
Unusual tiredness or weakness

Less common or rare

Blurred or double vision
Decreased urination
Numbness, tingling, pain, or weakness in hands or feet
Ringing or buzzing in ears or any loss of hearing
Seizures
Shortness of breath, troubled breathing, wheezing, or tightness in chest
Skin rash or itching
Unexplained sore throat and fever
Unusual bleeding or bruising

With spinal injection
Less common

Difficult urination
Numbness, tingling, pain, or weakness in hands or feet

Rare

Blurred vision or any change in vision

Other side effects may occur which usually do not require medical attention. These side effects may go away during treatment as your body adjusts to the medicine. However, check with your doctor if any of the following side effects continue or are bothersome:

With intravenous injection
More common

Diarrhea
Headache
Indigestion
Loss of appetite
Nausea or vomiting
Stomach pain
Unusual weight loss

With spinal injection
Less common

Back, leg, or stomach pain
Dizziness or lightheadedness
Headache
Nausea or vomiting

Other side effects not listed above may also occur in some patients. If you notice any other effects, check with your doctor.

AMPHOTERICIN B (Topical)
A commonly used brand name is Fungizone.

Amphotericin (am-foe-TER-i-sin) B belongs to the group of medicines called antifungals. Topical amphotericin B is applied to the skin and nails to treat some types of fungal infections. This medicine is available only with your doctor's prescription.

Before Using This Medicine

In order to decide on the best treatment for your medical problem, your doctor should be told:

—if you have ever had any unusual reaction to amphotericin B in the past. This medicine should not be used if you are allergic to it.

—if you are pregnant, if you intend to become pregnant, or if you are breast-feeding an infant, although amphotericin B has not been shown to cause problems.

Proper Use of This Medicine

To help clear up your infection completely, *keep using this medicine for the full time of treatment* even though your condition may have improved.

Apply enough amphotericin B to cover the affected area, and rub in gently.

Do not apply an occlusive dressing or airtight covering (for example, kitchen plastic wrap) over this medicine, since it may cause irritation of the skin. If you have any questions about this, check with your doctor.

If you miss a dose of this medicine, apply it as soon as possible. Then go back to your regular dosing schedule. If you have any questions about this, check with your doctor.

Precautions While Using This Medicine

To help cure the infection and to help prevent reinfection, good health habits are required. These include the following:

• Wash all towels and bedding after use.

• Use only freshly laundered clothes each time clothing is changed.

If you have any questions about this, check with your doctor, nurse, or pharmacist.

When amphotericin B is rubbed into the affected area, it may slightly stain the skin, especially if it is applied to affected areas on or around the nails.

If you are using the cream or lotion form of this medicine:

• If amphotericin B cream or lotion stains your clothing, the stain may be removed by hand-washing with soap and warm water.

If you are using the ointment form of this medicine:

• If amphotericin B ointment stains your clothing, the stain may be removed by applying a standard cleaning fluid.

Side Effects of This Medicine

Along with its needed effects, a medicine may cause some unwanted effects. Although not all of these side effects appear very often, when they do occur they may require medical attention. Check with your doctor if any of the following side effects occur:

Less common

Burning, itching, redness, or other sign of skin irritation not present before using this medicine

Rare

Skin rash

Other side effects may occur which usually do not require medical attention. These side effects may go away during treatment as your body adjusts to the medicine. However, check with your doctor if the following side effect continues or is bothersome:

Less common—for cream dosage form

Dryness of skin

Other side effects not listed above may also occur in some patients. If you notice any other effects, check with your doctor.

ANTHRALIN (Topical)

Some commonly used brand names are Anthra-Derm and Lasan.

Anthralin (AN-thra-lin) is applied to the skin to treat psoriasis. This medicine is available only with your doctor's prescription.

Before Using This Medicine

In order to decide on the best treatment for your medical problem, your doctor should be told:

—if you have ever had any unusual reaction to anthralin in the past. This medicine should not be used if you are allergic to it.

—if you are pregnant, if you intend to become pregnant, or if you are breast-feeding an infant, although anthralin has not been shown to cause problems.

—if you have kidney disease.

Proper Use of This Medicine

Use this medicine only as directed. Do not use more of it, do not use it more often, and do not use it for a longer period of time than your doctor ordered. To do so may increase the chance of side effects.

Anthralin may cause irritation of normal skin. Before applying this medicine to the affected areas, petrolatum may be applied to the skin or scalp around the affected areas for protection.

Apply a thin layer of ointment only to the affected area of the skin or scalp.

Immediately after applying the ointment, wash your hands to remove any medicine that may be on them.

Do not apply this medicine to blistered, raw, or oozing areas of the skin or scalp.

Keep this medicine away from the eyes.

If anthralin is applied to the skin at night, any ointment remaining on the affected areas the next morning should be removed with warm liquid petrolatum followed by a bath. If it is applied to the scalp at night, use a shampoo to clean the scalp the next morning.

If you miss a dose of this medicine, apply it as soon as possible. Then go back to your regular dosing schedule. But if it is almost time for your next dose, do not apply the missed dose at all. Instead, go back to your regular dosing schedule. If you have any questions about this, check with your doctor.

Precautions While Using This Medicine

Your doctor should check your progress at regular visits in order to make sure that anthralin does not cause kidney problems.

Anthralin may stain the skin, hair, or clothing:

• Avoid getting the medicine on your clothing.

• The stain on the skin or hair will wear off after you stop using this medicine.

• To prevent staining of the hands, plastic gloves may be worn when you apply this medicine.

• If the medicine is applied to the scalp at night, a plastic cap may be worn to prevent staining of the pillow.

Side Effects of This Medicine

Along with its needed effects, a medicine may cause some unwanted effects. Although not all of these side effects appear very often, when they do occur they may require medical attention. Check with your doctor if any of the following side effects occur:

Cloudy urine	Skin rash
Redness or other irritation of the skin not present before using this medicine	

Other side effects not listed above may also occur in some patients. If you notice any other effects, check with your doctor.

ANTICOAGULANTS (Systemic)

This information applies to the following medicines:

Coumarin Derivatives
Dicumarol (dye-KOO-ma-role)
Phenprocoumon (fen-proe-KOO-mon)
Warfarin (WAR-far-in)

Indandione Derivatives
Anisindione (an-iss-in-DYE-one)
Phenindione (fen-in-DYE-one)

This information does *not* apply to heparin.

Some commonly used   Generic names:
   brand names are:

Miradon	Anisindione
Dufalone*	Dicumarol
Danilone* Hedulin	Phenindione
Liquamar Marcumar*	Phenprocoumon
Athrombin-K	Warfarin Potassium
Coumadin Panwarfin Warfilone* Warnerin*	Warfarin Sodium

* Not available in the United States.

Anticoagulants decrease the clotting ability of the blood and therefore help to prevent harmful clots from forming in the blood vessels. They are given by mouth; warfarin is also given by injection. These medicines are sometimes called blood thinners, although they do not actually thin the blood. They also will not dissolve clots which already have formed. They are often used as treatment for certain blood vessel, heart, and lung conditions. Anticoagulants are available only with your doctor's prescription.

Before Using This Medicine

In order to decide on the best treatment for your medical problem, your doctor should be told:

—if you have ever had any unusual reaction to anticoagulants in the past.

—if you are pregnant or if you intend to become pregnant while using this medicine. Using anticoagulants during pregnancy may increase the chance of bleeding in both the baby and the mother. In addition, anticoagulants may cause birth defects if they are taken during the first 3 months of pregnancy.

—if you are breast-feeding an infant. Most anticoagulants pass into the breast milk and may cause bleeding problems in infants.

—if you have *any* other medical problems, since many medical problems affect the way your body responds to this medicine.

—if you have recently had any of the following conditions:

Changes in diet	Insertion of intrauterine device (IUD)
Childbirth	
Falls or blows to the body or head	
	Medical or dental surgery
Fever lasting more than a couple of days	Severe or continuing diarrhea
Heavy or unusual menstrual bleeding	Spinal anesthesia X-ray treatment

—if you are taking *any* medicine including over-the-counter (OTC) or nonprescription medicines, (aspirin, laxatives, and antacids, for example), since many medicines change the way this medicine affects your body. Always ask your doctor, nurse, or pharmacist, if starting or stopping any other medicine will change the way your anticoagulant works.

Proper Use of This Medicine

Take this medicine only as directed by your doctor. Do not take more or less of it, do not take it more often, and do not take it for a longer period of time than your doctor ordered.

Your doctor should check your progress at regular visits. A blood test must be taken regularly to see how fast your blood is clotting. This will help your doctor decide on the proper amount of anticoagulant you should be taking each day.

If you miss a dose of this medicine, take it as soon as possible. Then go back to your regular dosing schedule. If you do not remember until the next day, do not take the missed dose at all and do not double the next one. *Doubling the dose may cause bleeding.* Instead, go back to your regular dosing schedule. Be sure to give your doctor a record of any doses you miss. If you have any questions, check with your doctor.

Precautions While Using This Medicine

Tell all doctors and dentists you go to that you are taking this medicine.

Always check with your doctor, nurse, or pharmacist before you start or stop taking any other medicine. This includes any over-the-counter (OTC) or nonprescription medicine, even aspirin. Many medicines change the way this medicine affects your body. You may not be able to take the other medicine, or the dose of your anticoagulant may need to be changed.

Your doctor may want you to carry an identification card stating that you are using this medicine.

While you are taking this medicine, it is very important that you avoid sports and activities which may cause you to be injured. Report to your doctor any falls, blows to the body or head, or other injuries, since serious internal bleeding may occur without your knowing about it.

Take special care in brushing your teeth and in shaving. Use a soft tooth brush and floss gently. Also, it is best to use an electric shaver rather than a blade.

Drinking too much alcohol may change the way this anticoagulant affects your body. Generally, you should not take more than an occasional 1 or 2 drinks. You should not drink regularly on a daily basis or take more than 1 or 2 drinks at any time. If you have any questions, check with your doctor.

Eat a normal, balanced diet while you are taking this medicine. Do not diet or make other changes in your eating habits without your doctor's advice. Check with your doctor if you are unable to eat for several days or if you have continuing diarrhea or fever.

If you are taking anisindione tablets or phenindione tablets:

• Depending on your diet, this medicine may cause the urine to turn orange. Since it may be hard to tell the difference between blood in the urine and this normal coloration, check with your doctor if you notice any color change in your urine.

After you stop taking this medicine, your body will need time to recover before your blood clotting abilities return to normal. Your pharmacist or doctor can tell you how long this will take depending on which anticoagulant you were taking. Use the same caution during this period of time as you did while you were taking the anticoagulant.

Side Effects of This Medicine

Along with its needed effects, a medicine may cause some unwanted effects. Although not all of these side effects appear very often, when they do occur they may require medical attention. Check with your doctor if any of the following side effects occur:

Signs of bleeding inside the body

Abdominal pain or swelling	Coughing up blood
	Dizziness
Back pain or backaches	Severe or continuing headaches
Bloody or black tarry stools	Vomiting blood or material that looks like coffee grounds
Cloudy or bloody urine	
Constipation	

Other less common side effects

Diarrhea (more common for dicumarol)	Unexplained sore throat, fever, chills, or
Itching, skin rash, or hives	unusual tiredness or weakness
Nausea or vomiting	Unusual hair loss

If you are taking anisindione or phenindione:

• In addition to the side effects listed before, check with your doctor if any of the following side effects occur:

Dark urine
Swelling of feet or
  lower legs

Ulcers or sores in
  mouth or throat
Yellowing of eyes or
  skin

Since many things can affect the way your body reacts to this medicine, you should always watch for signs of unusual bleeding. Unusual bleeding may mean that your body is getting more medicine than it needs. Check with your doctor if any of the following signs of overdose occur:

Bleeding from gums
  when brushing
  teeth
Excessive bleeding
  or oozing from
  cuts or wounds

Unexplained bruis-
  ing or purplish
  areas on skin
Unexplained
  nosebleeds
Unusually heavy
  or unexpected
  menstrual
  bleeding

Other side effects may occur which usually do not require medical attention. These side effects may go away during treatment as your body adjusts to the medicine. However, check with your doctor if any of the following side effects continue or are bothersome:

More common

Bloated stomach
  or gas

Less common

Blurred vision
Loss of appetite

Stomach cramps

Other side effects not listed above may also occur in some patients. If you notice any other effects, check with your doctor.

ANTIDIABETICS, ORAL (Systemic)

This information applies to the following medicines:

Acetohexamide (a-seat-oh-HEX-a-mide)
Chlorpropamide (klor-PROE-pa-mide)
Tolazamide (tole-AZ-a-mide)
Tolbutamide (tole-BYOO-ta-mide)

Some commonly used brand names are:	Generic names:
Dimelor* Dymelor	Acetohexamide
Chloromide* Chloronase* Diabinese	Chlorpropamide

Tolinase	Tolazamide
Mobenol* Neo-Dibetic* Novobutamide* Oramide* Orinase Tolbutone*	Tolbutamide

*Not available in the United States.

This medicine belongs to a group of medicines called oral antidiabetics or oral hypoglycemics. They are taken by mouth to help reduce the amount of sugar present in the blood.

Oral antidiabetics are used to treat certain types of diabetes mellitus (sugar diabetes). They can usually be used only by adults who develop diabetes after 30 years of age and who do not require insulin shots (or who do not require more than 40 Units of insulin a day) to control their condition. This type of diabetic is said to have non-insulin-dependent diabetes mellitus (or NIDDM), sometimes known as maturity-onset or Type II diabetes. Oral antidiabetics do not help diabetic patients who have insulin-dependent diabetes mellitus (or IDDM), sometimes known as juvenile-onset or Type I diabetes.

Patients who are taking oral antidiabetic medicine may have to be switched to insulin if they:
—develop diabetic coma or ketoacidosis.
—have a severe injury or burn.
—develop a severe infection.
—are to have major surgery.
—are pregnant.

Oral antidiabetic medicines are available only with your doctor's prescription.

Before Using This Medicine

Importance of Diet—*Before prescribing medicine for your diabetes, your doctor will probably try to control your condition by prescribing a personal diet for you.* Such a diet is low in refined carbohydrates (foods such as sugar and candy used for quick energy). The daily number of calories in this diet should equal the number of calories used by your body each day. In addition, meals and snacks are arranged to meet the energy needs of your body at different times of the day.

Many diabetics are able to control their condition by carefully following their doctor's orders for proper diet and exercise. *Medicine is prescribed only when additional help is needed and is effective only when a schedule of diet and exercise is properly followed.*

Oral antidiabetic medicines are less effective if you are greatly overweight. It may be very important for you to go on a reducing diet. However, check with your doctor before going on any diet.

In order to decide on the best treatment for your medical problem, your doctor should be told:

—if you have ever had any unusual reaction to this medicine in the past. This medicine should not be taken if you are allergic to it.

—if you are pregnant or if you intend to become pregnant while using this medicine. Although medicines for diabetes taken by mouth have not been shown to cause birth defects or other problems, the chance always exists. Therefore, use by pregnant women should be carefully considered.

—if you are breast-feeding an infant. This medicine passes into the breast milk and may cause unwanted effects in infants of mothers taking it. Be sure you have discussed this with your doctor.

—if you have any of the following medical problems:

Kidney disease	Severe infection
Liver disease	Thyroid disease

—if you are now taking any of the following medicines or types of medicine:

Anticoagulants (blood thinners)	Oxyphenbutazone
	Oxytetracycline
Aspirin or other salicylates	Phenylbutazone
	Phenytoin (seizure
Chloramphenicol	medicine)
Cortisone-like medicines	Probenecid
	Propranolol
Dextrothyroxine	Sulfonamides (sulfa
Epinephrine	drugs)
Guanethidine	Thiazide diuretics
Insulin	(water pills)
Monoamine oxidase (MAO) inhibitors (medicine for depression)	Thyroid medicine

Proper Use of This Medicine

Take this medicine only as directed by your doctor. Do not take more or less of it than your doctor ordered, and take it at the same time each day.

Follow carefully the special diet your doctor gave you. This is the most important part of controlling your condition, and is necessary if the medicine is to work properly.

If you miss a dose of this medicine, take it as soon as possible. If it is almost time for your next dose, do not take the missed dose at all and do not double the next one. Instead, go back to your regular dosing schedule.

Precautions While Using This Medicine

Your doctor should check your progress at regular visits, especially during the first few weeks you take this medicine.

Avoid alcoholic beverages until you have discussed their use with your doctor. Some patients who drink alcohol while taking this medicine may suffer stomach pain, nausea, vomiting, dizziness, pounding headache, sweating, or flushing (redness of face and skin). In addition, alcohol may produce hypoglycemia (low blood sugar).

Before having any kind of surgery (including dental surgery) or emergency treatment, tell the doctor or dentist in charge that you are taking this medicine.

Your doctor may want you to carry an identification card or bracelet stating that you are using this medicine.

Do not take any other medicine, unless prescribed or approved by your doctor. This especially includes over-the-counter (OTC) or nonprescription medicine such as that for colds, cough, asthma, hay fever, or appetite control.

Eat or drink something containing sugar and check with your doctor right away if symptoms of low blood sugar (hypoglycemia) appear. Good sources of sugar are orange juice, corn syrup, honey, or sugar cubes or table sugar (especially if mixed or dissolved in water).

• *Signs of low blood sugar are:*

Anxiety	Headache
Chills	Nausea
Cold sweats	Nervousness
Cool pale skin	Rapid pulse
Drowsiness	Shakiness
Excessive hunger	Unusual tiredness or weakness

• *These signs may occur if you:*
—skip or delay meals.
—exercise much more than usual.
—cannot eat because of nausea and vomiting.
—drink a significant amount of alcohol.

• *Instruct someone with you to take you to your doctor or to a hospital right away if you think you are going to pass out.*

Even if these signs are corrected by sugar, it is very important to call your doctor or hospital emergency service right away. The blood sugar–lowering effects of this medicine may last for days and the signs may return often during this period of time.

Test for sugar in your urine as directed by your doctor. This is a convenient way to make sure your diabetes is being controlled and it provides an early warning when it is not.

While taking this medicine, use caution during exposure to the sun. Some people find their skin to be more sensitive to direct sunlight because of the medicine.

You may have read or heard about a study called the University Group Diabetes Program (UGDP). This study compared different treatments for diabetes, including one of the oral antidiabetic medicines (tolbutamide). The results of this study suggested that oral antidiabetics might increase the patient's risk of death from heart and blood vessel disease.

Other studies have not found this effect. In fact, some think that these medicines lower the risk of death from heart and blood vessel disease.

Although this disagreement has not yet been settled, you should keep three things in mind concerning this type of medicine:

• Your doctor prescribed this medicine only after considering the medicine's action and your needs.

• This medicine is used only after the diet prescribed for you did not control your diabetes.

• Your doctor will have you take this medicine only for a trial time to see if it will help your diabetes and will keep a close check on your health in general.

Side Effects of This Medicine

Along with its needed effects, a medicine may cause some unwanted effects. Although not all of these side effects appear very often, when they do occur they may require medical attention. Check with your doctor if any of the following side effects occur:

Rare

Dark urine	Unexplained sore
Fatigue	throat and fever
Itching of the skin	Unusual bleeding or
Light-colored stools	bruising
	Yellowing of the
	eyes or skin

Other side effects may occur which usually do not require medical attention. These side effects may go away during treatment as your body

adjusts to the medicine. However, check with your doctor if any of the following side effects continue or are bothersome:

More common

Diarrhea	Nausea and
Headache	vomiting
Heartburn	Stomach pain or
Loss of appetite	discomfort

Less common

Skin rash

Rare

Increased sensitivity of skin to sun

For patients taking chlorpropamide:
• Some patients who take chlorpropamide may retain or keep more body water than usual. Check with your doctor if any of the following signs of this condition occur:

Drowsiness	Swelling or puf-
Muscle cramps	finess of face,
Seizures	hands, or ankles
	Tiredness
	Weakness

Other side effects not listed above may also occur in some patients. If you notice any other effects, check with your doctor.

ANTIDYSKINETICS (Systemic)

This information applies to the following medicines:

Benztropine (BENZ-troe-peen)
Biperiden (bye-PER-i-den)
Cycrimine (SYE-kri-meen)
Ethopropazine (eth-oh-PROE-pa-zeen)
Procyclidine (proe-SYE-kli-deen)
Trihexyphenidyl (trye-hex-ee-FEN-i-dell)

This information does *not* apply to:

Amantadine	Haloperidol
Carbidopa and	Levodopa
Levodopa	Phenobarbital
Chlordiazepoxide	Propranolol
Diphenhydramine	

Some commonly used brand names are:	Generic names:
Bensylate* Cogentin	Benztropine
Akineton	Biperiden
Pagitane	Cycrimine
Parsidol Parsitan*	Ethopropazine

Kemadrin	Procyclidine
Aparkane* Artane Tremin	Trihexyphenidyl

*Not available in the United States.

This medicine belongs to the general class of medicines called antidyskinetics. It is used to treat Parkinson's disease, sometimes referred to as "shaking palsy." By improving muscle control and reducing stiffness, this medicine allows more normal movements of the body as the disease symptoms are reduced. This medicine is available only with your doctor's prescription.

Before Using This Medicine

In order to decide on the best treatment for your medical problem, your doctor should be told:

—if you have ever had any unusual reaction to antidyskinetics in the past. This medicine should not be taken if you are allergic to it.

—if you are pregnant, if you intend to become pregnant, or if you are breast-feeding an infant. Although antidyskinetics have not been shown to cause problems, the chance always exists.

—if you have any of the following medical problems:

Difficult urination	Intestinal blockage
Enlarged prostate	Kidney disease
Glaucoma	Liver disease
High blood pressure	Myasthenia gravis

—if you are taking any of the following medicines or types of medicine:

Amantadine	Medicine for
Antacids	diarrhea
Haloperidol	Other medicine for
Heart medicine	Parkinson's
Medicine for	disease
depression	Ulcer medicine

—if you are now taking central nervous system (CNS) depressants such as:

Antihistamines or	Prescription pain
medicine for hay	medicine
fever, other	Sedatives, tran-
allergies, or colds	quilizers, or
Barbiturates	sleeping medicine
Narcotics	Seizure medicine

—if you are now taking or have taken within the past 3 weeks monoamine oxidase (MAO) inhibitors such as:

Isocarboxazid	Phenelzine
Pargyline	Tranylcypromine

Proper Use of This Medicine

Take this medicine only as directed by your doctor. To lessen stomach upset, take this medicine immediately after meals or with food, unless your doctor has told you to take it on an empty stomach.

If you miss a dose of this medicine, take it as soon as possible. If it is within 2 hours of your next dose, do not take the missed dose at all and do not double the next one. Instead, go back to your regular dosing schedule. If you have any questions about this, check with your doctor.

Precautions While Using This Medicine

This medicine will add to the effects of alcohol and other medicines (CNS depressants) that slow down the nervous system. Some examples of CNS depressants are antihistamines or medicine for hay fever, other allergies, or colds; sedatives, tranquilizers, or sleeping medicine; prescription pain medicine or narcotics; barbiturates; medicine for seizures; tricyclic antidepressants (medicine for depression); or anesthetics, including some dental anesthetics. *Check with your doctor before taking any of the above while you are using this medicine.*

Do not take this medicine within 1 hour of taking antacid or medicine for diarrhea. Taking them too close together will make this medicine less effective.

This medicine may cause your eyes to become more sensitive to light than they are normally. Wearing sunglasses may help lessen the discomfort from bright light.

This medicine may cause some people to become drowsy, dizzy, or less alert than they are normally. *Make sure you know how you react to this medicine before you drive, use machines, or do other jobs that require you to be alert.*

This medicine will often reduce your tolerance of heat, since it makes you sweat less, causing your body temperature to increase. *Use extra care not to become overheated during exercise or hot weather while you are taking this medicine as this could possibly result in heat stroke.* Also, hot baths or saunas may make you feel dizzy or faint while you are taking this medicine.

Your mouth, nose, and throat may feel very dry while you are taking this medicine. *To help relieve mouth dryness, chew sugarless gum or dissolve bits of ice in your mouth.*

Side Effects of This Medicine

Along with its needed effects, a medicine may cause some unwanted effects. Although not all of these side effects appear very often, when they do occur they may require medical attention. Check with your doctor if any of the following side effects occur:

Less common

Constipation
Difficult urination

Rare

Eye pain
Skin rash

Other side effects may occur which usually do not require medical attention. These side effects may go away during treatment as your body adjusts to the medicine. However, check with your doctor if any of the following side effects continue or are bothersome:

More common

Bloated feeling	Headache
Dizziness	Rapid pulse
Dry mouth	Reduced sweating

Less common

Blurred vision	Mental confusion,
Drowsiness	especially in
Increased sensitivity	elderly
of eyes to light	Nausea and
	vomiting
	Nervousness
	Tiredness

Other side effects not listed above may also occur in some patients. If you notice any other effects, check with your doctor.

ANTIGLAUCOMA AGENTS, CHOLINERGIC (Ophthalmic)—Long-acting Cholinesterase Inhibitors

This information applies to the following medicines:

Demecarium (dem-e-KARE-ee-um)
Echothiophate (ek-oh-THYE-oh-fate)
Isoflurophate (eye-soe-FLURE-oh-fate)

Some commonly used brand names are:	Generic names:
Humorsol	Demecarium
Echodide Phospholine Iodide	Echothiophate
Floropryl	Isoflurophate

This medicine is used in the eye to treat certain types of glaucoma and other eye conditions. It is available only with your doctor's prescription.

Before Using This Medicine

In order to decide on the best treatment for your medical problem, your doctor should be told:

—if you have ever had any unusual reaction to this medicine in the past. This medicine should not be used if you are allergic to it.

—if you are pregnant, if you intend to become pregnant, or if you are breast-feeding an infant. Although cholinesterase inhibitors used in the eye have not been shown to cause problems, the chance always exists.

—if you have any of the following medical problems:

Asthma	Heart disease
Down's syndrome	Parkinsonism
(mongolism)	Stomach ulcer or
Epilepsy	other stomach
Eye disease	problems

—if you are now taking any of the following medicines or types of medicine:

Ambenonium	Pyridostigmine
Neostigmine	

—if you are now using echothiophate or isoflurophate eye medicine and are also using physostigmine eye drops or ointment.

Proper Use of This Medicine

It is very important that you use this medicine only as directed. Do not use more of it and do not use it more often than your doctor ordered. To do so may increase the chance of too much medicine being absorbed into the body and the chance of side effects.

If you miss a dose of this medicine and your dosing schedule is one dose to be applied:

Every other day—
Apply the missed dose as soon as possible if you remember it on the day it should be applied. Then go back to your regular dosing schedule. But if you do not remember the missed dose until the next day, apply it at that time. Then skip a day and start your dosing schedule again.

Once a day—
Apply the missed dose as soon as possible. Then go back to your regular dosing schedule. But if you do not remember the missed dose until the next day, do not apply it at all. Instead, apply your regularly scheduled dose.

More than once a day—
Apply the missed dose as soon as possible. Then go back to your regular dosing schedule. But if it is almost time for your next dose, do not apply the missed dose at all. Instead, apply your next dose at the regularly scheduled time. Then continue with your regular dosing schedule.

If your dosing schedule is different from any of the above and you miss a dose of this medicine, or if you have any questions, check with your doctor.

If you are using the eye-drop form of this medicine:

• How to apply this medicine: First, wash hands. With middle finger, apply pressure to the inside corner of the eye (and continue to apply pressure for 1 or 2 minutes after the medicine has been placed in the eye). Tilt head back and with the index finger of the same hand, pull lower eyelid away from eye to form a pouch. Drop the medicine into the pouch and gently close eyes. Do not blink. Keep eyes closed for 1 or 2 minutes to allow the medicine to be absorbed.

• Remove excess solution around the eye with a clean tissue, being careful not to touch the eye.

• Immediately after applying the eye drops, wash hands to remove any medicine that may be on them.

• To prevent contamination of the eye drops, do not touch the applicator tip to any surface (including the eye) and keep the container tightly closed.

If you are using the ointment form of this medicine:

• How to apply this medicine: First, wash hands. Pull lower eyelid away from eye to form a pouch. Squeeze a thin strip of ointment into the pouch. A 1/2-cm (approximately 1/4-inch) strip of ointment is usually enough unless otherwise directed by your doctor. Gently close eyes and keep them closed for 1 or 2 minutes to allow the medicine to be absorbed.

• Immediately after applying the eye ointment, wash hands to remove any medicine that may be on them.

• Since this medicine loses its effectiveness when exposed to moisture, do not wash the tip of the ointment tube or allow it to touch any moist surface.

• To prevent contamination of the eye ointment, do not touch the applicator tip to any surface (including the eye), wipe the tip of the ointment tube with a clean tissue, and keep the container tightly closed.

Precautions While Using This Medicine

Your doctor should check your eye pressure at regular visits.

If you will be using this medicine for a long period of time, your doctor should examine your eyes at regular visits.

Your doctor may want you to carry an identification card stating that you are using this medicine.

Before having any kind of surgery, (including dental surgery), tell the doctor in charge that you are using this medicine or have used it within the past month.

After you begin using this medicine, your vision may be blurred or there may be a change in your near or distant vision. This may require a change in your eyeglasses. *Make sure your vision is clear before you drive or do other jobs that require you to see well.*

Breathing in even small amounts of carbamate- or organophosphate-type insecticides or pesticides (for example, carbaryl [Sevin], demeton [Systox], diazinon, malathion, parathion, ronnel [Trolene]) may add to the effects of this medicine. Farmers, gardeners, residents of communities undergoing insecticide or pesticide spraying or dusting, workers in plants manufacturing such products, or other persons exposed to such poisons should protect themselves by wearing a mask over the nose and mouth, changing clothes frequently, and washing hands often while using this medicine.

Side Effects of This Medicine

Along with its needed effects, a medicine may cause some unwanted effects. Although not all of these side effects appear very often, when they do occur they may require medical attention. Check with your doctor if any of the following side effects occur:

Possible signs of too much medicine being absorbed into the body

Loss of bladder control	Unusual increase in sweating
Muscle weakness	Unusual tiredness or weakness
Nausea, vomiting, diarrhea, or stomach cramps or pain	Unusual watering of mouth
Shortness of breath, tightness in chest, or wheezing	Unusually slow or irregular heartbeat

Other side effects may occur which usually do not require medical attention. These side effects may go away during treatment as your body adjusts to the medicine. However, check with your doctor if any of the following side effects continue or are bothersome:

Blurred vision or change in near or distant vision	Eye pain Headache
Browache	Twitching of eyelids
Burning, redness, stinging, or other irritation of eyes	Watering of eyes

Other side effects not listed above may also occur in some patients. If you notice any other effects, check with your doctor.

ANTIHISTAMINES (Systemic)

This information applies to the following medicines:

Azatadine (a-ZA-ta-deen)
Bromodiphenhydramine (broe-moe-dye-fen-HYE-dra-meen)
Brompheniramine (brome-fen-EER-a-meen)
Carbinoxamine (kar-bi-NOX-a-meen)
Chlorpheniramine (klor-fen-EER-a-meen)
Clemastine (KLEM-as-teen)
Cyproheptadine (si-proe-HEP-ta-deen)
Dexchlorpheniramine (dex-klor-fen-EER-a-meen)
Dimenhydrinate (dye-men-HYE-dri-nate)
Dimethindene (dye-meth-IN-deen)
Diphenhydramine (dye-fen-HYE-dra-meen)
Diphenylpyraline (dye-fen-il-PEER-a-leen)
Doxylamine (dox-ILL-a-meen)
Pyrilamine (peer-ILL-a-meen)
Tripelennamine (tri-pel-ENN-a-meen)
Triprolidine (trye-PROE-li-deen)

This information does *not* apply to Hydroxyzine, Promethazine, or Trimeprazine

Some commonly used brand names and other names are:	Generic names:
Idulian* Optimine	Azatadine
Ambodryl Deserol*	Bromodiphenhy-dramine
Bromphen Dimetane Ilvin* Puretane Symptom 3	Brompheniramine
Allergefon* Clistin	Carbinoxamine

Chloramate Chlor-Trimeton Histalon* Histaspan Ibioton* Novopheniram* Phenetron Piriton* Teldrin	Chlorpheniramine
Tavegil* Tavist	Clemastine
Cyprodine Nuran* Periactin Vimicon*	Cyproheptadine
Polaramine	Dexchlorpheniramine
Dramamine Eldodram Gravol* Novodimenate* Travamine*	Dimenhydrinate
Dimethpyrindene Forhistal Triten	Dimethindene
Benadryl Bendylate Eldadryl Insomnal* Nautamine* Valdrene	Diphenhydramine
Diafen Hispril	Diphenylpyraline
Decapryn	Doxylamine
Allertoc Mepyramine Neo-Antergan* Thylogen	Pyrilamine
Benzoxal* PBZ Pyribenzamine Pyrizil*	Tripelennamine
Actidil Actidilon* Pro-Actidil*	Triprolidine

*Not available in the United States.

Antihistamines are used to relieve or prevent the symptoms of hay fever and other types of allergy. Some of the antihistamines are also used to prevent motion sickness, nausea, vomiting, and dizziness. In patients with Parkinson's disease, diphenhydramine may be used to decrease stiffness and tremors. In addition, since antihistamines may cause drowsiness as a side effect, some of them may be used to help people go to sleep.

Certain antihistamine preparations are available only with your doctor's prescription. Others are available without a prescription; however, your doctor may have special instructions on the proper dose of the medicine for your medical condition.

Before Using This Medicine

In order to decide on the best treatment for your medical problem, the following should be kept in mind and/or your doctor should be told:

—if you have ever had any unusual reaction to antihistamines in the past. This medicine should not be taken if you are allergic to it.

—if you are pregnant or if you intend to become pregnant. Although antihistamines have not been shown to cause problems in humans, the chance always exists.

—if you are breast-feeding an infant. Antihistamines may pass into the breast milk and cause unwanted effects in the infant.

—if you have any of the following medical problems:

Enlarged prostate	Overactive thyroid
Heart disease	Stomach ulcer
High blood pressure	Urinary tract
Increased eye	blockage
pressure	

—if you are now taking any central nervous system (CNS) depressants such as:

Barbiturates	Prescription pain
Medicine for	medicine
seizures	Sedatives, tran-
Narcotics	quilizers, or
Other antihis-	sleeping medicine
tamines or	Tricyclic an-
medicine for hay	tidepressants
fever, other	(medicine for
allergies,	depression)
or colds	

—if you are now taking or have taken within the past 2 weeks monoamine oxidase (MAO) inhibitors such as:

Isocarboxazid	Phenelzine
Pargyline	Tranylcypromine

Proper Use of This Medicine

Antihistamines are used to relieve or prevent the symptoms of your medical problem. Take them only as directed. Do not take more of them or take them more often than your doctor ordered.

Do not give this medicine to premature or newborn infants, unless otherwise directed by your doctor.

If you must take this medicine regularly and you miss a dose, take the missed dose as soon as possible. However, if it is almost time for your next dose, do not take the missed dose at all and do not double the next one. Instead, go back to your regular dosing schedule. If you have any questions about this, check with your doctor or pharmacist.

If you are taking this medicine by mouth:

• Take it with food or a glass of water or milk to lessen stomach irritation if necessary.

• If you are taking the long-acting tablet form of this medicine, the tablets are to be swallowed whole. Do not break, crush, or chew before swallowing.

If you are taking dimenhydrinate or diphenhydramine:

• If you are taking this medicine for motion sickness, take it at least 30 minutes before or, even better, 1 to 2 hours before you begin to travel.

If you are using the suppository form of this medicine:

• How to insert suppository: First remove foil wrapper and moisten the suppository with water. Lie down on side and push the suppository well up into the rectum with finger. If the suppository is too soft to insert because of storage in a warm place, before removing the foil wrapper chill the suppository in the refrigerator for 30 minutes or run cold water over it.

Precautions While Using This Medicine

This medicine will add to the effects of alcohol and other medicines (CNS depressants) that slow down the nervous system. Some examples of CNS depressants are other antihistamines or medicine for hay fever, other allergies, or colds; sedatives, tranquilizers, or sleeping medicine; prescription pain medicine or narcotics; barbiturates; medicine for seizures; tricyclic antidepressants (medicine for depression); or anesthetics, including some dental anesthetics. *Check with your doctor before taking any of the above while you are using this medicine.*

This medicine may cause some people to become drowsy or less alert than they are normally.

Even if taken at bedtime, it may cause some people to feel drowsy or less alert on arising. *Make sure you know how you react to this medicine before you drive, use machines, or do other jobs that require you to be alert.*

When taking antihistamines on a regular basis, make sure your doctor knows if you are taking large amounts of aspirin at the same time (as in arthritis). Effects of too much aspirin, such as ringing in the ears, may be covered up by the antihistamine.

Side Effects of This Medicine

Along with its needed effects, a medicine may cause some unwanted effects. Although not all of these side effects appear very often, when they do occur, they may require medical attention. Check with your doctor if any of the following side effects occur:

Rare

Unexplained sore throat and fever	Unusual weakness that continues
Unusual bleeding or bruising	

Other side effects may occur which usually do not require medical attention. These side effects may go away during treatment as your body adjusts to the medicine. However, check with your doctor if any of the following side effects continue or are bothersome:

More common

Drowsiness	Thickening of the bronchial secretions

Less common or rare

Blurred vision	Skin rash
Difficult or painful urination	Unusual increase in sweating
Dizziness	Unusually fast heartbeat
Dryness of mouth, nose, and throat	Upset stomach or stomach pain (more common with pyrilamine and tripelennamine)
Loss of appetite (increased appetite with cyproheptadine)	
Nervousness, restlessness, or trouble in sleeping (especially in children)	

Other side effects not listed above may also occur in some patients. If you notice any other effects, check with your doctor.

ANTIPYRINE, BENZOCAINE, AND GLYCERIN (Otic)

Some commonly used brand names are Auralgan and Aurasol.

Antipyrine (an-tee-PYE-reen), benzocaine (BEN-zoe-kane), and glycerin (GLI-ser-in) combination is used to help relieve the pain, swelling, and redness of some ear infections. It will not cure the infection itself. This medicine is available only with your doctor's prescription.

Before Using This Medicine

In order to decide on the best treatment for your medical problem, your doctor should be told:

—if you have had allergic reactions to antipyrine or glycerin or to benzocaine or other local anesthetics in the past.

—if you have a punctured ear drum.

Proper Use of This Medicine

You may warm the ear drops to body temperature (37 °C or 98.6 °F) by holding the bottle in your hand for a few minutes before applying.

To prevent contamination of the ear drops, do not touch the dropper to any surface (including the ear).

How to apply this medicine: Lie down or tilt the head so that the infected ear faces up. For adults, gently pull the ear lobe up and back to straighten the ear canal. (For children, gently pull the ear lobe down and back to straighten the ear canal.) Drop medicine into the ear canal. Keep ear facing up for several minutes to allow medicine to run to the bottom of the ear canal. A clean soft cotton plug may be gently inserted into the ear opening to prevent the medicine from leaking out.

Do not rinse dropper after use. Wipe the tip of the dropper with a clean tissue and keep the container tightly closed.

If you miss a dose of this medicine, apply it as soon as possible. Then go back to your regular dosing schedule. But if it is almost time for your next dose, do not apply the missed dose at all. Instead, go back to your regular dosing schedule. If you have any questions about this, check with your doctor.

Side Effects of This Medicine

Along with its needed effects, a medicine may cause some unwanted effects. The following side effects may go away during treatment as your body adjusts to the medicine; however, check with your doctor if either continues or is bothersome:

Itching or burning in the ear

Other side effects not listed above may also occur in some patients. If you notice any other effects, check with your doctor.

ANTITHYROID AGENTS (Systemic)

This information applies to the following medicines:

Methimazole (meth-IM-a-zole)
Propylthiouracil (proe-pill-thye-oh-YOOR-a-sill)

Some commonly used brand names and other names are:	Generic names:
Tapazole Thiamazole	Methimazole
Propacil Propyl-Thyracil	Propylthiouracil

Methimazole and propylthiouracil belong to the group of medicines known as antithyroid agents. They are used to treat conditions in which the thyroid gland produces too much thyroid hormone and also before thyroid surgery. Antithyroid agents may also be used for other conditions as determined by your doctor. Methimazole and propylthiouracil are available only with your doctor's prescription.

Before Using This Medicine

In order to decide on the best treatment for your medical problem, your doctor should be told:

—if you have ever had any unusual reaction to methimazole or propylthiouracil in the past. This medicine should not be taken if you are allergic to it.

—if you are pregnant or if you intend to become pregnant while using this medicine. Too much use of it during pregnancy may cause unwanted effects, including birth defects, in the baby. Be sure that you have discussed this with your doctor before taking this medicine.

—if you are breast-feeding an infant. This medicine passes into breast milk and may cause unwanted effects in infants of mothers taking this medicine.

—if you have any of the following medical problems:

Blood disease   Liver disease
Infection

—if you are now taking or have recently taken anticoagulants (blood thinners).

Proper Use of This Medicine

Use this medicine only as directed by your doctor. Do not use more or less of it and do not use it more often or for a longer period of time than your doctor ordered.

In order for it to work properly, *this medicine must be taken every day in regularly spaced doses, as ordered by your doctor.*

Food in your stomach may change the effects of this medicine. To make sure that you always get the same effects, try to take this medicine at the same time in relation to meals every day. That is, always take it with meals or always take it on an empty stomach.

If you miss a dose of this medicine, take it as soon as possible. If it is almost time for your next dose, take both doses together. Then go back to your regular dosing schedule. If you miss more than one dose or if you have any questions about this, check with your doctor.

Precautions While Using This Medicine

It is very important that your doctor check your progress at regular intervals.

It may take several days or weeks for this medicine to work. However, *do not stop taking this medicine without first checking with your doctor.* Some medical problems may require several years of continuous treatment.

Before having any kind of surgery (including dental surgery) or emergency treatment, *tell the doctor or dentist in charge that you are taking this medicine.*

Check with your doctor right away if you get an injury, infection, or illness of any kind. Your doctor may want you to stop taking this medicine.

Side Effects of This Medicine

Along with its needed effects, a medicine may cause some unwanted effects. Although not all of these side effects appear very often, when they do occur they may require medical attention. *Stop taking this medicine and check with your doctor immediately* if any of the following side effects occur:

Less common

| Unexplained fever, chills, or sore throat | Yellowing of eyes and skin |

Check with your doctor also if any of the following side effects occur:

Rare

Backache	Sleepiness
Changes in menstrual periods	Swelling of feet or lower legs
Coldness	Swollen lymph glands
Constipation	
Diarrhea	Tiredness
Dry, puffy skin	Unusual bleeding or bruising
Fever	
Headache	Unusual increase or decrease in urination
Irritability	
Listlessness	
Loss of hearing	Unusual weight gain
Muscle aches	Vomiting
Rapid or irregular heartbeat	Weakness

Other side effects may occur which usually do not require medical attention. These side effects may go away during treatment as your body adjusts to the medicine. However, check with your doctor if any of the following side effects continue or are bothersome:

More common

Itching

Less common

Dizziness	Numbness or tingling of fingers, toes, or face
Joint pain	
Loss of taste	
Nausea and vomiting	Skin rash
	Stomach pain

Rare

| Darkening of skin | Loss of hair |
| Lightening of hair color | Sore, red, watery eyes |

Other side effects not listed above may also occur in some patients. If you notice any other effects, check with your doctor.

APC (Systemic)

Some commonly used brand names are:

Acetophen	Asalco No. 1	Sal-Fayne
Aidant	Asphac-G	Salphenine
APAC	P-A-C	Tabloid APC
A.S.A. Compound	Compound Phencaset	

APC is a combination of aspirin (AS-pir-in), phenacetin (fe-NASS-e-tin), and caffeine (KAF-een). It is used for short periods of time (up to 10 days for adults and up to 5 days for children) to relieve pain and reduce fever. APC is taken by mouth in the form of capsules or tablets. This medicine is available without a prescription; however, the product's directions and warnings should be carefully followed. In addition, your doctor may have special instructions on the proper dose of APC for your medical condition.

Before Using This Medicine

In order to decide on the best treatment for your medical problem, your doctor should be told:

—if you have ever had any unusual reaction to acetaminophen, phenacetin, caffeine, aspirin or other salicylates including methyl salicylate (oil of wintergreen), or to other nonsteroidal anti-inflammatory agents such as fenoprofen, ibuprofen, indomethacin, naproxen, oxyphenbutazone, phenylbutazone, sulindac, or tolmetin.

—if you are pregnant or if you intend to become pregnant while using this combination medicine. Too much use of aspirin during the last 3 months of pregnancy may increase the length of pregnancy and may prolong labor. Aspirin taken during the last 2 weeks of pregnancy may cause the baby to have bleeding problems at birth. When phenacetin is used during pregnancy, it may cause side effects in the newborn infant. In addition, although aspirin, phenacetin, or caffeine has not been shown to cause birth defects in humans, the chance always exists.

—if you are breast-feeding an infant. Although aspirin, phenacetin, or caffeine has not been shown to cause problems, the chance always exists.

—if you have any of the following medical problems:

Anemia	Hemophilia or other bleeding problems
Asthma, allergies, and nasal polyps (history of)	Hodgkin's disease
	Hypoprothrombinemia
Glucose-6-phosphate dehydrogenase (G6PD) deficiency	Kidney disease
	Liver disease
	Ulcer or other stomach problems
Gout	Vitamin K deficiency

—if you are now taking any of the following medicines or types of medicine:

Antacids
Anticoagulants
(blood thinners)
Gout medicine
Inflammation
medicine (for
example, arthritis
medicine)
Insulin
Methotrexate

Oral hypoglycemics
(diabetes medicine
you take by
mouth)
Spironolactone
Urine acidifiers
(medicine to
make your
urine more acid)
Urine alkalizers
(medicine to
make your
urine less acid)
Vitamin C

Proper Use of This Medicine

Take this medicine with food or a full glass (8 ounces) of water or milk to lessen stomach irritation.

Do not use this medicine if it has a strong vinegar-like odor, since this means the aspirin in the product is breaking down. If you have any questions about this, check with your doctor or pharmacist.

Do not place tablets directly on tooth or gum surface as this may cause a burn.

Unless otherwise directed by your doctor:

• *Do not take more of this medicine than recommended on the package label.* If too much is taken, kidney damage may occur.

• Children up to 12 years of age should not take this medicine for more than 5 days in a row.

• Adults should not take this medicine for more than 10 days in a row.

If you have been directed to take this medicine for a longer period of time, it is important that your doctor check your progress at regular visits.

Keep this medicine out of the reach of children since overdose is very dangerous in young children.

Precautions While Using This Medicine

Check with your doctor:

—if your symptoms do not improve or if they become worse.

—if you are taking this medicine to bring down a fever, and the fever lasts for more than 3 days or returns.

Check the labels of all over-the-counter (OTC), nonprescription, and prescription medicines you now take. If any contain aspirin or other salicylates, or phenacetin be especially careful, since taking them while taking this medicine may lead to overdose. If you have any questions about this, check with your doctor or pharmacist.

Caution: Diabetics—This medicine contains aspirin and phenacetin which may cause false test results with urine sugar tests. If you have any questions about this, check with your doctor, nurse, or pharmacist, especially if your diabetes is not well controlled.

Stomach problems may be more likely to occur if you drink alcoholic beverages while being treated with this medicine. Check with your doctor if you have any questions about this.

If you plan to have surgery, including dental surgery, do not take this medicine for the 5 days before it, unless otherwise directed by your doctor. The aspirin in this product, if taken during this time, may cause bleeding problems.

Side Effects of This Medicine

Along with its needed effects, a medicine may cause some unwanted effects. Although not all of these side effects appear very often, when they occur they may require medical attention. When this medicine is used for short periods of time at low doses, side effects usually are rare. However, check with your doctor or pharmacist if any of the following occur:

Less common

Any loss of hearing
Bloody or black
tarry stools
Itching or skin rash
Nausea or vomiting

Stomach pain
Wheezing, tightness
in chest, or
shortness of
breath

Possible signs of overdose

Dizziness or
mental confusion
Nausea or vomiting
Rapid breathing

Ringing or buzzing
in ear (continu-
ing)
Severe or continuing
headache
Stomach pain

Possible side effects with long-term use

Bluish-colored
fingernails or
mucous mem-
branes
Cloudy urine

Swelling of feet or
lower legs
Unusual tiredness or
weakness

Other side effects may occur which usually do not require medical attention. These side effects may go away during treatment as your body adjusts to the medicine. However, check with your doctor or pharmacist if any of the following side effects continue or are bothersome:

Indigestion
Sleeplessness,
nervousness, or
jitters

Other side effects not listed above may also occur in some patients. If you notice any other effects, check with your doctor or pharmacist.

APC AND CODEINE (Systemic)
Some commonly used brand names are:
A.S.A. and Codeine Compound
P-A-C Compound with Codeine
Salatin with Codeine
Tabloid APC with Codeine

APC and codeine (KOE-deen) is a combination of pain relievers. APC is the short name for aspirin, phenacetin, and caffeine (AS-pir-in, fe-NASS-e-tin, and KAF-een). APC and codeine combination is available only with your doctor's prescription.

Before Using This Medicine
In order to decide on the best treatment for your medical problem, your doctor should be told:

—if you have ever had any unusual reaction to codeine, acetaminophen, phenacetin, caffeine, or aspirin or other salicylates including methyl salicylate (oil of wintergreen), or to other non-steroidal anti-inflammatory agents such as fenoprofen, ibuprofen, indomethacin, naproxen, oxyphenbutazone, phenylbutazone, sulindac, or tolmetin.

—if you are pregnant or if you intend to become pregnant while using this combination medicine. Too much use of aspirin during the last 3 months of pregnancy may increase the length of pregnancy and prolong labor. Aspirin taken during the last 2 weeks of pregnancy may cause the baby to have bleeding problems at birth. When phenacetin is used during pregnancy, it may cause side effects in the newborn infant. In addition, although aspirin, phenacetin, caffeine, or codeine has not been shown to cause birth defects in humans, the chance always exists.

—if you are breast-feeding an infant. Although aspirin, phenacetin, caffeine, and codeine have not been shown to cause problems, the chance always exists. Therefore, use by nursing mothers should be carefully considered.

—if you have any of the following medical problems:

Anemia	Gout
Asthma, allergies, and nasal polyps (history of)	Hemophilia or other bleeding problems
Brain disease or injury	Hodgkin's disease
	Hypoprothrombinemia
Colitis	Kidney disease
Emphysema, asthma, or chronic lung disease	Liver disease
	Ulcer or other stomach problems
Enlarged prostate or problems with urination	Underactive adrenal gland (Addison's disease)
Gallbladder disease or gallstones	Underactive thyroid
	Unusually slow or irregular heartbeat
Glucose-6-phosphate dehydrogenase (G6PD) deficiency	Vitamin K deficiency

—if you are now taking any of the following medicines or types of medicine:

Antacids	Prescription medicine for stomach cramps or spasms
Anticoagulants (blood thinners)	
Gout medicine	Spironolactone
Inflammation medicine (for example, arthritis medicine)	Urine acidifiers (medicine to make your urine more acid)
Insulin	Urine alkalizers (medicine to make your urine less acid)
Methotrexate	
Oral hypoglycemics (diabetes medicine you take by mouth)	Vitamin C

—if you are now taking other central nervous system (CNS) depressants such as:

Antihistamines or medicine for hay fever, other allergies, or colds	Sedatives, tranquilizers, or sleeping medicine
Barbiturates	Seizure medicine
Other narcotics	Tricyclic antidepressants (medicine for depression)
Other prescription pain medicine	

—if you are now taking or have taken within the past 2 weeks monoamine oxidase (MAO) inhibitors such as:

Isocarboxazid	Phenelzine
Pargyline	Tranylcypromine

Proper Use of This Medicine

Take this medicine with food or a full glass (8 ounces) of water or milk to lessen stomach irritation.

Do not use this medicine if it has a strong vinegar-like odor, since this means the aspirin in the product is breaking down. If you have any questions about this, check with your doctor or pharmacist.

Take this medicine only as directed by your doctor. Do not take more of it, do not take it more often, and do not take it for a longer period of time than your doctor ordered. If too much is taken, it may become habit-forming or cause kidney damage.

Keep this medicine out of the reach of children since overdose is very dangerous in young children.

Precautions While Using This Medicine

Check with your doctor if your symptoms do not improve or if they become worse.

Check the labels of all over-the-counter (OTC), nonprescription, and prescription medicines you now take. If any contain codeine or other narcotics, aspirin or other salicylates, or phenacetin be especially careful, since taking them while taking this medicine may lead to overdose. If you have any questions about this, check with your doctor or pharmacist.

Caution: Diabetics—This medicine contains aspirin and phenacetin which may cause false test results with urine sugar tests. If you have any questions about this, check with your doctor, nurse, or pharmacist, especially if your diabetes is not well controlled.

If you will be taking this medicine for a long period of time (for example, for several months at a time), your doctor should check your progress at regular visits.

Do not take this medicine for 5 days before having surgery, including dental surgery, unless otherwise directed by your doctor. The aspirin in this product, if taken during this time, may cause bleeding problems.

This medicine will add to the effects of alcohol and other medicines (CNS depressants) that slow down the nervous system. Some examples of CNS depressants are antihistamines or medicine for hay fever, other allergies, or colds; sedatives, tranquilizers, or sleeping medicine; prescription pain medicine or narcotics; barbiturates; medicine for seizures; tricyclic antidepressants (medicine for depression); or anesthetics, including some dental anesthetics. In addition, stomach problems may be more likely to occur if you drink alcoholic beverages while being treated with this medicine. *Check with your doctor before taking any of the above while you are using this medicine.*

This medicine may cause some people to become drowsy or less alert than they are normally. *Make sure you know how you react to this medicine before you drive, use machines, or do other jobs that require you to be alert.*

Dizziness, lightheadedness, or fainting may occur, especially when you get up from a lying or sitting position. Getting up slowly may help lessen this problem.

Nausea may occur, especially after the first couple of doses. This effect usually goes away if you lie down for awhile. However, if nausea or vomiting continues, check with your doctor.

Stomach problems may be more likely to occur if you drink alcoholic beverages while being treated with this medicine. Check with your doctor if you have any questions about this.

Side Effects of This Medicine

Along with its needed effects, a medicine may cause some unwanted effects. Although not all of these side effects appear very often, when they do occur they may require medical attention. Check with your doctor if any of the following side effects occur:

Any loss of hearing	Unusual excitement
Bloody or black	(especially in
tarry stools	children)
Itching or skin rash	Unusually slow
Nausea or vomiting	heartbeat
Shortness of breath	Wheezing or
Stomach pain	tightness
Troubled breathing	in chest

Possible signs of overdose

Dizziness or mental	Ringing or buzzing
confusion	in ear (con-
Nausea or vomiting	tinuing)
Rapid breathing	Severe or continuing
	headache
	Stomach pain

Possible side effects with long-term use of APC

Bluish-colored	Swelling of feet or
fingernails or	lower legs
mucous mem-	Unusual tiredness or
branes	weakness
Cloudy urine	

Other side effects may occur which usually do not require medical attention. These side effects may go away during treatment as your body adjusts to the medicine. However, check with your doctor if any of the following side effects continue or are bothersome:

More common

Constipation
Drowsiness

Less common

Difficult urination	Redness or flushing
Dizziness	of face
Feeling faint	Sleeplessness,
Frequent urge to	nervousness, or
urinate	jitters
Indigestion	Unusual increase in
Lightheadedness	sweating
Loss of appetite	Unusual tiredness or
	weakness

Other side effects not listed above may also occur in some patients. If you notice any other effects, check with your doctor.

APOMORPHINE (Systemic)

Apomorphine (a-poe-MOR-feen) is used in the emergency treatment of certain types of poisoning. It is given by injection to cause vomiting of the poison. This medicine is available only on prescription and should be administered only by or under the immediate supervision of a doctor.

Before Using This Medicine

In order to decide on the best treatment for your medical problem, your doctor should be told:

—if you have ever had any unusual reaction to codeine, hydromorphone, levorphanol, morphine, opium alkaloids, oxycodone, or oxymorphone.

—if you are pregnant, if you intend to become pregnant, or if you are breast-feeding an infant. Although apomorphine has not been shown to cause problems, the chance always exists.

—if you have heart disease.

—if you tend to vomit easily.

—if you are now taking an antiemetic (medicine for nausea or vomiting).

Proper Use of This Medicine

Before you receive an injection of this medicine, your doctor may want you to drink a full glass (8 ounces) of water. This is to help the medicine cause vomiting of the poison.

Side Effects of This Medicine

Along with its needed effects, a medicine may cause some unwanted effects. Although not all of these side effects appear very often, when they do occur they may require medical attention. Check with your doctor if any of the following side effects occur:

Shortness of breath	Unusually slow
or troubled	heartbeat
breathing	Vomiting (con-
	tinuing)

Other side effects may occur which usually do not require medical attention. These side effects may go away during treatment as your body adjusts to the medicine. However, check with your doctor if any of the following side effects continue or are bothersome:

More common

Drowsiness	Unusual tiredness or
Nausea	weakness
Unusual sweating	Unusual watering of
	mouth

Less common or rare

Dizziness or light-	Rapid or irregular
headedness	breathing
False sense of	Restlessness
well-being	Trembling
Feeling faint	Unusually fast
	heartbeat

Other side effects not listed above may also occur in some patients. If you notice any other effects, check with your doctor.

APPETITE SUPPRESSANTS (Systemic)

This information applies to the following medicines:

Benzphetamine (benz-FET-a-meen)
Chlorphentermine (klor-FEN-ter-meen)
Clortermine (klor-TER-meen)
Diethylpropion (dye-eth-il-PROE-pee-on)
Mazindol (MAY-zin-dole)
Phendimetrazine (fen-dye-MET-ra-zeen)
Phenmetrazine (fen-MET-ra-zeen)
Phentermine (FEN-ter-meen)

This information does not apply to fenfluramine.

Some commonly used brand names are:	Generic names:
Didrex	Benzphetamine
Pre-Sate	Chlorphentermine

Voranil	Clortermine
Dietec* Regibon* Tenuate Tepanil	Diethylpropion
Sanorex	Mazindol
Bontril PDM Phendiet Plegine	Phendimetrazine
Preludin	Phenmetrazine
Ionamin	Phentermine

* Not available in the United States.

Appetite suppressants are used in the short-term (a few weeks) treatment of obesity. For a few weeks (6 to 12), these medicines in combination with dieting can help patients lose weight. However, since their appetite-reducing effect is only temporary, they are useful only for the first few weeks of dieting until new eating habits are established. They are not effective for continuous use in diet control. These medicines are available only with your doctor's prescription.

Before Using This Medicine

In order to decide on the best treatment for your medical problem, your doctor should be told:

—if you have ever had any unusual reaction to amphetamine, dextroamphetamine, ephedrine, epinephrine, isoproterenol, metaproterenol, methamphetamine, norepinephrine (levarterenol), phenylephrine, phenylpropanolamine, pseudoephedrine, or terbutaline.

—if you are pregnant, if you intend to become pregnant, or if you are breast-feeding an infant. Although appetite suppressants in recommended doses have not been shown to cause problems in humans, the chance always exists.

—if you have any of the following medical problems:

Diabetes	Heart or blood
Epilepsy	vessel disease
Glaucoma	High blood pressure
	Overactive thyroid

—if you are now taking any of the appetite suppressants and are also taking any of the following medicines or types of medicine:

Guanethidine
Phenothiazines

—if you are now taking mazindol and are also taking medicine for asthma or other breathing problems (for example, epinephrine, isoproterenol).

—if you are now taking central nervous system (CNS) stimulants such as:

Caffeine	Medicine for nar-
Medicine for hyper-	colepsy (uncon-
active children	trolled desire
	for sleep
	or sudden
	attacks of sleep at
	irregular inter-
	vals)
	Other medicine for
	appetite control

—if you are now taking or have taken within the past 2 weeks monoamine oxidase (MAO) inhibitors such as:

Isocarboxazid	Phenelzine
Pargyline	Tranylcypromine

Proper Use of This Medicine

Take this medicine only as directed by your doctor. Do not take more of it, do not take it more often, and do not take it for a longer period of time than your doctor ordered. If too much is taken, it may become habit-forming.

If you think this medicine is not working as well after you have taken it for a few weeks, *do not increase the dose.* Instead, check with your doctor.

If you are taking the short-acting form of this medicine:

• Take the last dose for each day about 4 to 6 hours before bedtime to help prevent trouble in sleeping.

If you are taking the long-acting form of this medicine:

• Take the daily dose about 10 to 14 hours before bedtime to help prevent trouble in sleeping.

• These capsules or tablets are to be swallowed whole. Do not break, crush, or chew before swallowing.

If you are taking the appetite suppressant, mazindol:

• To help prevent trouble in sleeping, if you are taking this medicine in a:

—*1-mg tablet,* take the last dose for each day about 4 to 6 hours before bedtime.
—*2-mg tablet,* take the dose once each day about 10 to 14 hours before bedtime.

Precautions While Using This Medicine

Your doctor should check your progress at regular visits in order to make sure that this medicine does not cause unwanted effects.

If you will be taking this medicine in large doses for a long period of time, do not stop taking it without first checking with your doctor. Your doctor may want you to reduce gradually the amount you are taking before stopping completely.

Dryness of the mouth may occur while you are taking this medicine. Sucking on hard sugarless candy or ice chips or chewing sugarless gum may help relieve the dry mouth.

This medicine may cause some people to feel a false sense of well-being or to become dizzy, lightheaded, drowsy, or less alert than they are normally. *Make sure you know how you react to this medicine before you drive, use machines, or do other jobs that require you to be alert.*

Side Effects of This Medicine

Along with its needed effects, a medicine may cause some unwanted effects. Although not all of these side effects appear very often, when they do occur they may require medical attention. Check with your doctor if any of the following side effects occur:

Rare

> Mood or mental
> changes
> Skin rash or hives

Other side effects may occur which usually do not require medical attention. These side effects may go away during treatment as your body adjusts to the medicine. However, check with your doctor if any of the following side effects continue or are bothersome:

More common

False sense of well-being (less common with mazindol and phentermine)	Irritability Nervousness Restlessness Trouble in sleeping

Note: After such stimulant effects have worn off, drowsiness, trembling, unusual tiredness or weakness, or mental depression may occur.

Less common

Blurred vision Changes in sexual desire or decreased sexual ability Constipation (more common with mazindol) Diarrhea Difficult or painful urination	Dizziness or light-headedness Dryness of mouth (more common with mazindol) Frequent urge to urinate or increased urination Headache

Nausea or vomiting Stomach cramps or pain Unpleasant taste	Unusual sweating Unusually fast, pounding, or irregular heartbeat

Although not all of the side effects listed above have been reported for all of these medicines, they have been reported for at least one of them. However, since all of the appetite suppressants are very similar, any of the above side effects may occur with any of these medicines.

After you stop using this medicine, your body may need time to adjust. The length of time this takes depends on the amount of medicine you were using and how long you used it. During this period of time check with your doctor if you notice any of the following side effects:

Mental depression Nausea or vomiting Stomach cramps or pain	Trembling Unusual tiredness or weakness .

Other side effects not listed above may also occur in some patients. If you notice any other effects, check with your doctor.

ASPARAGINASE (Systemic)
A commonly used brand name is Elspar.

Asparaginase (a-SPARE-a-gin-ase) belongs to the group of drugs known as enzymes. It is used to treat some kinds of cancer by preventing the cancer cells from getting the materials they need to live. Asparaginase is available only from your doctor.

Before Using This Medicine

Asparaginase is a very strong medicine. In addition to its helpful effects in treating your medical problem, it has side effects that could be very serious. Make sure you have discussed the use of it with your doctor.

In order to decide on the best treatment for your medical problem, your doctor should be told:

—if you have ever had any unusual reaction to asparaginase in the past.

—if you are pregnant, if you intend to become pregnant, or if you are breast-feeding an infant. Although asparaginase has not been shown to cause problems, the chance always exists.

—if you have any of the following medical problems:

Diabetes	Kidney stones
Gout	Liver disease
Infection	Pancreatitis

—if you have ever been treated with asparaginase or had an allergic reaction to it.

—if you are taking gout medicine.

—if you have been treated with x-rays or cancer drugs by another doctor.

Proper Use of This Medicine

This medicine is usually given together with certain other medicines. If you are using a combination of drugs, it is important that you receive each medicine at the proper time. If you are taking some of these medicines by mouth, ask your doctor, nurse, or pharmacist to help you plan a way to remember to take them at the right time.

This medicine often causes nausea, vomiting, and loss of appetite. However, it is very important that you continue to receive the medicine, even if you begin to feel ill. After several doses, your stomach upset should lessen. If you have any questions about this, check with your doctor.

Precautions While Using This Medicine

It is very important that your doctor check your progress at regular visits.

While you are using this medicine, your doctor may want you to drink plenty of fluids and urinate often. This will help prevent kidney problems and keep your kidneys working well. If you have any questions about this, check with your doctor.

This medicine may cause some people to become drowsy or less alert than they are normally. *Make sure you know how you react to this medicine before you drive, use machines, or do other jobs that require you to be alert.* This effect may last several weeks after you have received the drug.

Side Effects of This Medicine

Along with its needed effects, a medicine may cause some unwanted effects. Although not all of these side effects appear very often, when they do occur they may require medical attention. Check with your doctor if any of the following side effects occur:

More common

Difficulty in breathing	Lightheadedness
Joint pain	Puffy face

Severe stomach pain with nausea and vomiting	Unusual bleeding or bruising
Skin rash or itching	Yellowing of the eyes and skin

Less common

Flank or stomach pain	Swelling of feet or lower legs
Shakiness or unusual body movements	Unexplained fever, chills or sore throat
Sore throat	Unusual thirst
Sores in the mouth or on the lips	Unusually frequent urination

Other side effects may occur which usually do not require medical attention. These side effects may go away during treatment as your body adjusts to the medicine. However, check with your doctor if any of the following side effects continue or are bothersome:

More common

Headache	Mild stomach cramps
Irritability	Nausea and vomiting
Loss of appetite	Weight loss

Less common

Drowsiness	Mental confusion
Hallucinations (seeing, hearing, or feeling things that are not there)	Mental depression
	Nervousness
	Tiredness

After you stop using this medicine, it may still produce some side effects that need attention. During this period of time, check with your doctor if you have severe stomach pain with nausea and vomiting.

Other side effects not listed above may also occur in some patients. If you notice any other effects, check with your doctor.

ASPIRIN AND CODEINE (Systemic)

A commonly used brand name is Empirin with Codeine.

Aspirin and codeine (AS-pir-in and KOE-deen) is a combination of pain relievers. It is available only with your doctor's prescription.

Before Using This Medicine

In order to decide on the best treatment for your medical problem, your doctor should be told:

—if you have ever had any unusual reaction to codeine or to aspirin or other salicylates including methyl salicylate (oil of wintergreen), or to other nonsteroidal anti-inflammatory agents such as fenoprofen, ibuprofen, indomethacin, naproxen, oxyphenbutazone, phenylbutazone, sulindac, or tolmetin.

—if you are pregnant or if you intend to become pregnant while using this medicine. Too much use of aspirin during the last 3 months of pregnancy may increase the length of pregnancy and may prolong labor. Also, aspirin taken during the last 2 weeks of pregnancy may cause the baby to have bleeding problems at birth. In addition, although aspirin and codeine have not been shown to cause birth defects in humans, the chance always exists.

—if you are breast-feeding an infant. Although aspirin and codeine have not been shown to cause problems, the chance always exists. Therefore, use by nursing mothers should be carefully considered.

—if you have any of the following medical problems:

Anemia	Hemophilia or other
Asthma, allergies,	bleeding problems
and nasal polyps	Hodgkin's disease
(history of)	Hypoprothrom-
Brain tumor	binemia
Colitis	Kidney disease
Emphysema,	Liver disease
asthma, or	Ulcer or other
chronic lung	stomach problems
disease	Underactive adrenal
Enlarged prostate or	gland (Addison's
problems with	disease)
urination	Underactive thyroid
Gallbladder disease	Unusually slow or
or gallstones	irregular heart-
Gout	beat
Head injury	Vitamin K deficiency

—if you are now taking any of the following medicines or types of medicine:

Antacids	Prescription
Anticoagulants	medicine for
(blood thinners)	stomach cramps
Gout medicine	or spasms
Inflammation	Spironolactone
medicine	Urine acidifiers
(for example,	(medicine to
arthritis	make your urine
medicine)	more acid)
Insulin	Urine alkalizers
Methotrexate	(medicine to
Oral hypoglycemics	make your urine
(diabetes medicine	less acid)
you take by	Vitamin C
mouth)	

—if you are now taking other central nervous system (CNS) depressants such as:

Antihistamines or	Sedatives, tran-
medicine for hay	quilizers,
fever, other	or sleeping
allergies,	medicine
or colds	Seizure medicine
Barbiturates	Tricyclic an-
Other narcotics	tidepressants
Other prescription	(medicine for
pain medicine	depression)

—if you are now taking or have taken within the past 2 weeks monoamine oxidase (MAO) inhibitors such as:

Isocarboxazid	Phenelzine
Pargyline	Tranylcypromine

Proper Use of This Medicine

Take this medicine with food or a full glass (8 ounces) of water or milk to lessen stomach irritation.

Do not use this medicine if it has a strong vinegar-like odor, since this means the aspirin is breaking down. If you have any questions about this, check with your doctor or pharmacist.

Keep this medicine out of the reach of children since overdose is especially dangerous in young children.

Take this medicine only as directed by your doctor. Do not take more of it, do not take it more often, and do not take it for a longer period of time than your doctor ordered. If too much is taken, it may become habit-forming.

Precautions While Using This Medicine

Check with your doctor if your symptoms do not improve or if they become worse.

Check the labels of all over-the-counter (OTC), nonprescription, and prescription medicines you now take. If any contain aspirin or other salicylates, or codeine be especially careful, since taking them while taking this medicine may lead to overdose. If you have any questions about this, check with your doctor or pharmacist.

Caution: Diabetics—This medicine contains aspirin which may cause false test results with urine sugar tests if you regularly take 8 or more tablets a day. Smaller doses or occasional use of aspirin usually do not affect urine sugar tests. If you have any questions about this, check with your doctor, nurse, or pharmacist, especially if your diabetes is not well controlled.

If you will be taking this medicine for a long period of time (for example, for several months at a time), your doctor should check your progress at regular visits.

Do not take this medicine for 5 days before having any kind of surgery, including dental surgery, unless otherwise directed by your doctor. Taking aspirin during this time may cause bleeding problems.

This medicine will add to the effects of alcohol and other medicines (CNS depressants) that slow down the nervous system. Some examples of CNS depressants are antihistamines or medicine for hay fever, other allergies, or colds; sedatives, tranquilizers, or sleeping medicine; prescription pain medicine or narcotics; barbiturates; medicine for seizures; tricyclic antidepressants (medicine for depression); or anesthetics, including some dental anesthetics. In addition, stomach problems may be more likely to occur if you drink alcoholic beverages while being treated with this medicine. *Check with your doctor before taking any of the above while you are using this medicine.*

This medicine may cause some people to become drowsy or less alert than they are normally. *Make sure you know how you react to this medicine before you drive, use machines, or do other jobs that require you to be alert.*

Dizziness, lightheadedness, or fainting may occur, especially when you get up from a lying or sitting position. Getting up slowly may help lessen this problem.

Nausea may occur, especially after the first couple of doses. This effect usually goes away if you lie down for awhile. However, if nausea or vomiting continues, check with your doctor.

Side Effects of This Medicine

Along with its needed effects, a medicine may cause some unwanted effects. Although not all of these side effects appear very often, when they do occur they may require medical attention. Check with your doctor if any of the following side effects occur:

More common

Nausea or vomiting
Stomach pain

Less common

Any loss of hearing	Itching or skin rash
Bloody or black tarry stools	Shortness of breath Troubled breathing

Unusual excitement (especially in children)	Unusually slow heartbeat Wheezing or tightness in chest

Possible signs of overdose

Dizziness or mental confusion	Ringing or buzzing in ear (continuing)
Rapid breathing	Severe or continuing headache

Other side effects may occur which usually do not require medical attention. These side effects may go away during treatment as your body adjusts to the medicine. However, check with your doctor if the following side effects continue or are bothersome:

More common

Constipation	Indigestion
Drowsiness	

Less common

Difficult urination	Loss of appetite
Dizziness	Redness or flushing of face
Feeling faint	
Frequent urge to urinate	Unusual increase in sweating
Lightheadedness	Unusual tiredness or weakness

Other side effects not listed above may also occur in some patients. If you notice any other effects, check with your doctor.

ATROPINE (Ophthalmic)

This information applies to the following medicines:

Atropine (A-troe-peen)
Homatropine (hoe-MA-troe-peen)
Scopolamine (skoe-POL-a-meen)

Some commonly used brand names are:	Generic names:
Atropisol BufOpto Atropine Isopto Atropine	Atropine
Homatrocel Isopto Homatropine	Homatropine
Isopto Hyoscine	Scopolamine

Ophthalmic atropine, homatropine, and scopolamine are used in the eye to dilate (enlarge) the pupil. They are used before eye examinations, before and after eye surgery, and to treat certain eye conditions. These medicines are available only with your doctor's prescription.

Before Using This Medicine

In order to decide on the best treatment for your medical problem, your doctor should be told:

—if you have ever had any unusual reaction to atropine, homatropine, or scopolamine in the past. This medicine should not be used if you are allergic to it.

—if you are pregnant, if you intend to become pregnant, or if you are breast-feeding an infant. Although atropine, homatropine, or scopolamine has not been shown to cause problems, the chance always exists.

—if you have any of the following medical problems:

Brain damage (in   Glaucoma
    children)   Spastic paralysis (in
Down's syndrome   children)
    (mongolism)

Proper Use of This Medicine

Use this medicine only as directed. Do not use more of it and do not use it more often than your doctor ordered. To do so may increase the chance of too much medicine being absorbed into the body and the chance of side effects. *This is especially important when this medicine is used in children, since overdose is very dangerous in children.*

If you miss a dose of this medicine and your dosing schedule is one dose to be applied:

Once a day—
    Apply the missed dose as soon as possible. Then go back to your regular dosing schedule. But if you do not remember the missed dose until the next day, do not apply it at all. Instead, apply your regularly scheduled dose.

More than once a day—
    Apply the missed dose as soon as possible. Then go back to your regular dosing schedule. But if it is almost time for your next dose, do not apply the missed dose at all. Instead, apply your next dose at the regularly scheduled time. Then continue with your regular dosing schedule.

If you have any questions about this, check with your doctor.

If you are using the eye-drop form of this medicine:
• How to apply this medicine: First, wash hands. With middle finger, apply pressure to the inside corner of the eye (and continue to apply pressure for 1 or 2 minutes after the medicine has been placed in the eye). Tilt head back and with the index finger of the same hand, pull lower eyelid away from eye to form a pouch. Drop the medicine into the pouch and gently close eyes. Do not blink. Keep eyes closed for 1 or 2 minutes to allow the medicine to be absorbed.

• To prevent contamination of the eye drops, do not touch the applicator tip to any surface (including the eye) and keep the container tightly closed.

If you are using the ointment form of this medicine:
• How to apply this medicine: First, wash hands. Pull lower eyelid away from eye to form a pouch. Squeeze a thin strip of ointment into the pouch. A 1/3- to 1/2-cm (approximately 1/8-inch in infants and young children and 1/4-inch in older children and adults) strip of ointment is usually enough unless otherwise directed by your doctor. Gently close eyes and keep them closed for 1 or 2 minutes to allow the medicine to be absorbed.

• To prevent contamination of the eye ointment, do not touch the applicator tip to any surface (including the eye), wipe the tip of the ointment tube with a clean tissue, and keep the tube tightly closed.

Precautions While Using This Medicine

After you apply this medicine to your eyes, your pupils will become unusually large. This will cause blurring of vision. It will also cause your eyes to become more sensitive to light than they are normally. Wearing sunglasses may help relieve the discomfort from bright light. These effects may continue for several days after you stop using this medicine. However, check with your doctor if they continue longer than:

—14 days if you are using atropine.
—3 days if you are using homatropine.
—7 days if you are using scopolamine.

Side Effects of This Medicine

Along with its needed effects, a medicine may cause some unwanted effects. Although not all of these side effects appear very often, when they do occur they may require medical attention. Check with your doctor if any of the following side effects occur:

Possible signs of too much medicine being absorbed into the body

Clumsiness or unsteadiness	Increased thirst or unusual dryness of mouth
Fever	
Flushing or redness of face	Mental confusion or unusual behavior
Hallucinations (seeing, hearing, or feeling things that are not there)	Skin rash Slurred speech Swollen stomach in infants

Unusual drowsiness,   Unusually fast
   tiredness, or   heartbeat
   weakness

Other side effects may occur which usually do not
require medical attention. These side effects
may go away during treatment as your body
adjusts to the medicine. However, check with
your doctor if any of the following side effects
continue or are bothersome:

Increased sensitivity   Irritation of eye not
   of eyes to light   present before
                     using this
                     medicine

Other side effects not listed above may also occur
in some patients. If you notice any other effects, check with your doctor.

AZATHIOPRINE (Systemic)
A commonly used brand name is Imuran.

Azathioprine (ay-za-THYE-oh-preen) belongs
to the group of medicines known as immunosup-
pressive agents. It is used in situations such as
transplants to reduce the body's natural immunity.
Azathioprine is available only with your doctor's
prescription.

Before Using This Medicine

Azathioprinc is a very strong medicine. In addition
to its helpful effects in treating your medical
problem, it has side effects that could be very
serious. Before you take this medicine, be sure
that you have discussed the use of it with your
doctor.

In order to decide on the best treatment for your
medical problem, your doctor should be told:

—if you have ever had any unusual reaction to
azathioprine in the past.

—if you are pregnant or if you intend to
become pregnant while using this medicine.
Azathioprine may cause birth defects. This can
happen if either the male or the female is using
it at the time of conception. The use of birth
control methods is recommended. If you have
any questions about this, check with your doctor.

—if you are breast-feeding an infant. Although
azathioprine has not been shown to cause problems, the chance always exists.

—if you have any of the following medical
problems:

Gout   Liver disease
Infection   Pancreatitis
Kidney disease

—if you have been treated with x-rays or
cancer drugs by another doctor.

Proper Use of This Medicine

Use this medicine only as directed by your doctor.
Do not use more or less of it, and do not use it
more often than your doctor ordered.

This medicine is sometimes given together with
certain other medicines. If you are using a combination of drugs, make sure that you take
each medicine at the proper time and do not
mix them. Ask your doctor, nurse, or pharmacist to help you plan a way to remember to
take your medicines at the right time.

*Do not stop taking this medicine without first
checking with your doctor.*

If you miss a dose of this medicine and your dosing
schedule is:
   Once a day—
      Do not take the missed dose at all and do
      not double the next one. Instead, go back to
      your regular dosing schedule and check
      with your doctor.
   Several times a day—
      Take the missed dose as soon as you
      remember it. If it is time for your next dose,
      take both doses together, then go back to
      your regular dosing schedule. If you miss
      more than one dose, check with your doc-
      tor.

Precautions While Using This Medicine

*It is very important that your doctor check your
progress at regular visits.*

Side Effects of This Medicine

Along with its needed effects, a medicine may
cause some unwanted effects. Although not all
of these side effects appear very often, when
they do occur they may require medical attention. Check with your doctor *immediately* if
any of the following side effects occur:

More common

Cold sores   Unusual bleeding or
Unexplained fever,   bruising
  chills, or sore   Unusual tiredness or
  throat   weakness

Less common

Diarrhea   Nausea and
Loss of appetite   vomiting
                   Yellowing of the
                   eyes and skin

Rare

Cough	Shortness of breath
Severe stomach pain with nausea and vomiting	Sores in the mouth and on the lips

Other side effects may occur which usually do not require medical attention. These side effects may go away during treatment as your body adjusts to the medicine. However, check with your doctor if any of the following side effects continue or are bothersome:

Rare

Joint pain	Skin rash
Loss of hair	

After you stop using this medicine, it may still produce some side effects that need attention. During this period of time check with your doctor if you notice any of the following:

Unexplained fever, chills, or sore throat	Unusual bleeding or bruising

Other side effects not listed above may also occur in some patients. If you notice any other effects, check with your doctor.

BACLOFEN (Systemic)
A commonly used brand name is Lioresal.

Baclofen (BAK-loe-fen) is a medicine used to help relax certain muscles in your body. It relieves the spasms, cramping, and tightness of muscles caused by medical problems such as multiple sclerosis. This medicine is available only with your doctor's prescription.

Before Using This Medicine

In order to decide on the best treatment for your medical problem, your doctor should be told:

—if you have ever had any unusual reaction to baclofen in the past. This medicine should not be taken if you are allergic to it.

—if you are pregnant or if you intend to become pregnant, or if you are breast-feeding an infant. Although this medicine has not been shown to cause problems in humans, the chance always exists.

—if you have any of the following medical problems:

Epilepsy	Stroke
Kidney disease	

—if you are taking any of the following medicines or types of medicine:

Insulin	
Oral hypoglycemics (diabetes medicine you take by mouth)	

—if you are now taking other central nervous system (CNS) depressants such as:

Antihistamines or medicine for hay fever, other allergies, or colds	Sedatives, tranquilizers, or sleeping medicine
Barbiturates	Seizure medicine
Narcotics	Tricyclic antidepressants
Pain medicine (prescription)	(medicine for depression)

—if you are now taking or have taken within the past 2 weeks monoamine oxidase (MAO) inhibitors such as:

Isocarboxazid	Phenelzine
Pargyline	Tranylcypromine

Proper Use of This Medicine

If you miss a dose of this medicine and remember within an hour or so of the missed dose, take it right away. Then go back to your regular dosing schedule. But if you do not remember until later, do not take the missed dose at all and do not double the next one. Instead, go back to your regular dosing schedule. If you have any questions about this, check with your doctor.

Precautions While Using This Medicine

Do not suddenly stop taking this medicine. Hallucinations (seeing, hearing, or feeling things that are not there) may occur if the medicine is stopped suddenly. Check with your doctor for the best way to reduce gradually the amount you are taking before stopping completely.

This medicine will add to the effects of alcohol and other medicines (CNS depressants) that slow down the nervous system. Some examples of CNS depressants are antihistamines or medicine for hay fever, other allergies, or colds; sedatives, tranquilizers, or sleeping medicine; prescription pain medicine or narcotics; barbiturates; medicine for seizures; tricyclic antidepressants (medicine for depression); or anesthetics, including some dental anesthetics. *Check with your doctor before taking any of the above while you are using baclofen.*

This medicine may cause some people to become drowsy or less alert than they are normally. *Make sure you know how you react to this medicine before you drive, use machines, or do other jobs that require you to be alert.*

Caution: Diabetics—This medicine may cause your blood sugar levels to rise. If you notice a change in the results of your urine sugar test or if you have any questions, check with your doctor.

Side Effects of This Medicine

Along with its needed effects, a medicine may cause some unwanted effects. Although not all of these side effects appear very often, when they do occur they may require medical attention. Check with your doctor if any of the following side effects occur:

Rare

Bloody or dark urine	Itching or skin rash
Chest pain	Mental depression
Fainting	
Hallucinations (seeing, hearing, or feeling things that are not there)	

Possible signs of overdose

Blurred vision or any change in vision	Unusual muscle weakness
Seizures	Vomiting
Shortness of breath or troubled breathing	

Other side effects may occur which usually do not require medical attention. These side effects may go away during treatment as your body adjusts to the medicine. However, check with your doctor if any of the following side effects continue or are bothersome:

More common

Dizziness	Mental confusion
Drowsiness	Nausea

Less common

Constipation	Headache
Frequent urge to urinate	Trouble in sleeping

Rare

Decreased sexual ability in males	Ringing or buzzing in ears
Diarrhea	Slurred speech
Difficult or painful urination	Stomach pain or discomfort
Loss of appetite	Stuffy nose
Muscle pain	Trembling
Pounding heartbeat	Weight gain

Other side effects not listed above may also occur in some patients. If you notice any other effects, check with your doctor.

BARBITURATES (Systemic)

This information applies to the following medicines:

Amobarbital (am-oh-BAR-bi-tal)
Butabarbital (byoo-ta-BAR-bi-tal)
Hexobarbital (hex-oh-BAR-bi-tal)
Mephobarbital (me-foe-BAR-bi-tal)
Metharbital (meth-AR-bi-tal)
Pentobarbital (pen-toe-BAR-bi-tal)
Phenobarbital (fee-noe-BAR-bi-tal)
Secobarbital (see-koe-BAR-bi-tal)
Secobarbital and Amobarbital (see-koe-BAR-bi-tal and am-oh-BAR-bi-tal)
Talbutal (TAL-byoo-tal)

Some commonly used brand names are:	Generic names:
Amytal Isobec*	Amobarbital
Buticaps Butisol	Butabarbital
Sombulex	Hexobarbital
Mebaral	Mephobarbital
Gemonil	Metharbital
Nembutal Nova-Rectal* Pentogen*	Pentobarbital
Eskabarb* Gardenal* Nova-Pheno* Sedadrops SK-Phenobarbital Solfoton	Phenobarbital
Secogen* Seconal Seral*	Secobarbital
Tuinal	Secobarbital and Amobarbital
Lotusate	Talbutal

*Not available in the United States.

Barbiturates (bar-BI-tyoo-rates) belong to the group of medicines called central nervous system (CNS) depressants. They are given by mouth, by injection, or rectally to treat insomnia or sleeplessness by helping patients fall asleep. Also, they are used to help calm or relax patients who are nervous or tense. Some of the barbiturates are used as anticonvulsants to help control convulsions or seizures in certain disorders or diseases, such as epilepsy. Barbiturates may also be used for other conditions as determined by your doctor. These medicines are available only with your doctor's prescription.

Before Using This Medicine

In order to decide on the best treatment for your medical problem, your doctor should be told:

—if you have ever had any unusual reaction to barbiturates.

—if you are pregnant or if you intend to become pregnant while using this medicine. Too much use of barbiturates during pregnancy may cause the baby to become dependent on the medicine. This may lead to withdrawal side effects after birth. In addition, use of this medicine during pregnancy may cause bleeding problems in the newborn infant. Also, use of barbiturates during late pregnancy may cause breathing problems in the newborn infant. Barbiturates taken for epilepsy during pregnancy may increase the chance of birth defects.

—if you are breast-feeding an infant. Barbiturates pass into the breast milk and may cause unwanted effects in infants of mothers taking this medicine.

—if you have any of the following medical problems:

Asthma (or history of), emphysema, or chronic lung disease	Kidney disease Liver disease Porphyria (or history of)
Hyperactivity (in children)	Underactive adrenal gland

—if you are now taking any central nervous system (CNS) depressants such as:

Antihistamines or medicine for hay fever, other allergies, or colds	Sedatives, tranquilizers, or sleeping medicine Seizure medicine
Narcotics Other barbiturates Prescription pain medicine	Tricyclic antidepressants (medicine for depression)

—if you are now taking or have taken within the past 2 weeks monoamine oxidase (MAO) inhibitors such as:

Isocarboxazid Pargyline	Phenelzine Tranylcypromine

—if you are now taking any of the following medicines or types of medicine:

Anticoagulants (blood thinners)	Digitalis Digitoxin
Contraceptives, oral (birth-control pills)	Doxycycline Estrogens Griseofulvin
Corticosteroids (cortisone-like medicines)	Phenytoin Quinidine
Cyclophosphamide	

Proper Use of This Medicine

Use this medicine only as directed by your doctor. Do not use more of it, do not use it more often, and do not use it for a longer period of time than your doctor ordered. If too much is used, it may become habit-forming.

Keep barbiturates out of the reach of children since overdose is especially dangerous in children.

If you are taking this medicine regularly (for example, every day as in epilepsy) and you miss a dose, take it right away if you remember within an hour or so of the missed dose. Then go back to your regular dosing schedule. But if you do not remember until later, do not take the missed dose at all and do not double the next one. Instead, go back to your regular dosing schedule. If you have any questions about this, check with your doctor.

If you are taking the *extended-release capsule or tablet* form of this medicine:

• These capsules or tablets are to be swallowed whole. Do not break, crush, or chew before swallowing.

If you are taking the *pediatric drop* form of this medicine:

• Do not use if solution is cloudy.

• This medicine is to be taken by mouth even though it may come in a dropper bottle. Measure the correct amount with the specially marked dropper. Each dose may be taken straight or mixed with water, milk, or fruit juices. Be sure to drink all of the liquid in order to get the full dose of medicine.

If you are using the *rectal suppository* form of this medicine:

• How to insert suppository: First remove the foil wrapper and moisten the suppository with water. Lie down on side and push the suppository well up into rectum with finger.

Precautions While Using This Medicine

If you will be using this medicine regularly for a long period of time:

• Your doctor should check your progress at regular visits.

• Do not stop using it without first checking with your doctor. Your doctor may want you to reduce gradually the amount you are using before stopping completely.

This medicine will add to the effects of alcohol and other medicines (CNS depressants) that slow down the nervous system. Some examples of CNS depressants are antihistamines or medicine for hay fever, other allergies, or colds; sedatives, tranquilizers, or sleeping medicine; prescription pain medicine or narcotics; barbiturates; medicine for seizures; tricyclic antidepressants (medicine for depression); or anesthetics, including some dental anesthetics. *Check with your doctor before taking any of the above while you are taking this medicine.*

If you think you may have taken an overdose, get emergency help at once. Taking an overdose of a barbiturate or taking alcohol or other CNS depressants with the barbiturate may lead to unconsciousness and possibly death. Some signs of an overdose are mental confusion, severe weakness, shortness of breath or troubled breathing, staggering, and unusually slow heartbeat.

This medicine may cause some people to become dizzy, lightheaded, drowsy, or less alert than they are normally. Even if taken at bedtime, it may cause some people to feel drowsy or less alert on arising. *Make sure you know how you react to this medicine before you drive, use machines, or do other jobs that require you to be alert.*

Side Effects of This Medicine

Along with its needed effects, a medicine may cause some unwanted effects. Although not all of these side effects appear very often, when they do occur they may require medical attention. Check with your doctor if any of the following side effects occur:

Less common or rare

Mental confusion or depression	Unusual excitement
Shortness of breath or troubled breathing	Unusual tiredness or weakness
Skin rash or hives	Unusually slow heart beat
Swelling of eyelids, face, or lips	Wheezing or tightness in chest
Unexplained sore throat and fever	Yellowing of eyes or skin
Unusual bleeding or bruising	

Other side effects may occur which usually do not require medical attention. These side effects may go away during treatment as your body adjusts to the medicine. However, check with your doctor if any of the following side effects continue or are bothersome:

More common

Clumsiness or unsteadiness	Drowsiness
Dizziness or lightheadedness	"Hangover" effect

Less common

Diarrhea	Nausea
Headache	Slurred speech
Joint or muscle pain	Vomiting

After you stop using this medicine, your body may need time to adjust. The length of time this takes depends on the amount of medicine you were using and how long you used it. During this period of time check with your doctor if you notice any of the following side effects:

Convulsions or seizures	Increased dreaming
Feeling faint	Nightmares
Hallucinations (seeing, hearing, or feeling things that are not there)	Trembling
	Trouble in sleeping
	Unusual restlessness
	Unusual weakness

Other side effects not listed above may also occur in some patients. If you notice any other effects, check with your doctor.

BECLOMETHASONE (Inhalation)

Some commonly used brand names are Beclovent and Vanceril.

Beclomethasone (be-kloe-METH-a-sone) is an adrenocorticoid (cortisone-like medicine). It belongs to the general family of medicines called steroids. This medicine is used to help prevent asthma attacks. It will not help an asthma attack that has already started. Adrenocorticoids are available only with your doctor's prescription.

Before Using This Medicine

In order to decide on the best treatment for your medical problem, your doctor should be told:

—if you have had any unusual reactions to steroids or aerosol spray inhalation medicines in the past.

—if you are pregnant, if you intend to become pregnant, or if you are breast-feeding an infant. Although beclomethasone has not been shown to cause problems in humans, the chance always exists.

—if you have an infection of the mouth, throat, or lungs.

Proper Use of This Medicine

Beclomethasone is used with a special inhaler and usually comes with patient directions. *Read the directions carefully before using.*

If you are also using a bronchodilator inhaler to help you breathe better, use it first, then wait several minutes before using this medicine. If your bronchodilator does not seem to be working, check with your doctor.

This medicine has to be taken every day in regularly spaced doses as ordered by your doctor. One to 4 weeks may pass before you feel its full effects.

Do not use this medicine more often than your doctor ordered. To do so may increase the chance of absorption through the lungs and the chance of side effects.

Container provides about 200 measured sprays.

Store away from heat and direct sunlight. Do not puncture, break, or burn container.

Gargling and rinsing your mouth after each dose may help prevent hoarseness and throat irritation.

If you miss a dose of this medicine, take it as soon as possible. If it is almost time for your next dose, do not take the missed dose at all and do not double the next one. Instead, go back to your regular dosing schedule. If you have any questions about this, check with your doctor.

Precautions While Using This Medicine

If you are also taking another adrenocortical steroid (for example, cortisone, prednisone) for your asthma along with this medicine, do not stop taking the other steroid without your doctor's advice, even if your asthma seems better. If your doctor tells you to reduce or stop taking your other steroid, check with him or her if you notice any of the following side effects:

Abdominal or back pain	Prolonged loss of appetite
Dizziness or fainting	Shortness of breath
Fever	Unusual tiredness
Muscle or joint pain	or weakness
Nausea or vomiting	Unusual weight loss

Also check with your doctor if you go through a period of unusual stress or if you have a severe asthma attack.

Check with your doctor:
—if signs of mouth, throat, or lung infection occur.
—if your symptoms do not improve.
—if your condition gets worse.

Side Effects of This Medicine

Along with its needed effects, a medicine may cause some unwanted effects. The following

side effects may go away during treatment as your body adjusts to the medicine; however, check with your doctor if they continue or are bothersome:

Cough	Throat irritation
Hoarseness	

Other side effects not listed above may also occur in some patients. If you notice any other effects, check with your doctor.

BELLADONNA ALKALOIDS AND BARBITURATES (Systemic)

This information applies to the following medicines:

Atropine (A-troe-peen), Hyoscyamine (hye-oh-SYE-a-meen), Scopolamine (skoe-POL-a-meen), and Butabarbital (byoo-ta-BAR-bi-tal)

Atropine, Hyoscyamine, Scopolamine, Butabarbital, Pentobarbital (pen-toe-BAR-bi-tal), and Phenobarbital (fee-noe-BAR-bi-tal)

Atropine, Hyoscyamine, Scopolamine, and Phenobarbital

Atropine and Phenobarbital

Belladonna and Amobarbital (am-oh-BAR-bi-tal)

Belladonna and Butabarbital

Belladonna and Phenobarbital

Hyoscyamine, Scopolamine, and Phenobarbital

Hyoscyamine and Butabarbital

Hyoscyamine and Phenobarbital

Some commonly used brand names are:	Generic names:
Minabel Omnibel Palbar	Atropine, Hyoscyamime, Scopolamine, and Butabarbital
Cyclo-Bell	Atropine, Hyoscyamine, Scopolamine, Butabarbital, Pentobarbital, and Phenobarbital
Barbidonna Donna-Sed Donnatal Donphen Hasp Hybephen Hyosophen Kinesed Sedralex Setamine Spalix Spasmolin Spasmophen Spasmorel Tri-Spas	Atropine, Hyoscyamine, Scopol- amine, and Phenobarbital

Alised Antrocol Atrobarb	Atropine and Phenobarbital
Amobell	Belladonna and Amobarbital
Butibel	Belladonna and Butabarbital
Belap Bellophen Bello-Phen Chardonna Donabarb Donnabarb Oxoids Phenobel Phenobella Sedajen Valaspas	Belladonna and Phenobarbital
Hybar	Hyoscyamine, Scopolamine, and Phenobar- bital
Cystospaz-SR	Hyoscyamine and Butabarbital

Anaspaz PB
Levsin-PB
Levsin
  w/Phenobarbital
Levsinex
  w/Phenobarbital
	Hyoscyamine and
	Phenobarbital

Belladonna alkaloids and barbiturates is a combination of medicines used to relieve cramping and spasms of the stomach, intestines, and bladder. It is used also to decrease the amount of acid formed in the stomach. This medicine is available only with your doctor's prescription.

Before Using This Medicine

In order to decide on the best treatment for your medical problem, your doctor should be told:

—if you have ever had an unusual reaction to atropine, belladonna, or barbiturates. This medicine should not be taken if you are allergic to it.

—if you are pregnant or if you intend to become pregnant while using this medicine. When used during pregnancy, barbiturates may cause difficulty in breathing and changes in blood clot formation in the newborn. Be

sure that you have discussed this with your doctor before taking this medicine. In addition, although belladonna alkaloids or barbiturates have not been shown to cause birth defects, the chance always exists.

—if you are breast-feeding an infant. Although belladonna alkaloids or barbiturates have not been shown to cause problems, the chance always exists.

—if you have any of the following medical problems:

Brain damage
  (children)
Chronic intestinal
  problems
Difficult urination
Glaucoma
Kidney disease
	Liver disease
	Lung disease
	Prostate enlarge-
	  ment
	Rapid heartbeat
	Spastic paralysis
	  (children)

—if you are now taking any of the following medicines or types of medicine:

Amantadine
Antacids
Anticoagulants
  (blood
  thinners)
Antidiarrhea
  medicine
Corticosteroids
  (cortisone-like
  medicine)
	Digitalis or
	  digitoxin (heart
	  medicine)
	Griseofulvin (fungus
	  medicine)
	Medicine for
	  Parkinson's
	  disease
	Other medicine for
	  intestinal or
	  stomach cramping
	Tetracycline
	Ulcer medicine

—if you are now taking any other central nervous system (CNS) depressants such as:

Antihistamines or
  medicine for hay
  fever, other
  allergies,
  or colds
Medicine for
  seizures
Narcotics
Other barbiturates
	Prescription pain
	  medicine
	Sedatives, tran-
	  quilizers,
	  or sleeping
	  medicine
	Tricyclic an-
	  tidepressants
	  (medicine for
	  depression)

—if you are now taking or have taken within the past 2 weeks monoamine oxidase (MAO) inhibitors such as:

Isocarboxazid Pargyline	Phenelzine Tranylcypromine

Proper Use of This Medicine

Take this medicine only as directed by your doctor. Do not take more or less of it, do not take it more often, and do not take it for a longer period of time than your doctor ordered.

Take this medicine about 1/2 to 1 hour before meals unless otherwise directed by your doctor.

If you miss a dose of this medicine, do not take the missed dose at all and do not double the next one. Instead, go back to your regular dosing schedule. If you have any questions about this, check with your doctor.

Precautions While Using This Medicine

This medicine will add to the effects of alcohol and other medicines (CNS depressants) that slow down the nervous system. Some examples of CNS depressants are antihistamines or medicine for hay fever, other allergies, or colds; sedatives, tranquilizers, or sleeping medicine; prescription pain medicine or narcotics; barbiturates; medicine for seizures; tricyclic antidepressants (medicine for depression); or anesthetics, including some dental anesthetics. *Check with your doctor before taking any of the above while you are using this medicine.*

Do not take this medicine within 1 hour of taking antacid or medicine for diarrhea. Taking them too close together will make the belladonna less effective.

This medicine may cause your eyes to become more sensitive to light than they are normally. Wearing sunglasses may help lessen the discomfort from bright light.

This medicine may cause some people to become drowsy, dizzy, or less alert than they are normally. *Make sure you know how you react to this medicine before you drive, use machines, or do other jobs that require you to be alert.*

Belladonna alkaloids will often make you sweat less, causing your body temperature to increase. *Use extra care not to become overheated during exercise or hot weather while you are taking this medicine,* as overheating could possibly result in heat stroke.

Your mouth, nose, and throat may feel very dry while you are taking this medicine. To help relieve mouth dryness, chew sugarless gum or dissolve bits of ice in your mouth.

Side Effects of This Medicine

Along with its needed effects, a medicine may cause some unwanted effects. Although not all of these side effects appear very often, when they do occur they may require medical attention. Check with your doctor if any of the following side effects occur:

Rare

Eye pain	Slurred speech
Hallucinations (seeing, hearing, or feeling things that are not there)	Unexplained sore throat and fever
Skin rash	Unusual bleeding or bruising
	Yellowing of eyes or skin

Other side effects may occur which usually do not require medical attention. These side effects may go away during treatment as your body adjusts to the medicine. However, check with your doctor if any of the following side effects continue or are bothersome:

More common

Constipation	Flushing of skin
Dizziness	Headache
Drowsiness	Mental confusion
Dryness of mouth, nose, throat, and skin	Rapid heartbeat
	Reduced sweating

Less common

Blurred vision	Increased sensitivity of eyes to sunlight
Clumsiness	
Decreased sexual ability	Nausea and vomiting
Difficult urination	Nervousness
	Reduced sense of taste

Other side effects not listed above may also occur in some patients. If you notice any other effects, check with your doctor.

BENZODIAZEPINES (Systemic)

This information applies to the following medicines:

Chlordiazepoxide (klor-dye-az-e-POX-ide)
Clorazepate (klor-AZ-e-pate)
Diazepam (dye-AZ-e-pam)
Flurazepam (flure-AZ-e-pam)
Lorazepam (lor-AZ-e-pam)
Oxazepam (ox-AZ-e-pam)
Prazepam (PRAZ-e-pam)

This information does not apply to clonazepam.

Some commonly used brand names are:	Generic names:
A-poxide	
C-Tran*	
Librium	
Nack*	
Novopoxide*	Chlordiazepoxide
Relaxil*	
SK-Lygen	

Tranxene	Clorazepate
D-Tran*	
E-Pam*	
Novodipam*	Diazepam
Valium	
Vivol*	
Dalmane	Flurazepam
Ativan	Lorazepam
Serax	Oxazepam
Verstran	Prazepam

* Not available in the United States.

Benzodiazepines (ben-zoe-dye-AZ-e-peens) are taken by mouth or given by injection. Some are used to relieve nervousness or tension. Others are used in the treatment of insomnia or sleeplessness. However, if used regularly (for example, every day) for insomnia or sleeplessness, they are usually not effective for more than a few weeks. Also, some of the benzodiazepines are used to relax muscles or relieve muscle spasm.

Benzodiazepines are usually not used for nervousness or tension caused by the stress of everyday life.

These medicines are available only with your doctor's prescription.

Before Using This Medicine

In order to decide on the best treatment for your medical problem, your doctor should be told:

—if you have ever had any unusual reaction to benzodiazepines.

—if you are pregnant or if you intend to become pregnant while using this medicine. Benzodiazepines may cause birth defects if taken during the first three months of pregnancy. In addition, too much use of this medicine during pregnancy may cause the baby to become dependent on the medicine. This may lead to withdrawal side effects after birth.

—if you are breast-feeding an infant. Benzodiazepines may pass into the breast milk and cause unwanted effects in infants of mothers taking this medicine.

—if you have any of the following medical problems:

Emphysema, asthma, bronchitis, or other chronic lung disease	Hyperactivity (in children)
	Kidney disease
Epilepsy	Liver disease
	Mental depression

Myasthenia gravis
Severe mental illness

—if you are now taking cimetidine.

—if you are now taking other central nervous system (CNS) depressants such as:

Antihistamines or medicine for hay fever, other allergies, or colds	Prescription pain medicine
	Seizure medicine
	Tricyclic antidepressants (medicine for depression)
Barbiturates	
Narcotics	
Other sedatives, tranquilizers, or sleeping medicine	

—if you are now taking or have taken within the past 2 weeks monoamine oxidase (MAO) inhibitors such as:

Isocarboxazid	Phenelzine
Pargyline	Tranylcypromine

Proper Use of This Medicine

Take this medicine only as directed by your doctor. Do not take more of it, do not take it more often, and do not take it for a longer period of time than your doctor ordered. If too much is taken, it may become habit-forming (causing mental or physical dependence).

If you are taking this medicine regularly (for example, every day) and you miss a dose, take it right away if you remember within an hour or so of the missed dose. Then go back to your regular dosing schedule. But if you do not remember until later, do not take the missed dose at all and do not double the next one. Instead, go back to your regular dosing schedule. If you have any questions about this, check with your doctor.

If you are taking flurazepam:

• *When you begin to take this medicine, 2 or 3 nights may pass before your sleeping problem improves.* It will take this long for the medicine to reach its full effect.

Precautions While Using This Medicine

If you will be taking this medicine regularly for a long period of time:

• Your doctor should check your progress at regular visits in order to make sure that the medicine does not cause unwanted effects.

• Check with your doctor at least every 4 months to make sure you need to continue taking this medicine (if you are taking flurazepam, check with your doctor every month).

If you will be taking this medicine in large doses or for a long period of time, do not stop taking it without first checking with your doctor. Your doctor may want you to reduce gradually the amount you are taking before stopping completely.

This medicine will add to the effects of alcohol and other medicines (CNS depressants) that slow down the nervous system. Some examples of CNS depressants are antihistamines or medicine for hay fever, other allergies, or colds; sedatives, tranquilizers, or sleeping medicine; prescription pain medicine or narcotics; barbiturates; medicine for seizures; tricyclic antidepressants (medicine for depression); or anesthetics, including some dental anesthetics. This effect may last for a few days after you stop taking this medicine. *Check with your doctor before taking any of the above while you are taking this medicine and also for a few days after you stop taking it.*

If you think you may have taken an overdose, get emergency help at once. Taking an overdose of a benzodiazepine or taking alcohol or other CNS depressants with the benzodiazepine may lead to unconsciousness and possibly death. Some signs of an overdose are mental confusion, severe drowsiness, severe weakness, shortness of breath or troubled breathing, staggering, and unusually slow heartbeat.

This medicine may cause some people to become dizzy, lightheaded, drowsy, or less alert than they are normally. Even if taken at bedtime, it may cause some people to feel drowsy or less alert on arising. *Make sure you know how you react to this medicine before you drive, use machines, or do other jobs that require you to be alert.*

Side Effects of This Medicine

Along with its needed effects, a medicine may cause some unwanted effects. Although not all of these side effects appear very often, when they do occur they may require medical attention. Check with your doctor if any of the following side effects occur:

Less common or rare

Continuing ulcers or sores in mouth or throat	Skin rash or itching Trouble in sleeping
Hallucinations (seeing, hearing, or feeling things that are not there)	Unexplained sore throat and fever Unusual excitement, nervousness, or irritability
Mental confusion or depression	

Unusually slow heartbeat, shortness of breath, or troubled breathing	Yellowing of eyes or skin

Other side effects may occur which usually do not require medical attention. These side effects may go away during treatment as your body adjusts to the medicine. However, check with your doctor if any of the following side effects continue or are bothersome:

More common

Clumsiness or unsteadiness	Dizziness or lightheadedness Drowsiness

Less common

Blurred vision	Nausea or vomiting
Constipation	Slurred speech
Diarrhea	Stomach pain
Headache	Unusual tiredness
Heartburn	or weakness

Although not all of the side effects listed above have been reported for all of these medicines, they have been reported for at least one of them. However, since all of the benzodiazepines are very similar, any of the above side effects may occur with any of these medicines.

After you stop using this medicine, your body may need time to adjust. If you took this medicine in high doses or for a long time, this may take up to 2 weeks. During this period of time check with your doctor if you notice any of the following side effects:

Convulsions or seizures	Trembling Trouble in sleeping
Mental confusion	Unusual irritability
Muscle cramps	Unusual nervousness
Nausea or vomiting	
Stomach cramps	Unusual sweating

For patients having diazepam injected:

• Check with your doctor if any of the following side effects occur: redness, swelling, or pain at the place of injection.

Other side effects not listed above may also occur in some patients. If you notice any other effects, check with your doctor.

BENZOYL PEROXIDE (Topical)

Some commonly used brand names are:

Benoxyl	Desquam-X	Persa-Gel
Benzac	Epi-Clear	Porox 7
Benzagel	Fostex BPO	Teen

Clear By	Panoxyl	Topex
Design	Persadox	Xerac BP
Dermodex		

Benzoyl peroxide (BEN-zoe-ill per-OX-ide) is applied to the skin to treat acne. Some of these preparations are available only with your doctor's prescription. Others are available without a prescription; however, your doctor may have special instructions on the proper use of benzoyl peroxide for your medical condition.

Before Using This Medicine

In order to decide on the best treatment for your medical problem, your doctor should be told:

—if you have ever had any unusual reaction to benzoyl peroxide in the past. This medicine should not be used if you are allergic to it.

—if you are pregnant, if you intend to become pregnant, or if you are breast-feeding an infant, although benzoyl peroxide has not been shown to cause problems.

—if you are now using any other topical acne preparation or preparation containing a peeling agent such as resorcinol, salicylic acid, sulfur, or tretinoin.

Proper Use of This Medicine

Use this medicine only as directed. Do not use more of it and do not use it more often than recommended on the label, unless otherwise directed by your doctor.

Keep this medicine away from the eyes, other mucous membranes such as the mouth, lips, and inside of the nose, and sensitive areas of the neck.

Do not apply this medicine to raw or irritated skin.

If you miss a dose of this medicine, apply or use it as soon as possible. Then go back to your regular dosing schedule. But if it is almost time for your next dose, do not apply or use the missed dose at all. Instead, go back to your regular dosing schedule. If you have any questions about this, check with your doctor or pharmacist.

If you are using the cream, gel, or lotion form of this medicine:
• Before applying, wash the affected area with nonmedicated soap and water or with a degreasing cleanser and then gently pat dry with a towel.
• Apply enough medicine to cover the affected areas, and rub in gently.

If you are using the cleansing lotion form of this medicine, use to wash the affected areas as directed.

Precautions While Using This Medicine

If your skin problem has not improved within 2 weeks, check with your doctor.

Do not use any other topical acne preparation or preparation containing a peeling agent (for example, resorcinol, salicylic acid, sulfur, or tretinoin) *on the same affected area as this medicine,* unless otherwise directed by your doctor. To do so may cause severe irritation of the skin.

This medicine may bleach hair or colored fabrics.

Side Effects of This Medicine

Along with its needed effects, a medicine may cause some unwanted effects. Although not all of these side effects appear very often, when they do occur they may require medical attention. Check with your doctor or pharmacist if either of the following side effects occurs:

Painful irritation   Skin rash
of skin

When you apply benzoyl peroxide, a mild stinging sensation, a feeling of warmth, or some reddening of the skin may be expected.

After you use this medicine for a few days, you may have some dryness and peeling of the skin.

Other side effects not listed above may also occur in some patients. If you notice any other effects, check with your doctor or pharmacist.

BETA-ADRENERGIC BLOCKING AGENTS
(Systemic)

This information applies to the following medicines:

Metoprolol (me-TOE-proe-lole)
Nadolol (nay-DOE-lole)
Propranolol (proe-PRAN-oh-lole)

Some commonly used brand names are: Generic names:

Lopressor	Metoprolol
Corgard	Nadolol
Inderal	Propranolol

These medicines belong to a group of medicines known as beta-adrenergic blocking agents, beta-blocking agents, or more commonly, beta-blockers. They are used to treat high blood pressure. Propranolol and nadolol are also used to relieve angina conditions. In addition, propranolol is useful in the treatment of certain heart conditions, in the prevention of migraine headaches, and in the treatment of certain other conditions as might be determined by your doctor.

Beta-blocking agents are available only with your doctor's prescription.

Before Using This Medicine

In order to decide on the best treatment for your medical problem, your doctor should be told:

—if you have ever had any unusual reaction to beta-blocker medicine in the past. This medicine should not be taken if you are allergic to it.

—if you are pregnant or if you intend to become pregnant while using this medicine. Use of propranolol during pregnancy may result in breathing problems and a lower heart rate in the newborn infant. Metoprolol and nadolol may also cause these problems but this has not yet been proven.

—if you are breast-feeding an infant. Although this medicine has not been shown to cause problems, the chance always exists.

—if you have any of the following medical problems:

Allergy, history of (asthma, eczema, hay fever, hives)	Emphysema
	Heart or blood vessel disease
Bradycardia (unusually slow heartbeat)	Kidney disease
	Liver disease
Diabetes mellitus (sugar diabetes)	Poor circulation in fingers and toes

—if you are now taking any of the following medicines or types of medicine:

Diabetes medicine	Isoproterenol
Epinephrine or phenylephrine	Medicine for asthma, bronchitis, or emphysema
Heart medicine	
	Reserpine

—if you are now taking or have taken within the past 2 weeks monoamine oxidase (MAO) inhibitors such as:

Isocarboxazid	Phenelzine
Pargyline	Tranylcypromine

Proper Use of This Medicine

Even if you feel well and do not notice any signs of medical problems, *take this medicine exactly as directed.* Do not miss any doses and do not take more medicine than your doctor ordered.

Ask your doctor about your personal pulse rate before and after taking beta-blocking agents. Then, while you are taking this medicine, check your pulse regularly. If it is much slower than your usual rate, check with your doctor. A pulse rate that is too slow may cause circulation problems.

Take this medicine with meals or immediately following meals unless your doctor tells you to take it on an empty stomach.

If you miss a dose of this medicine, take the missed dose as soon as possible. If the next scheduled dose is within 4 hours (8 hours when using nadolol), do not take the missed dose at all and do not double the next one. Instead, go back to your regular dosing schedule. If you have any questions about this, check with your doctor.

For patients taking this medicine for high blood pressure:

• Importance of Diet—When prescribing medicine for your condition, your doctor may also prescribe a personal diet for you. Such a diet may be low in sodium (salt) and/or calories to help you lose excess weight. Medicine is more effective when this diet is properly followed. Check with your doctor before going on any diet.

• Many patients who have high blood pressure will not notice any signs of the problem. In fact, many may feel normal. It is very important that you take your medicine exactly as directed and that you keep your doctor's appointments even if you feel well.

• Remember that this medicine will not cure your high blood pressure but it does control it. Therefore, you must continue to take it as directed if you expect to keep your blood pressure down. *You may have to take medicine for the rest of your life.* If high blood pressure is not treated, it can cause serious problems such as heart failure, blood vessel disease, stroke, or kidney disease.

Precautions While Using This Medicine

It is important that your doctor check your progress at regular visits. This will allow the dosage to be changed if needed and to make sure the medicine is working for you.

Do not stop taking this medicine without first checking with your doctor. Your doctor may want you to reduce gradually the amount you are taking before stopping completely. Some conditions may become worse when the medicine is stopped suddenly, and danger of heart attack is increased in some patients. Make sure that you have enough medicine on hand to last through weekends, holidays, or vacations. Do not miss any doses. You may want to carry an extra prescription in your wallet or purse in case of an emergency.

Your doctor may want you to carry a medical identification card stating that you are taking this medicine.

Before having any kind of surgery (including dental surgery) or emergency treatment, tell the doctor or dentist in charge that you are taking this medicine.

Caution: Diabetics—*This medicine may cause your blood sugar levels to fall.* Also, *this medicine may cover up signs of hypoglycemia (low blood sugar),* such as change in pulse rate or increased blood pressure. If you have any questions about this, check with your doctor.

This medicine may cause some people to become dizzy, lightheaded, drowsy, or less alert than they are normally. *Make sure you know how you react to this medicine before you drive, use machines, or do other jobs that require you to be alert.* If the problem continues or gets worse, check with your doctor.

Your eyes, mouth, and throat may feel very dry while you are taking this medicine. Chewing sugarless gum may help relieve mouth and throat dryness. The use of nonmedicated or plain eye drops (artificial tears) may be helpful for eye dryness.

This medicine will often make you more sensitive to cold. It tends to decrease blood circulation in the skin, fingers, and toes. Dress warmly during cold weather and be careful during prolonged exposure to cold such as in winter sports.

Chest pain resulting from exercise or physical exertion is usually reduced or prevented by this medicine. This may tempt a patient to be overly active. *Make sure you discuss with your doctor a safe amount of exercise for your medical problem.*

Side Effects of This Medicine

Along with its needed effects, a medicine may cause some unwanted effects. Although not all of these side effects appear very often, when they do occur they may require medical attention. Check with your doctor if any of the following side effects occur:

More common

Dizziness or lightheadedness	Unusually slow pulse

Less common

Breathing difficulty	Mental depression
Mental confusion, especially in elderly	Reduced alertness

Rare

Skin rash	Unusual bleeding and bruising
Unexplained fever and sore throat	

Other side effects may occur which usually do not require medical attention. These side effects may go away during treatment as your body adjusts to the medicine. However, check with your doctor if any of the following side effects continue or are bothersome:

More common

Cold hands and feet	Numbness and/or tingling of fingers and/or toes
Diarrhea	
Drowsiness (slight)	
Dryness of eyes, mouth, and/or skin	Unusual tiredness or weakness
Nausea	

Less common

Constipation	Headache
Hallucinations (seeing, hearing, or feeling things that are not there)	Nightmares and vivid dreams
	Sleeping problems

Other side effects not listed above may also occur in some patients. If you notice any other effects, check with your doctor.

BETHANECHOL (Systemic)
Some commonly used brand names are Duvoid, Myotonachol, and Urecholine.

Bethanechol (be-THAN-e-kole) is taken by mouth or given by injection to treat certain disorders of the urinary tract or bladder. It helps to cause urination and emptying of the bladder. This medicine is available only with your doctor's prescription.

Before Using This Medicine

In order to decide on the best treatment for your medical problem, your doctor should be told:

—if you have ever had any unusual reaction to bethanechol in the past. This medicine should not be taken if you are allergic to it.

—if you are pregnant, if you intend to become

pregnant, or if you are breast-feeding an infant. Although bethanechol has not been shown to cause problems in humans, the chance always exists.

—if you have any of the following medical problems:

Asthma	Overactive thyroid
Epilepsy	Parkinsonism
Heart or blood vessel disease	Recent bladder or intestinal surgery
High blood pressure	Stomach ulcer or other stomach problems
Intestinal blockage	Urinary tract blockage

—if you are now taking any of the following medicines:

Ambenonium	Procainamide
Mecamylamine	Pyridostigmine
Neostigmine	Quinidine

Proper Use of This Medicine

Take this medicine only as directed. Do not take more of it, do not take it more often, and do not take it for a longer period of time than your doctor ordered. To do so may increase the chance of side effects.

Take this medicine on an empty stomach (either 1 hour before or 2 hours after meals) to lessen the possibility of nausea and vomiting, unless otherwise directed by your doctor.

If you miss a dose of this medicine and you remember within an hour or so of the missed dose, take it right away. Then go back to your regular dosing schedule. But if you do not remember until 2 or more hours after the missed dose, do not take it at all and do not double the next one. Instead, go back to your regular dosing schedule. If you have any questions about this, check with your doctor.

Precautions While Using This Medicine

Dizziness, lightheadedness, or fainting may occur, especially when you get up from a lying or sitting position. Getting up slowly may help lessen this problem.

Side Effects of This Medicine

Along with its needed effects, a medicine may cause some unwanted effects. Although not all of these side effects appear very often, when they do occur they may require medical attention. Check with your doctor if any of the following side effects occur:

Rare—more common with the injection

Shortness of breath, wheezing, or tightness in chest

Other side effects may occur which usually do not require medical attention. These side effects may go away during treatment as your body adjusts to the medicine. However, check with your doctor if any of the following side effects continue or are bothersome:

Less common or rare—more common with the injection

Belching	Headache
Blurred vision or change in near or distant vision	Nausea or vomiting
	Redness or flushing of skin or feeling of warmth
Diarrhea	
Dizziness or lightheadedness	Stomach discomfort or pain
Feeling faint	Unusual increase in salivation or sweating
Frequent urge to urinate	

Other side effects not listed above may also occur in some patients. If you notice any other effects, check with your doctor.

BLEOMYCIN (Systemic)
A commonly used brand name is Blenoxane.

Bleomycin (blee-oh-MYE-sin) belongs to the general group of medicines called antineoplastics. It is used by injection to treat some kinds of cancer. Bleomycin is available only with a prescription and is to be administered only by or under the immediate supervision of your doctor.

Before Using This Medicine

Bleomycin is a very strong medicine. In addition to its helpful effects in treating your medical problem, it has side effects that could be very serious. Before you receive this medicine, be sure that you have discussed the use of it with your doctor.

In order to decide on the best treatment for your medical problem, your doctor should be told:

—if you have ever had any unusual reaction to bleomycin in the past.

—if you are pregnant or if you intend to become pregnant while using this medicine. This medicine may cause birth defects if either the male or female is taking it at the time of conception or if it is taken during pregnancy. Be sure that you have discussed this with your doctor before taking this medicine.

—if you are breast-feeding an infant. Although bleomycin has not been shown to cause problems, the chance always exists.

—if you have any of the following medical problems:

Kidney disease   Lung disease
Liver disease

—if you have been treated with x-rays or cancer drugs by another doctor.

Proper Use of This Medicine

This medicine is sometimes given together with certain other medicines. If you are using a combination of drugs, it is important that you receive each medicine at the proper time. If you are taking some of these medicines by mouth, ask your doctor, nurse, or pharmacist to help you plan a way to take them at the right time.

This medicine often causes vomiting and loss of appetite. However, it is very important that you continue to receive the medicine, even if you experience an upset stomach. If you have any questions about this, check with your doctor.

Precautions While Using This Medicine

It is very important that your doctor check your progress at regular visits.

Side Effects of This Medicine

Along with its needed effects, a medicine may cause some unwanted effects. Although not all of these side effects appear very often, when they do occur they may require medical attention. Check with your doctor *immediately* if any of the following side effects occur:

More common

Cough   Sores in the mouth
Shortness of breath   and on the lips

Less common

Faintness   Wheezing
Mental confusion

Rare

Blood in urine   Unexplained fever
Hearing problems   and sore throat
     (occurring
     after several days
     or weeks)
     Unusual bleeding or
     bruising

Other side effects may occur which usually do not require medical attention. These side effects may go away during treatment as your body adjusts to the medicine. However, check with your doctor if any of the following side effects continue or are bothersome:

More common

Darkening of the   Skin rash
   skin   Skin redness
Fever and chills   Skin tenderness
   (occurring within   Swelling of the
   3 to 6 hours   fingers
   after a dose)

Less common

Changes in finger-   Thickening or peel-
   nails or toenails   ing of skin
Headache   Vomiting and loss
Itching   of appetite
Loss of hair   Weight loss

Rare

Pain at the tumor   Swelling, stiffness,
   site   or pain in legs

After you stop receiving this medicine, it may still produce some side effects that need attention. During this period of time check with your doctor if you notice either of the following:

Cough
Shortness of breath

Other side effects not listed above may also occur in some patients. If you notice any other effects, check with your doctor.

BROMOCRIPTINE (Systemic)
A commonly used brand name is Parlodel.

Bromocriptine (broe-moe-KRIP-teen) is a medicine used to treat some menstrual problems. It is also used to stop milk production when mothers do not wish to breast-feed or when they have abnormal milk leakage. Bromocriptine may also be used for other conditions as determined by your doctor. It is available only with your doctor's prescription.

Before Using This Medicine

In order to decide on the best treatment for your medical problem, your doctor should be told:

—if you have ever had any unusual reaction to ergotamine or methysergide (used to treat migraine headaches) or to bromocriptine. This medicine should not be taken if you are allergic to it.

—if you intend to become pregnant while taking this medicine. Although this medicine has not been shown to cause birth defects or other problems in humans, the chance always exists.

—if you have liver disease.

—if you are now taking any of the following medicines or types of medicine:

Haloperidol	Oral contraceptives
Levodopa	(birth control
Medicine for high	pills)
blood pressure	Reserpine
Metoclopramide	Some tranquilizers
	(thioxanthenes)

—if you are now taking phenothiazine medicines such as:

Chlorpromazine	Prochlorperazine
Fluphenazine	Trifluoperazine
Perphenazine	Triflupromazine

—if you are now taking monoamine oxidase (MAO) inhibitors such as:

Isocarboxazid	Phenelzine
Pargyline	Tranylcypromine

Proper Use of This Medicine

If this medicine upsets your stomach, it may be taken with meals or milk. If stomach upset continues, check with your doctor.

If you miss a dose of this medicine, and remember it within 4 hours, take the missed dose when you remember it. However, if a longer time has passed, do not take the missed dose at all and do not double the next one. Instead, go back to your regular dosing schedule. If you have any questions about this, check with your doctor.

Precautions While Using This Medicine

It is important that your doctor check your progress at regular visits.

This medicine may cause some people to become dizzy or less alert than they are normally. *Make sure you know how you react to this medicine before you drive, use machines, or do other jobs that require you to be alert.*

For patients taking this medicine for menstrual problems:
• This medicine should not be taken if you are pregnant since it may cause you to have some other problems. It is best to use some type of birth control while you are taking it. However, do not use oral contraceptives ("the Pill") since they will prevent this medicine from working. Tell your doctor right away if you think you have become pregnant while taking this medicine.

Side Effects of This Medicine

Along with its needed effects, a medicine may cause some unwanted effects. Although not all of these side effects appear very often, when they do occur they may require medical attention. Check with your doctor if any of the following side effects occur:

More common

Dizziness or lightheadedness, especially when getting up from a lying or sitting position

Rare

Black tarry stools	Hallucinations (see-
Bloody vomit	ing, hearing, or
Fainting	feeling things that
	are not there)

Other side effects may occur which usually do not require medical attention. These side effects may go away during treatment as your body adjusts to the medicine. However, check with your doctor if any of the following side effects continue or are bothersome:

More common

Headache
Nausea

Less common

Constipation	Stomach pain
Diarrhea	Stuffy nose
Dry mouth	Tingling or pain in
Leg cramps at night	fingers and toes
Loss of appetite	when exposed to
	cold
	Vomiting

Other side effects not listed above may also occur in some patients. If you notice any other effects, check with your doctor.

BROMPHENIRAMINE, GUAIFENESIN, PHENYLEPHRINE, AND PHENYLPROPANOLAMINE (Systemic)

Some commonly used brand names are:
Dimetane Expectorant
Midatane Expectorant
Normatane Expectorant
Puretane Expectorant
Spentane Expectorant

Brompheniramine (brome-fen-IR-a-meen), guaifenesin (gwye-FEN-e-sin), phenylephrine (fen-ill-EF-rin), and phenylpropanolamine (fen-ill-proe-pa-NOLE-a-meen) is a combination antihistamine, cough reliever, and decongestant. It is used to treat nasal congestion (stuffy nose) and other symptoms of hay fever and other types of allergy. In addition, the guaifenesin acts to relieve cough by loosening mucus or phlegm ("flem") in the lungs. This medicine is available only with your doctor's prescription.

Before Using This Medicine

In order to decide on the best treatment for your medical problem, your doctor should be told:

—if you have ever had any unusual reaction to brompheniramine, guaifenesin, phenylephrine, phenylpropanolamine, or similar medicines in the past. This medicine should not be taken if you are allergic to it.

—if you are pregnant or if you intend to become pregnant while using this medicine. Although this medicine has not been shown to cause birth defects or other problems, the chance always exists.

—if you are breast-feeding an infant. Brompheniramine may pass into the breast milk and cause unwanted effects in the infant.

—if you have any of the following medical problems:

Diabetes	High blood pressure
Enlarged prostate	Overactive thyroid
Glaucoma	Stomach ulcer
Heart disease	Urinary tract blockage

—if you are now taking any of the following medicines or types of medicine:

Amphetamines	Tricyclic an-
Medicine for	tidepressants
asthma or	(medicine for
breathing prob-	depression)
lems	

—if you are now taking any central nervous system (CNS) depressants such as:

Antihistamines or	Narcotics
medicine for hay	Prescription pain
fever, other	medicine
allergies,	Sedatives, tran-
or colds	quilizers,
Barbiturates	or sleeping
Medicines for	medicine
seizures	

—if you are now taking or have taken within the past 2 weeks monoamine oxidase (MAO) inhibitors such as:

Isocarboxazid	Phenelzine
Pargyline	Tranylcypromine

Proper Use of This Medicine

Take brompheniramine, guaifenesin, phenyleph-rine, and phenylpropanolamine combination only as directed. Do not take more of it and do not take it more often than directed by your doctor. To do so may increase the chance of side effects.

Do not give this medicine to premature or newborn infants, unless otherwise directed by your doctor.

Take this medicine with food or a glass of water or milk to lessen stomach irritation, if necessary. Also, to help loosen mucus or phlegm ("flem") in the lungs, *drink a full glass (8 ounces) of water after each dose of this medicine.*

Precautions While Using This Medicine

The antihistamine in this medicine will add to the effects of alcohol and other medicines (CNS depressants) that slow down the nervous system. Some examples of CNS depressants are medicine for hay fever, other allergies, or colds; sedatives, tranquilizers, or sleeping medicine; prescription pain medicine or nar-cotics; barbiturates; medicine for seizures; tricyclic antidepressants (medicine for depres-sion); or anesthetics, including some dental anesthetics. *Check with your doctor before taking any of the above while you are using this medicine.*

Brompheniramine may cause some people to become drowsy, dizzy, or less alert than they are normally. *Make sure you know how you react to this medicine before you drive, use machines, or do other jobs that require you to be alert.*

Side Effects of This Medicine

Along with its needed effects, a medicine may cause some unwanted effects. Although not all of these side effects appear very often, when they do occur they may require medical atten-tion. Check with your doctor if any of the following side effects occur:

Rare

Unexplained sore	Unusual weakness
throat and fever	Unusually fast or
Unusual bleeding or	pounding heart-
bruising	beat

Other side effects may occur which usually do not require medical attention. These side effects may go away during treatment as your body adjusts to the medicine. However, check with your doctor if any of the following side effects continue or are bothersome:

More common

Drowsiness	Thickening of the bronchial secre-tions

Less common—more common with high doses

Diarrhea	Nausea, upset
Difficult or painful	stomach, or
urination	stomach pain
Dizziness	Nervousness,
Dryness of mouth,	restlessness, or
nose, or throat	trouble in sleep-
Headache	ing (especially
Loss of appetite	in children)
	Skin rash
	Unusual increase in
	sweating

Other side effects not listed above may also occur in some patients. If you notice any other effects check with your doctor.

BROMPHENIRAMINE, GUAIFENESIN, PHENYLEPHRINE, PHENYLPROPANOLAMINE, AND CODEINE (Systemic)

Some commonly used brand names are:

Dimetane Expectorant-DC
Midatane DC Expectorant
Normatane DC Expectorant
Puretane Expectorant DC
Spentane DC Expectorant

Brompheniramine (brome-fen-IR-a-meen), guaifenesin (gwye-FEN-e-sin), phenylephrine (fen-ill-EF-rin), phenylpropanolamine (fen-ill-proe-pa-NOLE-a-meen), and codeine (KOE-deen) is a combination antihistamine, cough reliever, and decongestant. It is used to treat nasal congestion (stuffy nose) and other symptoms of hay fever and other types of allergy, including relief of cough. This medicine is available only with your doctor's prescription.

Before Using This Medicine

In order to decide on the best treatment for your medical problem, your doctor should be told:

—if you have ever had any unusual reaction to brompheniramine, guaifenesin, phenylephrine, phenylpropanolamine, codeine, or similar medicines in the past. This medicine should not be taken if you are allergic to it.

—if you are pregnant or if you intend to become pregnant while using this medicine. Although this medicine has not been shown to cause birth defects, the chance always exists.

—if you are breast-feeding an infant. Brompheniramine may pass into the breast milk and cause unwanted effects in the infant. Codeine

passes into the breast milk. Although the amount of codeine in recommended doses of this medicine does not usually cause problems, the chance always exists.

—if you have any of the following medical problems:

Brain disease or in-	Kidney disease
jury	Liver disease
Colitis	Overactive or
Diabetes	underactive
Emphysema,	thyroid
asthma, or	Stomach ulcer
chronic lung	Underactive adrenal
disease	gland (Addison's
Enlarged prostate	disease)
Gall bladder disease	Unusually slow or
or gallstones	irregular heart-
Glaucoma	beat
Heart disease	Urinary tract
High blood pressure	blockage

—if you are now taking any of the following medicines or types of medicine:

Amphetamines	Prescription
Medicine for	medicine for
asthma or	stomach cramps
breathing prob-	or spasms
lems	Tricyclic an-
	tidepressants
	(medicine for
	depression)

—if you are now taking any central nervous system (CNS) depressants such as:

Antihistamines or	Narcotics
medicine for hay	Prescription pain
fever, other	medicine
allergies,	Sedatives, tran-
or colds	quilizers,
Barbiturates	or sleeping
Medicine for	medicine
seizures	

—if you are now taking or have taken within the past 2 weeks monoamine oxidase (MAO) inhibitors such as:

Isocarboxazid	Phenelzine
Pargyline	Tranylcypromine

Proper Use of This Medicine

Take brompheniramine, guaifenesin, phenylephrine, phenylpropanolamine, and codeine combination only as directed. Do not take more of it and do not take it more often than directed by your doctor. To do so may increase the chance of side effects. In addition, if too much is taken, the codeine in this medicine may become habit-forming.

Do not give this medicine to premature or newborn infants, unless otherwise directed by your doctor.

Take this medicine with food or a glass of water or milk to lessen stomach irritation, if necessary.

Precautions While Using This Medicine

The antihistamine in this medicine will add to the effects of alcohol and other medicines (CNS depressants) that slow down the nervous system. Some examples of CNS depressants are medicine for hay fever, other allergies, or colds; sedatives, tranquilizers, or sleeping medicine; prescription pain medicine or narcotics; barbiturates; medicine for seizures; tricyclic antidepressants (medicine for depression); or anesthetics, including some dental anesthetics. *Check with your doctor before taking any of the above while you are using this medicine.*

Both brompheniramine and codeine may cause some people to become drowsy, dizzy, or less alert than they are normally. *Make sure you know how you react to this medicine before you drive, use machines, or do other jobs that require you to be alert.*

Dizziness, lightheadedness, or fainting may occur, especially when you get up from a lying or sitting position. Getting up slowly may help. If the problem continues or gets worse, check with your doctor.

Side Effects of This Medicine

Along with its needed effects, a medicine may cause some unwanted effects. Although not all of these side effects appear very often, when they do occur they may require medical attention. Check with your doctor if any of the following side effects occur:

Rare

Unexplained sore throat and fever	Unusual weakness
Unusual bleeding or bruising	Unusually fast, slow, or pounding heartbeat

Other side effects may occur which usually do not require medical attention. These side effects may go away during treatment as your body adjusts to the medicine. However, check with your doctor if any of the following side effects continue or are bothersome:

More common

Constipation	Thickening of the bronchial secretions
Drowsiness	

Less common—more common with high doses

Diarrhea	Nausea, upset stomach, or stomach pain
Difficult or painful urination	
Dizziness or lightheadedness, especially when getting up from a lying or sitting position	Nervousness, restlessness, or trouble in sleeping (especially in children)
	Redness or flushing of face
Dryness of mouth, nose, or throat	Skin rash
Headache	Unusual increase in sweating
Loss of appetite	

Other side effects not listed above may also occur in some patients. If you notice any other effects, check with your doctor.

BROMPHENIRAMINE, PHENYLEPHRINE, AND PHENYLPROPANOLAMINE (Systemic)

Some commonly used brand names are:

Brompheniramine	Dimetapp
Compound	Eldatapp
Bromatapp	Puretapp

Brompheniramine (brome-fen-IR-a-meen), phenylephrine (fen-ill-EF-rin), and phenylpropanolamine (fen-ill-proe-pa-NOLE-a-meen) is a combination antihistamine and decongestant. It is used to treat nasal congestion (stuffy nose) and other symptoms of hay fever and other types of allergy. This medicine is available only with your doctor's prescription.

Before Using This Medicine

In order to decide on the best treatment for your medical problem, your doctor should be told:

—if you have ever had any unusual reaction to brompheniramine, phenylephrine, phenylpropanolamine, or similar medicines in the past. This medicine should not be taken if you are allergic to it.

—if you are pregnant or if you intend to become pregnant while using this medicine. Although this medicine has not been shown to cause birth defects or other problems, the chance always exists.

—if you are breast-feeding an infant. Brompheniramine may pass into the breast milk and cause unwanted effects in the infant.

—if you have any of the following medical problems:

Diabetes	High blood pressure
Enlarged prostate	Overactive thyroid
Glaucoma	Stomach ulcer
Heart disease	Urinary tract blockage

—if you are now taking any of the following medicines or types of medicine:

Amphetamines	Tricyclic an-
Medicine for	tidepressants
asthma or breath-	(medicine for
ing problems	depression)

—if you are now taking any central nervous system (CNS) depressants such as:

Antihistamines or	Narcotics
medicine for hay	Prescription pain
fever, other	medicine
allergies,	Sedatives, tran-
or colds	quilizers,
Barbiturates	or sleeping
Medicines for	medicine
seizures	

—if you are now taking or have taken within the past 2 weeks monoamine oxidase (MAO) inhibitors such as:

Isocarboxazid	Phenelzine
Pargyline	Tranylcypromine

Proper Use of This Medicine

Take brompheniramine, phenylephrine, and phenylpropanolamine combination only as directed. Do not take more of it and do not take it more often than recommended on the label, unless otherwise directed by your doctor. To do so may increase the chance of side effects.

Do not give this medicine to premature or newborn infants, unless otherwise directed by your doctor.

Take this medicine with food or a glass of water or milk to lessen stomach irritation, if necessary.

If you are taking the long-acting tablet form of this medicine, the tablets are to be swallowed whole. Do not break, crush, or chew before swallowing.

If you must take this medicine regularly and you miss a dose, take the missed dose as soon as possible. However, if it is almost time for your next dose, do not take the missed dose at all and do not double the next one. Instead, go back to your regular dosing schedule. If you have any questions about this, check with your doctor or pharmacist.

Precautions While Using This Medicine

The antihistamine in this medicine will add to the effects of alcohol and other medicines (CNS depressants) that slow down the nervous system. Some examples of CNS depressants are medicine for hay fever, other allergies, or colds; sedatives, tranquilizers, or sleeping medicine; prescription pain medicine or narcotics; barbiturates; medicine for seizures; tricyclic antidepressants (medicine for depression); or anesthetics, including some dental anesthetics. *Check with your doctor before taking any of the above while you are using this medicine.*

Brompheniramine may cause some people to become drowsy, dizzy, or less alert than they are normally. *Make sure you know how you react to this medicine before you drive, use machines, or do other jobs that require you to be alert.*

Side Effects of This Medicine

Along with its needed effects, a medicine may cause some unwanted effects. Although not all of these side effects appear very often, when they do occur they may require medical attention. Check with your doctor if any of the following side effects occur:

Rare

Tightness in chest	Unusual bleeding or
Unexplained sore	bruising
throat and fever	Unusual weakness
	Unusually fast or
	pounding heart-
	beat

Other side effects may occur which usually do not require medical attention. These side effects may go away during treatment as your body adjusts to the medicine. However, check with your doctor if any of the following side effects continue or are bothersome:

More common

Drowsiness	Thickening of the
	bronchial secre-
	tions

Less common—more common with high doses

Difficult or painful	Nausea, upset
urination	stomach, or
Dizziness	stomach pain
Dryness of mouth,	Nervousness,
nose, or throat	restlessness, or
Headache	trouble in sleep-
Loss of appetite	ing (especially in
	children)
	Skin rash
	Unusual increase in
	sweating

Other side effects not listed above may also occur in some patients. If you notice any other effects check with your doctor.

BUSULFAN (Systemic)
A commonly used brand name is Myleran.

Busulfan (byoo-SUL-fan) belongs to the group of medicines known as alkylating agents. It is used to treat some kinds of cancer as well as some noncancerous conditions. It is used also in some situations to reduce the body's natural immunity. Busulfan is available only with your doctor's prescription.

Before Using This Medicine
Busulfan is a very strong medicine. In addition to its helpful effects in treating your medical problem, it has side effects that could be very serious. Before you take this medicine, be sure that you have discussed the use of it with your doctor.

In order to decide on the best treatment for your medical problem, your doctor should be told:

—if you have ever had any unusual reaction to busulfan in the past.

—if you are pregnant or if you intend to have children. This medicine may cause birth defects if either the male or the female is taking it at the time of conception or if it is taken during pregnancy. It may also cause permanent sterility after it has been taken for a while. Be sure that you have discussed this with your doctor before taking this medicine.

—if you are breast-feeding an infant. Although busulfan has not been shown to cause problems, the chance always exists.

—if you have any of the following medical problems:

Blood disease	Infection
Gout	Kidney stones

—if you are taking gout medicine.

—if you have been treated with x-rays or cancer drugs by another doctor.

Proper Use of This Medicine
Use this medicine only as directed by your doctor. Do not use more or less of it, and do not use it more often than your doctor ordered. Take each dose at the same time of day to make sure it has the best effect.

This medicine sometimes causes nausea and vomiting. Even if you begin to feel ill, *do not stop using this medicine without first checking with your doctor.*

If you miss a dose of this medicine, do not take the missed dose at all and do not double the next one. Instead, go back to your regular dosing schedule. If you have any questions about this, check with your doctor.

Precautions While Using This Medicine
It is very important that your doctor check your progress at regular visits.

While you are using this medicine, your doctor may want you to drink plenty of fluids and urinate often. This will help prevent kidney problems and keep your kidneys working well. If you have any questions about this, check with your doctor.

Side Effects of This Medicine
Along with its needed effects, a medicine may cause some unwanted effects. Although not all of these side effects appear very often, when they do occur they may require medical attention. Check with your doctor if any of the following side effects occur:

More common
Unusual bleeding or bruising
Less common

Cough	Joint pain
Fever or chills	Shortness of breath
Flank or stomach pain	Swelling of feet or lower legs

Rare

Blurred vision	Unexplained fever, chills, or sore throat
Dryness, cracking, or sores on lips or in mouth	Yellowing of eyes or skin
Skin rash	

Other side effects may occur which usually do not require medical attention. These side effects may go away during treatment as your body adjusts to the medicine. However, check with your doctor if any of the following side effects continue or are bothersome:

Less common

Darkening of the skin	Loss of appetite
Diarrhea	Mental confusion
Dizziness	Nausea and vomiting
Fatigue	

Rare

Decreased sexual ability	Lack of sweating
	Loss of hair
Enlargement of breasts in males	Missing menstrual periods

After you stop using this medicine, it may still produce some side effects that need attention. During this period of time check with your doctor if you notice any unusual bleeding or bruising.

Other side effects not listed above may also occur in some patients. If you notice any other effects, check with your doctor.

BUTALBITAL AND APC (Systemic)

A commonly used brand name is Fiorinal.

Butalbital (byoo-TAL-bi-tal) and APC is a combined pain reliever, muscle relaxant, and tranquilizer. It is used to treat tension headaches. APC is the short name for aspirin, phenacetin, and caffeine (AS-pir-in, fe-NASS-e-tin, and KAF-een). Butalbital and APC combination is available only with your doctor's prescription.

Before Using This Medicine

In order to decide on the best treatment for your medical problem, your doctor should be told:

—if you have ever had any unusual reaction to barbiturates, acetaminophen, phenacetin, caffeine, or aspirin or other salicylates including methyl salicylate (oil of wintergreen), or to other nonsteroidal anti-inflammatory agents such as fenoprofen, ibuprofen, indomethacin, naproxen, oxyphenbutazone, phenylbutazone, sulindac, or tolmetin. This medicine should not be taken if you are allergic to it.

—if you are pregnant or if you intend to become pregnant while using this medicine. Too much use of aspirin during the last 3 months of pregnancy may increase the length of pregnancy and may prolong labor. Aspirin taken during the last 2 weeks of pregnancy may cause the baby to have bleeding problems at birth. When phenacetin or butalbital are used during pregnancy, it may cause side effects in the newborn infant. In addition, although aspirin, phenacetin, caffeine, and butalbital have not been shown to cause birth defects, the chance always exists.

—if you are breast-feeding an infant. Butalbital may cause side effects in infants of nursing mothers. Although aspirin, phenacetin, and caffeine have not been shown to cause problems, the chance always exists. Therefore, use by nursing mothers should be carefully considered.

—if you have any of the following medical problems:

Anemia	
Asthma, allergies, and nasal polyps (history of)	Hyperactivity (in children)
Emphysema or chronic lung disease	Hypoprothrombinemia
	Kidney disease
	Liver disease
Glucose-6-phosphate dehydrogenase (G6PD) deficiency	Porphyria (or history of)
	Ulcer or other stomach problems
Gout	Underactive adrenal gland (Addison's disease)
Hemophilia or other bleeding problems	
Hodgkin's disease	Vitamin K deficiency

—if you are now taking any of the following medicines or types of medicine:

Antacids	Insulin
Anticoagulants (blood thinners)	Methotrexate
	Oral hypoglycemics (diabetes medicine you take by mouth)
Contraceptives, oral (birth-control pills)	
Corticosteroids (cortisone-like medicines)	Phenytoin
	Quinidine
Cyclophosphamide	Spironolactone
Digitalis	Urine acidifiers (medicine to make your urine more acid)
Digitoxin	
Doxycycline	
Estrogens	Urine alkalizers (medicine to make your urine less acid)
Gout medicine	
Griseofulvin	
Inflammation medicine (for example, arthritis medicine)	Vitamin C

—if you are now taking any central nervous system (CNS) depressants such as:

Antihistamines or medicine for hay fever, other allergies, or colds	Sedatives, tranquilizers, or sleeping medicine
	Seizure medicine
Narcotics	Tricyclic antidepressants (medicine for depression)
Other barbiturates	
Other prescription pain medicine	

—if you are now taking or have taken within the past 2 weeks monoamine oxidase (MAO) inhibitors such as:

Isocarboxazid	Phenelzine
Pargyline	Tranylcypromine

Proper Use of This Medicine

Take this medicine with food or a full glass (8 ounces) of water or milk to lessen stomach irritation.

Do not use this medicine if it has a strong vinegar-like odor, since this means the aspirin in the product is breaking down. If you have any questions about this, check with your doctor or pharmacist.

Use this medicine only as directed by your doctor. Do not use more of it, do not use it more often, and do not use it for a longer period of time than your doctor ordered. If too much is used, it may become habit-forming or cause kidney damage.

Keep this medicine out of the reach of children since overdose is very dangerous in young children.

Precautions While Using This Medicine

Check the labels of all over-the-counter (OTC), nonprescription, and prescription medicines you now take. If any contain aspirin, phenacetin, or barbiturates be especially careful, since taking them while taking this medicine may lead to overdose. If you have any questions about this, check with your doctor or pharmacist.

Caution: Diabetics—This medicine contains aspirin and phenacetin which may cause false test results with urine sugar tests. If you have any questions about this, check with your doctor or pharmacist.

This medicine will add to the effects of alcohol and other medicines (CNS depressants) that slow down the nervous system. Some examples of CNS depressants are antihistamines or medicine for hay fever, other allergies, or colds; sedatives, tranquilizers, or sleeping medicine; prescription pain medicine or narcotics; barbiturates; medicine for seizures; tricyclic antidepressants (medicine for depression); or anesthetics, including some dental anesthetics. In addition, stomach problems may be more likely to occur if you drink alcoholic beverages while being treated with this medicine. *Check with your doctor before taking any of the above while you are using this medicine.*

This medicine may cause some people to become dizzy, lightheaded, drowsy, or less alert than they are normally. *Make sure you know how you react to this medicine before you drive, use machines, or do other jobs that require you to be alert.*

If you will be taking this medicine for a long period of time (for example, for several months at a time), it is important that your doctor check your progress at regular visits.

Do not take this medicine for 5 days before having surgery, including dental surgery, unless otherwise directed by your doctor. The aspirin in this product, if taken during this time, may cause bleeding problems.

Side Effects of This Medicine

Along with its needed effects, a medicine may cause some unwanted effects. Although not all of these side effects appear very often, when they do occur they may require medical attention. When this medicine is used for short periods of time at doses of not more than 6 capsules or tablets a day, side effects usually are rare. However, check with your doctor if any of the following side effects occur:

Less common

Any loss of hearing	Shortness of breath
Bloody or black tarry stools	or troubled breathing
Itching, skin rash, or hives	Unusual excitement
Mental confusion or depression	Unusually slow heartbeat
Nausea, vomiting, or stomach pain	Wheezing or tightness in chest

Rare

Swelling of eyelids, face, or lips	Unusual tiredness or weakness
Unexplained sore throat and fever	Yellowing of eyes or skin
Unusual bleeding or bruising	

Possible signs of overdose

Dizziness or mental confusion	Ringing or buzzing in ear (continuing)
Nausea or vomiting	
Rapid breathing	Severe or continuing headache (unexplained)
	Stomach pain

Possible side effects with long-term use of APC

Bluish-colored fingernails or mucous membranes	Swelling of feet or lower legs
Cloudy urine	Unusual tiredness or weakness

Other side effects may occur which usually do not require medical attention. These side effects may go away during treatment as your body

adjusts to the medicine. However, check with your doctor if any of the following side effects continue or are bothersome:

More common

Clumsiness or unsteadiness	Drowsiness
	Indigestion
Dizziness or light-headedness or feeling faint	

Less common

Diarrhea	Sleeplessness, nervousness, or jitters
Difficult urination	
Frequent urge to urinate	Slurred speech
Headache	Unusual increase in sweating
Joint or muscle pain	Unusual tiredness or weakness
Loss of appetite	
Redness or flushing of face	

Other side effects not listed above may also occur in some patients. If you notice any other effects, check with your doctor.

BUTALBITAL, APC, AND CODEINE
(Systemic)
A commonly used brand name is Fiorinal with Codeine.

Butalbital (byoo-TAL-bi-tal), APC, and codeine (KOE-deen) is a combination medicine used to relieve pain. APC is the short name for aspirin, phenacetin, and caffeine (AS-pir-in, fe-NASS-e-tin, and KAF-een). Butalbital, APC, and codeine combination is available only with your doctor's prescription.

Before Using This Medicine

In order to decide on the best treatment for your medical problem, your doctor should be told:

—if you have ever had any unusual reaction to barbiturates, codeine, acetaminophen, phenacetin, caffeine, or aspirin or other salicylates including methyl salicylate (oil of wintergreen), or to other nonsteroidal anti-inflammatory agents such as fenoprofen, ibuprofen, indomethacin, naproxen, oxyphenbutazone, phenylbutazone, sulindac, or tolmetin. This medicine should not be taken if you are allergic to it.

—if you are pregnant or if you intend to become pregnant while using this medicine. Too much use of aspirin during the last 3 months of pregnancy may increase the length of pregnancy and may prolong labor. Aspirin taken during the last 2 weeks of pregnancy may cause the baby to have bleeding problems at birth. When phenacetin or butalbital are used during pregnancy, they may cause side effects in the newborn infant. In addition, although aspirin, phenacetin, caffeine, butalbital, and codeine have not been shown to cause birth defects, the chance always exists.

—if you are breast-feeding an infant. Butalbital may cause side effects in infants of nursing mothers. Although aspirin, phenacetin, caffeine, and codeine have not been shown to cause problems, the chance always exists. Therefore, use by nursing mothers should be carefully considered.

—if you have any of the following medical problems:

Anemia	Hemophilia or other bleeding problems
Asthma, allergies, and nasal polyps (history of)	Hodgkin's disease
	Hyperactivity (in children)
Brain disease or injury	Hypoprothrombinemia
Colitis	Kidney disease
Emphysema, asthma or chronic lung disease	Liver disease
	Porphyria (or history of)
Enlarged prostate or problems with urination	Ulcer or other stomach problems
Gallbladder disease or gallstones	Underactive adrenal gland (Addison's disease)
Glucose-6-phosphate dehydrogenase (G6PD) deficiency	Underactive thyroid
	Unusually slow or irregular heartbeat
Gout	Vitamin K deficiency

—if you are now taking any of the following medicines or types of medicine:

Antacids	Inflammation medicine (for example, arthritis medicine)
Anticoagulants (blood thinners)	
Contraceptives, oral (birth-control pills)	Insulin
	Methotrexate
Corticosteroids (cortisone-like medicines)	Oral hypoglycemics (diabetes medicine you take by mouth)
Cyclophosphamide	
Digitalis	Phenytoin
Digitoxin	Prescription medicine for stomach cramps or spasms
Doxycycline	
Estrogens	
Gout medicine	Quinidine
Griseofulvin	

Spironolactone
Urine acidifiers
(medicine to
make your urine
more acid)

Urine alkalizers
(medicine to
make your urine
less acid)
Vitamin C

—if you are now taking any central nervous system (CNS) depressants such as:

Antihistamines or
medicine for
hay fever,
other allergies, or
colds
Other barbiturates
Other narcotics
Other prescription
pain medicine

Sedatives, tran-
quilizers,
or sleeping
medicine
Seizure medicine
Tricyclic an-
tidepressants
(medicine for
depression)

—if you are now taking or have taken within the past 2 weeks monoamine oxidase (MAO) inhibitors such as:

Isocarboxazid
Pargyline

Phenelzine
Tranylcypromine

Proper Use of This Medicine

Take this medicine with food or a full glass (8 ounces) of water or milk to lessen stomach irritation.

Do not use this medicine if it has a strong vinegar-like odor, since this means the aspirin in the product is breaking down. If you have any questions about this, check with your doctor or pharmacist.

Use this medicine only as directed by your doctor. Do not use more of it, do not use it more often, and do not use it for a longer period of time than your doctor ordered. If too much is used, it may become habit-forming or cause kidney damage.

Keep this medicine out of the reach of children since overdose is very dangerous in young children.

Precautions While Using This Medicine

Check the labels of all over-the-counter (OTC), nonprescription, and prescription medicines you now take. If any contain aspirin or other salicylates, phenacetin, barbiturates, or codeine or other narcotics, be especially careful, since taking them while taking this medicine may lead to overdose. If you have any questions about this, check with your doctor or pharmacist.

Caution: Diabetics—This medicine contains aspirin and phenacetin which may cause false test results with urine sugar tests. If you have any questions about this, check with your doctor or pharmacist.

This medicine will add to the effects of alcohol and other medicines (CNS depressants) that slow down the nervous system. Some examples of CNS depressants are antihistamines or medicine for hay fever, other allergies, or colds; sedatives, tranquilizers, or sleeping medicine; prescription pain medicine or narcotics; barbiturates; medicine for seizures; tricyclic antidepressants (medicine for depression); or anesthetics, including some dental anesthetics. In addition, stomach problems may be more likely to occur if you drink alcoholic beverages while being treated with this medicine. *Check with your doctor before taking any of the above while you are using this medicine.*

This medicine may cause some people to feel faint or become dizzy, lightheaded, drowsy, or less alert than they are normally. *Make sure you know how you react to this medicine before you drive, use machines, or do other jobs that require you to be alert.*

If you will be taking this medicine for a long period of time (for example, for several months at a time), your doctor should check your progress at regular visits.

Do not take this medicine for 5 days before having surgery, including dental surgery, unless otherwise directed by your doctor. The aspirin in this product, if taken during this time, may cause bleeding problems.

Dizziness, lightheadedness, or fainting may occur, especially when you get up from a lying or sitting position. Getting up slowly may help lessen this problem.

Nausea may occur, especially after the first couple of doses. This effect usually goes away if you lie down for awhile. However, if nausea or vomiting continues, check with your doctor.

Side Effects of This Medicine

Along with its needed effects, a medicine may cause some unwanted effects. Although not all of these side effects appear very often, when they do occur they may require medical attention. When this medicine is used for short periods of time at doses of not more than 6 capsules or tablets a day, side effects usually are rare. However, check with your doctor if any of the following side effects occur:

Less common

Any loss of hearing	Nausea, vomiting,
Bloody or black	or stomach pain
tarry stools	Shortness of breath
Itching, skin rash,	or troubled
or hives	breathing
Mental confusion or	Unusual excitement
depression	Wheezing or
	tightness
	in chest

Rare

Swelling of eyelids,	Unusual bleeding or
face, or lips	bruising
Unexplained sore	Unusual tiredness or
throat and fever	weakness
	Yellowing of eyes
	or skin

Possible signs of overdose

Dizziness or mental	Ringing or buzzing
confusion	in ear (continu-
Nausea or vomiting	ing)
Rapid breathing	Severe or continuing
	headache (un-
	explained)
	Stomach pain

Possible side effects with long-term use of APC

Bluish-colored	Swelling of feet or
fingernails or mu-	lower legs
cous membranes	Unusual tiredness or
Cloudy urine	weakness

Other side effects may occur which usually do not require medical attention. These side effects may go away during treatment as your body adjusts to the medicine. However, check with your doctor if any of the following side effects continue or are bothersome:

More common

Clumsiness or	Drowsiness
unsteadiness	Indigestion
Constipation	
Dizziness, light-	
headedness or	
feeling faint	

Less common

Diarrhea	Sleeplessness, ner-
Difficult urination	vousness, or jit-
Frequent urge	ters
to urinate	Slurred speech
Headache	Unusual increase in
Joint or muscle	sweating
pain	Unusual tiredness or
Loss of appetite	weakness
Redness or flushing	
of face	

Other side effects not listed above may also occur in some patients. If you notice any other effects, check with your doctor.

BUTORPHANOL (Systemic)
A commonly used brand name is Stadol.

Butorphanol (byoo-TOR-fa-nole) is a medicine used to relieve pain. It is used by injection and is available only with your doctor's prescription.

Before Using This Medicine

In order to decide on the best treatment for your medical problem, your doctor should be told:

—if you are pregnant or if you intend to become pregnant while using this medicine. Butorphanol crosses the placental barrier. Although it has not been shown to cause birth defects or other problems, the chance always exists. Therefore, use by pregnant women should be carefully considered.

—if you are breast-feeding an infant. Butorphanol may pass into breast milk. Although it has not been shown to cause problems, the chance always exists. Therefore, use by nursing mothers should be carefully considered.

—if you have any of the following medical problems:

Brain disease	Heart disease
or injury	Liver disease
Emphysema,	Narcotic
asthma, or	dependence or
chronic lung	addiction
disease	
Gallbladder disease	
or gallstones	

—if you are now taking any of the following medicines or types of medicine:

Methadone or other	Narcotics
narcotics when	Propoxyphene
used for the	
treatment of	
narcotic	
dependence	
or addiction	

—if you are now taking other central nervous system (CNS) depressants such as:

Antihistamines or	Sedatives, tran-
medicine for hay	quilizers,
fever, other	or sleeping
allergies, or	medicine
colds	Seizure medicine
Barbiturates	Tricyclic an-
Other prescription	tidepressants
pain medicine	(medicine for
	depression)

—if you are now taking or have taken within the past 2 weeks monoamine oxidase (MAO) inhibitors such as:

Isocarboxazid   Phenelzine
Pargyline   Tranylcypromine

Proper Use of This Medicine

Take this medicine only as directed by your doctor. Do not take more of it, do not take it more often, and do not take it for a longer period of time than your doctor ordered. If too much is taken, it may become habit-forming.

Precautions While Using This Medicine

If you will be taking this medicine for a long period of time (for example, for several months at a time), your doctor should check your progress at regular visits.

This medicine will add to the effects of alcohol and other medicines (CNS depressants) that slow down the nervous system. Some examples of CNS depressants are anesthetics, including dental anesthetics; antihistamines or medicine for hay fever, other allergies, or colds; barbiturates; medicine for seizures; narcotics; prescription pain medicine; sedatives, tranquilizers, or sleeping medicine; or tricyclic antidepressants (medicine for depression). *Check with your doctor before taking any of the above while you are using this medicine.*

This medicine may cause some people to become drowsy, dizzy, or lightheaded, or to feel a false sense of well-being. *Make sure you know how you react to this medicine before you drive, use machines, or do other jobs that require you to be alert and clear-headed.*

Nausea may occur, especially after the first couple of doses. This effect usually goes away if you lie down for a while. However, if nausea or vomiting continues, check with your doctor.

Side Effects of This Medicine

Along with its needed effects, a medicine may cause some unwanted effects. Although not all of these side effects appear very often, when they do occur they may require medical attention. Check with your doctor if any of the following side effects occur:

Less common

Hallucinations (see-   Mental confusion
  ing, hearing, or   Shortness of breath
  feeling things   Troubled breathing
  that are not
  there)

Other side effects may occur which usually do not require medical attention. These side effects

may go away during treatment as your body adjusts to the medicine. However, check with your doctor if any of the following side effects continue or are bothersome:

More common

Drowsiness

Less common

Blurred or double   False sense of well-
  vision   being
Dizziness or light-   Headache
  headedness   Nausea or vomiting

After you stop using this medicine, your body may need time to adjust. The length of time this takes depends on the amount of medicine you were using and how long you used it. During this period of time check with your doctor if you notice any of the following side effects:

Loss of appetite   Stomach cramps
Nervousness or rest-
  lessness

Other side effects not listed above may also occur in some patients. If you notice any other effects, check with your doctor.

CALCITONIN (Systemic)

A commonly used brand name is Calcimar.

Calcitonin (kal-si-TOE-nin) is given by injection to treat Paget's disease of bone. It may also be used for the treatment of too much calcium in the blood. This medicine is available only with your doctor's prescription.

Before Using This Medicine

In order to decide on the best treatment for your medical problem, your doctor should be told:

—if you have ever had any unusual reaction to calcitonin in the past. This medicine should not be used if you are allergic to it.

—if you are pregnant, if you intend to become pregnant, or if you are breast-feeding an infant. Although calcitonin has not been shown to cause problems in humans, the chance always exists.

—if you have a history of allergy.

—if you are now taking any of the following medicines or types of medicine:

Medicine contain-
  ing calcium
Vitamin D

Proper Use of This Medicine

Use this medicine only as directed by your doctor. Do not use more of it and do not use it more often than your doctor ordered.

This medicine is for injection only. If you will be giving yourself the injections, make sure you understand exactly how to give them. If you have any questions about this, check with your doctor.

If you miss a dose of this medicine and your dosing schedule is one dose to be given:

Every other day—
Give the missed dose as soon as possible if you remember it on the day it should be given. Then go back to your regular dosing schedule. But if you do not remember the missed dose until the next day, give it at that time. Then skip a day and start your dosing schedule again.

Once a day—
Give the missed dose as soon as possible. Then go back to your regular dosing schedule. But if you do not remember the missed dose until the next day, do not give it at all and do not double the next one. Instead, go back to your regular dosing schedule.

Twice a day—
If you remember within 2 hours or so of the missed dose, give it right away. Then go back to your regular dosing schedule. But if you do not remember the missed dose until later, do not give it at all and do not double the next one. Instead, go back to your regular dosing schedule.

If you have any questions about this, check with your doctor.

Precautions While Using This Medicine

Your doctor should check your progress at regular visits in order to make sure that this medicine does not cause unwanted effects.

If you are using this medicine for hypercalcemia (too much calcium in the blood), your doctor may want you to follow a low-calcium diet. If you have any questions about this, check with your doctor.

Side Effects of This Medicine

Along with its needed effects, a medicine may cause some unwanted effects. Although not all of these side effects appear very often, when they do occur they may require medical attention. Check with your doctor if the following side effect occurs:

Rare
Skin rash or hives

Other side effects may occur which usually do not require medical attention. These side effects may go away during treatment as your body adjusts to the medicine. However, check with your doctor if any of the following side effects continue or are bothersome:

More common
Nausea or vomiting   Pain, redness, soreness, or swelling at place of injection

Less common
Diarrhea   Flushing or redness of face or hands

Other side effects not listed above may also occur in some patients. If you notice any other effects, check with your doctor.

CALCITRIOL (Systemic)
A commonly used brand name is Rocaltrol.

Calcitriol (kal-si-TRYE-ole) is taken by mouth to treat hypocalcemia (not enough calcium in the blood) caused by kidney disease. It increases the amount of calcium in the blood. Calcitriol may also be used for other conditions as determined by your doctor. This medicine is available only with your doctor's prescription.

Before Using This Medicine

In order to decide on the best treatment for your medical problem, your doctor should be told:

—if you have ever had any unusual reaction to calcitriol in the past. This medicine should not be taken if you are allergic to it.

—if you are pregnant, if you intend to become pregnant, or if you are breast-feeding an infant. Although calcitriol has not been shown to cause problems in humans, the chance always exists.

—if you are now taking any of the following medicines or types of medicine:

Antacids containing   Dihydrotachysterol
   magnesium   Ergocalciferol
Cholecalciferol   Vitamin D
Cholestyramine
Digitalis glycosides
   (heart medicine)

—if you are now taking any nonprescription or over-the-counter (OTC) medicine.

Proper Use of This Medicine

Take this medicine only as directed. Do not take more of it and do not take it more often than your doctor ordered. To do so may increase the chance of overdose.

While you are taking this medicine, your doctor may want you to follow a special diet or take a calcium supplement. Be sure to follow instructions carefully. If you are already taking a calcium supplement or any medicine containing calcium, make sure your doctor knows.

If you miss a dose of this medicine, take it as soon as possible. Then go back to your regular dosing schedule. However, if you do not remember the missed dose until the next day, do not take it at all and do not double the next one. Instead, go back to your regular dosing schedule.

Precautions While Using This Medicine

Your doctor should check your progress at regular visits in order to make sure that this medicine does not cause unwanted effects.

Do not take antacids containing magnesium while you are taking this medicine. Taking these medicines together may cause unwanted effects.

Do not take any nonprescription or over-the-counter (OTC) medicine while you are taking this medicine, unless you have been told to do so by your doctor.

Side Effects of This Medicine

Along with its needed effects, a medicine may cause some unwanted effects. Although not all of these side effects appear very often, when they do occur they may require medical attention. Check with your doctor if any of the following side effects occur:

Possible signs of overdose

Bone pain	Nausea or vomiting
Cloudy urine	Severe stomach pain
Constipation	Unusual increase in
Headache (continu-	frequency of
ing)	urination,
High blood pressure	especially
Increased sensitivity	at night, or
of eyes to light	in amount
or irritation of	of urine
eyes	Unusual increase in
Irregular heartbeat	thirst
Itching of skin	Unusual tiredness or
Loss of appetite	weakness
Metallic taste in	Unusual weight loss
mouth	Unusually dry
Mood or mental	mouth
changes	
Muscle pain	

Other side effects not listed above may also occur in some patients. If you notice any other effects, check with your doctor.

CAPREOMYCIN (Systemic)
A commonly used brand name is Capastat.

Capreomycin (kap-ree-oh-MYE-sin) belongs to the general family of medicines called antibiotics. It is used to help the body overcome tuberculosis (TB). It is given by injection with one or more other medicines for TB. Capreomycin is available only with your doctor's prescription.

Before Using This Medicine

In order to decide on the best treatment for your medical problem, your doctor should be told:

—if you have ever had any unusual reaction to capreomycin. This medicine should not be taken if you are allergic to it.

—if you are pregnant, if you intend to become pregnant, or if you are breast-feeding an infant, although capreomycin has not been shown to cause problems in humans.

—if you have any of the following medical problems:

Eighth-cranial-nerve	Kidney disease
disease (loss of	Myasthenia gravis
hearing and/or	Parkinson's disease
balance)	

—if you are now taking any of the following medicines:

Amikacin	Kanamycin
Cephaloridine	Mercaptomerin
Cephalothin	Neomycin
Cisplatin	Paromomycin
Colistimethate	Polymyxin B
Colistin	Streptomycin
Ethacrynic acid	Tobramycin
Furosemide	Vancomycin
Gentamicin	

—if you have had any problems with this medicine in the past.

Precautions While Using This Medicine

If this medicine causes difficulty in breathing, drowsiness, irregular heartbeats, mood or mental changes, nausea, stomach pain or bloating, unusual tiredness or weakness, vomiting, or weak pulse, check with your doctor. These may be warning signs of more serious problems that could develop later.

Side Effects of This Medicine

Along with its needed effects, a medicine may cause some unwanted effects. Although not all of these side effects appear very often, when they do occur they may require medical attention. Check with your doctor if any of the following side effects occur:

More common

Blood in urine	Greatly increased or
Excessive thirst	decreased frequency of urination or amount of urine
	Loss of appetite

Less common

Clumsiness or unsteadiness	Ringing or buzzing sound or a feeling
Difficulty in breathing	of fullness in the ears
Dizziness	Stomach pain or
Drowsiness	bloating
Irregular heartbeats	Unusual tiredness or
Loss of hearing	weakness
Mood or mental changes	Vomiting
Muscle cramps or pain	Weak pulse
Nausea	

Other side effects may occur which usually do not require medical attention. These side effects may go away during treatment as your body adjusts to the medicine. However, check with your doctor if any of the following side effects continue or are bothersome:

Less common

Itching	Rash
Pain, hardness, unusual bleeding, or a sore at the place of injection	Redness
	Swelling
	Unexplained fever

Other side effects not listed above may also occur in some patients. If you notice any other effects, check with your doctor.

CARBACHOL (Ophthalmic)
Some commonly used brand names are:

Carbacel	Miostat
Isopto Carbachol	Murocarb

Carbachol (KAR-ba-kole) is used in the eye to treat glaucoma. Sometimes it is used in eye surgery. This medicine is available only with your doctor's prescription.

Before Using This Medicine

In order to decide on the best treatment for your medical problem, your doctor should be told:

—if you have ever had any unusual reaction to carbachol in the past. This medicine should not be used if you are allergic to it.

—if you are pregnant, if you intend to become pregnant, or if you are breast-feeding an infant. Although carbachol has not been shown to cause problems, the chance always exists.

—if you have any of the following medical problems:

Asthma	Stomach ulcer or
Heart disease	other stomach
Overactive thyroid	problems
Parkinson's disease	Urinary tract blockage

Proper Use of This Medicine

Use this medicine only as directed. Do not use more of it and do not use it more often than your doctor ordered. To do so may increase the chance of too much medicine being absorbed into the body and the chance of side effects.

How to apply this medicine: First, wash hands. With middle finger, apply pressure to the inside corner of the eye (and continue to apply pressure for 1 or 2 minutes after the medicine has been placed in the eye). Tilt head back and with the index finger of the same hand, pull lower eyelid away from eye to form a pouch. Drop the medicine into the pouch and gently close eyes. Do not blink. Keep eyes closed for 1 or 2 minutes to allow the medicine to be absorbed.

To prevent contamination of the eye drops, do not touch the applicator tip to any surface (including the eye) and keep the container tightly closed.

If you miss a dose of this medicine, apply it as soon as possible. Then go back to your regular dosing schedule. But if it is almost time for your next dose, do not apply the missed dose at all. Instead, apply your next dose at the regularly scheduled time. Then continue with your regular dosing schedule. If you have any questions about this, check with your doctor.

Precautions While Using This Medicine

Your doctor should check your eye pressure at regular visits.

For a short time after you apply this medicine, your vision may be blurred or there may be a change in your near or distant vision. *Make sure your vision is clear before you drive or do other jobs that require you to see well.*

Side Effects of This Medicine

Along with its needed effects, a medicine may cause some unwanted effects. Although not all of these side effects appear very often, when they do occur they may require medical attention. Check with your doctor if any of the following side effects occur:

Possible signs of too much medicine being absorbed into the body

Diarrhea, stomach cramps or pain, or vomiting	Shortness of breath, wheezing, or tightness in chest
Flushing or redness of face	Unusual increase in sweating
Frequent urge to urinate	Unusual watering of mouth

Other side effects may occur which usually do not require medical attention. These side effects may go away during treatment as your body adjusts to the medicine. However, check with your doctor if any of the following side effects continue or are bothersome:

Blurred vision or change in near or distant vision	Headache
	Irritation of eyes
Eye pain	Twitching of eyelids

Other side effects not listed above may also occur in some patients. If you notice any other effects, check with your doctor.

CARBOL-FUCHSIN (Topical)

Carbol-Fuchsin (kar-bol-FOOK-sin), also known as Castellani's (kas-tel-AN-eez) paint, belongs to the group of medicines called antifungals. It is applied to the skin and nails to treat some types of fungal infections. This medicine is available only with your doctor's prescription.

Before Using This Medicine

In order to decide on the best treatment for your medical problem, your doctor should be told:

—if you have ever had any unusual reaction to carbol-fuchsin in the past. This medicine should not be used if you are allergic to it.

—if you are pregnant, if you intend to become pregnant, or if you are breast-feeding an infant, although carbol-fuchsin has not been shown to cause problems.

Proper Use of This Medicine

To help clear up your infection completely, *keep using this medicine for the full time of treatment* even though your condition may have improved.

Carbol-fuchsin is a poison. Use only on the skin as directed.

Before applying this medicine, wash with soap and water the area to be treated, and dry thoroughly.

Using an applicator or swab, apply this medicine only to the affected area. Do not apply to large areas of the body, unless otherwise directed by your doctor.

When this medicine is applied to the fingers or toes, do not bandage them.

If you miss a dose of this medicine, apply it as soon as possible. Then go back to your regular dosing schedule. But if it is almost time for your next dose, do not apply the missed dose at all. Instead, go back to your regular dosing schedule. If you have any questions about this, check with your doctor.

Precautions While Using This Medicine

If your skin problem has not improved after you have used carbol-fuchsin for 1 week, check with your doctor.

To help cure the infection and to help prevent reinfection, good health habits are required. These include the following:
• Wash all towels and bedding after each use.

• Use only freshly laundered clothes each time clothing is changed.

If you have any questions about this, check with your doctor, nurse, or pharmacist.

This medicine will stain clothing. Avoid getting it on your clothes.

Side Effects of This Medicine

Along with its needed effects, a medicine may cause some unwanted effects. Although not all

of these side effects appear very often, when they do occur they may require medical attention. Check with your doctor if the following side effect occurs:

Irritation of skin not present before using this medicine

When this medicine is applied, a mild, temporary stinging may be expected.

Other side effects not listed above may also occur in some patients. If you notice any other effects, check with your doctor.

CARBOPROST (Systemic)
A commonly used brand name is Prostin/15M.

Carboprost (KAR-boe-prost) is given by injection to cause abortion. It is available only with your doctor's prescription and is to be administered only by or under the immediate care of your doctor.

Before Using This Medicine

In order to decide on the best treatment for your medical problem, your doctor should be told:

—if you have ever had any unusual reaction to carboprost in the past. This medicine should not be used if you are allergic to it.

—if you have any of the following medical problems:

Adrenal gland disease (history of)
High blood pressure (history of)
Anemia (history of)
Jaundice (history of)
Asthma (history of)
Kidney disease
Diabetes (history of)
Liver disease (or history of)
Epilepsy (history of)
Lung disease
Heart or blood vessel disease (or history of)
Uterus surgery (history of)

Side Effects of This Medicine

Along with its needed effects, a medicine may cause some unwanted effects. Although not all of these side effects appear very often, when they do occur they may require medical attention. Let the doctor or nurse know if any of the following side effects occur:

Less common or rare

Wheezing, troubled breathing, or tightness in chest

Other side effects may occur which usually do not require medical attention. These side effects usually go away after the medicine is stopped. However, let the doctor or nurse know if any of the following side effects continue or are bothersome:

More common

Diarrhea   Vomiting
Nausea

Less common

Chills or shivering
Fever

After this medicine is stopped, it may still produce some side effects that need attention. Check with your doctor if you notice any of the following:

Chills or shivering   Pain in lower abdomen
Fever
Foul-smelling   Unusual increase in
   vaginal discharge   uterine bleeding

Other side effects not listed above may also occur in some patients. If you notice any other effects, check with your doctor.

CARISOPRODOL (Systemic)

Some commonly used brand names are Rela, Soma, and Soprodol.

Carisoprodol (kar-eye-soe-PROE-dole) is a medicine used to help relax certain muscles in your body and relieve the pain and discomfort caused by strains, sprains, or other injury to your muscles. This medicine is available only with your doctor's prescription.

Before Using This Medicine

In order to decide on the best treatment for your medical problem, your doctor should be told:

—if you have had any unusual reaction to medicines like carisoprodol such as carbromal, mebutamate, meprobamate or tybamate.

—if you are pregnant or if you intend to become pregnant while taking this medicine. Carisoprodol has not been shown to cause problems in humans but the chance always exists.

—if you are breast-feeding an infant. Carisoprodol passes into breast milk and may cause unwanted side effects in infants of nursing mothers taking it.

—if you have any of the following medical problems:

Kidney disease   Porphyria
Liver disease

—if you are now taking other central nervous system (CNS) depressants such as:

Antihistamines or medicine for hay fever, other allergies, or colds
Barbiturates
Narcotics

Prescription pain medicine
Sedatives, tranquilizers or sleeping medicine
Seizure medicine
Tricyclic antidepressants (medicine for depression)

—if you are now taking or have taken within the past 2 weeks monoamine oxidase (MAO) inhibitors such as:

Isocarboxazid   Phenelzine
Pargyline   Tranylcypromine

Proper Use of This Medicine

If you miss a dose of this medicine and remember within an hour or so of the missed dose, take it right away. Then go back to your regular dosing schedule. But if you do not remember until later, do not take the missed dose at all and do not double the next one. Instead, go back to your regular dosing schedule. If you have any questions about this, check with your doctor.

Precautions While Using This Medicine

This medicine will add to the effects of alcohol and other medicines (CNS depressants) that slow down the nervous system. Some examples of CNS depressants are antihistamines or medicine for hay fever, other allergies, or colds; sedatives, tranquilizers, or sleeping medicine; prescription pain medicine or narcotics; barbiturates; medicine for seizures; tricyclic antidepressants (medicine for depression); or anesthetics, including some dental anesthetics. *Check with your doctor before taking any of the above while you are using this medicine.*

This medicine may cause some people to become drowsy or less alert than they are normally. *Make sure you know how you react to this medicine before you drive, use machines, or do other jobs that require you to be alert.*

Side Effects of This Medicine

Along with its needed effects, a medicine may cause some unwanted effects. Although not all of these side effects appear very often, when they do occur they may require medical attention. Check with your doctor if any of the following side effects occur:

Less common

Dizziness, lightheadedness, or fainting
Mental depression
Skin rash, hives, or itching

Unusually fast heartbeat
Wheezing, shortness of breath, or troubled breathing

Other side effects may occur which usually do not require medical attention. These side effects may go away during treatment as your body adjusts to the medicine. However, check with your doctor if any of the following side effects continue or are bothersome:

More common

Drowsiness

Less common

Clumsiness or unsteadiness
Headache
Hiccups
Nausea or vomiting
Sleeplessness

Stomach cramps or pain
Trembling
Unusual nervousness, restlessness, or irritability

Other side effects not listed above may also occur in some patients. If you notice any other effects, check with your doctor.

CARMUSTINE (Systemic)
A commonly used brand name is BiCNU.

Carmustine (kar-MUS-teen) belongs to the group of medicines known as alkylating agents. It is used by injection to treat some kinds of cancer. Carmustine is available only on prescription and is to be administered only by or under the immediate supervision of your doctor.

Before Using This Medicine

Carmustine is a very strong medicine. In addition to its helpful effects in treating your medical problem, it has side effects that could be very serious. Before you receive this medicine, be sure that you have discussed the use of it with your doctor.

In order to decide on the best treatment for your medical problem, your doctor should be told:

—if you have ever had any unusual reaction to carmustine in the past.

—if you are pregnant or if you intend to have children. This medicine may cause birth defects if either the male or female is taking it at the time of conception or if it is taken during pregnancy. It may also cause permanent sterility after it has been taken for a while. Be sure that you have discussed this with your doctor before taking this medicine.

—if you are breast-feeding an infant. Although carmustine has not been shown to cause problems, the chance always exists.

—if you have any of the following medical problems:

Blood disease   Kidney disease
Infection

—if you have been treated with x-rays or cancer drugs by another doctor.

Proper Use of This Medicine

This medicine is sometimes given together with certain other medicines. If you are using a combination of drugs, it is important that you receive each medicine at the proper time. If you are taking some of these medicines by mouth, ask your doctor, nurse, or pharmacist to help you plan a way to take them at the right time.

This medicine often causes nausea and vomiting, which usually last no longer than 4 to 6 hours. It is very important that you continue to receive the medicine, even if you begin to feel ill. Your doctor may prescribe a medicine to relieve stomach upset. If you have any questions about this, check with your doctor.

Precautions While Using This Medicine

It is very important that your doctor check your progress at regular visits.

Side Effects of This Medicine

Along with its needed effects, a medicine may cause some unwanted effects. Although not all of these side effects appear very often, when they do occur they may require medical attention. Check with your doctor if any of the following side effects occur:

More common
Unexplained fever,   Unusual bleeding or
  chills, or sore   bruising
  throat

Less common
Pain or redness at   Unusual tiredness or
  place of injection   weakness
Sores in the mouth
  and on lips

Rare
Cough   Unusual decrease in
Shortness of breath   urination
Swelling of feet   Yellowing of eyes
  or lower legs   and skin

Other side effects may occur which usually do not require medical attention. These side effects may go away during treatment as your body adjusts to the medicine. However, check with your doctor if any of the following side effects continue or are bothersome:

More common
Nausea and
  vomiting
Less common
Diarrhea   Dizziness
Difficulty in   Loss of appetite
  swallowing   Loss of hair
Difficulty in walk-   Skin rash and
  ing   itching
Discoloration of the
  skin along the
  vein of injection
Rare
Enlargement of breasts in males

This medicine may cause a temporary loss of hair in some people. After treatment with carmustine has ended, normal hair growth should return.

If carmustine accidentally seeps out of the vein into which it is injected, it may damage some tissues and cause scarring. Tell the doctor right away if you notice redness, pain, or swelling at the place of injection.

After you stop using this medicine, it may still produce some side effects that need attention. During this period of time check with your doctor if you notice any of the following:

Unexplained fever,   Unusual bleeding or
  chills, or sore   bruising
  throat

Other side effects not listed above may also occur in some patients. If you notice any other effects, check with your doctor.

CEPHALOSPORINS (Systemic)

This information applies to the following medicines:

Cefaclor (SEF-a-klor)
Cefadroxil (sef-a-DROX-ill)
Cefamandole (sef-a-MAN-dole)
Cefazolin (sef-A-zoe-lin)
Cefoxitin (se-FOX-i-tin)
Cephalexin (sef-a-LEX-in)
Cephaloglycin (sef-a-loe-GLYE-sin)
Cephaloridine (sef-a-LOR-i-deen)
Cephalothin (sef-A-loe-thin)
Cephapirin (sef-a-PYE-rin)
Cephradine (SEF-ra-deen)

Some commonly used brand names are:	Generic names:
Ceclor	Cefaclor
Duricef Ultracef	Cefadroxil
Mandol	Cefamandole
Ancef Kefzol	Cefazolin
Mefoxin	Cefoxitin
Ceporex* Keflex	Cephalexin
Kafocin	Cephaloglycin
Ceporan* Loridine	Cephaloridine
Ceporacin* Keflin Neutral	Cephalothin
Cefadyl	Cephapirin
Anspor Velosef	Cephradine

*Not available in the United States.

Cephalosporins (sef-a-loe-SPOR-ins) belong to the general family of medicines called antibiotics. They are given by mouth or by injection to help the body overcome infections. Cephaloglycin is given by mouth to help the body overcome infections of the urinary tract only. Cephalosporins are available only with your doctor's prescription.

Before Using This Medicine

In order to decide on the best treatment for your medical problem, your doctor should be told:

—if you have had severe allergic reactions to any of the cephalosporins, penicillins, penicillin-like medicines, or penicillamine.

—if you are pregnant, if you intend to become pregnant, or if you are breast-feeding an infant, although cephalosporins have not been shown to cause problems.

—if you have kidney disease.

—if you are taking any of the cephalosporins (except cephaloridine) and are also taking probenecid.

—if you are receiving cephaloridine or cephalothin by injection and are also receiving amikacin, colistin, ethacrynic acid, furosemide, gentamicin, kanamycin, neomycin, polymyxin B, streptomycin, or tobramycin.

Proper Use of This Medicine

Cephalosporins may be taken without regard to meals. However, if this medicine upsets your stomach, it may be taken with food.

If you are taking the oral liquid form of this medicine:

• This medicine is to be taken by mouth even though it may come in a dropper bottle. If this medicine does not come in a dropper bottle, use a specially marked measuring spoon or other device to measure each dose accurately since the average household teaspoon may not hold the right amount of liquid.

To help clear up your infection completely, *keep taking this medicine for the full time of treatment* even if you begin to feel better after a few days; *do not miss any doses.* This is especially important if you have a "strep" infection since serious heart problems could develop later if your infection is not completely cleared up.

If you do miss a dose of this medicine, take it as soon as possible. However, if it is almost time for your next dose and your dosing schedule is:

• 1 dose a day—Space the missed dose and the next dose 10 to 12 hours apart.

• 2 doses a day—Space the missed dose and the next dose 5 to 6 hours apart.

• 3 or more doses a day—Space the missed dose and the next dose 2 to 4 hours apart or double your next dose.

Then go back to your regular dosing schedule.

Precautions While Using This Medicine

If your symptoms do not improve within a few days or if they become worse, check with your doctor.

If you are receiving cephaloridine by injection and it causes difficult breathing, drowsiness, excessive thirst, greatly decreased frequency of urination or amount of urine, loss of appetite, or unusual tiredness or weakness, check with your doctor immediately.

Caution: Diabetics—This medicine may cause false test results with some urine sugar tests. Check with your doctor before changing your diet or the dosage of your diabetes medicine.

Side Effects of This Medicine

Along with its needed effects, a medicine may cause some unwanted effects. Although not all of these side effects appear very often, when they do occur they may require medical attention. Stop taking this medicine and check with your doctor if any of the following side effects occur:

Rare

> Severe stomach cramps, pain, and bloating
> Severe, watery diarrhea, which may be accompanied by blood, mucus, pus, or pieces of intestinal lining in the stool
> Unexplained fever

Other side effects may occur which usually do not require medical attention. These side effects may go away during treatment as your body adjusts to the medicine. However, check with your doctor if any of the following side effects continue or are bothersome:

More common (rare with cefoxitin)

Diarrhea	Stomach cramps or
Nausea	upset
	Vomiting

More common

Itching	Sore mouth or
Rash	tongue
Redness	Swelling

If you are taking cephaloglycin:

• Stop taking this medicine and check with your doctor if any of the following side effects occur:

More common

Bloody or black	Severe stomach
tarry stools	cramps,
Severe diarrhea	pain, and
	bloating

• Check with your doctor if any of the following side effects continue or are bothersome:

More common

Itching	Rash
Mild diarrhea	Redness
Mild stomach	Sore mouth or
cramps	tongue
or upset	Swelling
Nausea	Vomiting

If you are receiving cephaloridine by injection:

• In addition to the side effects mentioned above, check with your doctor if any of the following side effects occur:

Less common

Difficult breathing	Greatly decreased
Drowsiness	frequency of
Excessive thirst	urination or
	amount of urine
	Loss of appetite
	Unusual tiredness or
	weakness

Other side effects not listed above may also occur in some patients. If you notice any other effects, check with your doctor.

CHARCOAL, ACTIVATED (Oral)
Some commonly used brand names are Charcocaps, Charcodote, and Charcotabs.

Activated charcoal (AK-ti-vay-ted CHAR-kole) is taken by mouth in the emergency treatment of certain kinds of poisoning. It helps prevent the poison from being absorbed by the body. Ordinarily, this medicine should not be used in poisoning if corrosive agents such as alkalies (lye) and strong acids, cyanide, iron, ethyl alcohol, or methyl alcohol have been swallowed, since it will not prevent these poisons from being absorbed into the body.

This medicine may also be used to relieve diarrhea and intestinal gas or stomach discomfort.

Activated charcoal is available without a doctor's prescription; however, before using this medicine for poisoning, call your doctor, a poison control center, or an emergency room for advice. Also, your doctor may have special instructions on the proper use of this medicine for diarrhea or intestinal gas.

Before Using This Medicine

In order to decide on the best treatment for your medical problem, your doctor should be told:

—if you have ever had any unusual reaction to activated charcoal in the past. This medicine should not be taken if you are allergic to it.

—if you are pregnant, if you intend to become pregnant, or if you are breast-feeding an infant, although activated charcoal is not absorbed into the body and is not likely to cause problems.

—if you are now taking any other medicine (only for patients taking this medicine for stomach or intestinal problems).

Proper Use of This Medicine

Do not take this medicine mixed with ice cream or sherbert, since it may prevent the medicine from working properly.

For patients taking this medicine for poisoning:

• *Before taking this medicine in the treatment of poisoning, call your doctor, a poison control center, or an emergency room for advice.* It is a good idea to have these telephone numbers readily available.

• If you have been told to take both this medicine and ipecac syrup to treat the poisoning, *do not take this medicine until after you have taken the ipecac syrup to cause vomiting and the vomiting has stopped. This is usually about 30 minutes.* Taking them together may prevent the ipecac syrup from causing vomiting of the poison.

Precautions While Using This Medicine

For patients taking this medicine for stomach or intestinal problems:

• If you are taking this medicine for intestinal gas or stomach discomfort and your condition has not improved after 7 days, check with your doctor.

• If you are taking this medicine for diarrhea and your condition has not improved after 2 days or if you have fever with the diarrhea, check with your doctor.

• *If you are taking any other medicine, do not take it within 2 hours of the activated charcoal.* Taking them together may prevent the other medicine from being absorbed by your body. If you have any questions about this, check with your doctor or pharmacist.

Side Effects of This Medicine

This medicine will cause your stools to turn black. This is to be expected while you are taking this medicine.

There have not been any other side effects reported with this medicine. However, if you notice any other effects, check with your doctor.

CHLORAL HYDRATE (Systemic)
Some commonly used brand names are:

Aquachloral	Noctec
Chloralex*	Novochlorhydrate*
Chloralvan*	Oradrate
Cohidrate	

*Not available in the United States.

Chloral hydrate (klor-al HYE-drate) belongs to the group of medicines called sedatives and hypnotics. It is used in the treatment of insomnia or sleeplessness to help patients fall asleep and stay asleep through the night. Also, it is used to help calm or relax patients who are nervous or tense. This medicine is available only with your doctor's prescription.

Before Using This Medicine

In order to decide on the best treatment for your medical problem, your doctor should be told:

—if you have ever had any unusual reaction to chloral hydrate in the past. This medicine should not be used if you are allergic to it.

—if you are pregnant or if you intend to become pregnant while using this medicine. Too much use of chloral hydrate during pregnancy may cause the baby to become dependent on the medicine. This may lead to withdrawal side effects after birth.

—if you are breast-feeding an infant. Chloral hydrate passes into breast milk and may cause unwanted effects in infants of mothers taking this medicine.

—if you are taking this medicine by mouth or using the rectal suppository form of chloral hydrate and have any of the following medical problems:

Heart disease	Liver disease
Kidney disease	

—if you are taking this medicine by mouth and have gastritis or inflammation of the stomach.

—if you are using the rectal suppository form of chloral hydrate and have either of the following medical problems:

Colitis
Proctitis or inflam-
   mation of the
   rectum

—if you are now taking other central nervous system (CNS) depressants such as:

Antihistamines or medicine for hay fever, other allergies, or colds	Prescription pain medicine
	Seizure medicine
	Tricyclic antidepressants (medicine for depression)
Barbiturates	
Narcotics	
Other sedatives, tranquilizers, or sleeping medicine	

—if you are now taking or have taken within the past 2 weeks monoamine oxidase (MAO) inhibitors such as:

Isocarboxazid	Phenelzine
Pargyline	Tranylcypromine

—if you are now taking anticoagulants (blood thinners).

Proper Use of This Medicine

Use this medicine only as directed by your doctor. Do not use more of it, do not use it more often, and do not use it for a longer period of time than your doctor ordered. If too much is used, it may become habit-forming.

Keep this medicine out of the reach of children since overdose is especially dangerous in children.

If you miss a dose of this medicine, do not take the missed dose at all and do not double the next one. Instead, go back to your regular dosing schedule. If you have any questions about this, check with your doctor.

If you are taking the capsule form of chloral hydrate:

• Swallow the capsule whole. Do not chew since the medicine may cause a bad taste.

• Take this medicine with a full glass (8 ounces) of water, fruit juice, or ginger ale to lessen stomach upset.

If you are taking the oral liquid form of chloral hydrate:

• Take each dose of medicine mixed with 1/2 glass (4 ounces) of water, fruit juice, or ginger ale to improve flavor and lessen stomach upset.

If you are using the rectal suppository form of chloral hydrate:

• How to insert suppository: First remove the foil wrapper and moisten the suppository with water. Lie down on side and push the suppository well up into rectum with finger. If the suppository is too soft to insert because of storage in a warm place, before removing the foil wrapper chill the suppository in the refrigerator for 30 minutes or run cold water over it.

Precautions While Using This Medicine

If you will be using this medicine regularly for a long period of time:

• Your doctor should check your progress at regular visits in order to make sure that this medicine does not cause unwanted effects.

• Do not stop using it without first checking with your doctor. Your doctor may want you to reduce gradually the amount you are using before stopping completely.

This medicine will add to the effects of alcohol and other medicines (CNS depressants) that slow down the nervous system. Some examples of CNS depressants are antihistamines or medicine for hay fever, other allergies, or colds; sedatives, tranquilizers, or sleeping medicine; prescription pain medicine or narcotics; barbiturates; medicine for seizures; tricyclic antidepressants (medicine for depression); or anesthetics, including some dental anesthetics. *Check with your doctor before taking any of the above while you are using this medicine.*

If you think you may have taken an overdose, get emergency help at once. Taking an overdose of chloral hydrate or taking alcohol or other CNS depressants with chloral hydrate may lead to unconsciousness and possibly death. Some signs of an overdose are mental confusion, severe weakness, shortness of breath or troubled breathing, staggering, and unusually slow or irregular heartbeat.

This medicine may cause some people to become dizzy, lightheaded, drowsy, or less alert than they are normally. Even if taken at bedtime, it may cause some people to feel drowsy or less alert on arising. *Make sure you know how you react to this medicine before you drive, use machines, or do other jobs that require you to be alert.*

Side Effects of This Medicine

Along with its needed effects, a medicine may cause some unwanted effects. Although not all of these side effects appear very often, when they do occur they may require medical attention. Check with your doctor if any of the following side effects occur:

Less common

Skin rash or hives

Rare

Hallucinations (seeing, hearing, or feeling things that are not there)	Mental confusion Unusual excitement

Signs of overdose

Shortness of breath or troubled breathing	Unusually slow or irregular heart beat

Other side effects may occur which usually do not require medical attention. These side effects may go away during treatment as your body adjusts to the medicine. However, check with your doctor if any of the following side effects continue or are bothersome:

More common

Nausea Stomach pain	Vomiting

Less common

Clumsiness or unsteadiness Dizziness or lightheadedness	Drowsiness "Hangover" effect

After you stop using this medicine, your body may need time to adjust. The length of time this takes depends on the amount of medicine you were using and how long you used it. During this period of time check with your doctor if you notice any of the following side effects:

Hallucinations (seeing, hearing, or feeling things that are not there) Mental confusion Nausea or vomiting	Nervousness Restlessness Stomach pain Trembling Unusual excitement

Other side effects not listed above may also occur in some patients. If you notice any other effects, check with your doctor.

CHLORAMBUCIL (Systemic)
A commonly used brand name is Leukeran.

Chlorambucil (klor-AM-byoo-sill) belongs to the group of medicines called alkylating agents. It is used to treat some kinds of cancer as well as some noncancerous conditions. It is used also in some situations to reduce the body's natural immunity. Chlorambucil is available only with your doctor's prescription.

Before Using This Medicine

Chlorambucil is a very strong medicine. In addition to its helpful effects in treating your medical problem, it has side effects that could be very serious. Before you take this medicine, be sure that you have discussed the use of it with your doctor.

In order to decide on the best treatment for your medical problem, your doctor should be told:

—if you have ever had any unusual reaction to chlorambucil in the past.

—if you are pregnant or if you intend to have children. This medicine may cause birth defects if either the male or female is taking it at the time of conception or if it is taken during pregnancy. It may also cause permanent sterility after it has been taken for a while. Be sure that you have discussed this with your doctor before taking this medicine.

—if you are breast-feeding an infant. Although chlorambucil has not been shown to cause problems, the chance always exists.

—if you have any of the following medical problems:

Blood disease Gout	Infection Kidney stones

—if you are taking gout medicine.

—if you have been treated with x-rays or cancer drugs by another doctor.

Proper Use of This Medicine

Take this medicine only as directed by your doctor. Do not take more or less of it, and do not take it more often than your doctor ordered.

In order for this medicine to be most effective, it should be taken 1 hour before breakfast or 2 hours after the evening meal. Take it at the same time each day.

This medicine is sometimes given together with certain other medicines. If you are using a combination of drugs, make sure that you take each medicine at the proper time and do not mix them. Ask your doctor, nurse, or pharmacist to help you plan a way to remember to take your medicines at the right time.

This medicine sometimes causes nausea and vomiting. Even if you begin to feel ill, *do not stop using this medicine without first checking with your doctor.*

If you miss a dose of this medicine, do not take the missed dose at all and do not double the next one. Instead, go back to your regular dosing schedule and check with your doctor.

Precautions While Using This Medicine

It is very important that your doctor check your progress at regular visits.

While you are using this medicine, your doctor may want you to drink plenty of fluids and urinate often. This will help prevent kidney problems and keep your kidneys working well. If you have any questions about this, check with your doctor.

Side Effects of This Medicine

Along with its needed effects, a medicine may cause some unwanted effects. Although not all of these side effects appear very often, when they do occur they may require medical attention. Check with your doctor if any of the following side effects occur:

More common

Unusual bleeding or
bruising

Less common

Cough	Sores in the mouth
Flank or stomach	and on the lips
pain	Swelling of feet
Joint pain	or lower legs
Shortness of breath	Unexplained fever,
	chills, or sore
	throat
	Yellowing of eyes
	and skin

Rare

Blurred vision
Convulsions

Other side effects may occur which usually do not require medical attention. These side effects may go away during treatment as your body adjusts to the medicine. However, check with your doctor if any of the following side effects continue or are bothersome:

Less common

Nausea and
vomiting
Skin rash or itching

Rare

Changes in
menstrual period

This medicine may cause a temporary loss of hair in some people. After treatment with chlorambucil has ended, normal hair growth should return.

After you stop using this medicine, it may still produce some side effects that need attention. During this period of time check with your doctor if you notice any unusual bleeding or bruising.

Other side effects not listed above may also occur in some patients. If you notice any other effects, check with your doctor.

CHLORAMPHENICOL (Ophthalmic)

Some commonly used brand names are:

Chloromycetin	Ophthochlor
Chloroptic	Pentamycetin*
Econochlor	Sopamycetin*
Fenicol*	

*Not available in the United States.

Chloramphenicol (klor-am-FEN-i-kole) belongs to the general family of medicines called antibiotics. Chloramphenicol ophthalmic preparations are used to help the body overcome infections of the eye. They are available only with your doctor's prescription.

Before Using This Medicine

In order to decide on the best treatment for your medical problem, your doctor should be told:

—if you have ever had any unusual reaction to chloramphenicol. This medicine should not be taken if you are allergic to it.

—if you are pregnant, if you intend to become pregnant, or if you are breast-feeding an infant, although chloramphenicol ophthalmic preparations have not been shown to cause problems.

Proper Use of This Medicine

If you are using the eye drop form of this medicine:

• Although the bottle may not be full, it contains exactly the amount of medicine your doctor ordered.

• To prevent contamination of the eye drops, do not touch the applicator tip or dropper to any surface (including the eye), and keep the container tightly closed.

• How to apply this medicine: First, wash hands. Then tilt head back and pull lower eyelid away from eye to form a pouch. Drop medicine into the pouch and gently close eyes. Do not blink. Keep eyes closed for 1 or 2 minutes to allow medicine to come into contact with the infection.

• If you think you did not get the drop of medicine into your eye properly, use another drop.

If you are using the eye ointment form of this medicine:

• To prevent contamination of the eye ointment, do not touch the applicator tip to any surface (including the eye). After using, wipe the tip of the ointment tube with a clean tissue and keep the tube tightly closed.

• How to apply this medicine: First, wash hands. Then pull the lower eyelid away from eye to form a pouch. Squeeze a thin strip of ointment into the pouch. A 1-cm (approximately 1/3-inch) strip of ointment is usually enough unless otherwise directed by your doctor. Gently close eyes and keep them closed for 1 or 2 minutes to allow medicine to come into contact with the infection.

To help clear up your infection completely, *keep using this medicine for the full time of treatment,* even though your symptoms may have disappeared; *do not miss any doses.*

If you do miss a dose of this medicine, apply it as soon as possible. However, if it is almost time for your next application, skip the missed dose and go back to your regular dosing schedule.

Precautions While Using This Medicine

After application of this medicine to the eye, occasional stinging or burning may be expected.

After application, eye ointments usually cause your vision to blur for a few minutes.

If your symptoms do not improve within a few days or if they become worse, check with your doctor.

Side Effects of This Medicine

Along with its needed effects, a medicine may cause some unwanted effects. Although not all of these side effects appear very often, when they do occur they may require medical attention. Stop using this medicine and check with your doctor if any of the following side effects occur:

Very rare

Pale skin	Unusual bleeding or
Unexplained sore	bruising
throat or fever	Unusual tiredness or
	weakness

Other side effects not listed above may also occur in some patients.If you notice any other effects, check with your doctor.

CHLORAMPHENICOL (Otic)

A commonly used brand name is Chloromycetin.

Chloramphenicol (klor-am-FEN-i-kole) belongs to the general family of medicines called antibiotics. Chloramphenicol otic preparations are used to help the body overcome infections of the ear. They are available only with your doctor's prescription.

Before Using This Medicine

In order to decide on the best treatment for your medical problem, your doctor should be told:

—if you have ever had any unusual reaction to chloramphenicol. This medicine should not be taken if you are allergic to it.

—if you are pregnant, if you intend to become pregnant, or if you are breast-feeding an infant, although chloramphenicol otic preparations have not been shown to cause problems.

Proper Use of This Medicine

Before applying this medicine, wash the area to be treated (including the ear canal) with soap and water, and dry thoroughly. The ear canal should be dried with a sterile cotton applicator.

To prevent contamination of the ear drops, do not touch the dropper to any surface (including the ear), and keep the container tightly closed.

How to apply this medicine: Lie down or tilt the head so that the infected ear faces up. Gently pull the earlobe up and back for adults (down and back for children) to straighten the ear canal. Drop medicine into the ear canal. Keep ear facing up for 1 or 2 minutes to allow medicine to come into contact with the infection. A clean, soft cotton plug may be gently inserted into the ear opening to prevent the medicine from leaking out.

To help clear up your infection completely, *keep using this medicine for the full time of treatment,* even though your symptoms may have disappeared; *do not miss any doses.*

If you do miss a dose of this medicine, apply it as soon as possible. However, if it is almost time for your next application, skip the missed dose and go back to your regular dosing schedule.

Precautions While Using This Medicine

If your symptoms do not improve within a few days or if they become worse, check with your doctor.

Side Effects of This Medicine

Along with its needed effects, a medicine may cause some unwanted effects. Although not all of these side effects appear very often, when they do occur they may require medical attention. Check with your doctor if any of the following side effects occur:

Burning, itching, rash, redness, swelling, or other sign of irritation not present before you started using this medicine

Other side effects not listed above may also occur in some patients. If you notice any other effects, check with your doctor.

Clindamycin
Lincomycin
Oral anticoagulants (blood thinners you take by mouth)

Oral hypoglycemics (diabetes medicine you take by mouth)
Penicillins
Phenytoin

—if you are taking bone-marrow depressants such as:

Anticancer medicines
Colchicine
Gold salts

Oxyphenbutazone
Penicillamine
Phenylbutazone

—if you have taken this medicine or if you have had any problems with it in the past.

CHLORAMPHENICOL (Systemic)

Some commonly used brand names are:
Amphicol
Chloromycetin
Novochlorocap*
Pentamycetin*

---

*Not available in the United States.

Chloramphenicol (klor-am-FEN-i-kole) belongs to the general family of medicines called antibiotics. It is given by mouth or by injection to help the body overcome infections. Chloramphenicol is available only with your doctor's prescription.

Before Using This Medicine

In order to decide on the best treatment for your medical problem, your doctor should be told:

—if you have ever had any unusual reaction to chloramphenicol. This medicine should not be taken if you are allergic to it.

—if you are pregnant and within a week or two of your delivery date. Although chloramphenicol has not been shown to cause birth defects, it may cause gray skin color, low body temperature, bloated stomach, uneven breathing, and drowsiness in infants if taken within a week or two of your delivery date.

—if you are breast-feeding an infant. Chloramphenicol passes into the breast milk and may cause unwanted effects in infants of mothers taking this medicine.

—if you have either of the following medical problems:
Kidney disease
Liver disease

—if you are taking any of the following medicines or types of medicine:

Proper Use of This Medicine

Chloramphenicol is best taken with a full glass (8 ounces) of water on an empty stomach (either 1 hour before or 2 hours after meals), unless otherwise directed by your doctor.

If you are taking the oral liquid form of this medicine:

• Use a specially marked measuring spoon or other device to measure each dose accurately since the average household teaspoon may not hold the right amount of liquid.

To help clear up your infection completely, *keep taking this medicine for the full time of treatment* even if you begin to feel better after a few days; *do not miss any doses.*

If you do miss a dose of this medicine, take it as soon as possible. However, if it is almost time for your next dose and your dosing schedule is:

• 2 doses a day—Space the missed dose and the next dose 5 to 6 hours apart.

• 3 or more doses a day—Space the missed dose and the next dose 2 to 4 hours apart or double your next dose.

Then go back to your regular dosing schedule.

Do not save any unused part of this medicine for later use, unless otherwise directed by your doctor.

Precautions While Using This Medicine

If your symptoms do not improve within a few days or if they become worse, check with your doctor.

It is important that your doctor check your progress at regular visits.

Caution: Diabetics—This medicine may cause false test results with urine sugar tests. Check with your doctor before changing your diet or the dosage of your diabetes medicine.

If this medicine is being given to a child, especially a premature or newborn infant, and the child develops a gray skin color, low body temperature, bloated stomach, uneven breathing, and drowsiness, stop giving this medicine and check with your doctor immediately.

Side Effects of This Medicine

Along with its needed effects, a medicine may cause some unwanted effects. Although not all of these side effects appear very often, when they do occur they may require medical attention. Stop taking this medicine and check with your doctor if any of the following side effects occur:

Less common

Pale skin	Unusual bleeding or
Unexplained sore	bruising
throat or fever	Unusual tiredness or
	weakness

Rare

Eye pain, blurred	Numbness, tingling,
vision, or any loss	burning pain, or
of vision	weakness in the
	hands or feet

Other side effects may occur which usually do not require medical attention. These side effects may go away during treatment as your body adjusts to the medicine. However, check with your doctor if any of the following side effects continue or are bothersome:

Less common

Diarrhea	Vomiting
Nausea	

After you stop taking this medicine, some side effects may occur weeks or months later. During this period of time check with your doctor *immediately* if any of the following side effects occur:

Pale skin	Unusual bleeding or
Unexplained sore	bruising
throat or fever	Unusual tiredness or
	weakness

Other side effects not listed above may also occur in some patients. If you notice any other effects, check with your doctor.

CHLORAMPHENICOL (Topical)
A commonly used brand name is Chloromycetin.

Chloramphenicol (klor-am-FEN-i-kole) belongs to the general family of medicines called antibiotics. Chloramphenicol topical preparations are used to help the body overcome infections of the skin. Chloramphenicol is available only with your doctor's prescription.

Before Using This Medicine

In order to decide on the best treatment for your medical problem, your doctor should be told:

—if you have ever had any unusual reaction to chloramphenicol. This medicine should not be used if you are allergic to it.

—if you are pregnant, if you intend to become pregnant, or if you are breast-feeding an infant, although chloramphenicol topical preparations have not been shown to cause problems.

Proper Use of This Medicine

Before applying this medicine, wash the area to be treated with soap and water, and dry thoroughly.

To help clear up your infection completely, *keep using this medicine for the full time of treatment,* even though your symptoms may have disappeared; *do not miss any doses.* However, *do not use this medicine more often or for a longer period of time than your doctor ordered.*

If you do miss a dose of this medicine, apply it as soon as possible. However, if it is almost time for your next application, skip the missed dose and go back to your regular dosing schedule.

Precautions While Using This Medicine

If there is no improvement in your skin problem after you have used this medicine for 1 week or if it becomes worse, check with your doctor.

Side Effects of This Medicine

Along with its needed effects, a medicine may cause some unwanted effects. Although not all of these side effects appear very often, when they do occur they may require medical attention. Check with your doctor if any of the following side effects occur:

Burning, itching, rash, redness, swelling, or other sign of irritation not present before you started using this medicine

Other side effects not listed above may also occur in some patients. If you notice any other effects, check with your doctor.

CHLORDIAZEPOXIDE AND AMITRIPTYLINE (Systemic)

A commonly used brand name is Limbitrol

Chlordiazepoxide (klor-dye-az-e-POX-ide) and amitriptyline (a-mee-TRIP-ti-leen) is a combination of medicines used to treat depression that occurs with anxiety or nervous tension. This medicine is available only with your doctor's prescription.

Before Using This Medicine

In order to decide on the best treatment for your medical problem, your doctor should be told:

—if you have ever had any unusual reaction to benzodiazepines (such as chlordiazepoxide, clorazepate, diazepam, flurazepam, lorazepam, oxazepam, or prazepam) or to tricyclic antidepressants (such as amitriptyline, desipramine, doxepin, imipramine, nortriptyline, or protriptyline). This medicine should not be taken if you are allergic to it.

—if you are pregnant or if you intend to become pregnant while using this medicine. Benzodiazepines may cause birth defects if taken during the first 3 months of pregnancy. In addition, too much use of this medicine during pregnancy may cause the baby to become dependent on the medicine. This may lead to withdrawal side effects after birth.

—if you are breast-feeding an infant. Benzodiazepines may pass into the breast milk and cause unwanted effects in infants.

—if you have any of the following medical problems:

Alcoholism	Heart disease
Difficulty in	High blood pressure
urinating	Kidney disease
Emphysema,	Liver disease
asthma,	Myasthenia gravis
bronchitis, or	Thyroid disease
other chronic	Stomach or in-
lung disease	testinal problems
Enlarged prostate	
Epilepsy	
Glaucoma	

—if you are now taking *any* other medicines, including over-the-counter (OTC) or nonprescription medicine, especially the following:

Antihistamines or	Other medicine for
medicine for	depression
hay fever,	Other sedatives,
other allergies,	tranquilizers, or
or colds	sleeping medicine
Barbiturates	Prescription pain
Blood pressure	medicine
medicine	Seizure medicine
Estrogens	Thyroid medicine
Heart medicine	
Narcotics	

—if you are now taking or have taken within the past 2 weeks monoamine oxidase (MAO) inhibitors such as:

Isocarboxazid	Phenelzine
Pargyline	Tranylcypromine

Proper Use of This Medicine

Take this medicine only as directed by your doctor.

To reduce stomach upset, take this medicine immediately after meals or with food unless your doctor has told you to take it on an empty stomach.

Sometimes this medicine must be taken for several weeks before you begin to feel its full effects.

If you miss a dose of this medicine, do not take the missed dose at all and do not double the next one. Instead, go back to your regular dosing schedule. If you have any questions about this, check with your doctor.

Precautions While Using This Medicine

Your doctor should check your progress at regular visits.

Before having medical or dental surgery or emergency treatment, tell the doctor or dentist in charge that you are using this medicine.

This medicine will add to the effects of alcohol and other medicines (CNS depressants) that slow down the nervous system. Some examples of CNS depressants are antihistamines or medicine for hay fever, other allergies, or colds; sedatives, tranquilizers, or sleeping medicine; prescription pain medicine or narcotics; barbiturates; medicine for seizures; tricyclic antidepressants (medicine for depression); or anesthetics, including some dental anesthetics. This effect may last for a few days after you stop taking this medicine. *Check with your doctor before taking any of the above while you are using this medicine.*

This medicine may cause some people to become dizzy, lightheaded, drowsy, or less alert than they are normally. Even if taken at bedtime, it may cause some people to feel drowsy or less alert on arising. *Make sure you know how you react to this medicine before you drive, use machines, or do other jobs that require you to be alert.*

Dizziness, lightheadedness, or fainting may occur, especially when you get up from a lying or sitting position. Getting up slowly may help. If this problem continues or gets worse, check with your doctor.

If you will be taking this medicine in large doses or for a long period of time, do not stop taking it without first checking with your doctor. Your doctor may want you to reduce gradually the amount you are taking before stopping completely.

Side Effects of This Medicine

Along with its needed effects, a medicine may cause some unwanted effects. Although not all of these side effects appear very often, when they do occur they may require medical attention. Check with your doctor if any of the following side effects occur:

More common
    Blurred vision

Less common

Difficulty in urinating	Hallucinations (seeing, hearing, or feeling things that are not there)
Eye pain	
Fainting	Irregular heartbeat
	Shakiness

Rare

Seizures	Unexplained sore throat and fever
Skin rash and itching	Yellowing of eyes and skin

Other side effects may occur which usually do not require medical attention. These side effects may go away during treatment as your body adjusts to the medicine. However, check with your doctor if any of the following side effects continue or are bothersome:

More common

Bloating	Dizziness
Clumsiness or unsteadiness	Drowsiness
	Dry mouth
Constipation	Headache

Less common

Diarrhea	Tiredness or weakness
Nausea	

After you stop using this medicine, your body may need time to adjust. If you took this medicine in high doses or for a long time, this may take up to 2 weeks. During this period of time check with your doctor if you notice any of the following side effects:

Convulsions or seizures	Stomach cramps
	Trembling
Muscle cramps	Unusual sweating
Nausea or vomiting	

Other side effects not listed above may also occur in some patients. If you notice any other effects, check with your doctor.

CHLORDIAZEPOXIDE AND CLIDINIUM
(Systemic)
A commonly used brand name is Librax.

Chlordiazepoxide (klor-dye-az-e-POX-ide) and clidinium (kli-DI-nee-um) is a combination of medicines used to relax the digestive system and to reduce stomach acid. It is used to treat stomach and intestinal problems such as ulcers and colitis. This combination is available only with your doctor's prescription.

Before Using This Medicine

In order to decide on the best treatment for your medical problem, your doctor should be told:

—if you have ever had any unusual reaction to benzodiazepines such as chlordiazepoxide, clorazepate, diazepam, flurazepam, lorazepam, oxazepam, or prazepam. This medicine should not be taken if you are allergic to it.

—if you are pregnant or if you intend to become pregnant while using this medicine. Chlordiazepoxide may cause birth defects if taken during the first 3 months of pregnancy. In addition, too much use of this medicine during pregnancy may cause the baby to become dependent on the medicine. This may lead to withdrawal side effects after birth.

—if you have any of the following medical problems:

Difficult urination	Intestinal blockage
Emphysema, asthma, bronchitis, or other chronic lung disease	Kidney disease
	Liver disease
	Mental depression
	Myasthenia gravis
	Overactive thyroid
Enlarged prostate	Severe mental illness
Glaucoma	Severe ulcerative colitis
Hiatal hernia	
High blood pressure	

—if you are now taking any of the following medicines or types of medicine:

Amantadine	Medicine for
Haloperidol	parkinsonism
Heart medicine	Ulcer medicine
Medicine for diar- rhea	

—if you are now taking central nervous system (CNS) depressants such as:

Antihistamines or medicine for hay fever, other aller- gies, or colds	Prescription pain medicine
	Sedatives, tran- quilizers, or sleep-
Barbiturates	ing medicine
Narcotics	Seizure medicine
	Tricyclic an- tidepressants (medicine for depression)

—if you are now taking or have taken within the past 2 weeks monoamine oxidase (MAO) inhibitors such as:

Isocarboxazid	Phenelzine
Pargyline	Tranylcypromine

Proper Use of This Medicine

Take this medicine only as directed by your doctor. Do not take more of it, do not take it more often, and do not take it for a longer period of time than your doctor ordered. If too much is taken, it may become habit-forming.

Take this medicine about 1/2 to 1 hour before meals unless otherwise directed by your doctor.

If you miss a dose of this medicine, do not take the missed dose at all and do not double the next one. Instead, go back to your regular dosing schedule. If you have any questions about this, check with your doctor.

Precautions While Using This Medicine

If you will be taking this medicine regularly for a long period of time your doctor should check your progress at regular visits.

Do not take this medicine within an hour of taking antacid or medicine for diarrhea. Taking them too close together will make this medicine less effective.

This medicine may cause some people to become dizzy, lightheaded, drowsy, or less alert than they are normally. *Make sure you know how you react to this medicine before you drive, use machines, or do other jobs that require you to be alert.*

This medicine will add to the effects of alcohol and other medicines (CNS depressants) that slow down the nervous system. Some examples of CNS depressants are antihistamines or medicine for hay fever, other allergies, or colds; sedatives, tranquilizers, or sleeping medicine; prescription pain medicine or narcotics; barbiturates; medicine for seizures; tricyclic antidepressants (medicine for depression); or anesthetics, including some dental anesthetics. *Check with your doctor before taking any of the above while you are taking this medicine and also for a few days after you stop taking it.*

This medicine will often make you sweat less, causing your body temperature to increase. *Use extra care not to become overheated during exercise or hot weather while you are taking this medicine* as this could possibly result in heat stroke.

Your mouth, nose, and throat may feel very dry while you are taking this medicine. To help relieve mouth dryness, chew sugarless gum or dissolve bits of ice in your mouth.

Check with your doctor if you develop intestinal problems such as constipation. This is especially important if you are taking other medicine while you are taking chlordiazepoxide and clidinium. If not corrected, serious complications may result.

If you will be taking this medicine in large doses or for a long period of time, do not stop taking it without first checking with your doctor. Your doctor may want you to reduce gradually the amount you are taking before stopping completely.

Side Effects of This Medicine

Along with its needed effects, a medicine may cause some unwanted effects. Although not all of these side effects appear very often, when they do occur they may require medical attention. Check with your doctor if any of the following side effects occur:

More common

Blurred vision	Mental depression
Constipation	Skin rash or itching
Mental confusion	

Less common

Difficulty in urinating	Unusually slow heartbeat, shortness
Trouble in sleeping	of breath, or
Unusual excitement, nervousness, or irritability	troubled breath- ing

Rare

Eye pain	Yellowing of eyes
Unexplained sore	or skin
throat and fever	

Other side effects may occur which usually do not require medical attention. These side effects may go away during treatment as your body adjusts to the medicine. However, check with your doctor if any of the following side effects continue or are bothersome:

More common

Bloated feeling	Dry mouth
Dizziness	Headache
Drowsiness	Reduced sweating

Less common

Decreased sexual	Nausea
ability	Unusual tiredness or
	weakness

After you stop using this medicine, your body may need time to adjust. The length of time this takes depends on the amount of medicine you were using and how long you used it. During this period of time check with your doctor if you notice any of the following side effects:

Convulsions or	Nausea or vomiting
seizures	Stomach cramps
Muscle cramps	Trembling

Other side effects not listed above may also occur in some patients. If you notice any other effects, check with your doctor.

CHLOROXINE (Topical)

A commonly used brand name is Capitrol.

Chloroxine (klor-OX-een) is used in the treatment of dandruff and seborrheic dermatitis of the scalp. This medicine is available only with your doctor's prescription.

Before Using This Medicine

In order to decide on the best treatment for your medical problem, your doctor should be told:

—if you have ever had any unusual reaction to clioquinol (iodochlorhydroxyquin), iodoquinol (diiodohydroxyquin), or edetate disodium.

—if you are pregnant, if you intend to become pregnant, or if you are breast-feeding an infant, although chloroxine has not been shown to cause problems.

Proper Use of This Medicine

Wet the hair and scalp with lukewarm water. Apply enough chloroxine to the scalp to work up a lather, and rub it in well. Allow the lather to remain on the scalp for about 3 minutes, then rinse. Apply the medicine again and rinse thoroughly.

Do not use this medicine if blistered, raw, or oozing areas are present on your scalp, unless otherwise directed by your doctor.

Keep this medicine away from the eyes. If you should accidentally get some in your eyes, flush them thoroughly with water.

Precautions While Using This Medicine

This medicine may slightly discolor light-colored hair (for example, bleached, blond, or gray).

Side Effects of This Medicine

Along with its needed effects, a medicine may cause some unwanted effects. Although not all of these side effects appear very often, when they do occur they may require medical attention. Check with your doctor if any of the following side effects occur:

Irritation or burning Skin rash
of scalp not
present before
using this
medicine

Other side effects may occur which usually do not require medical attention. However, check with your doctor if either of the following side effects continues or is bothersome:

Dryness or in-
creased itching
of scalp

Other side effects not listed above may also occur in some patients. If you notice any other effects, check with your doctor.

CHLORPHENIRAMINE, PHENYLPROPANOLAMINE, AND ISOPROPAMIDE (Systemic)

Some commonly used brand names are Allernade, Capade, and Ornade.

Chlorpheniramine (klor-fen-IR-a-meen), phenylpropanolamine (fen-ill-proe-pa-NOLE-a-meen), and isopropamide (eye-soe-PROE-pa-mide) is a combination antihistamine, drying agent, and decongestant. It is used to treat nasal congestion (stuffy nose) and other symptoms of hay fever and other types of allergy. This medicine is available only with your doctor's prescription.

Before Using This Medicine

In order to decide on the best treatment for your medical problem, your doctor should be told:

—if you have ever had any unusual reaction to chlorpheniramine, isopropamide, phenylephrine, phenylpropanolamine, or similar medicines in the past or if you are allergic to iodine. This medicine should not be taken if you are allergic to it.

—if you are pregnant or if you intend to become pregnant while using this medicine. Although this medicine has not been shown to cause birth defects or other problems, the chance always exists.

—if you are breast-feeding an infant. Chlorpheniramine may pass into the breast milk and cause unwanted effects in the infant. In addition, both chlorpheniramine and isopropamide may decrease milk production.

—if you have any of the following medical problems:

Colitis	Intestinal blockage
Diabetes	Kidney disease
Enlarged prostate	Liver disease
Glaucoma	Myasthenia gravis
Heart disease	Overactive thyroid
Hiatal hernia	Stomach ulcer
High blood pressure	Urinary tract blockage

—if you are now taking any of the following medicines or types of medicine:

Amphetamines	Medicine for
Digitalis (heart medicine)	asthma or breathing problems
Guanethidine	Tricyclic antidepressants (medicine for depression)

—if you are now taking any central nervous system (CNS) depressants such as:

Antihistamines or medicine for hay fever, other allergies, or colds	Narcotics
	Prescription pain medicine
	Sedatives, tranquilizers, or sleeping medicine
Barbiturates	
Medicines for seizures	

—if you are now taking or have taken within the past 2 weeks monoamine oxidase (MAO) inhibitors such as:

Isocarboxazid	Phenelzine
Pargyline	Tranylcypromine

Proper Use of This Medicine

Take chlorpheniramine, phenylpropanolamine, and isopropamide combination only as directed. Do not take more of it and do not take it more often than recommended on the label, unless otherwise directed by your doctor. To do so may increase the chance of side effects.

Take this medicine with food or a glass of water or milk to lessen stomach irritation, if necessary.

If you must take this medicine regularly and you miss a dose, take the missed dose as soon as possible. However, if it is almost time for your next dose, do not take the missed dose at all and do not double the next one. Instead, go back to your regular dosing schedule. If you have any questions about this, check with your doctor or pharmacist.

Precautions While Using This Medicine

This medicine will add to the effects of alcohol and other medicines (CNS depressants) that slow down the nervous system. Some examples of CNS depressants are antihistamines or medicine for hay fever, other allergies, or colds; sedatives, tranquilizers, or sleeping medicine; prescription pain medicine or narcotics; barbiturates; medicine for seizures; tricyclic antidepressants (medicine for depression); or anesthetics, including some dental anesthetics. *Check with your doctor before taking any of the above while you are using this medicine.*

Both chlorpheniramine and isopropamide may cause some people to have blurred vision or to become drowsy, dizzy, or less alert than they are normally. *Make sure you know how you react to this medicine before you drive, use machines, or do other jobs that require you to be alert.*

Other people may become nervous or restless or may have trouble in sleeping from the phenylpropanolamine in this medicine. If you do have trouble in sleeping, *take the last dose of this medicine for each day a few hours before bedtime.* If you have any questions about this, check with your doctor.

This medicine will often make you sweat less, causing your body temperature to increase. *Use extra care not to become overheated during exercise or hot weather while you are taking this medicine,* since overheating could possibly result in heat stroke. Also, hot baths or saunas may make you feel dizzy or faint while you are taking this medicine.

Your mouth, nose, and throat may feel very dry while you are taking this medicine. To help relieve mouth dryness, chew sugarless gum or dissolve bits of ice in your mouth.

Side Effects of This Medicine

Along with its needed effects, a medicine may cause some unwanted effects. Although not all of these side effects appear very often, when they do occur they may require medical attention. Check with your doctor if any of the following side effects occur:

Rare

Tightness in chest	Unusual bleeding or
Unexplained sore	bruising
throat and fever	Unusual weakness
	Unusually fast or
	pounding heart-
	beat

With high doses

Irregular heartbeats
Mood or mental
changes

Other side effects may occur which usually do not require medical attention. These side effects may go away during treatment as your body adjusts to the medicine. However, check with your doctor if any of the following side effects continue or are bothersome:

More common

Blurred vision	Thickening of the
Drowsiness	bronchial
	secretions

Less common—more common with high doses

Difficult or painful	Nausea, upset
urination	stomach, or
Dizziness	stomach pain
Dryness of mouth,	Nervousness,
nose, or throat	restlessness, or
Headache	trouble in
Loss of appetite	sleeping (especial-
	ly in children)
	Skin rash

Other side effects not listed above may also occur in some patients. If you notice any other effects, check with your doctor.

CHLORZOXAZONE (Systemic)
A commonly used brand name is Paraflex.

Chlorzoxazone (klor-ZOX-a-zone) is a medicine that is used to help relax certain muscles in your body and relieve the pain and discomfort caused by strains, sprains, or other injury to your muscles. This medicine is available only with your doctor's prescription.

Before Using This Medicine

In order to decide on the best treatment for your medical problem, your doctor should be told:

—if you have ever had any unusual reaction to chlorzoxazone in the past. This medicine should not be taken if you are allergic to it.

—if you are pregnant, if you intend to become pregnant, or if you are breast-feeding an infant. Although chlorzoxazone has not been shown to cause problems, the chance always exists.

—if you have any of the following medical problems:

Allergies (asthma,	Liver disease or
eczema, hay	history of liver
fever, hives)	disease

—if you are now taking other central nervous system (CNS) depressants such as:

Antihistamines or	Sedatives, tran-
medicine for	quilizers,
hay fever, other	or sleeping
allergies, or colds	medicine
Barbiturates	Seizure medicine
Narcotics	Tricyclic an-
Prescription pain	tidepressants
medicine	(medicine for
	depression)

—if you are now taking or have taken within the past 2 weeks monoamine oxidase (MAO) inhibitors such as:

Isocarboxazid	Phenelzine
Pargyline	Tranylcypromine

Proper Use of This Medicine

If you miss a dose of this medicine and remember within an hour or so of the missed dose, take it right away. Then go back to your regular dosing schedule. But if you do not remember until later, do not take the missed dose at all and do not double the next one. Instead, go back to your regular dosing schedule. If you have any questions about this, check with your doctor.

Precautions While Using This Medicine

This medicine will add to the effects of alcohol and other medicines (CNS depressants) that slow down the nervous system. Some examples of CNS depressants are antihistamines or medicine for hay fever, other allergies, or colds; sedatives, tranquilizers, or sleeping medicine; prescription pain medicine or narcotics; barbiturates; medicine for seizures; tricyclic antidepressants (medicine for depression); or anesthetics, including some dental anesthetics. *Check with your doctor before taking any of the above while you are taking chlorzoxazone.*

This medicine may cause some people to become drowsy, dizzy, or less alert than they are normally. *Make sure you know how you react to this medicine before you drive, use machines, or do other jobs that require you to be alert.*

Side Effects of This Medicine

Along with its needed effects, a medicine may cause some unwanted effects. Although not all of these side effects appear very often, when they do occur they may require medical attention. Check with your doctor if any of the following side effects occur:

Rare

Bloody or black tarry stools	Unusual tiredness or weakness
Skin rash or itching	Yellowing of eyes or skin
Unexplained sore throat and fever	

Other side effects may occur which usually do not require medical attention. These side effects may go away during treatment as your body adjusts to the medicine. However, check with your doctor if any of the following side effects continue or are bothersome:

More common

Dizziness
Drowsiness

Less common

Constipation or diarrhea	Nausea or vomiting
Headache	Stomach cramps
Heartburn	Unusual excitement or nervousness
Lightheadedness	

In a few patients this medicine may cause the urine to turn orange or reddish purple. This will go away when you stop taking the medicine. If you have any questions about this, check with your doctor.

Other side effects not listed above may also occur in some patients. If you notice any other effects, check with your doctor.

CHLORZOXAZONE AND ACETAMINOPHEN
(Systemic)

Some commonly used brand names are:

Chlorofon-F	Miflex	Parafon Forte
Chlorzone Forte	Parachlor	Tuzon
Lobac		

Chlorzoxazone (klor-ZOX-a-zone) and acetaminophen (a-seat-a-MEE-noe-fen) is a combination medicine used to help relax certain muscles in your body and relieve the pain and discomfort caused by strains, sprains, or other injury to your muscles. This medicine is taken by mouth in the form of tablets and is available only with your doctor's prescription.

Before Using This Medicine

In order to decide on the best treatment for your medical problem, your doctor should be told:

—if you have ever had any unusual reaction to acetaminophen or chlorzoxazone. This medicine should not be taken if you are allergic to it.

—if you are pregnant, if you intend to become pregnant, or if you are breast-feeding an infant. Although chlorzoxazone and acetaminophen have not been shown to cause problems, the chance always exists.

—if you have any of the following medical problems:

Allergies (asthma, eczema, hay fever, hives)	Liver disease (severe)
Kidney disease (severe)	Virus infection of the liver

—if you are now taking other central nervous system (CNS) depressants such as:

Antihistamines or medicine for hay fever, other allergies, or colds	Sedatives, tranquilizers, or sleeping medicine
Barbiturates	Seizure medicine
Narcotics	Tricyclic antidepressants (medicine for depression)
Prescription pain medicine	

—if you are now taking or have taken within the past 2 weeks monoamine oxidase (MAO) inhibitors such as:

Isocarboxazid	Phenelzine
Pargyline	Tranylcypromine

Proper Use of This Medicine

If you miss a dose of this medicine and remember

within an hour or so of the missed dose, take it right away. Then go back to your regular dosing schedule. But if you do not remember until later, do not take the missed dose at all and do not double the next one. Instead, go back to your regular dosing schedule. If you have any questions about this, check with your doctor.

Precautions While Using This Medicine

If you will be taking this medicine for a long period of time (for example, for several months at a time), your doctor should check your progress at regular visits.

This medicine will add to the effects of alcohol and other medicines (CNS depressants) that slow down the nervous system. Some examples of CNS depressants are antihistamines or medicine for hay fever, other allergies, or colds; sedatives, tranquilizers, or sleeping medicine; prescription pain medicine or narcotics; barbiturates; medicine for seizures; tricyclic antidepressants (medicine for depression); or anesthetics, including dental anesthetics. Also, the risk of liver damage from acetaminophen may be greater if you use large amounts of alcoholic beverages with acetaminophen. *Check with your doctor before taking any of the above while you are taking this medicine.*

Check the labels of all over-the-counter (OTC), nonprescription, and prescription medicines you now take. If any contain acetaminophen be especially careful, since taking them while taking this medicine may lead to overdose. If you have any questions about this, check with your doctor, nurse, or pharmacist.

This medicine may cause some people to become drowsy, dizzy, or less alert than they are normally. *Make sure you know how you react to this medicine before you drive, use machines, or do other jobs that require you to be alert.*

Side Effects of This Medicine
Along with its needed effects, a medicine may cause some unwanted effects. Although not all of these side effects appear very often, when they do occur they may require medical attention. Check with your doctor if any of the following side effects occur:

Rare

Bloody or black tarry stools	Unusual bleeding or bruising
Skin rash or itching	
Unexplained sore throat and fever	Unusual tiredness or weakness
	Yellowing of eyes or skin

Possible signs of overdose of acetaminophen

Diarrhea	Stomach cramps or pain
Nausea or vomiting	

Other side effects may occur which usually do not require medical attention. These side effects may go away during treatment as your body adjusts to the medicine. However, check with your doctor if any of the following side effects continue or are bothersome:

More common

Dizziness
Drowsiness

Less common

Constipation or diarrhea	Nausea or vomiting
Headache	Stomach cramps
Heartburn	Unusual excitement or nervousness
Lightheadedness	

In a few patients this medicine may cause the urine to turn orange or reddish purple. This is not harmful and will go away when you stop taking the medicine. If you have any questions about this, check with your doctor.

Other side effects not listed above may also occur in some patients. If you notice any other effects, check with your doctor.

CHOLESTYRAMINE (Oral)
A commonly used brand name is Questran.

Cholestyramine (koe-LESS-tir-a-meen) is used to remove substances called bile acids from your body. With some liver problems, there is too much bile acid in your body and this can cause severe itching. Cholestyramine is also used to lower high cholesterol levels in the blood. This may help prevent medical problems caused by cholesterol clogging the blood vessels. Cholestyramine is available only with your doctor's prescription.

Before Using This Medicine
In order to decide on the best treatment for your medical problem, your doctor should be told:

—if you have ever had any unusual reaction to cholestyramine in the past. This medicine should not be taken if you are allergic to it.

—if you are pregnant, if you intend to become pregnant, or if you are breast-feeding an infant, although cholestyramine is not absorbed into the body and is not likely to cause problems.

—if you have any of the following medical problems:

Angina	Hemorrhoids
Bleeding problems	Kidney disease
Constipation	Stomach ulcer or
Gallstones	other stomach
Heart or blood	problems
vessel disease	

—if you are now taking any other medicines, especially:

Anticoagulants	Heart medicine
(blood thinners)	Thyroid medicine

Proper Use of This Medicine

Take this medicine exactly as directed by your doctor. Try not to miss any doses and do not take more medicine than your doctor ordered.

This medicine should never be taken in its dry form, since it could cause you to choke. Instead, always mix as follows:

• Place the medicine on the surface of a glassful (4 to 6 ounces or more) of water, milk, flavored drink, or your favorite juice or carbonated drink. If you use a carbonated drink, use a large glass to prevent too much foaming. Allow it to sit, without stirring, for 1 or 2 minutes to keep it from becoming lumpy when mixed. Then stir until it is completely mixed (it will *not* dissolve) before drinking. After drinking all the liquid containing the medicine, rinse the glass with a little more liquid and drink that also, to make sure you get all the medicine.

• You may also mix this medicine with milk in hot or regular breakfast cereals, or in thin soups such as tomato or chicken noodle soup. Or you may add it to some pulpy fruits such as crushed pineapple, pears, peaches, or fruit cocktail.

If you miss a dose of this medicine, take it as soon as possible. If it is almost time for your next dose, do not take the missed dose at all and do not double the next one. Instead, go back to your regular dosing schedule. If you have any questions about this, check with your doctor.

For patients taking this medicine for high cholesterol:

• Importance of Diet—Before prescribing medicine for your condition, your doctor will probably try to control your condition by prescribing a personal diet for you. Such a diet may be low in fats, sugars, and/or cholesterol. Many people are able to control their condition by carefully following their doctor's orders for proper diet and exercise. Medicine is prescribed only when additional help is needed. *Follow carefully the special diet your doctor gave you,* since the medicine is effective only when a schedule of diet and exercise is properly followed.

• Also, this medicine is less effective if you are greatly overweight. It may be very important for you to go on a reducing diet. However, check with your doctor before going on any diet.

• Remember that this medicine will not cure your cholesterol problem but it will help control it. Therefore, you must continue to take it as directed if you expect to lower your cholesterol level.

Precautions While Using This Medicine

It is very important that your doctor check your progress at regular visits. This will allow your doctor to see if the medicine is working properly and if you should continue to take it.

Do not take any other medicine unless prescribed by your doctor since cholestyramine may change the effect of other medicines.

Side Effects of This Medicine

Along with its needed effects, a medicine may cause some unwanted effects. Although not all of these side effects appear very often, when they do occur they may require medical attention. Check with your doctor if any of the following side effects occur:

More common
    Constipation
Rare

Black tarry stools	Unusual loss of
Severe stomach pain	weight
with nausea and	
vomiting	

Other side effects may occur which usually do not require medical attention. These side effects may go away during treatment as your body adjusts to the medicine. However, check with your doctor if any of the following side effects continue or are bothersome:

Less common

Belching	Heartburn or in-
Bloating	digestion
Diarrhea	Nausea or vomiting
	Stomach pain

Rare
    Rash or soreness of
    the skin, tongue,
    or around the
    anus

Other side effects not listed above may also occur in some patients. If you notice any other effects, check with your doctor.

CIMETIDINE (Systemic)
A commonly used brand name is Tagamet.

Cimetidine (sye-MET-i-deen) is a medicine used in the treatment of certain types of ulcers and in preventing their return. It is also used in some conditions in which the stomach produces too much acid. Cimetidine may also be used for other conditions as determined by your doctor. It is available only with your doctor's prescription.

Before Using This Medicine
In order to decide on the best treatment for your medical problem, your doctor should be told:

—if you have ever had any unusual reaction to cimetidine in the past. This medicine should not be taken if you are allergic to it.

—if you are pregnant, if you intend to become pregnant, or if you are breast-feeding an infant. Although cimetidine has not been shown to cause problems, the chance always exists.

—if you have kidney disease.

—if you are now taking any of the following medicines or types of medicine:

Anticoagulants (blood thinners)   Benzodiazepines (medicines for treating anxiety)

Proper Use of This Medicine
If you are taking several doses of cimetidine a day, take them with meals or shortly after meals and at bedtime, unless otherwise directed by your doctor. If you are taking a single daily dose, it is most often taken at bedtime.

Antacids may be taken with cimetidine to help relieve any stomach pain, unless your doctor has told you not to use them. You may want to use antacids since it may take several days or weeks for cimetidine to begin to relieve pain.

Take this medicine for the full time of treatment, even if you begin to feel better. Also, it is important that you keep your doctor's appointments for check-ups so that your doctor will be better able to tell you when to stop taking this medicine.

If you miss a dose of this medicine, take it as soon as possible. However, if it is almost time for your next dose do not take the missed dose at all and do not double the next one. Instead, go back to your regular dosing schedule. If you have any questions about this, check with your doctor.

Precautions While Using This Medicine
Cimetidine may cause some people to become dizzy or confused. *Be careful if you must drive, use machines, or do other jobs that require you to be alert and clear-headed.* If confusion occurs, check with your doctor.

Side Effects of This Medicine
Along with its needed effects, a medicine may cause some unwanted effects. Although not all of these side effects appear very often, when they do occur they may require medical attention. Check with your doctor if the following side effects occur:

Rare

Mental confusion	Unusual bleeding
Unexplained sore	or bruising
throat and fever	Unusual tiredness
	or weakness

Other side effects may occur which usually do not require medical attention. These side effects may go away during treatment as your body adjusts to the medicine. However, check with your doctor if any of the following side effects continue or are bothersome:

Less common

Diarrhea	Skin rash
Dizziness or	Swelling of the
headache	breasts
Muscle cramps or	or breast soreness
pains	

Some men who take cimetidine may notice a slight increase in the size of their breasts or some breast soreness. These side effects seem to be temporary and go away with continued use of cimetidine or after treatment has ended. If you have any questions about this, check with your doctor.

Other side effects not listed above may also occur in some patients. If you notice any other effects, check with your doctor.

CISPLATIN (Systemic)
A commonly used brand name is Platinol.

Cisplatin (SIS-pla-tin) belongs to the group of medicines known as alkylating agents. It is used by injection to treat some kinds of cancer. Cisplatin is available only on prescription and is to be administered only by or under the immediate supervision of your doctor.

Before Using This Medicine

Cisplatin is a very strong medicine. In addition to its helpful effects in treating your medical problem, it has some side effects that could be very serious. Before you receive this medicine be sure that you have discussed the use of it with your doctor.

In order to decide on the best treatment for your medical problem, your doctor should be told:

—if you have ever had any unusual reaction to cisplatin in the past.

—if you are pregnant or if you intend to have children while using this medicine. This medicine may cause birth defects if either the male or female is taking it at the time of conception or if it is taken during pregnancy. Be sure that you have discussed this with your doctor before taking this medicine.

—if you are breast-feeding an infant. Although cisplatin has not been shown to cause problems, the chance always exists.

—if you have any of the following medical problems:

Blood disease	Infection
Gout	Kidney disease
Hearing problems	Kidney stones

—if you are taking or have recently received either of the following medicines or types of medicine:

Aminoglycoside antibiotics (such as amikacin, gentamicin, kanamycin, streptomycin, tobramycin)	Gout medicine

—if you have been treated with x-rays or cancer drugs by another doctor.

Proper Use of This Medicine

This medicine is sometimes given together with certain other medicines. If you are using a combination of drugs, it is important that you receive each medicine at the proper time. If you are taking some of these medicines by mouth, ask your doctor, nurse, or pharmacist to help you plan a way to take them at the right time.

This medicine usually causes nausea and vomiting. However, it is very important that you continue to receive the medicine, even if you begin to feel ill. If you have any questions about this, check with your doctor.

Precautions While Using This Medicine

It is very important that your doctor check your progress at regular visits.

While you are receiving this medicine, your doctor may want you to drink plenty of fluids and urinate often. This will help prevent kidney problems and keep your kidneys working well. If you have any questions about this, check with your doctor.

Side Effects of This Medicine

Along with its needed effects, a medicine may cause some unwanted effects. Although not all of these side effects appear very often, when they do occur they may require medical attention. Check with your doctor *immediately* if any of the following side effects occur:

More common

Difficulty in hearing	
Flank or stomach pain	Unexplained fever, chills, or sore throat
Joint pain	
Ringing in the ears	Unusual bleeding or bruising
Swelling of feet or lower legs	

Less common

Loss of taste	Tremors
Numbness or tingling in the fingers, toes, or face	Unusually fast heartbeat
	Wheezing

Other side effects may occur which usually do not require medical attention. These side effects may go away during treatment as your body adjusts to the medicine. However, check with your doctor if any of the following side effects continue or are bothersome:

More common

Nausea and vomiting

Less common

Loss of appetite

Rare

Loss of hair

After you stop using this medicine, it may still produce some side effects that need attention. During this period of time check with your doctor if you notice any of the following side effects:

Difficulty in hearing	Unusual bleeding or bruising
Ringing in the ears	
Swelling of feet or lower legs	Unusual decrease in urination
Unexplained fever, chills, or sore throat	

Other side effects not listed above may also occur in some patients. If you notice any other effects, check with your doctor.

CLINDAMYCIN (Topical)
A commonly used brand name is Cleocin T.

Clindamycin (klin-da-MYE-sin) belongs to the general family of medicines called antibiotics. Clindamycin topical preparations are applied to the skin to help control acne. They may be used alone or with one or more other medicines which are applied to the skin or taken by mouth for acne. Clindamycin is available only with your doctor's prescription.

Before Using This Medicine

In order to decide on the best treatment for your medical problem, your doctor should be told:

—if you have had allergic reactions to any of the other clindamycins (by mouth or by injection) or lincomycin.

—if you are pregnant, if you intend to become pregnant, or if you are breast-feeding an infant, although clindamycin topical preparations have not been shown to cause problems.

—if you have stomach or intestinal disease, especially colitis.

—if you are now using either of the following medicines or types of medicine:

    Diarrhea medicine   Erythromycin
                          (topical)

Proper Use of This Medicine

It is important that you do not use this medicine more often than your doctor ordered.

Before applying this medicine, wash the area to be treated with soap and water, and dry thoroughly. After washing, it is best to wait 15 to 20 minutes before applying this medicine since it has an alcohol base.

How to apply this medicine:

• This medicine comes in a bottle with an applicator tip which may be used to apply the medicine directly to the skin.

• *Do not get this medicine in the eyes or on the mouth or lips*. This medicine contains alcohol and will sting or burn. In addition, it has an unpleasant taste. If this medicine does get in the eyes, wash them out carefully with large amounts of cool tap water.

• Apply a thin film of medicine to the affected area. Avoid using too much. Use the applicator with a dabbing motion instead of a rolling motion (like a roll-on deodorant, for example). If

the applicator tip becomes dry, turn the bottle upside down and press the tip several times to moisten it.

To help clear up your acne completely, *keep using this medicine for the full time of treatment,* even though your symptoms may have disappeared; *do not miss any doses.*

If you do miss a dose of this medicine, apply it as soon as possible. However, if it is almost time for your next application, skip the missed dose and go back to your regular dosing schedule.

Precautions While Using This Medicine

After application of this medicine to the skin, mild stinging or burning may be expected.

This medicine may cause the skin to become unusually dry. If this occurs, check with your doctor.

If your skin problem has not improved within 3 to 4 weeks, check with your doctor. However, it may take up to 8 to 12 weeks before full improvement is seen.

You may continue your normal use of cosmetics while you are using this medicine. However, it may be best not to use cosmetics too heavily or too often. If you have any questions about this, check with your doctor.

Side Effects of This Medicine

Along with its needed effects, a medicine may cause some unwanted effects. Although not all of these side effects appear very often, when they do occur they may require medical attention. Stop using this medicine and check with your doctor if any of the following side effects occur:

Less common

    Chapped skin
    Itching, rash, redness, swelling or other sign of irritation not present before you started using this medicine
    Mild diarrhea

Very rare

    Severe stomach cramps, pain, and bloating
    Severe, watery diarrhea, which may be accompanied by blood, mucus, pus, or pieces of intestinal lining in the stool
    Unexplained fever

Other side effects not listed above may also occur in some patients. If you notice any other effects, check with your doctor.

CLOFIBRATE (Systemic)
A commonly used brand name is Atromid-S.

Clofibrate (kloe-FYE-brate) is used to lower cholesterol and triglyceride (fat-like substances) levels in the blood. This may help prevent medical problems caused by such substances clogging the blood vessels. Clofibrate is available only with your doctor's prescription.

Before Using This Medicine

In addition to its helpful effects in treating your medical problem, this medicine may have some harmful effects.

You may have read or heard about a study called the WHO Study. This study compared the effects in patients who used clofibrate with effects in those who used a placebo (sugar pill). The results of this study suggested that clofibrate might increase the patient's risk of cancer, liver disease, and pancreatitis (inflammation of the pancreas), although it might also decrease the risk of heart attack. It may also increase the risk of gallstones and problems from gallbladder surgery.

Other studies have not found all of these effects.

Be sure you have discussed this with your doctor before taking this medicine.

Importance of Diet—Before prescribing medicine for your condition, your doctor will probably try to control your condition by prescribing a personal diet for you. Such a diet may be low in fats, sugars, and/or cholesterol. Many people are able to control their condition by carefully following their doctor's orders for proper diet and exercise. *Medicine is prescribed only when additional help is needed* and is effective only when a schedule of diet and exercise is properly followed.

Also, this medicine is less effective if you are greatly overweight. It may be very important for you to go on a reducing diet. However, check with your doctor before going on any diet.

In order to decide on the best treatment for your medical problem, your doctor should be told:

—if you have ever had any unusual reaction to clofibrate in the past. This medicine should not be taken if you are allergic to it.

—if you are pregnant or if you intend to become pregnant while using this medicine. Clofibrate may be harmful to your baby if you take it while you are pregnant or for up to several months before you become pregnant. Be sure that you have discussed this with your doctor before taking this medicine.

—if you are breast-feeding an infant. Although clofibrate has not been shown to cause problems, the chance always exists.

—if you have any of the following medical problems:

Gallstones	Liver disease
Heart disease	Stomach ulcer
Kidney disease	

—if you are now taking or have recently taken either of the following medicines or types of medicine:

Anticoagulants (blood thinners)	Furosemide (water pill)

Proper Use of This Medicine

Use this medicine only as directed by your doctor. Do not use more or less of it, and do not use it more often or for a longer period of time than your doctor ordered.

Follow carefully the special diet your doctor gave you. This is the most important part of controlling your condition, and is necessary if the medicine is to work properly.

Stomach upset may occur but usually lessens after a few doses. Take this medicine with food or immediately after meals to lessen possible stomach upset.

If you miss a dose of this medicine, take it as soon as possible. If it is almost time for your next dose, do not take the missed dose at all and do not double the next one. Instead, go back to your regular dosing schedule. If you have any questions about this, check with your doctor.

Precautions While Using This Medicine

It is very important that your doctor check your progress at regular visits. This will allow your doctor to see if the medicine is working properly to lower your cholesterol and triglyceride levels and if you should continue to take it.

Do not stop taking this medicine without first checking with your doctor. When you stop taking this medicine, your blood fat levels may increase again. Your doctor may want you to follow a special diet to help prevent this.

Side Effects of This Medicine

Along with its needed effects, a medicine may cause some unwanted effects. Although not all of these side effects appear very often, when

they do occur they may require medical attention. Check with your doctor *immediately* if any of the following side effects occur:

Rare

Chest pain	Severe stomach pain
Irregular heartbeat	with nausea and
	vomiting
	Shortness of
	breath

Check with your doctor also if any of the following side effects occur:

Rare

Blood in urine	Unusual decrease in
Swelling of feet	urination
or lower legs	Weight gain
Unexplained fever	
and chills or	
sore throat	

Other side effects may occur which usually do not require medical attention. These side effects may go away during treatment as your body adjusts to the medicine. However, check with your doctor if any of the following side effects continue or are bothersome:

More common

Nausea

Less common

Diarrhea	Vomiting
Stomach pain, gas,	
or heartburn	

Rare

Aching muscles	Increased appetite
Decreased sexual	Muscle cramping
ability	Sores in the mouth
Dizziness	and on the lips
Drowsiness	Swelling and pain
Dry, brittle hair or	where there are
loss of hair	sores on the skin
Dry skin, rash,	Tiredness or fatigue
or itching	Weakness
Headache	

Other side effects not listed above may also occur in some patients. If you notice any other effects, check with your doctor.

CLOMIPHENE (Systemic)

A commonly used brand name is Clomid.

Clomiphene (KLOE-mi-feen) is used as a fertility medicine in some women who are unable to become pregnant. It may also be used for other

conditions as determined by your doctor. Clomiphene is available only with your doctor's prescription.

Before Using This Medicine

If you become pregnant while using this medicine, there is a chance of a multiple birth (for example, twins, triplets) occurring. If you have any questions about this, check with your doctor.

In order to decide on the best treatment for your medical problem, your doctor should be told:

—if you have ever had any unusual reaction to clomiphene in the past. This medicine should not be taken if you are allergic to it.

—if you have any of the following medical problems:

Cyst on ovary	Mental depression
Fibroid tumors of	Unusual vaginal
the womb	bleeding
Liver disease	

Proper Use of This Medicine

Take this medicine only as directed by your doctor. If you are to begin on Day 5, count the first day of your menstrual period as Day 1. Beginning on Day 5, take one pill every day for as many days as your doctor ordered. To help you to remember to take your dose of medicine, take it at the same time every day.

If you miss a dose of this medicine, take it as soon as possible. If you do not remember until it is time for the next dose, take both doses together, then go back to your regular dosing schedule. If you miss more than one dose, check with your doctor.

Precautions While Using This Medicine

It is very important that your doctor check your progress at regular visits since you must stop taking this medicine if you become pregnant.

If your doctor has asked you to record your temperature daily, make sure that you do this every day so that you will know if you have begun to ovulate. It is important that intercourse take place at the correct time to give you the best chance of becoming pregnant. *Follow your doctor's instructions carefully.*

This medicine may cause vision problems, dizziness, or lightheadedness. *Make sure you know how you react to this medicine before you drive, use machines, or do other jobs that require you to be alert. This is especially important when the lighting is irregular.*

Side Effects of This Medicine

Along with its needed effects, a medicine may cause some unwanted effects. Although not all of these side effects appear very often, when they do occur they may require medical attention. When this medicine is used for short periods of time at low doses, side effects usually are rare. However, check with your doctor if any of the following side effects occur:

More common
Bloating
Stomach or pelvic
pain

Rare
Blurred vision
Decreased vision
Double vision
Seeing flashes
of light

Sensitivity of eyes
to light
Yellowing of eyes
and skin

Other side effects may occur which usually do not require medical attention. These side effects may go away during treatment as your body adjusts to the medicine. However, check with your doctor if any of the following side effects continue or are bothersome:

More common
Hot flashes

Less common
Breast discomfort
Headache

Nausea and
vomiting

Rare
Constipation or
diarrhea
Dizziness or
lightheadedness
Heavy menstrual
periods or
bleeding
between periods
Increased appetite
and weight gain

Loss of hair
Mental depression,
nervousness,
restlessness,
sleeplessness, or
tiredness
Skin rash and
itching
Unusually frequent
urination
Weight loss

Other side effects not listed above may also occur in some patients. If you notice any other effects, check with your doctor.

CLONIDINE (Systemic)
A commonly used brand name is Catapres.

Clonidine (KLOE-ni-deen) belongs to the general class of medicines called antihypertensives. It is used to treat high blood pressure. Clonidine may also be used for other conditions as deter-

mined by your doctor. Clonidine is available only with your doctor's prescription.

Before Using This Medicine

In order to decide on the best treatment for your medical problem, your doctor should be told:

—if you have ever had any unusual reaction to clonidine in the past. This medicine should not be taken if you are allergic to it.

—if you are pregnant, if you intend to become pregnant, or if you are breast-feeding an infant. Although clonidine has not been shown to cause problems in humans, the chance always exists.

—if you have any of the following medical problems:

Heart or blood
vessel disease
Kidney disease

Mental depression
(history of)
Raynaud's disease

—if you are now taking any of the following medicines or types of medicine:

Diuretics (water
pills)
Levodopa
Metoprolol
Nadolol
Other antihypertensives
(high blood
pressure
medicine)

Propranolol
Tricyclic antidepressants
(medicine for
depression)

—if you are now taking central nervous system (CNS) depressants such as:

Antihistamines or
medicine for hay
fever, other
allergies,
or colds
Barbiturates

Narcotics
Prescription pain
medicine
Sedatives, tranquilizers,
or sleeping
medicine
Seizure medicine

Proper Use of This Medicine

In order to help remember to take your medicine, try to get into the habit of taking it at the same time each day.

If you do miss a dose of this medicine, take it as soon as possible. Then go back to your regular dosing schedule. *If you miss more than one dose in a row check with your doctor right away.* If your body goes without this medicine for too long, your blood pressure may go up to a dangerously high level and some unpleasant effects may occur.

For patients taking this medicine for high blood pressure:

• Importance of Diet—In addition to prescribing medicine for your condition, your doctor will probably try to control your condition by prescribing a personal diet for you. Such a diet may be low in sodium (salt). Medicine is usually more effective when this diet is properly followed.

Also, it may be very important for you to go on a reducing diet. However, check with your doctor before going on any diet.

• Many patients who have high blood pressure will not notice any signs of the problem. In fact, many may feel normal. It is very important that you take your medicine exactly as directed and that you keep your doctor's appointments even if you feel well.

• Remember that this medicine will not cure your high blood pressure but it does control it. Therefore, you must continue to take it as directed if you expect to keep your blood pressure down. *You may have to take medicine for the rest of your life.* If high blood pressure is not treated, it can cause serious problems such as heart failure, blood vessel disease, stroke, or kidney disease.

Precautions While Using This Medicine

It is important that your doctor check your progress at regular visits.

Check with your doctor before you stop taking this medicine. Your doctor may want you to reduce gradually the amount you are taking before stopping completely.

Make sure that you have enough medicine on hand to last through weekends, holidays, or vacations. You should not miss taking any doses. You may want to ask your doctor for another prescription for clonidine to carry in your wallet or purse. You could then have it filled if you run out when you are away from home.

Clonidine will add to the effects of alcohol and other medicines (CNS depressants) that slow down the nervous system. Some examples of CNS depressants are antihistamines or medicine for hay fever, other allergies, or colds; sedatives, tranquilizers, or sleeping medicine; prescription pain medicine or narcotics; barbiturates; medicine for seizures; tricyclic antidepressants (medicine for depression); or anesthetics, including some dental anesthetics. *Check with your doctor before taking any of the above while you are using this medicine.*

Clonidine may cause some people to become drowsy or less alert than they are normally. This is more likely to happen when you begin to take it or when you increase the amount of medicine you are taking. *Make sure you know how you react to this medicine before you drive, use machines, or do other jobs that require you to be alert.*

Before having any kind of surgery (including dental surgery) or emergency treatment, *tell the doctor or dentist in charge that you are using this medicine.*

Dizziness, lightheadedness, or fainting may occur, especially when you get up from a lying or sitting position. Getting up slowly may help but if the problem continues or gets worse, check with your doctor.

The dizziness, lightheadedness, or fainting is also more likely to occur if you drink alcohol, stand for long periods of time, exercise, or if the weather is hot. *While you are taking this medicine, be careful in the amount of alcohol you drink. Also, use extra care during exercise or hot weather or if you must stand for long periods of time.* Check with your doctor if you have any questions about this.

Your mouth, nose, and throat may feel very dry while you are taking this medicine. To help relieve mouth dryness, chew sugarless gum or dissolve bits of ice in your mouth.

Do not take other medicines unless they have been discussed with your doctor. This especially includes over-the-counter (nonprescription) medicines for appetite control, asthma, colds, cough, hay fever, or sinus, since they may tend to increase your blood pressure.

Side Effects of This Medicine

Along with its needed effects, a medicine may cause some unwanted effects. Although not all of these side effects appear very often, when they do occur they may require medical attention. Check with your doctor if any of the following side effects occur:

Less common

Swelling of feet and
lower legs

Rare

Mental depression	Vivid dreams or
Paleness or cold	nightmares
feeling in finger-	
tips and toes	

Other side effects may occur which usually do not require medical attention. These side effects may go away during treatment as your body adjusts to the medicine. However, check with your doctor if any of the following side effects continue or are bothersome:

More common

Dizziness	Dry mouth
Drowsiness	

Less common

Constipation	Loss of appetite
Decreased sexual	Nausea or vomiting
ability	Painful salivary
Difficulty in sleep-	glands
ing	
Dizziness, light-	
headedness, or	
fainting, especial-	
ly when getting	
up from a lying	
or sitting position	

Rare

Headache	Swelling of the
Skin rash or hives	breasts

After you have been using this medicine for a while, it may cause unpleasant or even harmful effects if you stop taking it too suddenly. After you stop taking this medicine, check with your doctor if any of the following occur:

Anxiety	Rapid or irregular
Chest pain	heartbeat
Difficulty in sleep-	Restlessness
ing	Shaking or trembl-
Headache	ing of
Increased salivation	hands and fingers
Nausea	Stomach cramps
Nervousness	Sweating

Other side effects not listed above may also occur in some patients. If you notice any other effects, check with your doctor.

CLONIDINE AND CHLORTHALIDONE
(Systemic)
A commonly used brand name is Combipres.

Clonidine (KLOE-ni-deen) and chlorthalidone (klor-THAL-i-done) combinations are used in the treatment of high blood pressure. They are available only with your doctor's prescription.

Before Using This Medicine

In order to decide on the best treatment for your medical problem, your doctor should be told:

—if you are allergic to sulfonamides (sulfa drugs) or other thiazide diuretics (water pills). This medicine should not be taken if you are allergic to it.

—if you are pregnant or if you intend to become pregnant while using this medicine. When this medicine is used during pregnancy, it may cause side effects in the newborn infant. In addition, although this medicine has not been shown to cause birth defects, the chance always exists.

—if you are breast-feeding an infant. Although this medicine has not been shown to cause problems, the chance always exists.

—if you have any of the following medical problems:

Diabetes	Kidney disease
Gout	Liver disease
Heart or blood	Mental depression
vessel disease	(history of)
History of lupus	Pancreas disease
erythematosus	Problems with veins
	Raynaud's
	phenomenon

—if you are now taking any of the following medicines or types of medicine:

Colestipol	Nadolol
Corticosteroids	Oral anticoagulants
(cortisone-	(blood thinners
like medicines)	you take by
Corticotropin	mouth)
(ACTH)	Other diuretics
Diabetes medicine	(water pills)
Digitalis glycosides	or antihyper-
(heart medicine)	tensives (high
Gout medicine	blood pressure
Lithium	medicine)
Methenamine	Propranolol
Metoprolol	Tricyclic an-
	tidepressants
	(medicine for
	depression)

—if you are now taking central nervous system (CNS) depressants such as:

Antihistamines or	Prescription pain
medicine for hay	medicine
fever, other	Sedatives, tran-
allergies, or	quilizers,
colds	or sleeping
Barbiturates	medicine
Narcotics	Seizure medicine

Proper Use of This Medicine

This medicine may cause you to have an unusual feeling of tiredness when you begin to take it. You may also notice an increase in the amount of urine or in your frequency of urination.

After taking the medicine for a while, these effects should lessen. In general, in order to keep the increase in urine from affecting your sleep:

• If you are to take a single dose a day, take it in the morning after breakfast.

• If you are to take more than one dose a day, take the last dose no later than 6 p.m., unless otherwise directed by your doctor.

• However, it is best to plan your dose or doses according to a schedule that will least affect your personal activities and sleep. Ask your doctor, nurse, or pharmacist to help you plan the best time to take this medicine.

Importance of Diet—When prescribing medicine for your condition, your doctor may also prescribe a personal diet for you. Such a diet may be low in sodium (salt). Medicine is usually more effective when this diet is properly followed.

Also, it may be very important for you to go on a reducing diet. However, check with your doctor before going on any diet.

Many patients who have high blood pressure will not notice any signs of the problem. In fact, many may feel normal. It is very important that you take your medicine exactly as directed and that you keep your doctor's appointments even if you feel well.

Remember that this medicine will not cure your high blood pressure but it does control it. Therefore, you must continue to take it as directed if you expect to keep your blood pressure down. *You may have to take medicine for the rest of your life.* If high blood pressure is not treated, it can cause serious problems such as heart failure, blood vessel disease, stroke, or kidney disease.

In order to help remember to take your medicine, try to get into the habit of taking it at the same time each day.

If you do miss a dose of this medicine, take it as soon as possible. Then go back to your regular dosing schedule. *If you miss more than one dose in a row check with your doctor right away.* If your body goes without this medicine for too long, your blood pressure may go up to a dangerously high level.

Precautions While Using This Medicine

It is important that your doctor check your progress at regular visits.

This medicine may cause a loss of potassium from your body. To help prevent this, your doctor may want you to:

—eat or drink foods that have a high potassium content (for example, orange or other citrus fruit juices), or
—take a potassium supplement, or
—take another medicine to help prevent the loss of the potassium in the first place.

It is very important to follow these directions. Also, it is important not to change your diet on your own. This is more important if you are already on a special diet (as for diabetes), or if you are taking a potassium supplement or a medicine to reduce potassium loss. Extra potassium may not be necessary and, in some cases, too much potassium could be harmful.

Check with your doctor if you become sick and have severe or continuing vomiting or diarrhea. These problems may cause you to lose additional water and potassium.

Check with your doctor before you stop taking this medicine. Your doctor may want you to reduce gradually the amount you are taking before stopping completely.

Make sure that you have enough medicine on hand to last through weekends, holidays, or vacations. You should not miss taking any doses. You may want to ask your doctor for another prescription to carry in your wallet or purse. You could then have it filled if you run out when you are away from home.

Caution: Diabetics—Thiazide diuretics may raise blood sugar levels. While you are using this medicine, be especially careful in testing for sugar in your urine. If you have any questions about this, check with your doctor.

A few people who take this medicine may become more sensitive to sunlight than they are normally. When you begin to take this medicine, avoid too much sun or use of a sunlamp until you see how you react, especially if you tend to burn easily. If you have a severe reaction, check with your doctor.

This medicine will add to the effects of alcohol and other medicines (CNS depressants) that slow down the nervous system. Some examples of CNS depressants are antihistamines or medicine for hay fever, other allergies, or colds; sedatives, tranquilizers, or sleeping medicine; prescription pain medicine or narcotics; barbiturates; medicine for seizures; tricyclic antidepressants (medicine for depression); or anesthetics, including some dental anesthetics. *Check with your doctor before taking any of the above while you are using this medicine.*

This medicine may cause some people to become drowsy or less alert than they are normally. This is more likely to happen when you begin to take it or when you increase the amount of medicine you are taking. *Make sure you know how you react to this medicine before you drive, use machines, or do other jobs that require you to be alert.*

Before having any kind of surgery (including dental surgery) or emergency treatment, *make sure the doctor or dentist in charge knows that you are taking this medicine.*

Dizziness, lightheadedness, or fainting may occur, especially when you get up from a lying or sitting position. *Getting up slowly may help but if the problem continues or gets worse, check with your doctor.*

The dizziness, lightheadedness, or fainting is also more likely to occur if you drink alcohol, stand for long periods of time, exercise, or if the weather is hot. Drinking alcoholic beverages may also make the drowsiness worse. *While you are taking this medicine, be careful in the amount of alcohol you drink.* Also, use extra care during exercise or hot weather or if you must stand for long periods of time. Check with your doctor if you have any questions about this.

Your mouth, nose, and throat may feel very dry while you are taking this medicine. To help relieve mouth dryness, chew sugarless gum or dissolve bits of ice in your mouth.

Do not take other medicines unless they have been discussed with your doctor. This especially includes over-the-counter (nonprescription) medicines for appetite control, asthma, colds, cough, hay fever, or sinus, since they may tend to increase your blood pressure.

Side Effects of This Medicine

Along with its needed effects, a medicine may cause some unwanted effects. Although not all of these side effects appear very often, when they do occur they may require medical attention. *Check with your doctor if any of the following side effects occur, especially since some of them may mean that your body is losing too much potassium:*

Signs of too much potassium loss

Dryness of mouth	Muscle cramps or
Increased thirst	pain
Irregular heartbeats	Nausea or vomiting
Mood or mental	Unusual tiredness or
changes	weakness
	Weak pulse

Rare

Paleness or cold	Unusual bleeding or
feeling in finger-	bruising
tips and toes	Vivid dreams or
Severe stomach pain	nightmares
with nausea and	Yellowing of eyes or
vomiting	skin
Skin rash or hives	
Unexplained sore	
throat and fever	

Other side effects may occur which usually do not require medical attention. These side effects may go away during treatment as your body adjusts to the medicine. However, check with your doctor if any of the following side effects continue or are bothersome:

More common
    Constipation
    Drowsiness

Less common

Decreased sexual	Ear pain
ability	Headache
Diarrhea	Increased sensitivity
Difficulty in sleep-	to sunlight
ing	Loss of appetite
Dizziness or light-	
headedness when	
getting up	
from a lying	
or sitting position	

Other side effects not listed above may also occur in some patients. If you notice any other effects, check with your doctor.

CLOTRIMAZOLE (Topical)

Some commonly used brand names are Lotrimin and Mycelex.

Clotrimazole (kloe-TRIM-a-zole) belongs to the group of medicines called antifungals. It is applied to the skin to treat some types of fungal infections. This medicine is available only with your doctor's prescription.

Before Using This Medicine

In order to decide on the best treatment for your medical problem, your doctor should be told:

—if you have ever had any unusual reaction to clotrimazole in the past. This medicine should not be used if you are allergic to it.

—if you are pregnant, if you intend to become pregnant, or if you are breast-feeding an infant. Although only a very small amount of clotrimazole is absorbed into the body and has not been shown to cause problems, the chance always exists.

Proper Use of This Medicine

To help clear up your infection completely, *keep using this medicine for the full time of treatment* even though your condition may have improved.

Apply enough clotrimazole to cover the affected and surrounding skin areas, and rub in gently.

Keep this medicine away from the eyes.

When clotrimazole is used to treat certain types of fungal infections of the skin, an occlusive dressing or airtight covering (for example, kitchen plastic wrap) should *not* be applied over the medicine. To do so may cause irritation of the skin. *Do not apply an occlusive dressing over this medicine unless you have been directed to do so by your doctor.*

If you miss a dose of this medicine, apply it as soon as possible. Then go back to your regular dosing schedule. But if it is almost time for your next dose, do not apply the missed dose at all. Instead, go back to your regular dosing schedule. If you have any questions about this, check with your doctor.

Precautions While Using This Medicine

If your skin problem has not improved after you have used clotrimazole for 4 weeks, check with your doctor.

To help cure the infection and to help prevent reinfection, good health habits are required. These include the following:

• Wash all towels and bedding after each use.

• Use only freshly laundered clothes each time clothing is changed.

If you have any questions about this, check with your doctor, nurse, or pharmacist.

Side Effects of This Medicine

Along with its needed effects, a medicine may cause some unwanted effects. Although not all of these side effects appear very often, when they do occur they may require medical attention. Check with your doctor if any of the following side effects occur:

Skin rash or hives, blistering, burning, itching, peeling, stinging, or other sign of skin irritation not present before using this medicine

Other side effects not listed above may also occur in some patients. If you notice any other effects, check with your doctor.

CLOTRIMAZOLE (Vaginal)
A commonly used brand name is Gyne-Lotrimin.

Clotrimazole (kloe-TRIM-a-zole) belongs to the group of medicines called antifungals. It is used to treat fungal infections of the vagina. This medicine is available only with your doctor's prescription.

Before Using This Medicine

In order to decide on the best treatment for your medical problem, your doctor should be told:

—if you have ever had any unusual reaction to clotrimazole in the past. This medicine should not be used if you are allergic to it.

—if you are pregnant, if you intend to become pregnant, or if you are breast-feeding an infant. Although only a very small amount of clotrimazole is absorbed into the body and has not been shown to cause problems, the chance always exists.

Proper Use of This Medicine

Clotrimazole usually comes with patient directions. Read them carefully before using this medicine.

Use this medicine at bedtime, unless otherwise directed by your doctor.

Clotrimazole is usually inserted into the vagina with an applicator. However, if you are pregnant, check with your doctor before using the applicator to insert the vaginal cream or tablet.

To help clear up your infection completely, *keep using this medicine for the full time of treatment* even though your condition may have improved. Also, keep using this medicine even if you begin to menstruate during the time of treatment.

If you miss a dose of this medicine, insert it as soon as possible. Then go back to your regular dosing schedule. But if you do not remember the missed dose until the next day, do not insert the missed dose at all. Instead, go back to your regular dosing schedule. If you have any questions about this, check with your doctor.

Precautions While Using This Medicine

To help cure the infection and to help prevent reinfection, good health habits are required. These include the following:

- Wear cotton panties (or panties or pantyhose with cotton crotches) instead of synthetic (for example, nylon, rayon) underclothes.

- Wear freshly laundered underclothes.

If you have any questions about this, check with your doctor, nurse, or pharmacist.

If you have any questions about douching and intercourse during the time of treatment with clotrimazole, check with your doctor.

Since there may be some vaginal drainage while you are using this medicine, a sanitary napkin may be worn to protect your clothing.

Side Effects of This Medicine

Along with its needed effects, a medicine may cause some unwanted effects. Although not all of these side effects appear very often, when they do occur they may require medical attention. Check with your doctor if any of the following side effects occur:

Less common
 Vaginal burning or
 other irritation
 not present
 before using
 this medicine

Rare
 Skin rash

Other side effects may occur which usually do not require medical attention. These side effects may go away during treatment as your body adjusts to the medicine. However, check with your doctor if any of the following side effects continue or are bothersome:

Less common or rare
 Burning or irritation   Lower stomach
 in sexual partner   cramps or pain
 Increased frequency
 of urination

Other side effects not listed above may also occur in some patients. If you notice any other effects, check with your doctor.

COAL TAR (Topical)
Some commonly used brand names are:

DHS Tar	Pso-Rite	Tarpaste
Estar	Supertah	Tersa-Tar
Medotar	Tar Doak	Ul-Tar
Pentrax Tar	Tarbonis	Zetar

Coal tar is applied to the skin to treat eczema, psoriasis, seborrhea, and other skin disorders. Some of these preparations are available only with your doctor's prescription. Others are available without a prescription; however, your doctor may have special instructions on the proper use of coal tar for your medical condition.

Before Using This Medicine

In order to decide on the best treatment for your medical problem, your doctor should be told:

—if you have ever had any unusual reaction to coal tar in the past. This medicine should not be used if you are allergic to it.

—if you are pregnant, if you intend to become pregnant, or if you are breast-feeding an infant, although coal tar has not been shown to cause problems.

Proper Use of This Medicine

Use this medicine only as directed. Do not use more of it and do not use it more often than recommended on the label, unless otherwise directed by your doctor. To do so may increase the chance of side effects.

After applying this medicine, *protect the treated area from direct sunlight for at least 24 hours* since it may cause a severe reaction.

Do not apply this medicine to infected, blistered, raw, or oozing areas of the skin.

Keep this medicine away from the eyes. If you should accidentally get some in your eyes, flush them thoroughly with water at once.

If you miss a dose of this medicine, apply it as soon as possible. Then go back to your regular dosing schedule. But if it is almost time for your next dose, do not apply the missed dose at all. Instead, go back to your regular dosing schedule. If you have any questions about this, check with your doctor or pharmacist.

If you are using the cream or ointment form of this medicine:

• Apply enough medicine to cover the affected area, and rub in gently.

If you are using the gel form of this medicine:
• Apply enough gel to cover the affected area, and rub in gently. Allow the gel to remain on the affected area for 5 minutes, then remove excess gel by patting with a clean tissue.

If you are using the shampoo form of this medicine:
• Wet the scalp and hair with lukewarm water. Apply a generous amount of shampoo and rub into the scalp, then rinse. Apply the shampoo again, working up a rich lather, and allow to remain on the scalp for 5 minutes. Then rinse thoroughly.

If you are using the nonshampoo liquid form of this medicine:

• Some of these preparations are to be applied directly to dry or wet skin, some are to be added to lukewarm bath water, and some may be applied directly to dry or wet skin or added to lukewarm bath water. Make sure you know exactly how you should use this medicine. If you have any questions about this, check with your doctor or pharmacist.

• If this medicine is to be applied directly to the skin, apply enough to cover the affected area, and rub in gently.

• Some of these preparations contain alcohol and are flammable. Do not use near heat, near open flame, or while smoking.

Precautions While Using This Medicine
If this medicine is used on the scalp, it may temporarily discolor blond, bleached, or tinted hair.

Coal tar may stain the skin or clothing. Avoid getting it on your clothing. The stain on the skin will wear off after you stop using the medicine.

Side Effects of This Medicine
Along with its needed effects, a medicine may cause some unwanted effects. Although not all of these side effects appear very often, when they do occur they may require medical attention. Check with your doctor or pharmacist if either of the following side effects occurs:

Irritation of skin   Skin rash
not present
before using
this medicine

When you apply the gel or solution form of this medicine, a mild temporary stinging may be expected.

Other side effects not listed above may also occur in some patients. If you notice any other effects, check with your doctor or pharmacist.

CODEINE (Systemic)

Codeine (KOE-deen) is a medicine used to relieve pain. It is also used in some cases to prevent coughing. It is given in the form of tablets or by injection. Codeine is available only with your doctor's prescription. Since prescriptions cannot be refilled, a new prescription must be obtained from your doctor each time you need this medicine.

Before Using This Medicine
In order to decide on the best treatment for your medical problem, your doctor should be told:

—if you have ever had any unusual reaction to codeine in the past. This medicine should not be taken if you are allergic to it.

—if you are pregnant, if you intend to become pregnant, or if you are breast-feeding an infant. Although codeine has not been shown to cause problems, the chance always exists.

—if you have any of the following medical problems:

Brain disease or   Kidney disease
injury   Liver disease
Colitis   Underactive adrenal
Emphysema,   gland (Addison's
asthma, or   disease)
chronic lung   Underactive thyroid
disease   Unusually slow or
Enlarged prostate or   irregular heart-
problems with   beat
urination
Gallbladder disease
or gallstones

—if you are now taking other central nervous system (CNS) depressants such as:

Antihistamines or   Other prescription
medicine for hay   pain medicine
fever, other   Sedatives, tran-
allergies,   quilizers,
or colds   or sleeping
Barbiturates   medicine
Other narcotics   Seizure medicine
Tricyclic an-
tidepressants
(medicine for
depression)

—if you are now taking prescription medicine for stomach cramps or spasms.

—if you are now taking or have taken within the past 2 weeks monoamine oxidase (MAO) inhibitors such as:

Isocarboxazid	Phenelzine
Pargyline	Tranylcypromine

Proper Use of This Medicine

Take this medicine only as directed by your doctor. Do not take more of it, do not take it more often, and do not take it for a longer period of time than your doctor ordered. If too much is taken, it may become habit-forming.

Precautions While Using This Medicine

If you will be taking this medicine for a long period of time (for example, for several months at a time), your doctor should check your progress at regular visits.

This medicine will add to the effects of alcohol and other medicines (CNS depressants) that slow down the nervous system. Some examples of CNS depressants are antihistamines or medicine for hay fever, other allergies, or colds; sedatives, tranquilizers, or sleeping medicine; prescription pain medicine or narcotics; barbiturates; medicine for seizures; tricyclic antidepressants (medicine for depression); or anesthetics, including some dental anesthetics. *Check with your doctor before taking any of the above while you are taking this medicine.*

This medicine may cause some people to become drowsy or less alert than they are normally. *Make sure you know how you react to this medicine before you drive, use machines, or do other jobs that require you to be alert.*

Dizziness, lightheadedness, or fainting may occur, especially when you get up from a lying or sitting position. Getting up slowly may help lessen this problem.

Nausea may occur, especially after the first couple of doses. This effect usually goes away if you lie down for awhile. However, if nausea or vomiting continues, check with your doctor.

Side Effects of This Medicine

Along with its needed effects, a medicine may cause some unwanted effects. Although not all of these side effects appear very often, when they do occur they may require medical attention. Check with your doctor if any of the following side effects occur:

Shortness of breath	Unusually slow
Troubled breathing	heartbeat
Unusual excitement (especially in children)	

Other side effects may occur which usually do not require medical attention. These side effects may go away during treatment as your body adjusts to the medicine. However, check with your doctor if any of the following side effects continue or are bothersome:

More common

Constipation
Drowsiness

Less common

Difficult urination	Nausea or vomiting
Dizziness	Redness or
Feeling faint	flushing of face
Frequent urge to urinate	Unusual increase in sweating
Lightheadedness	Unusual tiredness or
Loss of appetite	weakness

Other side effects not listed above may also occur in some patients. If you notice any other effects, check with your doctor.

COLCHICINE (Systemic)
A commonly used brand name is Colsalide Improved.

Colchicine (KOL-chi-seen) is taken by mouth or given by injection to prevent or treat attacks of gout or gouty arthritis. It relieves inflammation, pain, and swelling. This medicine is available only with your doctor's prescription.

Before Using This Medicine

In order to decide on the best treatment for your medical problem, your doctor should be told:

—if you have ever had any unusual reaction to colchicine in the past. This medicine should not be taken if you are allergic to it.

—if you are pregnant or if you intend to become pregnant while using this medicine. Use of colchicine during pregnancy can cause harm to the baby.

—if you are breast-feeding an infant. Although colchicine has not been shown to cause problems, the chance always exists.

—if you have any of the following medical problems:

Blood disease
Heart disease
Intestinal disease
Kidney disease

Liver disease
Stomach ulcer or
other stomach
problems

Proper Use of This Medicine

If your doctor has told you to take colchicine only when a gout attack occurs:

• Start taking it at the first sign of the attack for best results.

• *Stop taking this medicine as soon as the gout pain is relieved or at the first sign of nausea, vomiting, stomach pain, or diarrhea.*

• If nausea, vomiting, stomach pain, or diarrhea continues, check with your doctor.

If your doctor has told you to take colchicine regularly to help prevent gout attacks:

• You should increase the dose you normally take at the first sign of an attack as advised by your doctor.

• *Stop taking the larger dose of medicine as soon as the gout pain is relieved or at the first sign of nausea, vomiting, stomach pain, or diarrhea.* If nausea, vomiting, stomach pain, or diarrhea continues, check with your doctor.

• After the gout attack is over, start taking colchicine again as ordered by your doctor.

If you are taking this medicine regularly and you miss a dose, take it as soon as possible. Then go back to your regular dosing schedule. If you do not remember the missed dose until it is almost time for your next dose, do not take the missed dose at all and do not double the next one. Instead, go back to your regular dosing schedule. If you have any questions about this, check with your doctor.

Precautions While Using This Medicine

If you will be taking colchicine for more than a few days at a time, your doctor should check your progress at regular visits.

Drinking too much alcohol may lessen the effects of colchicine. Therefore, *do not drink alcoholic beverages while you are taking this medicine,* unless you have first checked with your doctor.

Side Effects of This Medicine

Along with its needed effects, a medicine may cause some unwanted effects. Stop taking this medicine if any of the following side effects occur:

More common

Diarrhea
Nausea

Stomach pain
Vomiting

If any of these continue after you have stopped taking this medicine, check with your doctor.

Also, check with your doctor if any of the following side effects occur:

Rare

Redness, swelling,
or pain at place
of injection (for
the injection only)

With long-term use

Numbness, tingling,
pain, or weakness
in hands or feet
Skin rash

Unexplained sore
throat and fever
Unusual bleeding or
bruising
Unusual tiredness
or weakness

Other side effects may occur which usually do not require medical attention. However, check with your doctor if any of the following side effects continue or are bothersome:

Less common

Loss of appetite

With long-term use

Unusual loss of hair

Other side effects not listed above may also occur in some patients. If you notice any other effects, check with your doctor.

COLESTIPOL (Systemic)
A commonly used brand name is Colestid.

Colestipol (koe-LES-ti-pole) is used to lower high cholesterol levels in the blood. This may help prevent medical problems caused by cholesterol clogging the blood vessels. It may also be used for other conditions as determined by your doctor. Colestipol is available only with your doctor's prescription.

Before Using This Medicine

In order to decide on the best treatment for your medical problem, your doctor should be told:

—if you have ever had any unusual reaction to colestipol in the past. This medicine should not be taken if you are allergic to it.

—if you are pregnant, if you intend to become pregnant, or if you are breast-feeding an infant, although colestipol is not absorbed into the body and is not likely to cause problems.

—if you have any of the following medical problems:

Angina	Heart or blood
Bleeding problems	vessel disease
Constipation	Hemorrhoids
Gallstones	Stomach ulcer or
	other stomach
	problems

—if you are now taking any of the following medicines or types of medicine:

Anticoagulants	Tetracycline
(blood thinners)	Thiazide diuretics
Heart medicine	(water pills)
Penicillin	Any other medicine

Proper Use of This Medicine

Take this medicine exactly as directed by your doctor. Try not to miss any doses and do not take more medicine than your doctor ordered.

This medicine should never be taken in its dry form, since it could cause you to choke. Instead, always mix as follows:

• Add this medicine to a glassful (3 ounces or more) of water, milk, flavored drink, or your favorite juice or carbonated drink. If you use a carbonated drink, slowly mix in the powder in a large glass to prevent too much foaming. Stir until it is completely mixed (it will *not* dissolve) before drinking. After drinking all the liquid containing the medicine, rinse the glass with a little more liquid and drink that also, to make sure you get all the medicine.

• You may also mix this medicine with milk in hot or regular breakfast cereals, or in thin soups such as tomato or chicken noodle soup. Or you may add it to some pulpy fruits such as crushed pineapple, pears, peaches, or fruit cocktail.

If you miss a dose of this medicine, take it as soon as possible. If it is almost time for your next dose, do not take the missed dose at all and do not double the next one. Instead, go back to your regular dosing schedule. If you have any questions about this, check with your doctor.

For patients taking this medicine for high cholesterol:

• Importance of Diet—Before prescribing medicine for your condition, your doctor will probably try to control your condition by prescribing a personal diet for you. Such a diet may be low in fats, sugars, and/or cholesterol.

Many people are able to control their condition by carefully following their doctor's orders for proper diet and exercise. Medicine is prescribed only when additional help is needed and is effective only when a schedule of diet and exercise is properly followed.

Also, this medicine is less effective if you are greatly overweight. It may be very important for you to go on a reducing diet. However, check with your doctor before going on any diet.

• Remember that this medicine will not cure your cholesterol problem but it does help control it. Therefore, you must continue to take it as directed if you expect to lower your cholesterol level.

Precautions While Using This Medicine

It is very important that your doctor check your progress at regular visits. This will allow your doctor to see if the medicine is working properly to lower your cholesterol levels and if you should continue to take it.

Do not take any other medicine unless prescribed by your doctor since colestipol may interfere with other medicines.

Side Effects of This Medicine

Along with its needed effects, a medicine may cause some unwanted effects. Although not all of these side effects appear very often, when they do occur they may require medical attention. Check with your doctor if any of the following side effects occur:

More common

Constipation

Rare

Black tarry stools	Unusual loss of
Severe stomach pain	weight
with nausea and	
vomiting	

Other side effects may occur which usually do not require medical attention. These side effects may go away during treatment as your body adjusts to the medicine. However, check with your doctor if any of the following side effects continue or are bothersome:

Less common

Belching	Nausea or vomiting
Bloating	Stomach pain
Diarrhea	

Other side effects not listed above may also occur in some patients. if you notice any other effects, check with your doctor.

COLISTIN, NEOMYCIN, AND HYDROCORTISONE (Otic)
A commonly used brand name is Coly-Mycin S.

Colistin (koe-LIS-tin), neomycin (nee-oh-MYE-sin), and hydrocortisone (hye-droe-KOR-ti-sone) is a combination antibiotic and cortisone-like medicine. It is used to help the body overcome infections of the ear and to help provide relief from redness, irritation, and discomfort of certain ear problems. This medicine is available only with your doctor's prescription.

Before Using This Medicine
In order to decide on the best treatment for your medical problem, your doctor should be told:

—if you have had allergic reactions to any related antibiotics such as amikacin, colistin (by mouth or by injection), gentamicin, kanamycin, neomycin (by mouth or by injection), paromomycin, polymyxin B, streptomycin, or tobramycin.

—if you are pregnant, if you intend to become pregnant, or if you are breast-feeding an infant, although colistin, neomycin, and hydrocortisone otic preparations have not been shown to cause problems.

—if you have any other ear infection or problem (including punctured eardrum).

Proper Use of This Medicine
Before applying this medicine, wash the area to be treated (including the ear canal) with soap and water, and dry thoroughly. The ear canal should be dried with a sterile cotton applicator.

You may warm the ear drops to body temperature (37 °C or 98.6 °F), but no higher, by holding the bottle in your hand for a few minutes before applying. If this medicine gets too warm, it may break down and not work at all.

To prevent contamination of the ear drops, do not touch the dropper to any surface (including the ear), and keep the container tightly closed.

How to apply this medicine: Lie down or tilt the head so that the infected ear faces up. Gently pull the earlobe up and back for adults (down and back for children) to straighten the ear canal. Drop medicine into the ear canal. Keep ear facing up for about 5 minutes to allow medicine to come into contact with the infection. A clean, soft cotton plug may be gently inserted into the ear opening to prevent the medicine from leaking out. However, your doctor may want you to keep a cotton plug moistened with this medicine in your ear for the full time of treatment. If you have any questions about this, check with your doctor.

To help clear up your infection completely, *keep using this medicine for the full time of treatment,* even though your symptoms may have disappeared; *do not miss any doses.*

If you do miss a dose of this medicine, apply it as soon as possible. However, if it is almost time for your next application, skip the missed dose and go back to your regular dosing schedule.

Do not use this medicine for more than 10 days unless otherwise directed by your doctor.

Precautions While Using This Medicine
If your symptoms do not improve within 1 week or if they become worse, check with your doctor.

Side Effects of This Medicine
Along with its needed effects, a medicine may cause some unwanted effects. Although not all of these side effects appear very often, when they do occur they may require medical attention. Stop using this medicine and check with your doctor if any of the following side effects occur:

Itching, rash, redness, swelling, or other sign of irritation not present before you started using this medicine

Other side effects not listed above may also occur in some patients. If you notice any other effects, check with your doctor.

CROMOLYN (Inhalation)
A commonly used brand name is Intal.

Cromolyn (KROE-moe-lin) is a medicine used to prevent asthma attacks. It will not help an asthma attack that has already started. Cromolyn is available only with your doctor's prescription.

Before Using This Medicine
In order to decide on the best treatment for your medical problem, your doctor should be told:

—if you have had any unusual reactions to cromolyn, lactose, milk, or milk products in the past. This medicine should not be taken if you are allergic to it.

—if you are pregnant, if you intend to become pregnant, or if you are breast-feeding an infant. Although cromolyn has not been shown to cause problems, the chance always exists.

—if you have either of the following medical problems:

Kidney disease
Liver disease

Proper Use of This Medicine

This medicine is used with a special inhaler and usually comes with patient directions. Read the directions carefully before using.

Cromolyn must be inhaled every day in regularly spaced doses as ordered by your doctor. The medicine will not work if you swallow the capsules.

Up to 4 weeks may pass before you feel the full effects of the medicine.

If you are also using a bronchodilator inhaler to help you breathe better, use it first, then wait several minutes before using this medicine.

Gargling and rinsing your mouth after each dose may help prevent throat irritation, dryness of the mouth, and hoarseness.

If you miss a dose of this medicine and remember within an hour or so of the missed dose, take it right away. Then go back to your regular dosing schedule. But if you do not remember until later, do not take the missed dose at all and do not double the next one. Instead, go back to your regular dosing schedule. If you have any questions about this, check with your doctor.

Precautions While Using This Medicine

If you are also taking an adrenocortical steroid (for example, cortisone, prednisone) for your asthma along with this medicine, do not stop taking the steroid even if your asthma seems better unless told to do so by your doctor.

Check with your doctor if your symptoms do not improve or if your condition gets worse.

If this medicine is taken during an asthma attack, it may cause irritation and make the attack worse. Check with your doctor about using this medicine during asthma attacks.

Side Effects of This Medicine

Along with its needed effects, a medicine may cause some unwanted effects. Although not all of these side effects appear very often, when they do occur they may require medical attention. Check with your doctor if any of the following side effects occur:

Less common

Chest tightness	Nausea or vomiting
Difficult or painful urination	Severe or continuing headache
Dizziness	Skin rash or itching
Frequent urge to urinate	Swelling of the lips and eyes
Increased wheezing	Trouble in swallowing
Joint pain or swelling	Troubled breathing
Muscle pain or weakness	

Other side effects may occur which usually do not require medical attention. These side effects may go away during treatment as your body adjusts to the medicine. However, check with your doctor if any of the following side effects continue or are bothersome:

More common
Cough
Hoarseness

Less common

Dryness of the mouth	Throat irritation
Stuffy nose	Watering of the eyes

Other side effects not listed above may also occur in some patients. If you notice any other effects, check with your doctor.

CYCLANDELATE (Systemic)
A commonly used brand name is Cyclospasmol.

Cyclandelate (sye-KLAN-de-late) belongs to the group of medicines called vasodilators. Vasodilators increase the size of blood vessels. Cyclandelate is used to treat problems resulting from poor blood circulation. It is available only with your doctor's prescription.

Before Using This Medicine

In order to decide on the best treatment for your medical problem, your doctor should be told:

—if you have ever had any unusual reaction to cyclandelate in the past. This medicine should not be taken if you are allergic to it.

—if you are pregnant, if you intend to become pregnant, or if you are breast-feeding an infant. Although cyclandelate has not been shown to cause problems, the chance always exists.

—if you have any of the following medical problems:

Angina (chest pain)	Hardening of the arteries
Bleeding problems	
Glaucoma	

—if you have recently had a heart attack or stroke.

—if you smoke.

Proper Use of This Medicine

If this medicine upsets your stomach, it may be taken with meals, milk, or antacids.

If you miss a dose of this medicine, take it as soon as you remember. If it is almost time for your next dose, do not take the missed dose at all and do not double the next one. Instead, go back to your regular dosing schedule. If you have any questions about this, check with your doctor.

Precautions While Using This Medicine

It may take some time for this medicine to work. If you feel that the medicine is not working, do not stop taking it on your own. Instead, check with your doctor.

The helpful effects of this medicine may be decreased if you smoke.

Dizziness may occur, especially when you get up from a lying or sitting position or climb stairs. Getting up slowly may help. If this problem continues or gets worse, check with your doctor.

Side Effects of This Medicine

Along with its needed effects, a medicine may cause some unwanted effects. No serious side effects have been reported for this medicine. However, the following side effects may occur in some patients. Check with your doctor if they continue or are bothersome:

Belching, heartburn, nausea, or stomach pain	Rapid heartbeat
	Tingling sensation in face, fingers, or toes
Dizziness	
Flushing of the face	Unusual sweating
Headache	Weakness

Other side effects not listed above may also occur in some patients. If you notice any other effects, check with your doctor.

CYCLOBENZAPRINE (Systemic)
A commonly used brand name is Flexeril.

Cyclobenzaprine (sye-kloe-BEN-za-preen) is a medicine that is used to help relax certain muscles in your body. It also relieves the pain and discomfort caused by strains, sprains, or other injury to your muscles. Cyclobenzaprine is taken by mouth and is available only with your doctor's prescription.

Before Using This Medicine

In order to decide on the best treatment for your medical problem, your doctor should be told:

—if you have ever had any unusual reaction to cyclobenzaprine in the past. This medicine should not be taken if you are allergic to it.

—if you are pregnant or if you intend to become pregnant while using this medicine. Although cyclobenzaprine has not been shown to cause birth defects or other problems in humans, the chance always exists.

—if you are breast-feeding an infant. Although cyclobenzaprine has not been shown to cause problems, the chance always exists.

—if you have any of the following medical problems:

Glaucoma	Overactive thyroid
Heart or blood vessel disease	Problems with urination

—if you are now taking other central nervous system (CNS) depressants such as:

Antihistamines or medicine for hay fever, other allergies, or colds	Prescription pain medicine
Barbiturates	Sedatives, tranquilizers, or sleeping medicine
Narcotics	Seizure medicine
	Tricyclic antidepressants (medicine for depression)

—if you are now taking any of the following medicines or types of medicine:

Clonidine	Prescription medicine for stomach cramps or spasms
Guanethidine	

—if you are now taking or have taken within the past 2 weeks monoamine oxidase (MAO) inhibitors such as:

Isocarboxazid	Phenelzine
Pargyline	Tranylcypromine

Proper Use of This Medicine

If you miss a dose of this medicine and remember within an hour or so of the missed dose, take it right away. Then go back to your regular dosing schedule. But if you do not remember until later, do not take the missed dose at all and do

not double the next one. Instead, go back to your regular dosing schedule. If you have any questions about this, check with your doctor.

Precautions While Using This Medicine

This medicine will add to the effects of alcohol and other medicines (CNS depressants) that slow down the nervous system. Some examples of CNS depressants are antihistamines or medicine for hay fever, other allergies, or colds; sedatives, tranquilizers, or sleeping medicine; prescription pain medicine or narcotics; barbiturates; medicine for seizures; tricyclic antidepressants (medicine for depression); or anesthetics, including some dental anesthetics. *Check with your doctor before taking any of the above while you are using this medicine.*

This medicine may cause some people to have blurred vision or to become drowsy, dizzy, or less alert than they are normally. *Make sure you know how you react to this medicine before you drive, use machines, or do other jobs that require you to be alert.*

Dryness of the mouth may occur while you are taking this medicine. Sucking on hard candy or ice chips or chewing gum may help relieve the dry mouth.

Side Effects of This Medicine

Along with its needed effects, a medicine may cause some unwanted effects. Although not all of these side effects appear very often, when they do occur they may require medical attention. Check with your doctor if any of the following side effects occur:

Rare

Clumsiness or unsteadiness	Itching or skin rash
Hallucinations (seeing, hearing, or feeling things that are not there)	Mental confusion or depression
	Problems in urinating
	Swelling of face, lips, or tongue
	Troubled breathing

Other side effects may occur which usually do not require medical attention. These side effects may go away during treatment as your body adjusts to the medicine. However, check with your doctor if any of the following side effects continue or are bothersome:

More common

Dizziness	Dry mouth
Drowsiness	

Less common

Bad taste in the mouth	Sleeplessness
Blurred vision	Unusual tiredness or weakness
Indigestion	Unusually fast heartbeat
Nausea	
Numbness, tingling, pain, or weakness in hands or feet	

Other side effects not listed above may also occur in some patients. If you notice any other effects, check with your doctor.

CYCLOPENTOLATE (Ophthalmic)

Some commonly used brand names are Cyclogyl and Mydplegic*.

---

*Not available in the United States.

Cyclopentolate (sye-kloe-PEN-toe-late) is used in the eye to dilate (enlarge) the pupil. It is used before eye examinations and to treat certain eye conditions. This medicine is available only with your doctor's prescription.

Before Using This Medicine

In order to decide on the best treatment for your medical problem, your doctor should be told:

—if you have ever had any unusual reaction to cyclopentolate in the past. This medicine should not be used if you are allergic to it.

—if you are pregnant, if you intend to become pregnant, or if you are breast-feeding an infant. Although cyclopentolate has not been shown to cause problems, the chance always exists.

—if you have any of the following medical problems:

Brain damage (in children)	Spastic paralysis (in children)
Down's syndrome (mongolism)	

Proper Use of This Medicine

Use this medicine only as directed. Do not use more of it and do not use it more often than your doctor ordered. To do so may increase the chance of too much medicine being absorbed into the body and the chance of side effects. *This is especially important when this medicine is used in children, since overdose is very dangerous in children.*

How to apply this medicine: First, wash hands. With middle finger, apply pressure to the inside corner of the eye (and continue to apply pressure for 1 or 2 minutes after the medicine has been placed in the eye). Tilt head back and with the index finger of the same hand, pull lower eyelid away from eye to form a pouch. Drop the medicine into the pouch and close eyes. Do not blink. Keep eyes closed for 1 or 2 minutes to allow the medicine to be absorbed.

To prevent contamination of the eye drops, do not touch the applicator tip to any surface (including the eye) and keep the container tightly closed.

If you miss a dose of this medicine, apply it as soon as possible. Then go back to your regular dosing schedule. But if it is almost time for your next dose, do not apply the missed dose at all. Instead, apply your next dose at the regularly scheduled time. Then continue with your regular dosing schedule. If you have any questions about this, check with your doctor.

Precautions While Using This Medicine

After you apply this medicine to your eyes, your pupils will become unusually large. This will cause blurring of vision. It will also cause your eyes to become more sensitive to light than they are normally. Wearing sunglasses may help relieve the discomfort from bright light. If these side effects continue for longer than 36 hours after you have stopped using this medicine, check with your doctor.

Side Effects of This Medicine

Along with its needed effects, a medicine may cause some unwanted effects. Although not all of these side effects appear very often, when they do occur they may require medical attention. Check with your doctor if any of the following side effects occur:

Possible signs of too much medicine being absorbed into the body

Clumsiness or unsteadiness	Mental confusion
Fever	Skin rash
Flushing or redness of face	Slurred speech
	Swollen stomach in infants
Hallucinations (seeing, hearing, or feeling things that are not there)	Unusual behavior, especially in children
Increased thirst or unusual dryness of mouth	Unusual drowsiness, tiredness, or weakness
	Unusually fast heartbeat

Other side effects may occur which usually do not require medical attention. These side effects may go away during treatment as your body adjusts to the medicine. However, check with your doctor if the following side effect continues or is bothersome:

Increased sensitivity of eyes to light

When you apply this medicine to the eye, some burning may be expected.

Other side effects not listed above may also occur in some patients. If you notice any other effects, check with your doctor.

CYCLOPHOSPHAMIDE (Systemic)

Some commonly used brand names are Cytoxan and Procytox*.

---

*Not available in the United States.

Cyclophosphamide (sye-kloe-FOSS-fa-mide) belongs to the group of medicines called alkylating agents. It is used to treat some kinds of cancer as well as some noncancerous conditions. It is used also in some situations to reduce the body's natural immunity. Cyclophosphamide is available only with your doctor's prescription.

Before Using This Medicine

Cyclophosphamide is a very strong medicine. In addition to its helpful effects in treating your medical problem, it has side effects that could be very serious. Before you take this medicine, be sure that you have discussed the use of it with your doctor.

In order to decide on the best treatment for your medical problem, your doctor should be told:

—if you have ever had any unusual reaction to cyclophosphamide in the past.

—if you are pregnant or if you intend to have children. This medicine may cause birth defects if either the male or female is taking it at the time of conception or if it is taken during pregnancy. It may also cause permanent sterility after it has been taken for a while. Be sure that you have discussed this with your doctor before taking this medicine.

—if you are breast-feeding an infant. Although cyclophosphamide has not been shown to cause problems, the chance always exists.

—if you have any of the following medical problems:

Blood disease	Kidney disease
Gout	Kidney stones
Infection	Liver disease

—if you are now taking or have recently taken any of the following medicines or types of medicines:

Allopurinol or other medicine for gout	Chloramphenicol
Barbiturates	Cortisone or cortisone-like medicines

—if you have been treated with x-rays or cancer drugs by another doctor.

Proper Use of This Medicine

Take this medicine only as directed by your doctor. Do not take more or less of it, and do not take it more often than your doctor ordered.

This medicine works best and is less likely to cause problems if taken first thing in the morning. However, your doctor may want you to take it with food in smaller doses over the day to lessen stomach upset. If you have any questions about this, check with your doctor.

This medicine is sometimes given together with certain other medicines. If you are using a combination of drugs, make sure that you take each medicine at the proper time and do not mix them. Ask your doctor, nurse, or pharmacist to help you plan a way to remember to take your medicines at the right time.

This medicine often causes nausea, vomiting, and loss of appetite. However, it is very important that you continue to use the medicine even if you begin to feel ill. If this medicine is being given to a child, tell your doctor if it causes nausea and vomiting. Your doctor may want to change the dose of the medicine. *Do not stop taking this medicine without first checking with your doctor.*

If you miss a dose of this medicine, do not take the missed dose at all and do not double the next one. Instead, go back to your regular dosing schedule and check with your doctor.

Precautions While Using This Medicine

It is very important that your doctor check your progress at regular visits.

While you are using this medicine, it is important that you drink plenty of fluids and urinate

often. This will help prevent kidney problems and keep your kidneys working well. Adults or children over 100 pounds (45 kg) in weight should drink 7 to 12 cups (up to 3 quarts) of fluids a day. Smaller children should drink 1 to 2 quarts of fluids a day, depending on weight. If you have any questions about this, check with your doctor.

Before having any kind of surgery, including dental surgery, or emergency treatment, make sure the doctor or dentist in charge knows that you are taking this medicine.

Side Effects of This Medicine

Along with its needed effects, a medicine may cause some unwanted effects. Although not all of these side effects appear very often, when they do occur they may require medical attention. *Stop taking this medicine and check with your doctor* if the following side effects occur:

Blood in urine
Painful urination

Check with your doctor also if any of the following side effects occur:

More common

Missing menstrual periods	Unexplained fever, chills, or sore throat

Less common

Cough	Swelling of feet or lower legs
Dizziness, mental confusion, or agitation	Tiredness or weakness
Flank or stomach pain	Unusual bleeding or bruising
Joint pain	Unusually rapid heartbeat
Shortness of breath	

Rare

Black tarry stools	
Redness, swelling, or pain at the place of injection	Unusual thirst Unusually frequent urination
Sores in the mouth and on the lips	Yellowing of eyes and skin

Other side effects may occur which usually do not require medical attention. These side effects may go away during treatment as your body adjusts to the medicine. However, check with your doctor if any of the following side effects continue or are bothersome:

More common

Darkening of skin and fingernails	Loss of appetite Loss of hair Nausea and vomiting

Less common

Flushing or redness of the face	Swollen lips
Headache	Unusual increase in sweating
Skin rash, hives, or itching	

This medicine may cause a temporary loss of hair in some people. After treatment with cyclophosphamide has ended, normal hair growth should return, although the new hair may be a slightly different color or texture.

After you stop using this medicine, it may still produce some side effects that need attention. During this period of time check with your doctor if you notice the following side effect:

Blood in urine

Other side effects not listed above may also occur in some patients. If you notice any other effects, check with your doctor.

CYCLOSERINE (Systemic)
A commonly used brand name is Seromycin.

Cycloserine (sye-kloe-SER-een) belongs to the general family of medicines called antibiotics. It is given by mouth to help the body overcome tuberculosis (TB) and infections of the urinary tract. When cycloserine is used for TB, it is given with one or more other medicines for TB. Cycloserine is available only with your doctor's prescription.

Before Using This Medicine

In order to decide on the best treatment for your medical problem, your doctor should be told:

—if you have ever had any unusual reaction to cycloserine. This medicine should not be taken if you are allergic to it.

—if you are pregnant, if you intend to become pregnant, or if you are breast-feeding an infant, although cycloserine has not been shown to cause problems.

—if you have any of the following medical problems:

Alcoholism	Mental disorders such as depression, psychosis, severe anxiety
Convulsive disorders such as seizures or epilepsy	
	Severe kidney disease

—if you are now taking either of the following medicines:

Ethionamide
Isoniazid

Proper Use of This Medicine

Cycloserine may be taken after meals if it upsets your stomach.

To help clear up your infection completely, *it is very important that you keep taking this medicine for the full time of treatment* even if you begin to feel better after a few weeks. If you are taking this medicine for TB, you may have to take it every day for as long as 1 to 2 years or more. *It is important that you do not miss any doses.*

If you do miss a dose of this medicine, take it as soon as possible. However, if it is almost time for your next dose, do not take the missed dose or double your next dose. Instead, go back to your regular dosing schedule.

Your doctor may also want you to take some other medicines (for example, seizure medicine, a sedative, or vitamin B_6) to help prevent or lessen some of the side effects of cycloserine. If so, *it is very important to take these medicines every day along with cycloserine.* If you have any questions about this, check with your doctor.

Precautions While Using This Medicine

If your symptoms do not improve within 2 to 3 weeks or if they become worse, check with your doctor.

It is very important that your doctor check your progress at regular visits.

If cycloserine causes you to feel very depressed or to have thoughts of suicide, check with your doctor immediately. Your doctor will probably want to change your medicine.

This medicine may cause some people to become dizzy or drowsy. *Make sure you know how you react to this medicine before you drive, use machines, or do other jobs that require you to be alert.* If these reactions are especially bothersome, check with your doctor.

Some of cycloserine's side effects (for example, seizures) may be more likely to occur if you drink alcoholic beverages regularly while you are taking this medicine. Therefore, *you should not drink alcoholic beverages while you are taking this medicine.*

Side Effects of This Medicine

Along with its needed effects, a medicine may cause some unwanted effects. Although not all of these side effects appear very often, when they do occur they may require medical attention. Stop taking this medicine and check with your doctor if any of the following side effects occur:

More common

Anxiety	Nightmares
Confusion	Other mood or
Depression	mental changes
Dizziness	Speech problems
Drowsiness	Thoughts of suicide
Muscle twitching or	Unusual irritable
trembling	feeling
Nervousness	Unusual restlessness

Less common

Blurred vision or	Numbness, tingling,
any loss of	burning pain, or
vision, with or	weakness in the
without eye pain	hands or feet
Increased sensitivity	Rash
to sunlight	Yellowing of eyes or
	skin

Rare

Seizures

Other side effects may occur which usually do not require medical attention. These side effects may go away during treatment as your body adjusts to the medicine. However, check with your doctor if any of the following side effects continue or are bothersome:

More common

Headache

Less common

Pale skin	Unusual tiredness
Unusual bleeding	or weakness
or bruising	

Other side effects not listed above may also occur in some patients. If you notice any other effects, check with your doctor.

CYTARABINE (Systemic)
A commonly used brand name is Cytosar-U

Cytarabine (sye-TARE-a-been) belongs to the group of medicines called antimetabolites. It is used by injection to treat some kinds of cancer as well as some noncancerous conditions. Cytarabine is available only on prescription and is to be administered only by or under the immediate supervision of your doctor.

Before Using This Medicine

Cytarabine is a very strong medicine. In addition to its helpful effects in treating your medical problems, it has side effects that could be very serious. Before you receive this medicine, be sure that you have discussed the use of it with your doctor.

In order to decide on the best treatment for your medical problem, your doctor should be told:

—if you have ever had any unusual reaction to cytarabine in the past.

—if you are pregnant or if you intend to have children. This medicine may cause birth defects if either the male or female is taking it at the time of conception or if it is taken during pregnancy. It may also cause permanent sterility after it has been taken for a while. Be sure that you have discussed this with your doctor before taking this medicine.

—if you are breast-feeding an infant. Although cytarabine has not been shown to cause problems, the chance always exists.

—if you have any of the following medical problems:

Blood disease	Kidney disease
Gout	Kidney stones
Infection	Liver disease

—if you are taking gout medicine.

—if you have been treated with x-rays or cancer drugs by another doctor.

Proper Use of This Medicine

This medicine is sometimes given together with certain other medicines. If you are using a combination of drugs, it is important that you receive each medicine at the proper time. If you are taking some of these medicines by mouth, ask your doctor, nurse, or pharmacist to help you plan a way to take them at the right time.

This medicine often causes nausea and vomiting. However, it is very important that you continue to receive the medicine even if you begin to feel ill. If you have any questions about this, check with your doctor.

Precautions While Using This Medicine

It is very important that your doctor check your progress at regular visits.

While you are using this medicine, your doctor may want you to drink plenty of fluids and urinate often. This will help prevent kidney problems and keep your kidneys working well. If you have any questions about this, check with your doctor.

Side Effects of This Medicine

Along with its needed effects, a medicine may cause some unwanted effects. Although not all of these side effects appear very often, when they do occur they may require medical attention. Check with your doctor if any of the following side effects occur:

More common

Unexplained fever and chills	Unusual bleeding or bruising
Unexplained sore throat	

Less common

Flank or stomach pain	Swelling of feet and lower legs
Joint pain	Yellowing of eyes and skin
Sores in the mouth and on the lips	

Rare

Black tarry stools	Pain at place of injection
Cough	
Difficulty in swallowing	Shortness of breath
Heartburn	Unusual decrease in urination

Other side effects may occur which usually do not require medical attention. These side effects may go away during treatment as your body adjusts to the medicine. However, check with your doctor if any of the following side effects continue or are bothersome:

More common

Fainting spells	Nausea and vomiting
Headache	
Irregular heartbeat	Tiredness
	Weakness

Less common

Diarrhea	Skin rash

Rare

Chest pain	Loss of hair
Dizziness	Skin freckling
Loss of appetite	Stomach pain

After you stop using this medicine, it may still produce some side effects that need attention. During this period of time check with your doctor if you notice any of the following:

Unexplained fever and chills	Unusual bleeding or bruising
Unexplained sore throat	

Other side effects not listed above may also occur in some patients. If you notice any other effects, check with your doctor.

DACARBAZINE (Systemic)
A commonly used brand name is DTIC-Dome.

Dacarbazine (da-KAR-ba-zeen) belongs to the group of medicines called alkylating agents. It is used by injection to treat some kinds of cancer. Dacarbazine is available only from your doctor.

Before Using This Medicine

Dacarbazine is a very strong medicine. In addition to its helpful effects in treating your medical problem, it has side effects that could be very serious. Before you receive this medicine, be sure that you have discussed the use of it with your doctor.

In order to decide on the best treatment for your medical problem, your doctor should be told:

—if you have ever had any unusual reaction to dacarbazine in the past.

—if you are pregnant or if you intend to have children. This medicine may cause birth defects if either the male or female is taking it at the time of conception or if it is taken during pregnancy. It may also cause permanent sterility after it has been taken for awhile. Be sure that you have discussed this with your doctor before taking this medicine.

—if you are breast-feeding an infant. Although dacarbazine has not been shown to cause problems, the chance always exists.

—if you have any of the following medical problems:

Blood disease	Kidney disease
Gout	Liver disease
Infection	

—if you are now taking allopurinol.

—if you have been treated with x-rays or cancer drugs by another doctor.

Proper Use of This Medicine

This medicine is sometimes given together with certain other medicines. If you are using a combination of drugs, it is important that you receive each medicine at the proper time. If you are taking some of these medicines by mouth, ask your doctor, nurse, or pharmacist to help you plan a way to remember to take them at the right time.

This medicine often causes nausea, vomiting, and loss of appetite. The injection may also cause a feeling of burning or pain. However, it is very important that you continue to receive the medicine, even if you begin to feel ill. After 1 or 2 days, your stomach upset should lessen. You may want to avoid eating heavy meals for 4 to 6 hours before receiving a dose to help lessen stomach upset. Also, your doctor may prescribe a medicine for relief. If you have any questions about this, check with your doctor.

Precautions While Using This Medicine

It is very important that your doctor check your progress at regular visits.

Side Effects of This Medicine

Along with its needed effects, a medicine may cause some unwanted effects. Although not all of these side effects appear very often, when they do occur they may require medical attention. Check with your doctor if any of the following side effects occur:

More common

Redness, swelling, or pain at the place of injection	Unexplained fever, chills, or sore throat
	Unusual bleeding or bruising

Rare

Sores in the mouth and on the lips

Other side effects may occur which usually do not require medical attention. These side effects may go away during treatment as your body adjusts to the medicine. However, check with your doctor if any of the following side effects continue or are bothersome:

More common

Loss of appetite
Nausea and vomiting

Less common

Blurred vision	Headache
Confusion	Joint or muscle pain
Feelings of uneasiness	Loss of hair
Flushing of the face	Numbness of the face

Rare

Diarrhea

This medicine may cause a temporary loss of hair in some people. After treatment with dacarbazine has ended, normal hair growth should return.

If dacarbazine accidentally seeps out of the vein into which it is injected, it may damage some tissues and cause scarring. Tell the doctor right away if you notice redness, pain, or swelling at the site of injection.

After you stop using this medicine, it may still produce some side effects that need attention. During this period of time check with your doctor if you notice unusual bleeding or bruising.

Other side effects not listed above may also occur in some patients. If you notice any other effects, check with your doctor.

DACTINOMYCIN (Systemic)
A commonly used brand name is Cosmegen.

Dactinomycin (dak-ti-noe-MYE-sin) belongs to the group of medicines known as antineoplastics. It is used by injection to treat some kinds of cancer as well as some noncancerous conditions. Dactinomycin is available only with a prescription and is to be administered only by or under the immediate supervision of your doctor.

Before Using This Medicine

Dactinomycin is a very strong medicine. In addition to its helpful effects in treating your medical problem, it has side effects that could be very serious. Before you receive this medicine, be sure that you have discussed the use of it with your doctor.

In order to decide on the best treatment for your medical problem, your doctor should be told:

—if you have ever had any unusual reaction to dactinomycin in the past.

—if you are pregnant or if you intend to have children. This medicine may cause birth defects if either the male or female is taking it at the time of conception or if it is taken during pregnancy. It may also cause permanent sterility after it has been taken for a while. Be sure that you have discussed this with your doctor before taking this medicine.

—if you are breast-feeding an infant. Although dactinomycin has not been shown to cause problems, the chance always exists.

—if you have any of the following medical problems:

Blood disease	Infection
Chicken pox	Kidney disease
Gout	Liver disease

—if you are taking gout medicine.

—if you have been treated with x-rays or cancer drugs by another doctor.

Proper Use of This Medicine

This medicine is sometimes given together with certain other medicines. If you are using a combination of drugs, it is important that you receive each medicine at the proper time. If you are taking some of these medicines by mouth, ask your doctor, nurse, or pharmacist to help you plan a way to remember to take them at the right time.

This medicine often causes nausea and vomiting. However, it is very important that you continue to receive the medicine, even if you begin to feel ill. Your doctor may prescribe a medicine to relieve stomach upset. If you have any questions about this, check with your doctor.

Precautions While Using This Medicine

It is very important that your doctor check your progress at regular visits.

Side Effects of This Medicine

Along with its needed effects, a medicine may cause some unwanted effects. Although not all of these side effects appear very often, when they do occur they may require medical attention. Check with your doctor *immediately* if any of the following side effects occur:

More common

Black tarry stools	Sores in the mouth
Continuing stomach	and on the lips
pain	Unexplained fever,
Diarrhea	chills, or sore
Difficulty in	throat
swallowing	Unusual bleeding or
Heartburn	bruising

Rare

Joint pain	Wheezing
Pain at place of	Yellowing of eyes
injection	and skin
Swelling of feet or	
lower legs	

Other side effects may occur which usually do not require medical attention. These side effects may go away during treatment as your body adjusts to the medicine. However, check with your doctor if any of the following side effects continue or are bothersome:

More common

Acne	Nausea and
Darkening of the	vomiting
skin	Skin problems
Loss of hair	Tiredness

This medicine often causes a temporary loss of hair. After treatment with dactinomycin has ended, normal hair growth should return.

If dactinomycin accidentally seeps out of the vein into which it is injected, it may damage some tissues and cause scarring. Tell the doctor right away if you notice redness, pain, or swelling at the site of injection.

After you stop using this medicine, it may still produce some side effects that need attention. During this period of time check with your doctor if you notice any of the following:

Black tarry stools	Unexplained fever,
Diarrhea	chills, or sore
Sores in the mouth	throat
and on the lips	Unusual bleeding or
Stomach pain	bruising
	Yellowing of eyes
	and skin

Other side effects not listed above may also occur in some patients. If you notice any other effects, check with your doctor.

DANAZOL (Systemic)

Some commonly used brand names are Cyclomen* and Danocrine.

*Not available in the United States.

Danazol (DA-na-zole) is used to treat endometriosis and a certain type of breast disease called fibrocystic breast disease. This medicine is available only with your doctor's prescription.

Before Using This Medicine

In order to decide on the best treatment for your medical problem, your doctor should be told:

—if you have ever had any unusual reaction to danazol in the past. This medicine should not be taken if you are allergic to it.

—if you are breast-feeding an infant. Although danazol has not been shown to cause problems in humans, the chance always exists.

—if you have any of the following medical problems:

Epilepsy	Liver disease
Heart disease	Migraine headaches
Kidney disease	

Proper Use of This Medicine

In order for this medicine to help you, *it must be taken regularly for the full time of treatment* as ordered by your doctor.

If you miss a dose of this medicine, take it as soon as possible. Then go back to your regular dosing schedule. However, if you do not remember the missed dose until it is almost time for your next dose, do not take the missed dose at all and do not double the next one. Instead, go back to your regular dosing schedule. If you have any questions about this, check with your doctor.

Precautions While Using This Medicine

Your doctor should check your progress at regular visits in order to make sure that this medicine does not cause unwanted effects.

During the time you are taking danazol, your menstrual period may not be regular or you may not have a menstrual period at all. This is to be expected when taking this medicine. If regular menstruation does not begin within 60 to 90 days after you stop taking this medicine, check with your doctor.

If you suspect that you may have become pregnant, stop taking this medicine and check with your doctor. Continued use of danazol during pregnancy may cause unwanted effects in the baby.

Side Effects of This Medicine

Along with its needed effects, a medicine may cause some unwanted effects. Although not all of these side effects appear very often, when they do occur they may require medical attention. Check with your doctor if any of the following side effects occur:

More common

Acne or increased oiliness of skin or hair	Swelling of feet or lower legs
Decrease in breast size	Unnatural hair growth
Hoarseness or deepening of voice	Unusual weight gain

Rare

Enlarged clitoris	Yellowing of eyes or skin

Other side effects may occur which usually do not require medical attention. These side effects may go away during treatment as your body adjusts to the medicine. However, check with your doctor if any of the following side effects continue or are bothersome:

Less common

Burning, dryness, or itching of vagina or vaginal bleeding	Mood or mental changes
Flushing or redness of skin	Nervousness
	Unusual sweating

Other side effects not listed above may also occur in some patients. If you notice any other effects, check with your doctor.

DANTROLENE (Systemic)
A commonly used brand name is Dantrium.

Dantrolene (DAN-troe-leen) is a medicine used to help relax certain muscles in your body. It relieves the spasms, cramping, and tightness of muscles caused by certain medical problems such as multiple sclerosis. This medicine is available only with your doctor's prescription.

Before Using This Medicine

In order to decide on the best treatment for your medical problem, your doctor should be told:

—if you have ever had any unusual reaction to dantrolene in the past. This medicine should not be taken if you are allergic to it.

—if you are pregnant, if you intend to become pregnant, or if you are breast-feeding an infant. Although dantrolene has not been shown to cause problems, the chance always exists.

—if you have any of the following medical problems:

Emphysema, asthma, bronchitis, or other chronic lung disease	Liver disease, such as hepatitis or cirrhosis, or history of liver disease
Heart disease	

—if you are a female over 35 years of age and are taking estrogens (for example, birth control pills).

—if you are now taking any other central nervous system (CNS) depressants such as:

Antihistamines or medicine for hay fever, other allergies, or colds	Sedatives, tranquilizers, or sleeping medicine
Barbiturates	Seizure medicine
Narcotics	Tricyclic antidepressants (medicine for depression)
Prescription pain medicine	

—if you are now taking or have taken within the past 2 weeks monoamine oxidase (MAO) inhibitors such as:

Isocarboxazid   Phenelzine
Pargyline   Tranylcypromine

Proper Use of This Medicine

Use this medicine only as directed by your doctor. Do not use more of it and do not use it more often than your doctor ordered. To do so may increase the chance of side effects.

If you miss a dose of this medicine and remember within an hour or so of the missed dose, take it right away. Then go back to your regular dosing schedule. But if you do not remember until later, do not take the missed dose at all and do not double the next one. Instead, go back to your regular dosing schedule. If you have any questions about this, check with your doctor.

Precautions While Using This Medicine

If you will be taking this medicine for a long period of time (for example, for several months at a time), your doctor should check your progress at regular visits.

This medicine will add to the effects of alcohol and other medicines (CNS depressants) that slow down the nervous system. Some examples of CNS depressants are antihistamines or medicine for hay fever, other allergies, or colds; sedatives, tranquilizers, or sleeping medicine; prescription pain medicine or narcotics; barbiturates; medicine for seizures; tricyclic antidepressants (medicine for depression); or anesthetics, including some dental anesthetics. *Check with your doctor before taking any of the above while you are using this medicine.*

This medicine may cause some people to become drowsy, dizzy, or less alert than they are normally. *Make sure you know how you react to this medicine before you drive, use machines, or do other jobs that require you to be alert.*

Some people who take dantrolene may become more sensitive to sunlight than they are normally. When you first begin taking this medicine, avoid too much sun or too much use of a sunlamp until you see how you react, especially if you tend to burn easily. If you have a severe reaction, check with your doctor.

Side Effects of This Medicine

Along with its needed effects, a medicine may cause some unwanted effects. Although not all of these side effects appear very often, when they do occur they may require medical attention. Check with your doctor if any of the following side effects occur:

Less common

Bloody or black   Mental depression
  tarry stools   or confusion
Bloody or dark   Pain or burning
  urine   while urinating
Chest pain   Yellowing of eyes
Convulsions or   or skin
  seizures
Itching or skin rash

Other side effects may occur which usually do not require medical attention. These side effects may go away during treatment as your body adjusts to the medicine. However, check with your doctor if any of the following side effects continue or are bothersome:

More common

Diarrhea   Drowsiness
Dizziness or   Muscle weakness
  lightheadedness   Nausea
                       Unusual tiredness

Less common

Blurred vision or   Increased sensitivity
  any change in   of skin to
  vision   sunlight
Chills and fever   Muscle aches or
Decreased sexual   pains
  ability   Nervousness or
Difficulty in   sleeplessness
  swallowing   Slurring of speech
Frequent urge to   or other speech
  urinate or dif-   problems
  ficult urination   Stomach cramps or
                          discomfort
                       Unusually fast
                          heartbeat

Other side effects not listed above may also occur in some patients. If you notice any other effects, check with your doctor.

DAPSONE (Systemic)
A commonly used brand name is Avlosulfon.

Dapsone (DAP-sone), a sulfone, belongs to the general family of medicines called anti-infectives. It is given by mouth to help the body overcome leprosy (Hansen's disease) and to help control dermatitis herpetiformis, a skin problem. It may be given alone or with one or more other medicines for leprosy. Dapsone is available only with your doctor's prescription.

Before Using This Medicine

In order to decide on the best treatment for your medical problem, your doctor should be told:

—if you have had allergic reactions to sulfoxone, furosemide, or thiazide diuretics (water pills), oral hypoglycemics (diabetes medicine you take by mouth), glaucoma medicine you take by mouth (for example, acetazolamide, dichlorphenamide, ethoxzolamide, methazolamide), or any other sulfonamides (sulfa medicines).

—if you are pregnant or if you intend to become pregnant, although dapsone has not been shown to cause problems.

—if you are breast-feeding an infant. Dapsone passes into the breast milk and may be used to help prevent leprosy in an infant whose mother has leprosy. However, dapsone may cause problems in an infant with glucose-6-phosphate dehydrogenase (G6PD) deficiency.

—if you have any of the following medical problems:

Glucose-6-phosphate dehydrogenase (G6PD) deficiency	Liver disease
	Methemoglobin reductase deficiency
Kidney disease	Severe anemia

—if you are now taking dapsone for leprosy and are also taking aminobenzoic acid (PABA).

—if you are now taking either probenecid or rifampin.

—if you have had any problems with this medicine in the past.

Proper Use of This Medicine

To help clear up your leprosy completely or to keep it from coming back, *it is very important that you keep taking this medicine for the full time of treatment* even if you begin to feel better after a few weeks or months. You may have to take it every day for as long as 3 years or more, or for life. *It is important that you do not miss any doses.*

If you are taking this medicine for leprosy and you do miss a dose, take it as soon as possible. However, if it is almost time for your next dose, space the missed dose and the next dose 10 to 12 hours apart. Then go back to your regular dosing schedule.

If you are taking this medicine for dermatitis herpetiformis, you may skip a missed dose if it does not make your symptoms come back or get worse. If your symptoms do come back or get worse, take the missed dose as soon as possible. Then go back to your regular dosing schedule.

If you are taking this medicine for dermatitis herpetiformis, your doctor may want you to follow a gluten-free diet. If you have any questions about this, check with your doctor.

Precautions While Using This Medicine

If this medicine causes back, leg, or stomach pains; loss of appetite; pale skin; unexplained sore throat or fever; unusual tiredness or weakness; or yellowing of eyes or skin, stop taking it and check with your doctor as soon as possible.

If your symptoms of leprosy do not improve within 2 to 3 months (or within a few days for dermatitis herpetiformis) or if they become worse, check with your doctor.

It is very important that your doctor check your progress at regular visits.

Side Effects of This Medicine

Along with its needed effects, a medicine may cause some unwanted effects. Although not all of these side effects appear very often, when they do occur they may require medical attention. Stop taking this medicine and check with your doctor if any of the following side effects occur:

More common

Back, leg, or stomach pains	Skin rash
	Unexplained fever
Loss of appetite	Unusual tiredness or weakness
Pale skin	

Rare

Bluish fingernails, lips, or skin	Numbness, tingling, pain, burning, or weakness in hands or feet
Difficult breathing	
Itching, dryness, redness, scaling, or peeling of the skin, or loss of hair	Unexplained sore throat
	Yellowing of eyes or skin

Other side effects may occur which usually do not require medical attention. These side effects may go away during treatment as your body adjusts to the medicine. However, check with your doctor if any of the following side effects continue or are bothersome:

Rare

Dizziness	Nausea
Headache	Vomiting
Lightheadedness	

Other side effects not listed above may also occur in some patients. If you notice any other effects, check with your doctor.

DAUNORUBICIN (Systemic)

Daunorubicin (daw-noe-ROO-bi-sin) belongs to the general group of medicines known as antineoplastics. It is used by injection to treat some kinds of cancer. Daunorubicin is available only with a prescription and is to be administered only by or under the immediate supervision of your doctor.

Before Using This Medicine

Daunorubicin is a very strong medicine. In addition to its helpful effects in treating your medical problem, it has side effects that could be very serious. Before you receive this medicine, be sure that you have discussed the use of it with your doctor.

In order to decide on the best treatment for your medical problem, your doctor should be told:

—if you have ever had any unusual reaction to daunorubicin in the past.

—if you are pregnant or if you intend to have children. This medicine may cause birth defects if either the male or female is taking it at the time of conception or if it is taken during pregnancy. It may also cause permanent sterility after it has been taken for a while. Be sure that you have discussed this with your doctor before taking this medicine.

—if you are breast-feeding an infant. Although daunorubicin has not been shown to cause problems, the chance always exists.

—if you have any of the following medical problems:

Gout	Kidney disease
Heart disease	Kidney stones
Infection	Liver disease

—if you are taking gout medicine.

—if you have been treated with x-rays or cancer drugs by another doctor.

Proper Use of This Medicine

This medicine is sometimes given together with certain other medicines. If you are using a combination of drugs, it is important that you receive each medicine at the proper time. If you are taking some of these medicines by mouth, ask your doctor, nurse, or pharmacist to help you plan a way to take them at the right time.

This medicine often causes nausea and vomiting. However, it is very important that you continue to receive it, even if you begin to feel ill. Your doctor may prescribe a medicine to relieve stomach upset. If you have any questions about this, check with your doctor.

Precautions While Using This Medicine

It is very important that your doctor check your progress at regular visits.

While you are using this medicine, your doctor may want you to drink plenty of fluids and urinate often. This will help prevent kidney problems and keep your kidneys working well. If you have any questions about this, check with your doctor.

Daunorubicin causes the urine to turn reddish in color, which may stain clothes. This is not blood. It is perfectly normal and lasts for only 1 or 2 days after each dose is given.

Side Effects of This Medicine

Along with its needed effects a medicine may cause some unwanted effects. When some of these effects appear, it may mean that the amount of medicine you are receiving needs to be changed. Other side effects may require medical attention. Check with your doctor *immediately* if any of the following side effects occur:

More common

Fever and chills	Swelling of feet and
Irregular heartbeat	lower legs
Shortness of breath	Unexplained fever,
Sores in the mouth	chills, or sore
and on the lips	throat

Less common

Flank pain	Stomach pain
Joint pain	Unusual bleeding or
Pain at the injection	bruising
site	

Rare

Skin rash or itching

Other side effects may occur which usually do not require medical attention. These side effects may go away during treatment as your body

adjusts to the medicine. However, check with your doctor if any of the following side effects continue or are bothersome:

More common
   Loss of hair
   Nausea and
     vomiting
Less common or rare
   Darkening or
     redness of
     the skin
   Diarrhea

This medicine often causes a temporary and total loss of hair. After treatment with daunorubicin has ended, normal hair growth should return.

If daunorubicin accidentally seeps out of the vein into which it is injected, it may damage some tissues and cause scarring. Tell the doctor right away if you notice redness, pain, or swelling at the site of injection.

After you stop using this medicine, it may still produce some side effects that need attention. During this period of time check with your doctor if you notice any of the following side effects:

   Irregular heartbeat   Swelling of feet and
   Shortness of breath   lower legs

Other side effects not listed above may also occur in some patients. If you notice any other effects, check with your doctor.

DESONIDE AND ACETIC ACID (Otic)
A commonly used brand name is Tridesilon.

Desonide (DESS-oh-nide) and acetic acid (a-SEE-tik AS-id) combination is used to treat certain infections of the ear canal. It also helps relieve the redness, itching, and swelling that may accompany these infections. Desonide is an adrenocorticoid (cortisone-like medicine) and belongs to the general family of medicines called steroids. Desonide and acetic acid combination is available only with your doctor's prescription.

Before Using This Medicine

In order to decide on the best treatment for your medical problem, your doctor should be told:

   —if you have ever had any unusual reaction to steroids in the past. This medicine should not be used if you are allergic to it.

—if you have any of the following medical problems:
   Any other ear infec-   Punctured ear drum
     tion or condition

Proper Use of This Medicine

Do not use any leftover medicine for future ear problems without first checking with your doctor. This medicine should not be used on many kinds of bacterial, viral, or fungal infections.

Before applying this medicine, wash the area to be treated (including the ear canal) with soap and water, and dry thoroughly. The ear canal should be dried with a sterile cotton applicator.

To prevent contamination of the ear drops, do not touch the dropper to any surface (including the ear), and keep the container tightly closed.

How to apply this medicine: Lie down or tilt the head so that the infected ear faces up. For adults, gently pull the ear lobe up and back to straighten the ear canal. (For children, gently pull the ear lobe down and back to straighten the ear canal.) Drop medicine into the ear canal. Keep ear facing up for several minutes to allow medicine to run to the bottom of the ear canal. A clean, soft cotton plug may be gently inserted into the ear opening to prevent the medicine from leaking out.

If you miss a dose of this medicine, apply it as soon as possible. Then go back to your regular dosing schedule. But if it is almost time for your next dose, do not apply the missed dose at all. Instead, go back to your regular dosing schedule. If you have any questions about this, check with your doctor.

Precautions While Using This Medicine

If your symptoms have not improved after 5 to 7 days, or if your ear problem becomes worse, check with your doctor.

Side Effects of This Medicine

After application of this medicine to the ear, occasional stinging, itching, or burning may be expected. If this continues or is bothersome, check with your doctor.

There have not been any other common or important side effects reported with this medicine. However, if you notice any other effects, check with your doctor.

DEXAMETHASONE (Nasal)
A commonly used brand name is Decadron.

Dexamethasone (dex-a-METH-a-sone) is an adrenocorticoid (cortisone-like medicine). It belongs to the general family of medicines called steroids. Cortisone-like medicines are used nasally to help relieve the stuffy nose, irritation, and discomfort of many nasal problems. Adrenocorticoids for use in the nose are available only with your doctor's prescription.

Before Using This Medicine

In order to decide on the best treatment for your medical problem, your doctor should be told:

—if you have had any unusual reactions to aerosol spray inhalation or nasal medicines in the past. This medicine should not be used if you are allergic to it.

—if you are pregnant, if you intend to become pregnant, or if you are breast-feeding an infant. Although nasal adrenocorticoids have not been shown to cause birth defects or other problems in humans, the chance always exists.

—if you have an infection of the nose, sinuses, or throat or if you have a fungal infection.

Proper Use of This Medicine

This medicine usually comes with patient directions. Read them carefully before using.

Do not use this medicine more often or for a longer period of time than your doctor ordered. To do so may increase the chance of absorption through the lining of the nose and the chance of side effects.

This medicine is used with a special inhaler. Save your inhaler, since refill units may be available at lower cost.

Container provides about 170 measured sprays.

Store away from heat and direct sunlight. Do not puncture, break, or burn container.

Check with your doctor before using this medicine for nasal problems, other than the one for which it was prescribed, since it should not be used on many bacterial, viral, or fungal nasal infections.

If you miss a dose of this medicine and remember within an hour or so of the missed dose, take it right away. Then go back to your regular dosing schedule. But if you do not remember until later, do not take the missed dose at all and do not double the next one. Instead, go back to your regular dosing schedule. If you have any questions about this, check with your doctor.

Precautions While Using This Medicine

Check with your doctor:

—if signs of a nose, sinus, or throat infection occur.

—if your symptoms do not improve.

—if your condition gets worse.

This medicine may be absorbed through the lining of the nose and can affect growth. Therefore, children using it should be followed closely by their doctor.

Side Effects of This Medicine

Along with its needed effects, a medicine may cause some unwanted effects. Although not all of these side effects appear very often, when they do occur they may require medical attention. Check with your doctor if any of the following side effects occur:

Less common or rare

Continuing stuffy nose	Tightness in chest
Loss of sense of smell	Unexplained nosebleeds
Shortness of breath	Wheezing

Other side effects may occur which usually do not require medical attention. These side effects may go away during treatment as your body adjusts to the medicine. However, check with your doctor if either of the following side effects continues or is bothersome:

More common

Dryness or irritation of the nose

Other side effects not listed above may also occur in some patients. If you notice any other effects, check with your doctor.

DEXBROMPHENIRAMINE AND PSEUDOEPHEDRINE (Systemic)
Some commonly used brand names are Disophrol and Drixoral.

Dexbrompheniramine (dex-brom-fen-EER-a-meen) and pseudoephedrine (soo-doe-e-FED-rin) is a combination antihistamine and decongestant. It is used to treat nasal congestion (stuffy nose) and other symptoms of hay fever and other types of allergy. This medicine is available only with your doctor's prescription.

Before Using This Medicine

In order to decide on the best treatment for your medical problem, your doctor should be told:

—if you have ever had any unusual reaction to dexbrompheniramine, pseudoephedrine, or similar medicines in the past. This medicine should not be taken if you are allergic to it.

—if you are pregnant or if you intend to become pregnant while using this medicine. Although this medicine has not been shown to cause birth defects or other problems, the chance always exists.

—if you are breast-feeding an infant. Both dexbrompheniramine and pseudoephedrine pass into the breast milk and may cause unwanted effects in the infant.

—if you have any of the following medical problems:

Diabetes	High blood pressure
Enlarged prostate	Overactive thyroid
Glaucoma	Stomach ulcer
Heart or blood vessel disease	Urinary tract blockage

—if you are now taking any of the following medicines or types of medicine:

Alkavervir	Nadolol
Amphetamines	Propranolol
Digitalis glycosides (heart medicine)	Protoveratrine A
	Reserpine
Guanethidine	Tricyclic an-
Mecamylamine	tidepressants
Medicine for asthma or breathing prob- blems	(medicine for depression)
	Veratrum viride
Methyldopa	alkaloids
Metoprolol	

—if you are now taking any central nervous system (CNS) depressants such as:

Antihistamines or medicine for hay fever, other allergies, or colds	Narcotics
	Prescription pain medicine
	Sedatives, tran- quilizers,
Barbiturates	or sleeping
Medicines for seizures	medicine

—if you are now taking or have taken within the past 2 weeks monoamine oxidase (MAO) inhibitors such as:

Isocarboxazid	Phenelzine
Pargyline	Tranylcypromine

Proper Use of This Medicine

Take dexbrompheniramine and pseudoephedrine combination only as directed. Do not take more of it and do not take it more often than recommended on the label, unless otherwise directed by your doctor. To do so may increase the chance of side effects.

Take this medicine with food or a glass of water or milk to lessen stomach irritation, if necessary.

The tablets are to be swallowed whole so that they will be longacting. Do not break, crush, or chew before swallowing.

If you must take this medicine regularly and you miss a dose, take the missed dose as soon as possible. However, if it is almost time for your next dose, do not take the missed dose at all and do not double the next one. Instead, go back to your regular dosing schedule. If you have any questions about this, check with your doctor or pharmacist.

Precautions While Using This Medicine

The antihistamine in this medicine will add to the effects of alcohol and other medicines (CNS depressants) that slow down the nervous system. Some examples of CNS depressants are other antihistamines or medicine for hay fever, other allergies, or colds; sedatives, tranquilizers, or sleeping medicine; prescription pain medicine or narcotics; barbiturates; medicine for seizures; tricyclic antidepressants (medicine for depression); or anesthetics, including some dental anesthetics. *Check with your doctor before taking any of the above while you are using this medicine.*

Dexbrompheniramine may cause some people to become drowsy, dizzy, or less alert than they are normally. *Make sure you know how you react to this medicine before you drive, use machines, or do other jobs that require you to be alert.*

Other people may become nervous or restless or may have trouble in sleeping due to the pseudoephedrine in this medicine. If you do have trouble in sleeping, take the last dose of this medicine for each day a few hours before bedtime. If you have any questions about this, check with your doctor.

Side Effects of This Medicine

Along with its needed effects, a medicine may cause some unwanted effects. Although not all of these side effects appear very often, when they do occur they may require medical attention. Check with your doctor if any of the following side effects occur:

Rare

Unexplained sore throat and fever	Unusual bleeding or bruising
	Unusual weakness

With high doses

Hallucinations (seeing, hearing, or feeling things that are not there)	Unusually slow heartbeat, shortness of breath, or troubled breathing
Irregular heartbeat	

Other side effects may occur which usually do not require medical attention. These side effects may go away during treatment as your body adjusts to the medicine. However, check with your doctor if any of the following side effects continue or are bothersome:

More common

Drowsiness	Thickening of the bronchial secretions

Less common—more common with high doses

Difficult or painful urination	Nervousness, restlessness, or trouble in sleeping (especially in children)
Dizziness	
Dryness of mouth, nose, or throat	
Headache	Skin rash
Loss of appetite	Unusual increase in sweating
Nausea, upset stomach, or stomach pain	Unusual paleness
	Unusually fast or pounding heartbeat

Other side effects not listed above may also occur in some patients. If you notice any other effects, check with your doctor.

DIAZOXIDE (Oral)
A commonly used brand name is Proglycem.

Diazoxide (dye-az-OX-ide) when taken by mouth is used in the treatment of hypoglycemia (low blood sugar). Diazoxide is available only with your doctor's prescription.

Before Using This Medicine

In order to decide on the best treatment for your medical problem, your doctor should be told:

—if you are allergic to sulfonamides (sulfa drugs) or thiazide diuretics.

—if you are pregnant or if you intend to become pregnant while using this medicine.

Too much use of diazoxide during pregnancy may cause unwanted effects in the baby. Be sure that you have discussed this with your doctor before taking this medicine. In addition, although diazoxide has not been shown to cause birth defects in humans, they have occurred in animals and the chance always exists.

—if you are breast-feeding an infant. Although diazoxide has not been shown to cause problems, the chance always exists.

—if you have any of the following medical problems:

Angina	Kidney disease
Diabetes	Liver disease
Gout	Heart or blood vessel disease

—if you have had a recent heart attack or stroke.

—if you are now taking any of the following medicines or types of medicine:

Antihypertensives (high blood pressure medicine)	Medicines to improve blood circulation
Asthma medicine	Oral anticoagulants (blood thinners you take by mouth)
Cold remedies	
Diuretics (water pills)	
Gout medicine	Phenytoin
	Propranolol

Proper Use of This Medicine

Take this medicine only as directed by your doctor. Do not take more or less of it than your doctor ordered, and take it at the same time each day.

Follow carefully the special diet your doctor gave you. This is an important part of controlling your condition, and is necessary if the medicine is to work properly.

Test for sugar in your urine as directed by your doctor. This is a convenient way to make sure your condition is being controlled and it provides an early warning when it is not. Two urine tests for sugar are widely used: the tablet urine test and the paper-strip urine test. The results of these two tests are read differently. For example, a 3-plus reading of a tablet urine test is not equal to a 3-plus reading of a paper-strip urine test. Do not change from one test to the other unless told to do so by your doctor. In addition, your doctor may instruct you to test your urine for acetone.

If you miss a dose of this medicine, take it as soon as possible. If it is almost time for your next dose, do not take the missed dose at all and do

not double the next one. Instead, go back to your regular dosing schedule. If you have any questions about this, check with your doctor.

Precautions While Using This Medicine

It is very important that your doctor check your progress at regular visits, especially during the first few weeks of treatment.

Do not take any other medicine, unless prescribed or approved by your doctor, since some may interfere with this medicine's effects. This especially includes over-the-counter (OTC) or nonprescription medicine such as that for colds, cough, asthma, hay fever, or appetite control.

Check with your doctor right away if signs of high blood sugar (hyperglycemia) occur. These signs usually include:

Drowsiness	Increased urination
Flushed, dry skin	Loss of appetite
Fruit-like breath odor	Unusual thirst

These signs may occur if the dose of the medicine is too high, or if you have a fever or infection or are experiencing unusual stress.

Check with your doctor also if these signs of low blood sugar (hypoglycemia) occur:

Anxiety	Nausea
Chills	Nervousness
Cold sweats	Rapid pulse
Cool pale skin	Shakiness
Drowsiness	Unusual tiredness
Excessive hunger	or weakness
Headache	

Signs of both low blood sugar and high blood sugar must be corrected before they progress to a more serious condition. In either situation, you should check with your doctor immediately.

Side Effects of This Medicine

Along with its needed effects, a medicine may cause some unwanted effects. Although not all of these side effects appear very often, when they do occur they may require medical attention. Check with your doctor if any of the following side effects occur:

More common

Swelling of hands, feet, or lower legs	Unusual decrease in urination
	Unusual weight gain

Less common

Rapid or irregular heartbeat

Rare

Chest pain	Skin rash
Confusion	Unusual bleeding or
Fever	bruising
Numbness of the hands	

Other side effects may occur which usually do not require medical attention. These side effects may go away during treatment as your body adjusts to the medicine. However, check with your doctor if any of the following side effects continue or are bothersome:

Less common

Changes in ability to taste	Loss of appetite
Constipation	Nausea and vomiting
Increased hair growth on forehead, back, arms, and legs	Stiffness
	Stomach pain
	Trembling and shaking of hands and fingers

This medicine may cause a temporary increase in hair growth in some people. After treatment with diazoxide has ended, normal hair growth should return.

Other side effects not listed above may also occur in some patients. If you notice any other effects, check with your doctor.

DICYCLOMINE (Systemic)
Some commonly used brand names are:

Bentyl	Cyclobec*
Bentylol*	Dyspas

*Not available in the United States.

Dicyclomine (dye-SYE-kloe-meen) belongs to the general family of medicines called antispasmodics. It helps to decrease stomach cramps and cramping or spasms of the intestines and bladder. Dicyclomine is available only with your doctor's prescription.

Before Using This Medicine

In order to decide on the best treatment for your medical problem, your doctor should be told:

—if you have ever had any unusual reaction to this medicine in the past. This medicine should not be taken if you are allergic to it.

—if you are pregnant, if you intend to become pregnant, or if you are breast-feeding an infant. Although dicyclomine has not been shown to cause problems, the chance always exists.

—if you have any of the following medical problems:

Difficult urination	Intestinal blockage
Enlarged prostate	Kidney disease
Glaucoma	Liver disease
Heart disease	Myasthenia gravis
Hiatal hernia	Overactive thyroid
	Severe ulcerative colitis

—if you are now taking any of the following medicines or types of medicine:

Amantadine	Medicine for sleep
Antacids	Medicine for
Antihistamines	Parkinson's
Haloperidol	disease
Medicine for	Medicine for ulcers
depression	Nerve medicine
Medicine for diar-	Sedatives or tran-
rhea	quilizers

—if you are now taking or have taken within the past 2 weeks monoamine oxidase (MAO) inhibitors such as:

Isocarboxazid	Phenelzine
Pargyline	Tranylcypromine

Proper Use of This Medicine

Take this medicine exactly as directed by your doctor. Do not take more or less of it, do not take it more often, and do not take it for a longer period of time than your doctor ordered.

If this medicine upsets your stomach, take it with food or milk, unless otherwise directed by your doctor.

If you miss a dose of this medicine, do not take the missed dose at all and do not double the next one. Instead, go back to your regular dosing schedule. If you have any questions about this, check with your doctor.

Precautions While Using This Medicine

This medicine will add to the effects of alcohol and other medicines (CNS depressants) that slow down the nervous system. Some examples of CNS depressants are antihistamines or medicine for hay fever, other allergies, or colds; sedatives, tranquilizers, or sleeping medicine; prescription pain medicine or narcotics; barbiturates; medicine for seizures; tricyclic antidepressants (medicine for depression); or anesthetics, including some dental anesthetics. *Check with your doctor before*

taking any of the above while you are using this medicine.

This medicine may cause some people to become drowsy or less alert than they are normally. *Make sure you know how you react to this medicine before you drive, use machines, or do other jobs that require you to be alert.*

Check with your doctor if you develop intestinal problems such as constipation. This is especially important if you are taking other medicine while taking dicyclomine.

Although this side effect does not occur often, this medicine may make you sweat less, causing your body temperature to increase. Use extra care not to become overheated during exercise or hot weather while you are taking this medicine, as overheating could possibly result in heat stroke. Also, hot baths or saunas may make you feel dizzy or faint while you are taking this medicine.

Do not take this medicine within 1 hour of taking antacids or medicine for diarrhea. Taking them too close together will make this medicine less effective.

Side Effects of This Medicine

Along with its needed effects, a medicine may cause some unwanted effects. Although not all of these side effects appear very often, when they do occur they may require medical attention. Check with your doctor if any of the following side effects occur:

More common

Constipation

Less common

Difficult urination

Rare

Skin rash

Other side effects may occur which usually do not require medical attention. These side effects may go away during treatment as your body adjusts to the medicine. However, check with your doctor if any of the following side effects continue or are bothersome:

More common

Bloated feeling	Headache
Dizziness	

Less common

Decreased sexual ability	Nausea and vomiting
Drowsiness	Nervousness
Mental confusion (especially in elderly)	

Rare

    Decreased sweating   Rapid pulse
    Dry mouth

Other side effects not listed above may also occur in some patients. If you notice any other effects, check with your doctor.

DIGITALIS MEDICINES (Systemic)

This information applies to the following medicines:

Digitalis (di-ji-TAL-iss)
Digitoxin (di-ji-TOX-in)
Digoxin (di-JOX-in)
Gitalin (JI-tal-in)
Lanatoside C (lan-AT-oh-side C)
Ouabain (WAH-bane)

Some commonly used brand names and other names are:	Generic names:
Cedilanid-D	Deslanoside
Digifortis Pil-Digis	Digitalis
Crystodigin Purodigin	Digitoxin
Lanoxin	Digoxin
Gitaligin	Gitalin
Cedilanid	Lanatoside C
Strophanthin-G	Ouabain

These medicines are used to improve the strength and efficiency of the heart, or in some cases, to control the rate of the heartbeat. This leads to better blood circulation and reduced swelling of hands and ankles in patients having such a problem. Digitalis medicines are available only with your doctor's prescription.

Before Using This Medicine

In order to decide on the best treatment for your medical problem, your doctor should be told:

—if you have ever had any unusual reaction to digitalis medicine in the past. This medicine should not be taken if you are allergic to it.

—if you are pregnant, if you intend to become pregnant, or if you are breast-feeding an infant. Although this medicine has not been shown to cause problems, the chance always exists.

—if you have any of the following medical problems:

Emphysema or other severe lung disease	Hypokalemia (too little potassium in the blood)
Hypercalcemia (too much calcium in the blood)	Kidney disease Thyroid disease

—if you are now taking any of the following medicines or types of medicine:

Antacids	Diuretics (water pills)
Asthma or hay fever medicine	Ephedrine or epinephrine
Blood pressure medicine	Medicine for sinus congestion
Cholestyramine	Neomycin
Diarrhea medicine	Reducing or diet medicine

—if you are now taking or have taken within the past 2 weeks any of the following medicines or types of medicine:

Amphotericin B	Phenobarbital or phenylbutazone or rifampin (does not apply to patients taking digoxin)
Any digitalis medicines or other heart medicines, especially quinidine	
Corticosteroids (cortisone-like medicine)	Potassium supplements Thyroid medicine

Proper Use of This Medicine

To keep your heart working properly, *take this medicine exactly as directed even though you may feel well.* Do not miss taking any of the doses and do not take more medicine than ordered.

Ask your doctor about your personal pulse rate. Then, while you are taking this medicine, check your pulse regularly. If it is much slower than usual or if it changes in rhythm or force, check with your doctor. Such changes may mean that side effects are developing.

To help you remember to take your dose of medicine, try to take it at the same time every day.

If you miss a dose of this medicine, do not take the missed dose at all and do not double the next one. Instead, go back to your regular dosing schedule. If you have any questions about this, check with your doctor.

For patients taking the liquid form of digoxin:

•This medicine is to be taken by mouth even though it may come in a dropper bottle. The amount you should take is to be measured with the specially marked dropper.

Precautions While Using This Medicine

Do not stop taking this medicine without first checking with your doctor.

Keep this medicine out of the reach of children since digitalis medicines are an important cause of accidental poisoning in children.

Before having any kind of surgery (including dental surgery) or emergency treatment, tell the doctor or dentist in charge that you are using this medicine.

Your doctor may want you to carry a medical identification card or bracelet stating that you are using this medicine.

Do not take any other medicine unless ordered by your doctor. Many over-the-counter (OTC) or nonprescription medicines contain ingredients which interfere with digitalis medicines or which may make your condition worse. They include antacids; asthma remedies; cold, cough, or sinus preparations; medicine for diarrhea; and reducing or diet medicines.

For patients taking the tablet or capsule forms of this medicine:

• Caution—This medicine may look like other tablets or capsules you now take. It is very important that you do not get the medicines mixed up since this may have serious results. Ask your pharmacist for ways to avoid mix-ups with medicines that look alike.

Side Effects of This Medicine

Along with its needed effects, a medicine may cause some unwanted effects. Although not all of these side effects appear very often, when they do occur they may require medical attention. Check with your doctor if any of the following side effects occur:

More common

Loss of appetite	Unusual tiredness
Lower stomach pain	or weakness
Nausea or vomiting	Unusually slow or
	uneven pulse

Less common

Blurred vision or	Diarrhea
"yellow vision"	Mental depression
(yellow halo seen	or confusion
around objects)	(especially in
	elderly patients)

Rare

Drowsiness	Skin rash or
Headache	hives

Other side effects not listed above may also occur in some patients. If you notice any other effects, check with your doctor.

DIMETHYL SULFOXIDE (Topical)
A commonly used brand name is Rimso-50.

Dimethyl sulfoxide (dye-METH-il sul-FOX-ide) is instilled into the bladder to relieve the symptoms of the bladder condition called interstitial cystitis. This medicine is available only with your doctor's prescription.

Before Using This Medicine

In order to decide on the best treatment for your medical problem, your doctor should be told:

—if you have ever had any unusual reaction to dimethyl sulfoxide in the past. This medicine should not be used if you are allergic to it.

—if you are pregnant, if you intend to become pregnant, or if you are breast-feeding an infant. Although dimethyl sulfoxide has not been shown to cause birth defects in humans, the chance always exists.

—if you are now taking any other medicine.

Side Effects of This Medicine

Along with its needed effects, a medicine may cause some unwanted effects. Although not all of these side effects appear very often, when they do occur they may require medical attention. Check with your doctor if any of the following side effects occur:

Nasal congestion	Skin rash, hives,
Shortness of breath	or itching
or troubled	Swelling of face
breathing	

Some patients may have some discomfort during the time this medicine is being instilled into the bladder. However, the discomfort usually becomes less each time the medicine is used.

Dimethyl sulfoxide may cause you to have a garlic-like taste within a few minutes after the medicine is instilled into the bladder. This effect may last for several hours. It may also cause your breath and skin to have a garlic-like odor which may last up to 72 hours.

Other side effects not listed above may also occur in some patients. If you notice any other effects, check with your doctor.

DINOPROST (Intra-amniotic)
A commonly used brand name is Prostin F$_2$ Alpha.

Dinoprost (DYE-noe-prost) is given by injection to cause abortion. It is available only with your doctor's prescription and is to be administered only by or under the immediate care of your doctor.

Before Using This Medicine

In order to decide on the best treatment for your medical problem, your doctor should be told:

—if you have ever had any unusual reaction to dinoprost in the past. This medicine should not be used if you are allergic to it.

—if you have any of the following medical problems:

Asthma (history of)	High blood pressure
Epilepsy	Lung disease
Glaucoma	Uterus surgery
Heart or blood	(history of)
vessel disease	

Side Effects of This Medicine

Along with its needed effects, a medicine may cause some unwanted effects. Although not all of these side effects appear very often, when they do occur they may require medical attention. Let the doctor or nurse know if any of the following side effects occur:

Less common or rare

Seizures	Wheezing, troubled breathing, or tightness in chest

Other side effects may occur which usually do not require medical attention. These side effects usually go away after the medicine is stopped. However, let the doctor or nurse know if any of the following side effects continue or are bothersome:

More common

Diarrhea	Vomiting
Nausea	

After this medicine is stopped, it may still produce some side effects that need attention. Check with your doctor if you notice any of the following side effects:

Chills or shivering	Pain in lower abdomen
Fever	
Foul-smelling vaginal discharge	Unusual increase in uterine bleeding

Other side effects not listed above may also occur in some patients. If you notice any other effects, check with your doctor.

DINOPROSTONE (Vaginal)
A commonly used brand name is Prostin E$_2$.

Dinoprostone (dye-noe-PROST-one) suppositories are inserted into the vagina of pregnant women to produce abortion. They are available only with your doctor's prescription and are to be administered only by or under the immediate care of your doctor.

Before Using This Medicine

In order to decide on the best treatment for your medical problem, your doctor should be told:

—if you have ever had any unusual reaction to dinoprostone in the past. This medicine should not be used if you are allergic to it.

—if you have any of the following medical problems:

Anemia (history of)	Inflammation or infection of cervix or vagina
Asthma (history of)	
Diabetes (history of)	
Epilepsy (history of)	Jaundice (history of)
Heart or blood vessel disease (or history of)	Kidney disease (or history of)
High blood pressure (history of)	Liver disease (or history of)
	Lung disease
	Uterus surgery (history of)

Proper Use of This Medicine

After the suppository is inserted into the vagina, remain lying down for at least 10 minutes so that the medicine can be absorbed.

Side Effects of This Medicine

Along with its needed effects, a medicine may cause some unwanted effects. Although not all of these side effects appear very often, when they do occur they may require medical attention. Let the doctor or nurse know if any of the following side effects occur:

Less common or rare

 Wheezing, troubled breathing,
  or tightness in chest

Other side effects may occur which usually do not require medical attention. These side effects usually go away after the medicine is stopped. However, let the doctor or nurse know if any of the following side effects continue or are bothersome:

More common

Diarrhea	Nausea
Fever	Vomiting

Less common

 Chills or shivering
 Headache

After this medicine is stopped it may still produce some side effects that need attention. Check with your doctor if any of the following side effects occur:

Chills or shivering	Pain in lower ab-
Fever	domen
Foul-smelling	Unusual increase in
vaginal discharge	uterine bleeding

Other side effects not listed above may also occur in some patients. If you notice any other effects, check with your doctor.

DIONE-TYPE ANTICONVULSANTS
(Systemic)

This information applies to the following medicines:

Paramethadione (par-a-meth-a-DYE-one)
Trimethadione (trye-meth-a-DYE-one)

Some commonly used brand names are:	Generic names:
Paradione	Paramethadione
Tridione	Trimethadione

This medicine belongs to the general family of medicines called anticonvulsants. It is used to control certain seizures in the treatment of epilepsy. This medicine is available only with your doctor's prescription.

Before Using This Medicine

In order to decide on the best treatment for your medical problem, your doctor should be told:

 —if you have had any unusual reaction to anticonvulsant medicines in the past. This medicine should not be taken if you are allergic to it.

 —if you are pregnant or if you intend to become pregnant while using this medicine. This medicine may cause birth defects if taken during pregnancy, and may cause bleeding problems in the newborn infant.

 —if you are breast-feeding an infant. Although these anticonvulsants have not been shown to cause problems, the chance always exists.

 —if you have any of the following medical problems:

Blood disease	Kidney disease
Diseases of the eye	Liver disease
or optic nerve	

 —if you are now taking medicine for mental depression or mental illness.

 —if you are taking other anticonvulsant medicine.

Proper Use of This Medicine

This medicine must be taken every day in regularly spaced doses as ordered by your doctor.

If this medicine upsets your stomach, take it with food or milk unless otherwise directed by your doctor.

If you miss a dose of this medicine, take it as soon as possible. If it is almost time for your next dose, do not take the missed dose at all and do not double the next one. Instead, go back to your regular dosing schedule.

Precautions While Using This Medicine

It is very important that your doctor check your progress at regular visits, especially during the first few months you take this medicine.

If you have been taking this medicine regularly, do not stop taking it without first checking with your doctor. Your doctor may want you to reduce gradually the amount you are taking before stopping completely in order to reduce the possibility of seizures.

This medicine may cause your eyes to become more sensitive to bright light than they are normally, making it difficult for you to see well. Wearing sunglasses may help. It may also be difficult to see in light that changes in brightness. If you notice this effect, be especially careful when driving at night.

This medicine may cause some people to become drowsy or less alert than they are normally. *Make sure you know how you react to this medicine before you drive, use machines, or do other jobs that require you to be alert.* After you have taken this medicine for a while, this effect may not be so bothersome.

Side Effects of This Medicine

Along with its needed effects, a medicine may cause some unwanted effects. Although not all of these side effects appear very often, when they do occur they may require medical attention. Check with your doctor if any of the following side effects occur:

Rare

Fluid buildup in body causing puffy face, hands, legs, and feet
Skin rash
Swollen glands
Unexplained sore throat and fever

Unusual bleeding or bruising, such as recurring nosebleeds or bleeding gums
Yellowing of eyes and skin

Other side effects may occur which usually do not require medical attention. These side effects may go away during treatment as your body adjusts to the medicine. However, check with your doctor if any of the following side effects continue or are bothersome:

More common

Changes in vision
Dizziness
Drowsiness

Headache
Increased sensitivity of eyes to light

Less common

Itchy skin
Nausea or vomiting

Unusual tiredness or weakness

Other side effects not listed above may also occur in some patients. If you notice any other effects, check with your doctor.

DIPHENOXYLATE AND ATROPINE
(Systemic)

Some commonly used brand names are Colonil, Lomotil, and SK-Diphenoxylate.

Diphenoxylate (dye-fen-OX-i-late) and atropine (A-troe-peen) is a combination medicine used along with other measures to treat severe diarrhea. This medicine is available only with your doctor's prescription.

Before Using This Medicine

In order to decide on the best treatment for your medical problem, your doctor should be told:

—if you have ever had any unusual reaction to diphenoxylate and atropine in the past. This medicine should not be taken if you are allergic to it.

—if you are pregnant, if you intend to become pregnant, or if you are breast-feeding an infant. Although this medicine has not been shown to cause problems, the chance always exists.

—if you have any of the following medical problems:

Addison's disease
Alcoholism
Colitis
Difficult urination
Emphysema, asthma, bronchitis, or other chronic lung disease
Enlarged prostate
Gallbladder disease or gallstones

Glaucoma
Heart disease
Hiatal hernia
High blood pressure
Kidney disease
Liver disease
Myasthenia gravis
Overactive or underactive thyroid

—if you are now taking any of the following medicines or types of medicine:

Amantadine
Haloperidol

Heart medicine
Ulcer medicine

—if you are now taking other central nervous system (CNS) depressants such as:

Antihistamines or medicine for hay fever, other allergies, or colds
Barbiturates
Other narcotics
Prescription pain medicine

Sedatives, tranquilizers, or sleeping medicine
Seizure medicine
Tricyclic antidepressants (medicine for depression)

Proper Use of This Medicine

Take this medicine only as directed by your doctor. Do not take more of it, do not take it more often, and do not take it for a longer period of time than your doctor ordered. If too much is taken, it may become habit-forming, or may cause overdose in a child.

Keep this medicine out of the reach of children since overdose is especially dangerous in children.

If this medicine upsets your stomach, your doctor may want you to take it with food.

If you miss a dose of this medicine, do not take the missed dose at all and do not double the next one. Instead, go back to your regular dosing schedule. If you have any questions about this, check with your doctor.

For patients taking the liquid form of this medicine:
- This medicine is to be taken by mouth even though it may come in a dropper bottle. The amount to be taken is to be measured with the specially marked dropper.

Precautions While Using This Medicine

If you will be taking this medicine regularly for a long period of time:
- Your doctor should check your progress at regular visits.
- Do not stop taking it without first checking with your doctor. Your doctor may want you to reduce gradually the amount you are taking before stopping completely.

Check with your doctor if your diarrhea does not stop after a few days or if you develop a fever.

This medicine will add to the effects of alcohol and other medicines (CNS depressants) that slow down the nervous system. Some examples of CNS depressants are antihistamines or medicine for hay fever, other allergies, or colds; sedatives, tranquilizers, or sleeping medicine; prescription pain medicine or narcotics; barbiturates; medicine for seizures; tricyclic antidepressants (medicine for depression); or anesthetics, including some dental anesthetics. *Check with your doctor before taking any of the above while you are taking this medicine.*

This medicine may cause some people to become dizzy, drowsy, or less alert than they are normally. Even if taken at bedtime, it may cause some people to feel drowsy or less alert on arising. *Make sure you know how you react to this medicine before you drive, use machines, or do other jobs that require you to be alert.*

Before having any kind of surgery (including dental surgery), tell the doctor or dentist in charge that you are using this medicine.

Side Effects of This Medicine

Along with its needed effects, a medicine may cause some unwanted effects. Although not all of these side effects appear very often, when they do occur they may require medical attention. *When this medicine is used for short periods of time at low doses, side effects usually are rare.* However, check with your doctor *immediately* if any of the following side effects occur:

Bloating	Nausea and
Constipation	vomiting
Loss of appetite	Stomach pain

Check with your doctor immediately also if the following effects occur, since they may indicate an overdose:

Loss of con-	Shallow breathing
sciousness	Unusual excitement
Pinpoint pupils	

Other side effects may occur which usually do not require medical attention. These side effects may go away during treatment as your body adjusts to the medicine. However, check with your doctor if any of the following side effects continue, worsen, or are bothersome:

Less common or rare

Blurred vision	Numbness of hands
Dizziness, depres-	or feet
sion, drowsiness	Rapid heartbeat
Dryness of skin and	Restlessness
mouth	Skin rash or itching
Fever	Swelling of the
Flushing	gums
Headache	Unusual decrease in
	urination

After you stop using this medicine, your body may need time to adjust. The length of time this takes depends on the amount of medicine you were using and how long you used it. During this period of time check with your doctor if you notice any of the following side effects:

Muscle cramps	Stomach cramps
Nausea and	Unusual sweating
vomiting	
Shaking or trem-	
bling	

Other side effects not listed above may also occur in some patients. If you notice any other effects, check with your doctor.

DIPIVEFRIN (Ophthalmic)
A commonly used brand name is Propine.

Dipivefrin (dye-PI-ve-frin) is used in the eye to treat certain types of glaucoma. This medicine is available only with your doctor's prescription.

Before Using This Medicine

In order to decide on the best treatment for your medical problem, your doctor should be told:

—if you have ever had any unusual reaction to dipivefrin in the past. This medicine should not be used if you are allergic to it.

—if you are pregnant, if you intend to become pregnant, or if you are breast-feeding an infant. Although dipivefrin has not been shown to cause problems, the chance always exists.

Proper Use of This Medicine

Use this medicine only as directed. Do not use more of it and do not use it more often than your doctor ordered. To do so may increase the chance of too much medicine being absorbed into the body and the chance of side effects.

How to apply this medicine: First, wash hands. With middle finger, apply pressure to the inside corner of the eye (and continue to apply pressure for 1 or 2 minutes after the medicine has been placed in the eye). Tilt head back and with the index finger of the same hand, pull lower eyelid away from eye to form a pouch. Drop the medicine into the pouch and gently close eyes. Do not blink. Keep eyes closed for 1 or 2 minutes to allow the medicine to be absorbed.

To prevent contamination of the eye drops, do not touch the applicator tip to any surface (including the eye). Also, keep the container tightly closed.

If you miss a dose of this medicine, apply the missed dose as soon as possible. Then go back to your regular dosing schedule. But if it is almost time for your next dose, do not apply the missed dose at all. Instead, apply your next dose at the regularly scheduled time. Then continue with your regular dosing schedule. If you have any questions about this, check with your doctor.

Precautions While Using This Medicine

Your doctor should check your eye pressure at regular visits.

Side Effects of This Medicine

Along with its needed effects, a medicine may cause some unwanted effects. Although not all of these side effects appear very often, when they do occur they may require medical attention. Check with your doctor if any of the following side effects occur:

Rare—Possible signs of too much medicine being absorbed into the body

Unusually fast or irregular heartbeat

Other side effects may occur which usually do not require medical attention. These side effects may go away during treatment as your body adjusts to the medicine. However, check with your doctor if any of the following side effects continue or are bothersome:

More common

Burning, stinging, or other irritation of eye

Other side effects not listed above may also occur in some patients. If you notice any other effects, check with your doctor.

DIPYRIDAMOLE (Systemic)
A commonly used brand name is Persantine.

Dipyridamole (dye-peer-ID-a-mole) is used to help prevent or reduce the occurrence of angina attacks. It will not relieve the pain of an attack that has already started. Dipyridamole may also be used for other conditions as determined by your doctor. Dipyridamole is available only with your doctor's prescription.

Before Using This Medicine

In order to decide on the best treatment for your medical problem, your doctor should be told:

—if you have ever had any unusual reaction to dipyridamole in the past. This medicine should not be taken if you are allergic to it.
—if you are pregnant, if you intend to become pregnant, or if you are breast-feeding an infant. Although dipyridamole has not been shown to cause problems, the chance always exists.

Proper Use of This Medicine

Dipyridamole must be taken in regularly spaced doses, as ordered by your doctor.

This medicine works best when taken with a full glass (8 ounces) of water at least 1 hour before meals.

Sometimes dipyridamole must be taken regularly for 2 or 3 months before it reaches its full effect in the treatment of angina.

If you miss a dose of this medicine, take it as soon as possible unless it is within 4 hours of your next scheduled dose. Then go back to your regular dosing schedule. Do not double doses. If you have any questions about this, check with your doctor.

Precautions While Using This Medicine

Dipyridamole is used to prevent angina attacks. *Do not take this medicine to relieve the pain of an attack* that has already started, because it works too slowly. Check with your doctor if you need a fast-acting medicine such as nitroglycerin to relieve the pain of an angina attack.

Dizziness, lightheadedness, or fainting may occur, especially when you get up from a lying or sitting position. Getting up slowly may help. If this problem continues or gets worse, check with your doctor.

Side Effects of This Medicine

Along with its needed effects, a medicine may cause some unwanted effects. The following side effects may go away during treatment as your body adjusts to the medicine; however, check with your doctor if they continue or are bothersome:

Dizziness, light-headedness, or fainting	Nausea or vomiting
	Skin rash
	Stomach cramping
Flushing	Weakness
Headache	

Other side effects not listed above may also occur in some patients. If you notice any other effects, check with your doctor.

DISOPYRAMIDE (Systemic)
Some commonly used brand names are Norpace and Rythmodan*.

---

* Not available in the United States.

Disopyramide (dye-soe-PEER-a-mide) is used to return irregular heartbeats to a normal rhythm and to slow an overactive heart. This allows the heart to work more efficiently. Disopyramide is available only with your doctor's prescription.

Before Using This Medicine

In order to decide on the best treatment for your medical problem, your doctor should be told:

—if you have ever had any unusual reaction to disopyramide in the past. This medicine should not be taken if you are allergic to it.

—if you are pregnant, if you intend to become pregnant, or if you are breast-feeding an infant. Although disopyramide has not been shown to cause problems, the chance always exists.

—if you have any of the following medical problems:

Difficult urination	Kidney disease
Enlarged prostate	Liver disease
Glaucoma	Myasthenia gravis

—if you are now taking any of the following medicines:

Anticoagulant medicine (blood thinners)	Medicine for angina or blood pressure (such as propranolol) Other heart medicine

Proper Use of This Medicine

Take this medicine exactly as directed by your doctor even though you may feel well. Do not miss any doses and do not take more medicine than ordered.

Do not stop taking this medicine without first checking with your doctor, as stopping dosage suddenly may cause a serious change in heart function.

If you miss a dose of this medicine, take it as soon as possible unless it is within 4 hours of your next scheduled dose. Do not double doses. Instead, go back to your regular dosing schedule. If you have any questions about this, check with your doctor or pharmacist.

Precautions While Using This Medicine

Your doctor should check your progress at regular visits to make sure the medicine is helping your heart properly.

This medicine may cause hypoglycemia (low blood sugar) in some people. Eat or drink a food containing sugar and *call your doctor right away if these symptoms appear:*

Anxiety	Nausea
Chills	Nervousness
Cold sweats	Rapid pulse
Cool, pale skin	Shakiness
Drowsiness	Unusual tiredness or weakness
Excessive hunger	

Dizziness, lightheadedness, or fainting may occur, especially when you get up from a lying or sitting position. This is due to lowered blood pressure. Getting up slowly may help. This effect does not occur often at the doses disopyramide is usually used; however, *make sure you know how you react to this medicine before you drive, use machines, or do other jobs that require you to be alert.* If the problem continues or gets worse, check with your doctor.

Caution—Avoid alcoholic beverages until you have discussed their use with your doctor. Alcohol may make the low blood sugar effect worse and/or increase the possibility of dizziness or fainting.

Your eyes, mouth, and nose may feel very dry while you are taking this medicine, especially during the first few weeks. To help relieve mouth dryness, chew sugarless gum or dissolve bits of ice in your mouth.

Side Effects of This Medicine

Along with its needed effects, a medicine may cause some unwanted effects. Although not all

of these side effects appear very often, when they do occur they may require medical attention. Check with your doctor if any of the following side effects occur:

More common
Difficult urination

Less common

Chest pains	Unexplained short-
Dizziness,	ness of breath
lightheaded-	Unusual change in
ness, or fainting	heartbeat—to
Mental confusion	very fast or very
Muscle weakness	slow
Swelling of ankles	Weight gain (rapid)
and feet	

Rare

Eye pain	Unexplained fever
Mental depression	and sore throat
	Yellowing of eyes
	and skin

Other side effects may occur which usually do not require medical attention. These side effects may go away during treatment as your body adjusts to the medicine. However, check with your doctor if any of the following side effects continue or are bothersome:

More common
Dry mouth

Less common

Bloating—gas	Headache
Blurred vision	Loss of appetite
Constipation	Nervousness
Dry eyes and nose	

Rare

Decreased sexual	Sleeplessness
ability	

Other side effects not listed above may also occur in some patients. If you notice any other effects, check with your doctor.

DISULFIRAM (Systemic)
A commonly used brand name is Antabuse.

Disulfiram (dye-SUL-fi-ram) is used to help overcome your drinking problem. It is not a cure for alcoholism, but rather will discourage you from drinking. Disulfiram is available only with your doctor's prescription.

Before Using This Medicine

In order to decide on the best treatment for your medical problem, your doctor should be told:

—if you have had any allergic reactions to disulfiram, rubber, pesticides, or fungicides.

—if you are pregnant, if you intend to become pregnant, or if you are breast-feeding an infant. Although disulfiram has not been shown to cause problems, the chance always exists.

—if you have any of the following medical problems:

Brain damage	Liver disease or
Diabetes mellitus	cirrhosis of
(sugar diabetes)	the liver
Epilepsy	Severe mental illness
Heart disease	Skin allergy
Kidney disease	Underactive thyroid

—if you are now taking any of the following medicines or types of medicine:

Anticoagulants	Isoniazid
(blood thinners)	Phenytoin

—if you are now taking or have taken within the past several days either of the following medicines:

Metronidazole
Paraldehyde

Proper Use of This Medicine

Before you take the first dose of this medicine, *make sure you have not taken any alcoholic beverage or alcohol-containing product or medicine* (for example, tonics, elixirs, and cough syrups) *during the past 12 hours.* If you are not sure about the alcohol content of medicines you may have taken, check with your doctor or pharmacist.

Take this medicine every day as directed by your doctor. The medicine is usually taken each morning. However, if it makes you drowsy, ask your doctor if you may take it at bedtime instead.

Precautions While Using This Medicine

Do not drink any alcohol, even small amounts, while you are taking this medicine because it may make you very sick. This includes alcohol-containing products or medicines such as elixirs, tonics, sauces, vinegars, cough syrups, mouth washes, or gargles. Also, do not apply to your skin any alcohol-containing liniments or lotions such as rubbing alcohol, back rubs, after-shave lotions, cologne, toilet waters, or after-bath preparations because the alcohol they contain may be absorbed into your body.

Some of the symptoms you may experience if you use any alcohol while taking this medicine are throbbing headache, nausea and vomiting, mental confusion, unusually fast or pounding heartbeat, dizziness or fainting, flushing or redness of face, sweating, troubled breathing, chest pain, weakness, or blurred vision. These symptoms will last as long as there is any alcohol left in your system, from 30 minutes to several hours. If you have a severe reaction or have taken a large enough amount of alcohol, heart attack, unconsciousness, convulsions, and death may occur.

Your doctor may want you to carry an identification card stating that you are using this medicine. This card should list the symptoms most likely to occur if alcohol is taken, and the doctor, clinic, or hospital to be contacted in case of an emergency. These cards may be available from the manufacturer. Ask your doctor or pharmacist if you have any questions about this.

If you will be taking this medicine for a long period of time (for example, for several months at a time), your doctor should check your progress at regular visits.

Before buying or using any liquid prescription or nonprescription medicine, check with your pharmacist to see if it contains any alcohol.

This medicine may cause some people to become drowsy or less alert than they are normally. *Make sure you know how you react to this medicine before you drive, use machines, or do other jobs that require you to be alert.*

Side Effects of This Medicine

Along with its needed effects, a medicine may cause some unwanted effects. Although not all of these side effects appear very often, when they do occur they may require medical attention. Check with your doctor if any of the following side effects occur:

Less common

Eye pain, tenderness, or any change in vision	Numbness, tingling, pain, or weakness in hands or feet
Mood or mental changes	

Rare

Yellowing of eyes or skin

Other side effects may occur which usually do not require medical attention. These side effects may go away during treatment as your body adjusts to the medicine. However, check with your doctor if any of the following side effects continue or are bothersome:

More common

Drowsiness

Less common or rare

Decreased sexual ability	Skin rash
	Stomach discomfort
Headache	Unusual tiredness
Metallic- or garlic-like taste in mouth	

Other side effects not listed above may also occur in some patients. If you notice any other effects, check with your doctor.

DOXAPRAM (Systemic)
A commonly used brand name is Dopram.

Doxapram (DOX-a-pram) is given by injection to stimulate or increase breathing in certain conditions. This medicine is available only with your doctor's prescription.

Before Using This Medicine

In order to decide on the best treatment for your medical problem, your doctor should be told:

—if you have ever had any unusual reaction to doxapram in the past. This medicine should not be used if you are allergic to it.

—if you are pregnant, if you intend to become pregnant, or if you are breast-feeding an infant. Although doxapram has not been shown to cause problems, the chance always exists.

—if you have any of the following medical problems:

Asthma or lung disease	Heart disease
	High blood pressure
Epilepsy	Overactive thyroid

—if you are now taking either of the following medicines or types of medicine:

Amphetamines
Medicine for
  asthma or breath-
  ing problems

—if you are now taking or have taken within the past 2 weeks monoamine oxidase (MAO) inhibitors such as:

Isocarboxazid	Phenelzine
Pargyline	Tranylcypromine

Side Effects of This Medicine

Along with its needed effects, a medicine may cause some unwanted effects. Although not all of these side effects appear very often, when they do occur they may require medical attention. Check with your doctor if any of the following side effects occur:

Less common or rare

Chest pain or tightness in chest	Wheezing or troubled or unusually fast breathing
Redness, swelling, or pain at place of injection	

Possible signs of overdose

Convulsions or seizures	Unusual increase in reflexes
Uncontrolled trembling or movements of the body	

Other side effects may occur which usually do not require medical attention. These side effects may go away during treatment as your body adjusts to the medicine. However, check with your doctor if any of the following side effects continue or are bothersome:

Less common

Coughing	Headache
Diarrhea	Mental confusion
Dizziness or lightheadedness	Nausea or vomiting
	Unusual increase in sweating
Feeling of unusual warmth	Urination problems

Other side effects not listed above may also occur in some patients. If you notice any other effects, check with your doctor.

DOXORUBICIN (Systemic)

Doxorubicin (dox-oh-ROO-bi-sin) belongs to the general group of medicines known as antineoplastics. It is used by injection to treat some kinds of cancer. Doxorubicin is available only with a prescription and is to be administered only by or under the immediate supervision of your doctor.

Before Using This Medicine

Doxorubicin is a very strong medicine. In addition to its helpful effects in treating your medical problem, it has side effects that could be very serious. Before you receive this medicine, be sure that you have discussed the use of it with your doctor.

In order to decide on the best treatment for your medical problem, your doctor should be told:

—if you have ever had any unusual reaction to doxorubicin in the past.

—if you are pregnant or if you intend to have children. This medicine may cause birth defects if either the male or female is taking it at the time of conception or if it is taken during pregnancy. It may also cause permanent sterility after it has been taken for a while. Be sure that you have discussed this with your doctor before taking this medicine.

—if you are breast-feeding an infant. Although doxorubicin has not been shown to cause problems, the chance always exists.

—if you have any of the following medical problems:

Gout	Kidney stones
Heart disease	Liver disease

—if you are taking gout medicine.

—if you have been treated with x-rays or cancer drugs by another doctor.

Proper Use of This Medicine

This medicine is sometimes given together with certain other medicines. If you are using a combination of drugs, it is important that you receive each medicine at the proper time. If you are taking some of these medicines by mouth, ask your doctor, nurse, or pharmacist to help you plan a way to take them at the right time.

This medicine often causes nausea and vomiting. However, it is very important that you continue to receive it, even if you begin to feel ill. Your doctor may prescribe a medicine to relieve stomach upset. If you have any questions about this, check with your doctor.

Doxorubicin causes the urine to turn reddish in color, which may stain clothes. This is not blood. It is perfectly normal and only lasts for 1 or 2 days after each dose is given.

Precautions While Using This Medicine

It is very important that your doctor check your progress at regular visits.

While you are using this medicine, your doctor may want you to drink plenty of fluids and urinate often. This will help prevent kidney problems and keep your kidneys working well. If you have any questions about this, check with your doctor.

Side Effects of This Medicine

Along with its needed effects, a medicine may cause some unwanted effects. Although not all of these side effects appear very often, when they do occur they may require medical attention. Check with your doctor *immediately* if any of the following side effects occur:

More common

Irregular heartbeat	Swelling of feet and lower legs
Shortness of breath	
Sores in the mouth and on the lips	Unexplained fever, chills, or sore throat

Less common

Flank pain	Stomach pain
Joint pain	Unusual bleeding or
Pain at the place	bruising
of injection	

Rare

Skin rash or itching
Wheezing

Other side effects may occur which usually do not require medical attention. These side effects may go away during treatment as your body adjusts to the medicine. However, check with your doctor if any of the following side effects continue or are bothersome:

More common

Loss of hair
Nausea and
vomiting

Less common

Darkening of the	Darkening or
soles, palms, or	redness of the
nails	skin
	Diarrhea

Rare

Sore, red eyes
Watery eyes

This medicine often causes a temporary and total loss of hair. After treatment with doxorubicin has ended, normal hair growth should return.

If doxorubicin accidentally seeps out of the vein into which it is injected, it may damage some tissues and cause scarring. Tell the doctor right away if you notice redness, pain, or swelling at the place of injection.

After you stop using this medicine, it may still produce some side effects that need attention. During this period of time check with your doctor if you notice any of the following side effects:

Dizziness	Swelling of feet and
Drowsiness	lower legs
Headache	Unusual tiredness or
Irregular heartbeat	weakness
Mental confusion	

Other side effects not listed above may also occur in some patients. If you notice any other effects, check with your doctor.

DOXYLAMINE AND PYRIDOXINE (Systemic)
A commonly used brand name is Bendectin.

Doxylamine and pyridoxine (dox-IL-a-meen and peer-i-DOX-een) is a combination medicine used to prevent nausea and vomiting. It is used most often for the nausea and vomiting of pregnancy (morning sickness). This medicine is available only with your doctor's prescription.

Before Using This Medicine

The use of any medicine during pregnancy must be carefully considered. Although doxylamine and pyridoxine combination has not been shown to increase the likelihood of birth defects or other problems, the chance always exists. Therefore, use this medicine only when absolutely necessary. Some women find that eating a few crackers in the morning may relieve morning sickness; also, getting more rest or drinking very hot or very cold drinks may help.

In order to decide on the best treatment for your medical problem, your doctor should be told:

—if you have ever had any unusual reaction to doxylamine or to antihistamines in the past. This medicine should not be taken if you are allergic to it.

—if you are breast-feeding an infant. Doxylamine may pass into the breast milk and cause unwanted effects in the infant.

—if you have any of the following medical problems:

Enlarged prostate	Overactive thyroid
Heart disease	Stomach ulcer
High blood pressure	Urinary tract
Increased eye	blockage
pressure	

—if you are now taking levodopa.

—if you are now taking any central nervous system (CNS) depressants such as:

Antihistamines or	Prescription pain
medicine for hay	medicine
fever, other	Sedatives, tran-
allergies,	quilizers,
or colds	or sleeping
Barbiturates	medicine
Medicine for	Tricyclic an-
seizures	tidepressants
Narcotics	(medicine for
	depression)

—if you are now taking or have taken within the past 2 weeks monoamine oxidase (MAO) inhibitors such as:

Isocarboxazid	Phenelzine
Pargyline	Tranylcypromine

Proper Use of This Medicine

Doxylamine and pyridoxine combination is used to relieve or prevent nausea and vomiting. Take it only as directed. Do not take more of it and do not take it more often than your doctor ordered.

Take this medicine with food or a glass of water or milk to lessen stomach irritation, if necessary.

If you are taking this medicine for the nausea and vomiting of pregnancy:

• Take this medicine at bedtime and swallow the tablets whole. The special coating on the tablet delays the medicine's action until the morning hours. In some cases, your doctor may tell you to take additional doses during the day.

• Remember, it is best to take no medicine during pregnancy unless really necessary. If you have any questions about this, check with your doctor.

Precautions While Using This Medicine

Doxylamine and pyridoxine combination will add to the effects of alcohol and other medicines (CNS depressants) that slow down the nervous system. Some examples of CNS depressants are antihistamines or medicine for hay fever, other allergies, or colds; sedatives, tranquilizers, or sleeping medicine; prescription pain medicine or narcotics; barbiturates; medicine for seizures; tricyclic antidepressants (medicine for depression); or anesthetics, including some dental anesthetics. *Check with your doctor before taking any of the above while you are using this medicine.*

This medicine may cause some people to become drowsy or less alert than they are normally. Even if taken at bedtime, it may cause some people to feel drowsy or less alert on arising. *Make sure you know how you react to this medicine before you drive, use machines, or do other jobs that require you to be alert.*

When taking doxylamine and pyridoxine combination on a regular basis, make sure your doctor knows if you are taking large amounts of aspirin at the same time (as in arthritis). Effects of too much aspirin, such as ringing in the ears, may be covered up by this medicine.

Side Effects of This Medicine

Along with its needed effects, a medicine may cause some unwanted effects. Although not all of these side effects appear very often, when they do occur they may require medical attention. Check with your doctor if any of the following side effects occur:

Rare

Unexplained sore throat and fever	Unusual bleeding or bruising

Unusual weakness
that continues

Other side effects may occur which usually do not require medical attention. These side effects may go away during treatment as your body adjusts to the medicine. However, check with your doctor if they continue or are bothersome:

More common

Drowsiness	Thickening of the bronchial secretions

Less common or rare

Blurred vision	Nervousness, restlessness, or trouble in sleeping
Difficult or painful urination	
Dizziness	Skin rash
Dryness of mouth, nose, and throat	Unusual increase in sweating
Loss of appetite	Unusually fast heartbeat
	Upset stomach or stomach pain

Other side effects not listed above may also occur in some patients. If you notice any other effects, check with your doctor.

DROCODE, PROMETHAZINE, AND APC
(Systemic)

A commonly used brand name is Synalgos-DC.

Drocode (DROE-kode), promethazine (proe-METH-a-zeen), and APC is a combination of pain relievers along with a mild sedative used to calm or relax patients. APC is the short name for aspirin (AS-pir-in), phenacetin (fe-NASS-e-tin), and caffeine (KAF-een). Drocode, promethazine, and APC combination is taken by mouth in the form of capsules and is available only with your doctor's prescription.

Before Using This Medicine

In order to decide on the best treatment for your medical problem, your doctor should be told:

—if you have ever had any unusual reaction to codeine, drocode (dihydrocodeine), promethazine or other phenothiazines, phenacetin, caffeine, or aspirin, other salicylates including methyl salicylate (oil of wintergreen), or other nonsteroidal anti-inflammatory agents such as fenoprofen, ibuprofen, indomethacin, naproxen, oxyphenbutazone, phenylbutazone, sulindac, or tolmetin.

—if you are pregnant or if you intend to become pregnant while using this combination medicine. Too much use of aspirin during the last 3 months of pregnancy may increase the length of pregnancy and may prolong labor. Aspirin taken during the last 2 weeks of pregnancy may cause the baby to have bleeding problems at birth. When phenacetin is used during pregnancy, it may cause side effects in the newborn infant. In addition, although drocode, promethazine, aspirin, phenacetin, or caffeine has not been shown to cause birth defects in humans, the chance always exists.

—if you are breast-feeding an infant. Although drocode, promethazine, aspirin, phenacetin, or caffeine has not been shown to cause problems, the chance always exists.

—if you have any of the following medical problems:

Anemia	Hemophilia or other
Asthma, allergies,	bleeding problems
and nasal polyps	High blood pressure
(history of)	Hodgkin's disease
Brain disease or	Hypoprothrom-
injury	binemia
Colitis	Kidney disease
Emphysema,	Liver disease
asthma, or	Overactive or
chronic lung	underactive
disease	thyroid
Enlarged prostate or	Reye's syndrome
problems with	Ulcer or other
urination	stomach problems
Gallbladder disease	Underactive adrenal
or gallstones	gland (Addison's
Glaucoma	disease)
Glucose-6-	Unusually slow or
phosphate	irregular heart-
dehydrogenase	beat
(G6PD) deficiency	Vitamin K deficiency
Gout	
Heart disease	

—if you are now taking any of the following medicines or types of medicine:

Anticoagulants	Insulin
(blood thinners)	Medicine for epilepsy
Epinephrine	(anticonvulsants)
Gout medicine	Methotrexate
Guanethidine (high	Oral hypoglycemics
blood pressure	(diabetes medicine
medicine)	you take by
Inflammation	mouth)
medicine	Prescription
(for example,	medicine for
arthritis medicine)	stomach cramps
	or spasms

—if you are now taking any of the following medicines that may affect hearing:

Amikacin	Gentamicin
Aspirin or other	Kanamycin
salicylates	Mercaptomerin
Capreomycin	Neomycin
Cephaloridine	Polymyxins
Cephalothin	Streptomycin
Cisplatin	Tobramycin
Ethacrynic acid	Vancomycin
Furosemide	Viomycin

—if you are now taking central nervous system (CNS) depressants such as:

Antihistamines or	Other sedatives,
medicine for hay	tranquilizers, or
fever, other	sleeping medicine
allergies,	Seizure medicine
or colds	Tricyclic an-
Barbiturates	tidepressants
Other narcotics	(medicine for
Other prescription	depression)
pain medicine	

—if you are now taking or have taken within the past 2 weeks monoamine oxidase (MAO) inhibitors such as:

Isocarboxazid	Phenelzine
Pargyline	Tranylcypromine

Proper Use of This Medicine

Take this medicine with food or a full glass (8 ounces) of water or milk to lessen stomach irritation.

Do not use this medicine if it has a strong vinegar-like odor, since this means the aspirin in the product is breaking down. If you have any questions about this, check with your doctor or pharmacist.

Take this medicine only as directed by your doctor. Do not take more of it, do not take it more often, and do not take it for a longer period of time than your doctor ordered. If too much is taken, it may become habit-forming or cause kidney damage.

Keep this medicine out of the reach of children since overdose is very dangerous in young children.

Precautions While Using This Medicine

Check the labels of all over-the-counter (OTC), nonprescription, and prescription medicines you now take. If any contain drocode (dihydrocodeine), aspirin, phenacetin, or promethazine be especially careful, since taking them while taking this medicine may lead to overdose. Also, make sure your doctor knows if you are taking large amounts of aspirin (as in arthritis). Effects of too much aspirin, such as dizziness or ringing in the ears, may be covered up by the promethazine in this medicine. If you have any questions, check with your doctor or pharmacist.

Caution: Diabetics—This medicine contains aspirin and phenacetin which may cause false test results with urine sugar tests. If you have any questions about this, check with your doctor, nurse, or pharmacist, especially if your diabetes is not well controlled.

If you will be taking this medicine for a long period of time (for example, for several months at a time), your doctor should check your progress at regular visits.

This medicine will add to the effects of alcohol and other medicines (CNS depressants) that slow down the nervous system. Some examples of CNS depressants are antihistamines or medicine for hay fever, other allergies, or colds; sedatives, tranquilizers, or sleeping medicine; prescription pain medicine or narcotics; barbiturates; medicine for seizures; tricyclic antidepressants (medicine for depression); or anesthetics, including dental anesthetics. In addition, stomach problems may be more likely to occur if you drink alcoholic beverages while being treated with this medicine. *Check with your doctor before taking any of the above while you are taking this medicine.*

This medicine may cause some people to become drowsy, dizzy, lightheaded, or less alert than they are normally. *Make sure you know how you react to this medicine before you drive, use machines, or do other jobs that require you to be alert.*

Dizziness, lightheadedness, or fainting may occur, especially when you get up from a lying or sitting position. Getting up slowly may help lessen this problem.

The promethazine in this medicine may cause a few people to become more sensitive to sunlight than they are normally. When you first begin taking this medicine, avoid too much sun or too much use of a sunlamp until you see how you react. If you have a severe reaction, check with your doctor.

Nausea may occur, especially after the first couple of doses. This effect usually goes away if you lie down for a while. However, if nausea or vomiting continues, check with your doctor.

Do not take this medicine for 5 days before having any kind of surgery, including dental surgery, unless otherwise directed by your doctor. The aspirin in this product, if taken during this time, may cause bleeding problems.

Side Effects of This Medicine

Along with its needed effects, a medicine may cause some unwanted effects. Although not all of these side effects appear very often, when they do occur they may require medical attention. Check with your doctor if any of the following side effects occur:

Less common

Any loss of hearing	Troubled breathing
Bloody or black tarry stools	Unusually slow heartbeat
Itching or skin rash	Wheezing or tightness
Shortness of breath	in chest
Stomach pain	

Rare

Unexplained fever and sore throat

Possible side effects with long-term use of APC

Bluish-colored fingernails or mucous membranes	Swelling of feet or lower legs
Cloudy urine	Unusual tiredness or weakness

Other side effects may occur which usually do not require medical attention. These side effects may go away during treatment as your body adjusts to the medicine. However, check with your doctor if any of the following side effects continue or are bothersome:

More common

Constipation	Lightheadedness
Dizziness	Nausea or vomiting
Drowsiness	Thickening of the bronchial secretions

Less common or rare

Blurred vision	Nervousness, restlessness, or trouble in sleeping
Difficult or painful urination	
Dryness of mouth, nose, and throat	Redness or flushing of face
Feeling faint	
Frequent urge to urinate	Ringing or buzzing in ear
Headache	Unusual increase in sweating
Indigestion	
Loss of appetite	Unusual tiredness or weakness
	Unusually fast heartbeat

Other side effects not listed above may also occur in some patients. If you notice any other effects, check with your doctor.

EPHEDRINE (Systemic)
Some commonly used brand names are Ectasule Minus and Ephedsol.

Ephedrine (e-FED-rin) is taken by mouth or given by injection to treat bronchial asthma, chronic bronchitis, emphysema, and other lung diseases. It relieves wheezing, shortness of breath, and troubled breathing. This medicine may be used also for the relief of nasal congestion in hay fever or other allergies. Some of these preparations are available only with your doctor's prescription. Others are available without a prescription; however, your doctor may have special instructions on the proper dose of ephedrine for your medical condition.

Before Using This Medicine

In order to decide on the best treatment for your medical problem, your doctor should be told:

—if you have ever had any unusual reaction to medicines like ephedrine such as amphetamines, epinephrine, isoproterenol, metaproterenol, norepinephrine (levarterenol), phenylephrine, phenylpropanolamine, pseudoephedrine, or terbutaline.

—if you are pregnant or if you intend to become pregnant. Although ephedrine has not been shown to cause problems, the chance always exists.

—if you are breast-feeding an infant. Ephedrine passes into the breast milk and may cause unwanted effects in infants of mothers taking this medicine.

—if you have any of the following medical problems:

Diabetes	Heart or blood
Enlarged prostate	vessel disease
Glaucoma	High blood pressure
	Overactive thyroid

—if you are now taking any of the following medicines or types of medicine:

Amphetamines	Medicine for hay
Digitalis glycosides	fever or other
(heart medicine)	allergies (in-
Ergonovine	cluding nose
Guanethidine	drops or sprays)
Medicine for	Methylergonovine
asthma or	Reserpine
breathing prob-	Tricyclic an-
lems	tidepressants
	(medicine for
	depression)

—if you are now taking or have taken within the past 2 weeks monoamine oxidase (MAO) inhibitors such as:

Isocarboxazid	Phenelzine
Pargyline	Tranylcypromine

Proper Use of This Medicine

Take this medicine only as directed. Do not take more of it and do not take it more often than recommended on the label, unless otherwise directed by your doctor.

To help prevent trouble in sleeping, *take the last dose of medicine for each day a few hours before bedtime.* If you have any questions about this, check with your doctor.

If you miss a dose of this medicine and you remember within an hour or so of the missed dose, take it right away. Then go back to your regular dosing schedule. But if you do not remember until later, do not take the missed dose at all and do not double the next one. Instead, go back to your regular dosing schedule. If you have any questions about this, check with your doctor.

If you are taking the extended-release capsule form of this medicine:

• Swallow the capsule whole.

• Do not crush, break, or chew before swallowing.

• If the capsule is too large to swallow, you may mix the contents of the capsule with applesauce, jelly, honey, or syrup and swallow without chewing.

Side Effects of This Medicine

Along with its needed effects, a medicine may cause some unwanted effects. Although not all of these side effects appear very often, when they do occur they may require medical attention. Check with your doctor if any of the following side effects occur:

Rare

Chest pain or irregular heartbeat

With high doses

Hallucinations (seeing, hearing, or feeling things that are not there)	Mood or mental changes

Other side effects may occur which usually do not require medical attention. These side effects may go away during treatment as your body adjusts to the medicine. However, check with your doctor if any of the following side effects continue or are bothersome:

More common

Nervousness	Trouble in sleeping
Restlessness	

Less common

Difficult or painful urination	Trembling
	Troubled breathing
Dizziness or light-headedness	Unusual increase in sweating
Feeling of warmth	Unusual paleness
Headache	Unusually fast or pounding heart-beat
Loss of appetite	
Nausea or vomiting	
	Weakness

Other side effects not listed above may also occur in some patients. If you notice any other effects, check with your doctor.

EPINEPHRINE (Ophthalmic)

This information applies to the following medicines:

Epinephrine (ep-i-NEF-rin)
Epinephryl Borate (ep-i-NEF-rill BOR-ate)

Some commonly used brand names are:	Generic names:
Epifrin	Epinephrine
Epitrate	
Glaucon	
Murocoll	
Mytrate	
Epinal	Epinephryl Borate
Eppy/N	

Ophthalmic epinephrine is used in the eye to treat certain types of glaucoma. It may also be used in eye surgery. This medicine is available only with your doctor's prescription.

Before Using This Medicine

In order to decide on the best treatment for your medical problem, your doctor should be told:

—if you have ever had any unusual reaction to epinephrine in the past. This medicine should not be used if you are allergic to it.

—if you are pregnant, if you intend to become pregnant, or if you are breast-feeding an infant. Although ophthalmic epinephrine has not been shown to cause problems, the chance always exists.

—if you have any of the following medical problems:

Diabetes	High blood pressure
Eye disease	Overactive thyroid
Heart or blood vessel disease	

—if you are now taking any of the following medicines or types of medicine:

Digitalis glycosides (heart medicine)	Tricyclic antidepressants (medicine for depression)

Proper Use of This Medicine

Use this medicine only as directed. Do not use more of it and do not use it more often than your doctor ordered. To do so may increase the chance of too much medicine being absorbed into the body and the chance of side effects.

How to apply this medicine: First, wash hands. With middle finger, apply pressure to the inside corner of the eye (and continue to apply pressure for 1 or 2 minutes after the medicine has been placed in the eye). Tilt head back and with the index finger of the same hand, pull lower eyelid away from eye to form a pouch. Drop the medicine into the pouch and gently close eyes. Do not blink. Keep eyes closed for 1 or 2 minutes to allow the medicine to be absorbed.

To prevent contamination of the eye drops, do not touch the applicator tip to any surface (including the eye) and keep the container tightly closed.

If you miss a dose of this medicine, apply the missed dose as soon as possible. Then go back to your regular dosing schedule. But if it is almost time for your next dose, do not apply the missed dose at all. Instead, apply your next dose at the regularly scheduled time. Then continue with your regular dosing schedule. If you have any questions about this, check with your doctor.

If you are using epinephrine ophthalmic solution:

• Do not use if the solution turns pinkish or brownish in color, or if it becomes cloudy.

If you are using epinephryl borate ophthalmic solution:

• The color of this solution may vary from colorless to amber yellow. Do not use if the solution turns dark brown or becomes cloudy.

Precautions While Using This Medicine

Your doctor should check your eye pressure at regular visits.

Side Effects of This Medicine

Along with its needed effects, a medicine may cause some unwanted effects. Although not all of these side effects appear very often, when they do occur they may require medical attention. Check with your doctor if any of the following side effects occur:

Possible signs of too much medicine being absorbed into the body

Feeling faint	Unusual trembling
Unusual increase in sweating	Unusually fast, irregular, or pounding heartbeat
Unusual paleness	

Other side effects may occur which usually do not require medical attention. These side effects may go away during treatment as your body adjusts to the medicine. However, check with your doctor if any of the following side effects continue or are bothersome:

More common

Browache	Irritation of eye
Headache	Watering of eyes

Less common

Blurred or decreased vision
Eye pain

When you apply this medicine to the eye, some stinging or burning may be expected.

Other side effects not listed above may also occur in some patients. If you notice any other effects, check with your doctor.

EPINEPHRINE (Systemic)

This information applies to the following medicines:

Epinephrine (ep-i-NEF-rin)
Racepinephrine (race-ep-i-NEF-rin)

Some commonly used brand names are:	Generic names:
Adrenalin	Epinephrine
AsthmaHaler	
Bronitin	
Bronkaid	
Medihaler-Epi	
Primatene	

AsthmaNefrin	Racepinephrine
microNEFRIN	
Vaponefrin	

Epinephrine is used in the treatment of bronchial asthma, chronic bronchitis, emphysema, and other lung diseases. It relieves wheezing, shortness of breath, and troubled breathing. Also, epinephrine injection may be used in the emergency treatment of allergic reactions to insect stings, medicines, foods, or other substances. Epinephrine injection and some of the epinephrine inhalation preparations are available only with your doctor's prescription. Other epinephrine inhalation preparations are available without a prescription; however, your doctor may have special instructions on the proper dose of this medicine for your medical condition.

Before Using This Medicine

In order to decide on the best treatment for your medical problem, your doctor should be told:

—if you have ever had any unusual reaction to medicines like epinephrine such as amphetamines, ephedrine, isoproterenol, metaproterenol, norepinephrine, (levarterenol), phenylephrine, phenylpropanolamine, psuedoephedrine, or terbutaline.

—if you are pregnant or if you intend to become pregnant while using this medicine. Use of epinephrine during pregnancy may cause unwanted effects in the baby.

—if you are breast-feeding an infant. Epinephrine passes into the breast milk and may cause unwanted effects in infants of mothers using epinephrine.

—if you have any of the following medical problems:

Brain damage	High blood pressure
Diabetes	Overactive thyroid
Glaucoma	Parkinson's disease
Heart or blood vessel disease	

—if you are now taking any of the following medicines or types of medicine:

Amphetamines	Medicine for asthma or breathing problems
Diabetes medicine you take by mouth	
	Methylergonovine
Digitalis glycosides (heart medicine)	Phenoxybenzamine
	Phentolamine
Ergonovine	Propranolol
Guanethidine	Sedatives or tranquilizers such as phenothiazine medicines
Insulin	
Medicine for angina attacks (for example, nitroglycerin)	
	Tolazoline
	Tricyclic antidepressants (medicine for depression)

Proper Use of This Medicine

Do not use if the solution turns pinkish to brownish in color or if it becomes cloudy.

Use this medicine only as directed. Do not use more of it and do not use it more often than recommended on the label, unless otherwise directed by your doctor. To do so may increase the chance of side effects.

If you are using the inhalation form of this medicine:

• *Do not use this medicine without a doctor's prescription, unless your medical problem has been diagnosed as asthma by a doctor.*

• Some of these preparations may come with patient directions. Read them carefully before using this medicine.

• If you are using this medicine in a nebulizer or in a combination nebulizer and respirator, make sure you understand exactly how to use it. If you have any questions about this, check with your doctor or pharmacist.

• If you are using the inhalation aerosol form of this medicine:

—Keep spray away from the eyes.

—*Do not take more than 2 inhalations of this medicine at any one time,* unless otherwise directed by your doctor. Allow 1 to 2 minutes after the first inhalation to make certain that a second inhalation is necessary.

—Save your applicator. Refill units of this medicine may be available.

—Store away from heat and direct sunlight. Do not puncture, break, or burn the container.

If you are using the injection form of this medicine:

• This medicine is for injection only. If you will be giving yourself the injections, make sure you understand exactly how to give them. If you have any questions about this, check with your doctor.

Precautions While Using This Medicine

Caution: Diabetics—This medicine may cause your blood sugar levels to rise. If you notice a change in the results of your urine sugar test or if you have any questions, check with your doctor.

If you are using the inhalation form of this medicine:

• *If you still have trouble breathing 20 minutes after using this medicine, or if your condition*

gets worse, stop using the medicine and check with your doctor at once.

• Dryness of the mouth and throat may occur after using this medicine. Rinsing the mouth with water after each dose may help prevent the dryness.

Side Effects of This Medicine

Along with its needed effects, a medicine may cause some unwanted effects. Although not all of these side effects appear very often, when they do occur they may require medical attention. Check with your doctor if either of the following side effects occurs:

Rare

Chest pain
Irregular heartbeat

Other side effects may occur which usually do not require medical attention. These side effects may go away during treatment as your body adjusts to the medicine. However, check with your doctor if any of the following side effects continue or are bothersome:

More common with the injection—rare with recommended doses of inhalation

Headache	Unusually fast or
Nervousness	pounding heart-
Restlessness	beat

Less common with the injection—rare with recommended doses of inhalation

Dizziness or light-	Trouble in sleeping
headedness	Troubled breathing
Flushing or redness	Unusual increase in
of face or skin	sweating
Nausea or vomiting	Unusual paleness
Trembling	Weakness

With inhalation only

Coughing or other	Dryness of mouth
bronchial irrita-	and throat
tion (with high	
doses)	

Other side effects not listed above may also occur in some patients. If you notice any other effects, check with your doctor.

ERGOLOID MESYLATES (Systemic)
A commonly used brand name is Hydergine.

Ergoloid mesylates (er-goe-loid MESS-i-lates) are used to treat some changes in mood, dizziness, and other problems that may be due to poor blood circulation to the brain, as well as for some other medical problems. This medicine is different from other ergot alkaloids such as ergotamine and methysergide. It is not useful for treating migraine headache. This medicine is available only with your doctor's prescription.

Before Using This Medicine

In order to decide on the best treatment for your medical problem, your doctor should be told:

—if you have ever had any unusual reaction to ergot alkaloids in the past. This medicine should not be taken if you are allergic to it.

—if you have any of the following medical problems:

Liver disease   Slow pulse
Low blood pressure

—if you are taking medicines containing ergotamine or methysergide for treatment of migraine headaches.

Proper Use of This Medicine

Take this medicine only as directed by your doctor. Do not take more or less of it, and do not take it more often or for a longer period of time than your doctor ordered.

If you miss a dose of this medicine, do not take the missed dose at all and do not double the next one. Instead, go back to your regular dosing schedule. If you have any questions about this, or if you miss more than one dose, check with your doctor.

For patients taking the sublingual (under-the-tongue) tablets:

• Dissolve the tablet under your tongue. The sublingual tablet should not be chewed or swallowed since it works much faster when absorbed through the lining of the mouth. Do not eat, drink, or smoke while a tablet is dissolving.

Precautions While Using This Medicine

It is important that your doctor check your progress at regular visits.

While you are taking this medicine, do not expose your body to very cold temperatures for long periods of time. The medicine may lessen your body's ability to adjust to the cold.

It may take several weeks for this medicine to work. However, *do not stop taking this medicine without first checking with your doctor.*

Side Effects of This Medicine

Along with its needed effects, a medicine may cause some unwanted effects. No serious side effects have been reported for this medicine.

However, the following side effects may occur in some patients. Check with your doctor if they continue or are bothersome, especially since some may indicate that you are taking too much medicine:

Rare

Dizziness or light-headedness when getting up from a lying or sitting position	Loss of appetite
	Nausea and vomiting
	Skin rash
	Soreness under the tongue
Drowsiness	
Fever	Stomach cramps

Signs of overdose

Blurred vision	Flushing
Dizziness	Headache
Fainting	Nasal stuffiness

Other side effects not listed above may also occur in some patients. If you notice any other effects, check with your doctor.

ERGONOVINE (Systemic)

This information applies to the following medicines:

Ergonovine (er-goe-NOE-veen)
Methylergonovine (meth-ill-er-go-NOE-veen)

Some commonly used brand names are:	Generic names:
Ergotrate	Ergonovine
Methergine	Methylergonovine

This medicine is usually given to stop excessive bleeding that sometimes occurs after a baby is delivered. It is available only on prescription and is to be administered only by or under the supervision of your doctor.

Before Using This Medicine

In order to decide on the best treatment for your medical problem, your doctor should be told:

—if you have ever taken ergotamine or methysergide and had an unusual reaction to it. This medicine should not be taken if you are allergic to it.

—if you are breast-feeding an infant. This medicine passes into the breast milk and may cause unwanted effects in infants of mothers taking large doses of it. Be sure you have discussed this with your doctor before taking this medicine.

—if you have any of the following medical problems:

Angina (chest pain)	High blood pressure
Blood vessel disease	Infection
Hardening of the arteries	Kidney disease
	Liver disease

Proper Use of This Medicine

Take this medicine only as directed by your doctor. Do not take more of it, do not take it more often, and do not take it for a longer period of time than your doctor ordered. If too much is taken, it may cause serious effects such as nausea and vomiting; cold, painful hands or feet; or even gangrene.

If you miss a dose of this medicine, do not take the missed dose at all and do not double the next one. Instead, go back to your regular dosing schedule. If you have any questions about this, check with your doctor.

Precautions While Using This Medicine

If you have an infection or illness of any kind, check with your doctor before taking this medicine, since you may be more sensitive to the effects of it.

Side Effects of This Medicine

Along with its needed effects, a medicine may cause some unwanted effects. Although not all of these side effects appear very often, when they do occur they may require medical attention. Check with your doctor if any of the following side effects occur:

Rare

Numb, cold hands or feet	Shortness of breath
	Sudden severe headache

Other side effects may occur which usually do not require medical attention. These side effects may go away during treatment as your body adjusts to the medicine. However, check with your doctor if any of the following side effects continue or are bothersome:

More common

Nausea and vomiting

Less common

Chest pain	Dizziness
Confusion	Ringing in the ears
Cramping	Unusual sweating
Diarrhea	

Other side effects not listed above may also occur in some patients. If you notice any other effects, check with your doctor.

***

ERGOTAMINE (Systemic)
Some commonly used brand names are:

Ergomar	Gynergen
Ergostat	Medihaler
	Ergotamine

Ergotamine (er-GOT-a-meen) is used to treat migraine headaches and some kinds of throbbing headaches. It is not used to prevent headaches, but is used to treat an attack once it has started. This medicine is available only with your doctor's prescription.

Before Using This Medicine

In order to decide on the best treatment for your medical problem, your doctor should be told:

—if you have ever had any unusual reaction to ergotamine in the past. This medicine should not be taken if you are allergic to it.

—if you are pregnant or if you intend to become pregnant while using this medicine. Too much use of ergotamine during pregnancy may cause unwanted effects in the baby. Be sure that you have discussed this with your doctor before taking this medicine. In addition, although ergotamine has not been shown to cause birth defects, the chance always exists.

—if you are breast-feeding an infant. Ergotamine passes into the breast milk and may cause unwanted effects in infants of mothers taking large doses of it. Be sure you have discussed this with your doctor before taking this medicine.

—if you have any of the following medical problems:

Angina	Infection
Hardening of the arteries	Kidney disease
	Liver disease
Heart disease	Problems with veins
High blood pressure	Severe itching

For patients using ergotamine tartrate inhalation aerosol:

In order to decide on the best treatment for your medical problem, your doctor should be told:

—if you have had any unusual reactions to aerosol spray inhalation medicines in the past.

—if you have an infection of the mouth, throat, or lungs.

Proper Use of This Medicine

Take this medicine only as directed by your doctor. If the amount you are to take does not relieve your headache, do not take more than your doctor ordered. Instead, check with your doctor. Taking too much of this medicine or taking it too frequently may cause serious effects such as nausea and vomiting; cold, painful hands or feet; or even gangrene.

This medicine works best if you:

- *Take it at the first sign of headache.*

- *Lie down in a quiet, dark room for at least 2 hours after taking it.*

For patients using the inhalation form of this medicine:

- This medicine usually comes with patient directions. Read them carefully before using this medicine.

- This medicine is used with a special inhaler. Save your inhaler. Refill units of the medicine may be available at lower cost.

- Container provides about 300 measured sprays.

- Store away from heat and direct sunlight. Do not puncture, break, or burn container.

Precautions While Using This Medicine

If you have been taking this medicine regularly, *do not stop taking it without first checking with your doctor.* Your doctor may want you to reduce gradually the amount you are using before stopping completely. If you stop taking it suddenly, your headaches may return or worsen.

Since drinking alcoholic beverages may make headaches worse, it is best to avoid alcohol while you are suffering from them. If you have any questions about this, check with your doctor.

Since smoking may increase some of the harmful effects of this medicine, it is best to avoid smoking while you are using it. If you have any questions about this, check with your doctor.

Avoid prolonged exposure to very cold temperatures while you are using this medicine, since cold may increase the harmful effects of the medicine.

If you have an infection or illness of any kind, check with your doctor before taking this medicine, since you may be more sensitive to the effects of it.

For patients using the inhalation form of this medicine:

- If signs of a mouth, throat, or lung infection occur, if your condition gets worse, or if your symptoms do not improve, check with your doctor.

- Cough, hoarseness, or throat irritation may occur. Gargling and rinsing your mouth after each dose may help prevent the hoarseness and irritation; however, check with your doctor if these or any other side effects continue or are bothersome.

Side Effects of This Medicine

Along with its needed effects, a medicine may cause some unwanted effects. Although not all of these side effects appear very often, when they do occur they may require medical attention. Check with your doctor *immediately* if any of the following side effects occur:

Extreme thirst	Red or violet
Numbness and	blisters on skin
tingling of	of hands or feet
fingers, toes, or	Stomach pain or
face	bloating

Check with your doctor also if the following side effects occur:

More common

Itching	Pale or cold hands
Pain in arms, legs,	or feet
or lower back	Swelling
	Weakness in the
	legs

Uncommon or rare

Anxiety or confu-	Unusually fast or
sion	slow
Changes in vision	heartbeat
Chest pain	

Other side effects may occur which usually do not require medical attention. These side effects may go away during treatment as your body adjusts to the medicine. However, check with your doctor if any of the following side effects continue or are bothersome:

More common

Diarrhea	Headache
Dizziness	Nausea and
	vomiting

After you stop using this medicine, your body may need time to adjust. The length of time this takes depends on the amount of medicine you were using and how long you used it. During this period of time check with your doctor if your headaches begin again or worsen.

Other side effects not listed above may also occur in some patients. If you notice any other effects, check with your doctor.

ERGOTAMINE, BELLADONNA ALKALOIDS, AND PHENOBARBITAL
(Systemic)

Some commonly used brand names are Bellergal and Bellergal-S.

Ergotamine (er-GOT-a-meen), belladonna alkaloids (bell-a-DON-a AL-ka-loids), and phenobarbital (feen-oh-BAR-bi-tal) is a combination medicine used for a variety of problems including menstrual and stomach problems and some kinds of throbbing headaches. It is available only with your doctor's prescription.

Before Using This Medicine

In order to decide on the best treatment for your medical problem, your doctor should be told:

—if you have ever had an unusual reaction to ergot medicines, atropine, belladonna, or barbiturates. This medicine should not be taken if you are allergic to it.

—if you are pregnant or if you intend to become pregnant while using this medicine. Too much use of it during pregnancy may cause unwanted effects in the baby. Be sure that you have discussed this with your doctor before taking this medicine. In addition, although this medicine has not been shown to cause birth defects, the chance always exists.

—if you are breast-feeding an infant. This medicine passes into the breast milk and may cause unwanted effects in infants of mothers taking large doses of it. Be sure you have discussed this with your doctor before taking this medicine.

—if you have any of the following medical problems:

Angina	High blood pressure
Asthma (or history	(severe)
of), emphysema,	Infection
or chronic lung	Intestinal disease
disease	Kidney disease
Blood vessel disease	Liver disease
Brain damage (in	Porphyria
children)	Prostate enlarge-
Difficult urination	ment
Glaucoma	Severe itching
Hardening of the	Spastic paralysis (in
arteries	children)
Heart disease	Underactive adrenal
	gland

—if you are now taking any of the following medicines or types of medicine:

Amantadine	Anticoagulants
Antacids	(blood thinners)

Corticosteroids	Haloperidol
(cortisone-like	Medicine for diar-
medicine)	rhea
Digitalis or digitox-	Medicine for in-
in (heart	testinal or
medicine)	stomach cramping
Doxycycline or	Medicine for
other tetracyclines	Parkinson's
Griseofulvin (fungus	disease
medicine)	Phenothiazines (like
	chlorpromazine)
	Ulcer medicine

—if you are now taking any other central nervous system (CNS) depressants such as:

Antihistamines or	Prescription pain
medicine for hay	medicine
fever, other	Sedatives, tran-
allergies,	quilizers, or
or colds	sleeping medicine
Medicine for	Tricyclic an-
seizures	tidepressants
Narcotics	(medicine for
Other barbiturates	depression)

—if you are now taking or have taken within the past 2 weeks monoamine oxidase (MAO) inhibitors such as:

Isocarboxazid	Phenelzine
Pargyline	Tranylcypromine

Proper Use of This Medicine

Take this medicine only as directed by your doctor. If the amount you are to take does not seem to work, do not take more than your doctor ordered. Instead, check with your doctor. Taking too much of this medicine or taking it too frequently may cause serious effects such as nausea and vomiting; cold, painful hands or feet; or even gangrene. Also, if too much is used, it may become habit-forming.

Keep this medicine out of the reach of children since overdose is especially dangerous in children.

If you miss a dose of this medicine, do not take the missed dose at all and do not double the next one. Instead, go back to your regular dosing schedule. If you have any questions about this, check with your doctor.

Precautions While Using This Medicine

If you have been taking this medicine regularly, *do not stop taking it without first checking with your doctor.* Your doctor may want you to reduce gradually the amount you are using before stopping completely.

This medicine will add to the effects of alcohol and other medicines (CNS depressants) that slow down the nervous system. Some examples of

CNS depressants are antihistamines or medicine for hay fever, other allergies, or colds; sedatives, tranquilizers, or sleeping medicine; prescription pain medicine or narcotics; barbiturates; medicine for seizures; tricyclic antidepressants (medicine for depression); or anesthetics, including some dental anesthetics. *Check with your doctor before taking any of the above while you are taking this medicine.*

This medicine may cause some people to become drowsy, dizzy, or less alert than they are normally. *Make sure you know how you react to this medicine before you drive, use machines, or do other jobs that require you to be alert.*

Since smoking may increase some of the harmful effects of this medicine, it is best to avoid smoking while you are using it. If you have any questions about this, check with your doctor.

Avoid prolonged exposure to very cold temperatures while you are using this medicine, since cold may increase the harmful effects of the medicine.

If you have an infection or illness of any kind, check with your doctor before taking this medicine, since you may be more sensitive to the effects of it.

Do not take antacid or medicine for diarrhea within 1 hour of taking this medicine. Taking them too close together will make the belladonna less effective.

This medicine may cause your eyes to become more sensitive to light than they are normally. Wearing sunglasses may help lessen the discomfort from bright light.

Belladonna alkaloids will often make you sweat less, causing your body temperature to increase. *Use extra care not to become overheated during exercise or hot weather while you are taking this medicine,* as overheating could possibly result in heat stroke.

Your mouth, nose, and throat may feel very dry while you are taking this medicine. To help relieve mouth dryness, chew sugarless gum or dissolve bits of ice in your mouth.

Side Effects of This Medicine

Along with its needed effects, a medicine may cause some unwanted effects. Although not all of these side effects appear very often, when they do occur they may require medical attention. Check with your doctor *immediately* if any of the following side effects occur:

Blurred vision	Mental confusion,
Extreme drowsiness,	especially in the
or irritability	elderly
Extreme thirst	Mental depression
Fever	Numbness and
Flushing of skin	tingling of
Hallucinations (see-	fingers, toes,
ing, hearing, or	or face
feeling things	Rapid heartbeat
that are not	Shortness of breath
there)	or troubled
	breathing
	Stomach pain or
	bloating

Check with your doctor also if any of the following side effects occur:

More common

Pain in arms, legs,	Swelling of feet
or lower back	and lower legs
Pale or cold hands	Unusual excitement
or feet	Weakness in the
Skin rash or	legs
itching	

Less common or rare

Chest pain	Yellowing of eyes or
	skin

Other side effects may occur which usually do not require medical attention. These side effects may go away during treatment as your body adjusts to the medicine. However, check with your doctor if any of the following side effects continue or are bothersome:

More common

Clumsiness or	Dizziness or light-
unsteadiness	headedness
Constipation	Drowsiness
	"Hangover" effect
	Headache

Less common

Decreased sexual	Nausea and
ability	vomiting
Difficult urination	Nervousness
Dryness of mouth	Reduced sense of
or skin	taste
Increased sensitivity	Reduced sweating
of eyes to	
sunlight	

After you stop taking this medicine, your body may need time to adjust. The length of time this takes depends on the amount of medicine you were taking and how long you took it. During this period of time check with your doctor if your headaches begin again or worsen.

Other side effects not listed above may also occur in some patients. If you notice any other effects, check with your doctor.

ERGOTAMINE AND CAFFEINE (Systemic)
Some commonly used brand names are:

Cafergot	Ergocaffein
Cafermine	Lanatrate
Cafetrate	Migrastat
Ergocaf	

Ergotamine (er-GOT-a-meen) and caffeine (KAF-een) is a combination medicine used to treat migraine headaches and some kinds of throbbing headaches. It is not used to prevent headaches, but is used to treat an attack once it has started. This medicine is available only with your doctor's prescription.

Before Using This Medicine

In order to decide on the best treatment for your medical problem, your doctor should be told:

—if you have ever had any unusual reaction to ergotamine in the past. This medicine should not be taken if you are allergic to it.

—if you are pregnant or if you intend to become pregnant while using this medicine. Too much use of it during pregnancy may cause unwanted effects in the baby. Be sure that you have discussed this with your doctor before taking this medicine. In addition, although this medicine has not been shown to cause birth defects, the chance always exists.

—if you are breast-feeding an infant. This medicine passes into the breast milk and may cause unwanted effects in infants of mothers taking large doses of it. Be sure you have discussed this with your doctor before taking this medicine.

—if you have any of the following medical problems:

Angina	Infection
Blood vessel disease	Kidney disease
Hardening of the arteries	Liver disease
	Severe itching
Heart disease	Stomach ulcer
High blood pressure	

Proper Use of This Medicine

Take this medicine only as directed by your doctor. If the amount you are to take does not relieve your headache, do not take more than your doctor ordered. Instead, check with your doctor. Taking too much of this medicine or taking it too often may cause serious effects such as nausea and vomiting; cold, painful hands or feet; or even gangrene.

This medicine works best if you:

• *Take it at the first sign of headache or migraine attack.*

• *Lie down in a quiet, dark room for at least 2 hours after taking it.*

For patients using the rectal suppository form of this medicine:

• How to insert suppository: First remove the foil wrapper and moisten the suppository with water. Lie down on side and push the suppository well up into rectum with finger. If suppository is too soft to insert because of storage in a warm place, before removing the foil wrapper chill the suppository in the refrigerator for 30 minutes or run cold water over it.

Precautions While Using This Medicine

If you have been taking this medicine regularly, *do not stop taking it without first checking with your doctor.* Your doctor may want you to reduce gradually the amount you are using before stopping completely. If you stop taking it suddenly, your headaches may return or worsen.

Since drinking alcoholic beverages may make headaches worse, it is best to avoid alcohol while you are suffering from them. If you have any questions about this, check with your doctor.

Since smoking may increase some of the harmful effects of this medicine, it is best to avoid smoking while you are using it. If you have any questions about this, check with your doctor.

Avoid prolonged exposure to very cold temperatures while you are using this medicine, since cold may increase the harmful effects of the medicine.

If you have an infection or illness of any kind, check with your doctor before taking this medicine, since you may be more sensitive to the effects of it.

Side Effects of This Medicine

Along with its needed effects, a medicine may cause some unwanted effects. Although not all of these side effects appear very often, when they do occur they may require medical attention. Check with your doctor *immediately* if any of the following side effects occur:

Extreme thirst	Red or violet blisters on skin of hands or feet
Numbness and tingling of fingers, toes, or face	
	Stomach pain or bloating

Check with your doctor also if the following side effects occur:

More common

Itching	Pale or cold hands
Pain in arms, legs,	or feet
or lower back	Swelling of feet and
	lower legs
	Weakness in the legs

Less common or rare

Anxiety or confu-	Chest pain
sion	Unusually fast or
Changes in vision	slow heartbeat

Other side effects may occur which usually do not require medical attention. These side effects may go away during treatment as your body adjusts to the medicine. However, check with your doctor if any of the following side effects continue or are bothersome:

More common

Diarrhea	Headache
Dizziness	Nausea and
	vomiting

After you stop using this medicine, your body may need time to adjust. The length of time this takes depends on the amount of medicine you were using and how long you used it. During this period of time check with your doctor if your headaches begin again or worsen.

Other side effects not listed above may also occur in some patients. If you notice any other effects, check with your doctor.

ERGOTAMINE, CAFFEINE, BELLADONNA ALKALOIDS, AND PENTOBARBITAL
(Systemic)
A commonly used brand name is Cafergot-PB.

Ergotamine (er-GOT-a-meen), caffeine (KAF-een), belladonna alkaloids (bell-a-DON-a AL-ka-loids), and pentobarbital (pen-toe-BAR-bi-tal) is a combination medicine used as needed to treat migraine headaches and some kinds of throbbing headaches. It is not used to prevent headaches, but is used to treat an attack once it has started. It is available only with your doctor's prescription.

Before Using This Medicine

In order to decide on the best treatment for your medical problem, your doctor should be told:

—if you have ever had an unusual reaction to atropine, belladonna, barbiturates, or ergot medicines in the past. This medicine should not be taken if you are allergic to it.

—if you are pregnant or if you intend to become pregnant while using this medicine. Too much use of it during pregnancy may cause unwanted effects in the baby. Be sure that you have discussed this with your doctor before taking this medicine. In addition, although this medicine has not been shown to cause birth defects, the chance always exists.

—if you are breast-feeding an infant. This medicine passes into the breast milk and may cause unwanted effects in infants of mothers taking large doses of it. Be sure you have discussed this with your doctor before taking this medicine.

—if you have any of the following medical problems:

Angina	High blood pressure
Asthma (or history	Infection
of), emphysema,	Intestinal disease
or chronic lung	Kidney disease
disease	Liver disease
Blood vessel disease	Prostate enlarge-
Brain damage	ment
(children)	Severe itching
Difficult urination	Spastic paralysis
Glaucoma	(children)
Hardening of the	Stomach ulcer
arteries	Underactive adrenal
Heart disease	gland

—if you are now taking any of the following medicines or types of medicine:

Amantadine	Doxycycline or
Antacids	other tetracyclines
Anticoagulants	Griseofulvin (fungus
(blood thinners)	medicine)
Corticosteroids	Medicine for diar-
(cortisone-like	rhea
medicine)	Medicine for
Digitalis or digitox-	Parkinson's
in (heart	disease
medicine)	Medicine for in-
	testinal or
	stomach cramping
	Ulcer medicine

—if you are now taking any other central nervous system (CNS) depressants such as:

Antihistamines or	Prescription pain
medicine for hay	medicine
fever, other	Sedatives, tran-
allergies,	quilizers,
or colds	or sleeping
Medicine for	medicine
seizures	Tricyclic an-
Narcotics	tidepressants
Other barbiturates	(medicine for
	depression)

—if you are now taking or have taken within

the past 2 weeks monoamine oxidase (MAO) inhibitors such as:

Isocarboxazid	Phenelzine
Pargyline	Tranylcypromine

Proper Use of This Medicine

Take this medicine only as directed by your doctor. If the amount you are to take does not relieve your headache, do not take more than your doctor ordered. Instead, check with your doctor. Taking too much of this medicine or taking it too often may cause serious effects such as nausea and vomiting; cold, painful hands or feet; or even gangrene. Also, if too much is used, it may become habit-forming.

Keep this medicine out of the reach of children since overdose is especially dangerous in children.

This medicine works best if you:
• *Take it at the first sign of headache or migraine attack.*

• *Lie down in a quiet, dark room for at least 2 hours after taking it.*

For patients using the rectal suppository form of this medicine:

• How to insert suppository—First remove the foil wrapper and moisten the suppository with water. Lie down on side and push the suppository well up into rectum with finger. If suppository is too soft to insert because of storage in a warm place, before removing the foil wrapper chill the suppository in the refrigerator for 30 minutes or run cold water over it.

Precautions While Using This Medicine

If you have been taking this medicine regularly, *do not stop taking it without first checking with your doctor.* Your doctor may want you to reduce gradually the amount you are using before stopping completely. If you stop using it suddenly, your headaches may return or worsen.

This medicine will add to the effects of alcohol and other medicines (CNS depressants) that slow down the nervous system. Some examples of CNS depressants are antihistamines or medicine for hay fever, other allergies, or colds; sedatives, tranquilizers, or sleeping medicine; prescription pain medicine or narcotics; barbiturates; medicine for seizures; tricyclic antidepressants (medicine for depression); or anesthetics, including dental anesthetics. *Check with your doctor before*

taking any of the above while you are taking this medicine.

This medicine may cause some people to become drowsy, dizzy, or less alert than they are normally. *Make sure you know how you react to this medicine before you drive, use machines, or do other jobs that require you to be alert.*

Since smoking may increase some of the harmful effects of this medicine, it is best to avoid smoking while you are using it. If you have any questions about this, check with your doctor.

Avoid prolonged exposure to very cold temperatures while you are using this medicine, since cold may increase the harmful effects of the medicine.

If you have an infection or illness of any kind, check with your doctor before taking this medicine, since you may be more sensitive to the effects of it.

Do not take antacid or medicine for diarrhea within 1 hour of taking this medicine. Taking them too close together will make the belladonna less effective.

This medicine may cause your eyes to become more sensitive to light than they are normally. Wearing sunglasses may help lessen the discomfort from bright light.

Belladonna alkaloids will often make you sweat less, causing your body temperature to increase. *Use extra care not to become overheated during exercise or hot weather while you are taking this medicine,* as overheating could possibly result in heat stroke.

Your mouth, nose, and throat may feel very dry while you are taking this medicine. To help relieve mouth dryness, chew sugarless gum or dissolve bits of ice in your mouth.

Side Effects of This Medicine

Along with its needed effects, a medicine may cause some unwanted effects. Although not all of these side effects appear very often, when they do occur they may require medical attention. Check with your doctor *immediately* if any of the following side effects occur:

Blurred vision	Hallucinations (see-
Extreme drowsiness	ing, hearing, or
or irritability	feeling things
Extreme thirst	that are not
Fever	there)
Flushing of skin	

Mental confusion, especially in the elderly
Mental depression
Numbness and tingling of fingers, toes, or face
Rapid heartbeat

Red or violet blisters on skin of hands or feet
Shortness of breath or troubled breathing
Stomach pain or bloating

Check with your doctor also if any of the following side effects occur:

More common

Pain in arms, legs, or lower back
Pale or cold hands or feet
Skin rash or itching

Swelling of feet and lower legs
Unusual excitement
Weakness in the legs

Less common or rare

Chest pain

Yellowing of eyes or skin

Other side effects may occur which usually do not require medical attention. These side effects may go away during treatment as your body adjusts to the medicine. However, check with your doctor if any of the following side effects continue or are bothersome:

More common

Clumsiness or unsteadiness
Constipation
Dizziness or lightheadedness
Drowsiness

Dryness of mouth or skin
"Hangover" effect
Headache
Reduced sweating

Less common

Decreased sexual ability
Difficult urination
Increased sensitivity of eyes to sunlight

Nausea and vomiting
Nervousness
Reduced sense of taste

After you stop taking this medicine, your body may need time to adjust. The length of time this takes depends on the amount of medicine you were taking and how long you took it. During this period of time check with your doctor if your headaches begin again or worsen.

Other side effects not listed above may also occur in some patients. If you notice any other effects, check with your doctor.

ERYTHROMYCIN (Ophthalmic)
A commonly used brand name is Ilotycin.

Erythromycin (eh-rith-roe-MYE-sin) belongs to the general family of medicines called antibiotics. Erythromycin ophthalmic preparations are used to help the body overcome infections of the eye. They are available only with your doctor's prescription.

Before Using This Medicine

In order to decide on the best treatment for your medical problem, your doctor should be told:

—if you have had allergic reactions to any of the other erythromycins.

—if you are pregnant, if you intend to become pregnant, or if you are breast-feeding an infant, although erythromycin ophthalmic preparations have not been shown to cause problems.

Proper Use of This Medicine

To prevent contamination of the eye ointment, do not touch the applicator tip to any surface (including the eye). After using, wipe the tip of the ointment tube with a clean tissue and keep the tube tightly closed.

How to apply this medicine: First, wash hands. Then pull the lower eyelid away from eye to form a pouch. Squeeze a thin strip of ointment into the pouch. A 1-cm (approximately 1/3-inch) strip of ointment is usually enough unless otherwise directed by your doctor. Gently close eyes and keep them closed for 1 or 2 minutes to allow medicine to come into contact with the infection.

To help clear up your infection completely, *keep using this medicine for the full time of treatment,* even though your symptoms may have disappeared; *do not miss any doses.*

If you do miss a dose of this medicine, apply it as soon as possible. However, if it is almost time for your next application, skip the missed dose and go back to your regular dosing schedule.

Precautions While Using This Medicine

After application, eye ointments usually cause your vision to blur for a few minutes.

If your symptoms do not improve within a few days or if they become worse, check with your doctor.

Side Effects of This Medicine

There have not been any common or important side effects reported with this medicine. However, if you notice any side effects, check with your doctor.

ERYTHROMYCIN (Topical)
A commonly used brand name is Ilotycin.

Erythromycin (eh-rith-roe-MYE-sin) belongs to the general family of medicines called antibiotics. Erythromycin topical preparations are used to help the body overcome infections of the skin. Erythromycin is available only with your doctor's prescription.

Before Using This Medicine

In order to decide on the best treatment for your medical problem, your doctor should be told:

—if you have had allergic reactions to any of the other erythromycins.

—if you are pregnant, if you intend to become pregnant, or if you are breast-feeding an infant, although erythromycin topical preparations have not been shown to cause problems.

—if you are now using clindamycin (topical).

Proper Use of This Medicine

Before applying this medicine, wash the area to be treated with soap and water, and dry thoroughly.

To help clear up your infection completely, *keep using this medicine for the full time of treatment,* even though your symptoms may have disappeared; *do not miss any doses.*

If you do miss a dose of this medicine, apply it as soon as possible. However, if it is almost time for your next application, skip the missed dose and go back to your regular dosing schedule.

Precautions While Using This Medicine

If there is no improvement in your skin problem after using this medicine for 1 week or if it becomes worse, check with your doctor.

Side Effects of This Medicine

There have not been any common or important side effects reported with this medicine. However, if you notice any effects, check with your doctor.

ERYTHROMYCINS (Systemic)

Some commonly used brand names are:	Generic names:
E-Mycin	
Erythromid*	
Ilotycin	
Novorythro*	Erythromycin
Robimycin	
RP-Mycin	

Ilosone	Erythromycin Estolate
E.E.S. E-Mycin E Pediamycin Wyamycin E	Erythromycin Ethylsuccinate
Ilotycin	Erythromycin Gluceptate
Erythrocin	Erythromycin Lactobionate
Bristamycin Erypar Erythrocin Ethril Pfizer-E SK-Erythromycin Wyamycin S	Erythromycin Stearate

*Not available in the United States.

Erythromycins (eh-rith-roe-MYE-sins) belong to the general family of medicines called antibiotics. They are given by mouth or by injection to help the body overcome infections. Erythromycins are also used to prevent "strep" infections in patients with a history of rheumatic heart disease who may be allergic to penicillin. They may also be used in Legionnaires' disease. Erythromycins are available only with your doctor's prescription.

Before Using This Medicine

In order to decide on the best treatment for your medical problem, your doctor should be told:

—if you have had allergic reactions to any of the erythromycins.

—if you are pregnant, if you intend to become pregnant, or if you are breast-feeding an infant, although erythromycins have not been shown to cause problems.

—if you have liver disease.

—if you are now taking any of the following medicines or types of medicine:

Aminophylline	Oxtriphylline
Clindamycin	Penicillins
Lincomycin	Theophylline

—if you have had any problems with this medicine in the past (erythromycin estolate).

Proper Use of This Medicine

Generally, erythromycins are best taken with a full glass (8 ounces) of water on an empty stomach (for example, 1 hour before or 3 to 4 hours after meals), unless otherwise directed by your doctor. However, certain brands of erythromycin enteric-coated tablets, as well as erythromycin estolate and erythromycin ethylsuccinate, may be taken without regard to meals. In addition, certain brands of erythromycin stearate tablets may be taken on an empty stomach or immediately before meals. If you have any questions about this, check with your doctor or pharmacist.

If you are taking the liquid form of this medicine:

• This medicine is to be taken by mouth even though it may come in a dropper bottle. If this medicine does not come in a dropper bottle, use a specially marked measuring spoon or other device to measure each dose accurately since the average household teaspoon may not hold the right amount of liquid.

If you are taking the chewable tablet form of this medicine:

• Tablets must be chewed or crushed before they are swallowed.

If you are taking the enteric-coated tablet form of this medicine:

• Swallow tablets whole. Do not break or crush. If you are not sure about the tablet you are taking, check with your pharmacist.

To help clear up your infection completely, *keep taking this medicine for the full time of treatment* even if you begin to feel better after a few days; *do not miss any doses.* This is especially important if you have a "strep" infection since serious heart problems could develop later if your infection is not completely cleared up.

If you do miss a dose of this medicine, take it as soon as possible. However, if it is almost time for your next dose and your dosing schedule is:

• 2 doses a day—Space the missed dose and the next dose 5 to 6 hours apart.

• 3 or more doses a day—Space the missed dose and the next dose 2 to 4 hours apart or double your next dose.

Then go back to your regular dosing schedule.

Precautions While Using This Medicine

If your symptoms do not improve within a few days or if they become worse, check with your doctor.

If this medicine causes dark or amber urine, pale stools, stomach pain, unusual tiredness or weakness, or yellowing of eyes or skin, stop taking it and check with your doctor immediately.

Side Effects of This Medicine

Along with its needed effects, a medicine may cause some unwanted effects. Although not all of these side effects appear very often, when they do occur they may require medical attention. Stop taking this medicine and check with your doctor *immediately* if any of the following side effects occur:

Less common with erythromycin estolate (rare with other erythromycins)

Dark or amber urine	Unusual tiredness or weakness
Pale stools	Yellowing of eyes or skin
Stomach pain	

Other side effects may occur which usually do not require medical attention. These side effects may go away during treatment as your body adjusts to the medicine. However, check with your doctor if any of the following side effects continue or are bothersome:

Less common with all erythromycins

Diarrhea	Stomach cramping and discomfort
Nausea	
Sore mouth or tongue	Vomiting

Other side effects not listed above may also occur in some patients. If you notice any other effects, check with your doctor.

ESTROGENS (Systemic)

This information applies to the following medicines:

Chlorotrianisene (klor-oh-trye-AN-i-seen)
Diethylstilbestrol (dye-eth-il-stil-BESS-trole)
Estradiol (ess-tra-DYE-ole)
Conjugated Estrogens (ESS-troe-jenz)
Esterified Estrogens
Estrone
Estropipate (ess-troe-PI-pate)
Ethinyl Estradiol (ETH-in-il ess-tra-DYE-ole)
Quinestrol (quin-ESS-trole)

Some commonly used brand names and other names are:	Generic names:
TACE	Chlorotrianisene
DES Stilphostrol	Diethylstilbestrol
Delestrogen Estrace	Estradiol

Progynon

Premarin	Conjugated Estrogens
Amnestrogen	Esterified Estrogens
Theelin	Estrone
Ogen Piperazine Estrone Sulfate	Estropipate
Estinyl Feminone	Ethinyl Estradiol
Estrovis	Quinestrol

Estrogens (ESS-troe-jenz) are often called female hormones. They are produced by the body and are necessary for the normal sexual development of the female and for the regulation of the menstrual cycle during the childbearing years.

Estrogens are prescribed for several reasons:

—for the proper regulation of the menstrual cycle

—to prevent pregnancy when used as birth control pills

—in the treatment of selected cases of breast cancer

—to provide additional hormone when the body does not produce enough of its own, as during the menopause or following certain kinds of surgery

—in the treatment of men suffering from certain kinds of breast cancer or cancer of the prostate

Estrogens are usually taken by mouth as tablets or capsules because this method is easier and less costly than injection. However, to suit the individual needs of the patient, they are sometimes given by injection intravenously to produce a rapid effect, or intramuscularly for a more lasting effect.

There is no medical evidence to support the belief that the use of estrogens will keep the patient feeling young, keep the skin soft, or delay the appearance of wrinkles. Nor has it been proven that the use of estrogens during the menopause will relieve emotional and nervous symptoms.

Estrogens are available only with your doctor's prescription.

Before Using This Medicine

In using estrogens, the following points should be kept in mind:

• Estrogens are very useful medicines. However, in addition to their helpful effects in treating your medical problem, they sometimes have side effects that could be very serious. A paper called "Information for the Patient" is given to you with your prescription. Read this carefully.

• The prolonged use of estrogens has been reported to increase the risk of endometrial cancer (cancer of the uterus lining) in women after the menopause. This risk seems to increase the longer estrogens are taken and the higher their dose. The risk is greatly reduced when lower doses are used and when they are used for no more than 3 out of every 4 weeks. When estrogens are used in this manner for less than 1 year, there is less risk.

Note: If the uterus has been removed by surgery (total hysterectomy), there is no risk of endometrial cancer.

In order to decide on the best treatment for your medical problem, your doctor should be told:

—if you have ever had any unusual reaction to estrogens in the past. This medicine should not be taken if you are allergic to it.

—if you are pregnant or if you intend to become pregnant. Estrogens may cause birth defects if taken during pregnancy. Also, daughters of women who took diethylstilbestrol (DES) during pregnancy have developed unwanted changes in reproductive organs; and in rare cases, cancer of the vagina and/or uterine cervix has developed after childbearing age has been reached.

—if you are breast-feeding an infant. Estrogens pass into the breast milk and may cause unwanted effects in infants of mothers taking this medicine.

—if you have any of the following medical problems:

Asthma	Kidney disease
Blood clots (or history of)	Liver disease (such as jaundice or
Cancer (or history of)	porphyria)
	Lumps in breasts
Changes in vaginal bleeding	Mental depression Migraine headaches
Diabetes	Stroke (or history
Endometriosis	of)
Epilepsy	Thyroid disease
Gallbladder disease	Tumors or growths
Heart or circulation disease	in uterus (not cancerous)
High blood pressure	

—if you are now taking any of the following medicines or types of medicine:

Carbamazepine	Phenobarbital
Oral anticoagulants (blood thinners you take by mouth)	Phenytoin Primidone Rifampin

Tricyclic anti-
depressants
(medicine
for depression)

Proper Use of This Medicine

Take this medicine only as directed by your doctor. Do not take more of it and do not take it for a longer period of time than your doctor ordered. Try to take the medicine at the same time each day to reduce the possibility of side effects and to allow it to work better.

Nausea may occur during the first few weeks after you start taking this medicine. This effect usually disappears with continued use. If the nausea is bothersome, it can usually be prevented or reduced by taking each dose with food or immediately after food.

If you miss a dose of this medicine, take it as soon as possible. If it is almost time for your next dose, do not take the missed dose at all and do not double the next one. Instead, go back to your regular dosing schedule. If you have any questions about this, check with your doctor.

Precautions While Using This Medicine

It is very important that your doctor check your progress at regular visits. These visits will usually be every 6 to 12 months, unless your doctor requires them more often.

Tell the doctor or dentist in charge that you are taking this medicine before any kind of surgery (including dental surgery) or emergency treatment, since this medicine may change your blood-clotting ability.

While taking this medicine, use caution during exposure to the sun or sunlamps. Some people may find that their skin will sunburn more easily. Also, they may develop brown, blotchy spots on exposed areas. These spots usually disappear gradually when the medicine is stopped.

If you suspect that you may have become pregnant, stop taking the medicine immediately and check with your doctor. Continued use of this medicine during pregnancy may cause birth defects in the child. It may also increase the risk of vaginal cancer developing in daughters when they reach childbearing age.

Do not give this medicine to anyone else. Your doctor has prescribed it only for you after studying your health record and the results of your physical examination. Estrogens may be dangerous for other people because of differences in their health and body make-up.

Side Effects of This Medicine

Along with their needed effects, estrogens may cause some unwanted effects such as blood clots and problems of the breasts, gallbladder, liver, and uterus.

The following side effects may be caused by blood clots but rarely occur; however, if they do occur, they require immediate medical attention. If your doctor is not available, go to the nearest hospital emergency room.

Pains in chest, groin, or legs (especially in calves of legs)	Sudden loss of coordination
Severe, sudden headache	Sudden loss of vision or change in vision
Slurring of speech (sudden)	Sudden shortness of breath

Other side effects which may occur and require medical attention (but usually not on an emergency basis) are:

Less common or rare

Changes in vaginal bleeding (spotting, breakthrough bleeding, prolonged bleeding, or complete stoppage of bleeding)	Lumps in breast Mental depression Pains in stomach or side Skin rash Vaginal discharge (thick, white, and curd-like)
Increased blood pressure	Yellowing of eyes and skin

Other side effects may occur which usually do not require medical attention. These side effects may go away during treatment as your body adjusts to the medicine. However, check with your doctor if any of the following side effects continue or are bothersome:

More common

Cramps of lower stomach	Swelling and increased tenderness of breasts in males or females
Loss of appetite	
Nausea	
	Swelling of ankles and feet

Less common

Brown, blotchy spots on exposed skin	Diarrhea (mild) Dizziness Increased skin sensitivity to sun
Changes in sexual interest (usually decreased in males and increased in females)	Irritability Some loss of scalp hair Vomiting

Other side effects not listed above may also occur in some patients. If you notice any other effects, check with your doctor.

ESTROGENS (Vaginal)

This information applies to the following medicines:

Dienestrol (dye-en-ESS-trole)
Diethylstilbestrol (dye-eth-il-stil-BESS-trole)
Conjugated Estrogens (ESS-troe-jenz)
Estropipate (ess-troe-PI-pate)

Some commonly used brand names and other names are:	Generic names:
DV Cream	Dienestrol
DES	Diethylstilbestrol
Premarin	Conjugated Estrogens
Ogen Piperazine Estrone Sulfate	Estropipate

Estrogens (ESS-troe-jenz) are often called female hormones. They are produced by the body and are necessary for the normal sexual development of the female and for the regulation of the menstrual cycle during the childbearing years.

Uncomfortable changes may occur in vaginal tissues when the body does not produce enough estrogens, as during the menopause or following certain kinds of surgery. In order to relieve such uncomfortable conditions, estrogens are sometimes prescribed for vaginal use in the form of special creams or suppositories.

When used vaginally or on the skin, most estrogens are absorbed into the blood stream and produce many of the same effects in the body as when they are taken by mouth.

Estrogens for vaginal use are available only with your doctor's prescription.

Before Using This Medicine

Since vaginal estrogens may be absorbed into the body, the following points should be kept in mind:

• Estrogens are very useful medicines. However, in addition to their helpful effects in treating your medical problem, they sometimes have side effects that could be very serious. A paper called "Information for the Patient" is given to you with your prescription. Read this carefully.

• The prolonged use of estrogens has been reported to increase the risk of endometrial cancer (cancer of the uterus lining) in women after the menopause. This risk seems to increase the longer estrogens are used and the higher their dose. The risk is greatly reduced when lower doses are used and when they are used for no more than 3 out of every 4 weeks. When estrogens are used in this manner for less than 1 year, there is less risk.

Note: If the uterus has been removed by surgery (total hysterectomy), there is no risk of endometrial cancer.

• Cigarette smoking during the time estrogens are taken may cause increased risk of serious side effects affecting the heart and/or blood circulation. The risk increases as the amount of smoking and the age of the smoker increase. Women aged 39 to 45 may be at greater risk when they smoke and use estrogens.

In order to decide on the best treatment for your medical problem, your doctor should be told:

—if you have ever had any unusual reaction to estrogens in the past. This medicine should not be taken if you are allergic to it.

—if you are pregnant or if you intend to become pregnant. Estrogens may cause birth defects if taken during pregnancy. In rare cases, daughters of women who took diethylstilbestrol (DES) during pregnancy have developed cancer of the vagina and uterine cervix upon reaching childbearing age.

—if you are breast-feeding an infant. Estrogens pass into the breast milk and may cause unwanted effects in infants of mothers taking this medicine.

—if you have any of the following medical problems:

Asthma	High blood pressure
Blood clots (or history of)	Kidney disease
	Liver disease
Cancer (or history of)	(such as jaundice or porphyria)
Changes in vaginal bleeding	Lumps in breast
Diabetes	Mental depression
Endometriosis	Migraine headaches
Epilepsy	Thyroid disease
Gallbladder disease	Tumors or growths
Heart or circulation disease	in uterus (not cancerous)

—if you are now taking any of the following medicines or types of medicine:

Carbamazepine	Primidone
Oral anticoagulants (blood thinners you take by mouth)	Rifampin
	Tricyclic antidepressants (medicine for depression)
Phenobarbital	
Phenytoin	

Proper Use of This Medicine

Use this medicine only as directed. Do not use more of it and do not use it for a longer period of time than your doctor ordered.

This medicine is often used at bedtime to increase effectiveness through better absorption. To protect your clothing while using this medicine, you may find sanitary napkins helpful.

Nausea may rarely occur during the first few weeks after you start using this medicine. This effect usually disappears with continued use. If the nausea is bothersome, it can usually be prevented or reduced if you eat a solid breakfast or a mid-morning snack.

Vaginal creams and some vaginal suppositories are inserted with a plastic dose applicator. Directions for using the applicator are included with your medicine. If you do not receive the directions or do not understand them, ask your doctor, pharmacist, or nurse for information or additional explanation.

If you miss a dose of this medicine and do not remember it until the next day, do not use the missed dose at all. Instead, go back to your regular dosing schedule. If you have any questions about this, check with your doctor.

Precautions While Using This Medicine

It is very important that your doctor check your progress at regular visits. These visits will usually be every 6 to 12 months, unless your doctor requires them more often.

Before having any kind of surgery (including dental surgery) or emergency treatment, tell the doctor or dentist in charge that you are using this medicine, since this medicine may change your blood-clotting ability.

While using this medicine, use caution during exposure to the sun or sunlamps. Some people may find that their skin will sunburn more easily. Also, they may develop brown, blotchy spots on exposed areas. These spots usually disappear gradually when the medicine is stopped.

If you suspect that you may have become pregnant, stop using the medicine immediately and check with your doctor. Continued use of this medicine during pregnancy may cause birth defects in the child. It may also increase the risk of vaginal cancer developing in daughters when they reach childbearing age.

Do not give this medicine to anyone else. Your doctor has prescribed it only for you after studying your health record and the results of your physical examination. Estrogens may be dangerous for other people because of differences in their health and body make-up.

Side Effects of This Medicine

Along with their needed effects, estrogens sometimes cause some unwanted effects such as blood clots and problems of the breasts, gallbladder, liver, and uterus; however, when used vaginally, the possibility of side effects may be lessened because the time of treatment is usually short.

The following side effects may be caused by blood clots but rarely occur; however, if they do occur, they require immediate medical attention. If your doctor is not available, go to the nearest hospital emergency room.

Pains in chest, groin, or legs (especially in calves of legs)	Sudden loss of coordination
Severe, sudden headache	Sudden loss of vision or change in vision
Slurred speech (sudden)	Sudden shortness of breath

Other serious side effects which may occur and require medical attention (but usually not on an emergency basis) are:

Less common or rare

Changes in vaginal bleeding (spotting, breakthrough bleeding, prolonged bleeding, or complete stoppage of bleeding)	Lumps in breasts
	Mental depression
	Pains in stomach or side
	Skin rash
	Vaginal discharge (thick, white, and curd-like)
Increased blood pressure	Yellowing of eyes or skin

Other side effects may occur which usually do not require medical attention. These side effects may go away during treatment as your body adjusts to the medicine. However, check with your doctor if any of the following side effects continue or are bothersome:

More common

Cramps of lower stomach	Swelling of ankles and feet
Loss of appetite	Swelling and increased tenderness of breasts
Nausea	

Less common

Brown, blotchy spots on exposed skin	Changes in sexual interest (usually increased in females)

Diarrhea (mild)   Irritability
Dizziness   Some loss of scalp
Increased skin sensi-   hair
tivity to sun   Vomiting

Other side effects not listed above may also occur in some patients. If you notice any other effects, check with your doctor.

ESTROGENS AND PROGESTINS (Systemic)
Oral Contraceptives

This information applies to the following medicines:

Ethynodiol (e-thye-noe-DYE-ole) Diacetate and Ethinyl Estradiol
(ETH-in-il ess-tra-DYE-ole)
Ethynodiol Diacetate and Mestranol (MES-tranole)
Norethindrone (nor-eth-IN-drone) and Ethinyl Estradiol
Norethindrone and Mestranol
Norethindrone Acetate and Ethinyl Estradiol
Norethynodrel (nor-e-THYE-noe-drel) and Mestranol
Norgestrel (nor-JESS-trel) and Ethinyl Estradiol

For information about Norethindrone or Norgestrel when used as single-ingredient oral contraceptives, see *Progestins (Systemic)*.

Some commonly used brand names are:	Generic names:
Demulen	Ethynodiol Diacetate and Ethinyl Estradiol
Ovulen	Ethynodiol Diacetate and Mestranol
Ovcon Brevicon Modicon	Norethindrone and Ethinyl Estradiol
Norinyl Ortho-Novum	Norethindrone and Mestranol
Norlestrin Loestrin	Norethindrone Acetate and Ethinyl Estradiol
Enovid	Norethynodrel and Mestranol
Ovral Lo-Ovral	Norgestrel and Ethinyl Estradiol

Oral contraceptives are known also as the Pill, OC's, BC's, BC tablets, or birth control pills.

They usually contain two types of female hormones, estrogens (ESS-troe-jenz) and progestins (proe-JESS-tins). When taken by mouth on a regular schedule, they change the hormone balance of the body which prevents pregnancy.

Sometimes these preparations are used in the treatment of conditions that benefit from added hormones; however, they have no effect on venereal disease.

Oral contraceptives are available only with your doctor's prescription.

Before Using This Medicine

In order to make the use of oral contraceptives (birth control tablets) as safe and reliable as possible, you should understand how and when to take them and what effects may be expected. A paper with information for the patient will be given to you with your filled prescription, and will provide many details concerning the use of oral contraceptives. Read this paper carefully and ask your doctor, nurse, or pharmacist if you need additional information or explanation.

In order to decide on the best treatment for your medical problem, your doctor should be told:

—if you have ever had any unusual reaction to estrogens or progestins in the past. This medicine should not be taken if you are allergic to it.

—if you smoke cigarettes.

—if you suspect that you are pregnant. Oral contraceptives may cause birth defects if taken during pregnancy. Also, daughters of women who took diethylstilbestrol (DES) during pregnancy have developed unwanted changes in reproductive organs; and in rare cases, cancer of the vagina and/or uterine cervix has developed after childbearing age has been reached. It is not yet known if the estrogens in oral contraceptives also cause this effect, but the chance does exist.

—if you are breast-feeding an infant. The estrogens in oral contraceptives pass into the breast milk and may cause unwanted effects in infants of mothers taking this medicine.

—if you have any of the following medical problems:

Asthma   Epilepsy
Blood clots (or   Gallbladder disease
history of)   Heart or circulation
Cancer (or history   disease
of)   High blood pressure
Changes in vaginal   Kidney disease
bleeding   Liver disease
Diabetes   (such as jaundice
Endometriosis   or porphyria)

Lumps in breasts
Mental depression
Migraine headaches
Stroke (or history
of)

Thyroid disease
Tumors or growths
in uterus (not
cancerous)

—if you are now taking any of the following medicines or types of medicine:

Carbamazepine
Oral anticoagulants
(blood thinners
you take by
mouth)

Phenobarbital
Phenytoin
Primidone
Rifampin

Proper Use of This Medicine

Take this medicine only as directed by your doctor. This medicine must be taken exactly on schedule to prevent pregnancy. Try to take the medicine at the same time each day, 24 hours apart, to reduce the possibility of side effects and to provide the best protection.

Nausea may occur during the first few weeks after you start taking this medicine. This effect usually disappears with continued use. If the nausea is bothersome, it can usually be prevented or reduced by taking each dose with food or immediately after food.

For missed doses:
• If you are using a 21-day schedule and you miss a dose of this medicine for one day, take the missed tablet as soon as you remember. If it is not remembered until the next day, take the missed tablet plus the tablet that is regularly scheduled for that day. This means that you will take 2 tablets on the same day. Then go back to your regular dosing schedule.

• If you are using a 21-day schedule and you miss a dose for 2 days in a row, take 2 tablets a day for each of the next 2 days, then go back to your regular dosing schedule. In addition, you should use a second method of birth control to make sure that you are fully protected for the rest of the cycle.

• If you are using a 21-day schedule and you miss a dose for 3 days or more in a row, stop taking the medicine completely and use another method of birth control until your period begins or until your doctor determines that you are not pregnant. Then restart protection with a new cycle of tablets.

• If you are using a 28-day schedule and you miss any of the first 21 (active) tablets, follow the instructions for the 21-day schedule depending on how many doses you have missed. If you miss any of the last 7 (inactive) tablets, there is no danger of pregnancy. However, the first tablet (active) of the next month's cycle

must be taken on the regularly scheduled day, in spite of any missed doses, if pregnancy is to be avoided. The active and inactive tablets are colored differently for your convenience.

Precautions While Using This Medicine

It is very important that your doctor check your progress at regular visits. These visits will usually be every 6 to 12 months, unless your doctor requires them more often.

When you begin to use oral contraceptives, your body will require several days to adjust before pregnancy will be prevented; therefore, you should *use a second method of birth control for the first cycle (or 3 weeks)* to ensure full protection.

Tell the doctor or dentist in charge that you are taking this medicine before any kind of surgery (including dental surgery) or emergency treatment, since this medicine may change your blood-clotting ability.

Vaginal bleeding of various amounts may occur between your regular menstrual periods (sometimes called spotting when slight, or breakthrough bleeding when heavier), during the first 2 months of use. If this should occur:

• Continue on your regular dosing schedule.

• The bleeding usually stops within 1 week.

• Check with your doctor if the bleeding continues for more than 1 week.

• After you have been taking oral contraceptives on schedule and for more than 2 months, check with your doctor.

Missed menstrual periods may occur:

—if you have not taken the medicine exactly as scheduled. Pregnancy must be considered a possibility.

—if the medicine is not properly adjusted for your needs.

—if you have taken oral contraceptives for a long time, usually 2 or more years, and stop their use.

Check with your doctor if you miss any menstrual periods so that the cause may be determined.

Cigarette smoking during the use of oral contraceptives has been found to increase the risk of serious side effects affecting the heart and/or blood circulation. The risk increases as the age of the patient and the amount of smoking increase. This risk may be greater in women 39 to 45 years of age. *To reduce the risk of serious side effects, do not smoke cigarettes while using oral contraceptives.* Discuss smoking and oral contraceptive use with your doctor.

While taking this medicine, use caution during exposure to the sun or sunlamps. Some people may find that their skin will sunburn more easily. Also, they may develop brown, blotchy spots on exposed areas. These spots usually disappear gradually when the medicine is stopped.

If you suspect that you may have become pregnant, stop taking this medicine immediately and check with your doctor. Continued use of this medicine during pregnancy may cause birth defects in the child. It may also increase the risk of vaginal cancer developing in daughters when they reach childbearing age.

The hormones in oral contraceptives may cause birth defects. Since it takes a while for the effects of this medicine to wear off, birth defects may occur even though the tablets are no longer being used. Therefore, *when you stop using oral contraceptives, it is very important that you wait at least 3 months before becoming pregnant. Be sure to use another method of birth control during that time.*

Caution: Your doctor has prescribed this medicine only for you after studying your health record and the results of your physical examination. Use of the tablets by other persons may be dangerous because of differences in health and body make-up. Therefore, do not give your oral contraceptives to anyone else (and do not take tablets prescribed for someone else). Also, check with your doctor before taking any left-over oral contraceptives from an old prescription, especially after a pregnancy. This medicine may be dangerous if your health has changed since your last physical examination.

Since one of the most important factors in the proper use of oral contraceptives is taking every dose exactly on schedule, you should never let your tablet supply run out. Always keep 1 extra month's supply of tablets on hand. To keep the extra month's supply from becoming too old, use it next, after the pills now being used, and replace the extra supply each month on a regular schedule. The tablets will keep well when kept dry and at room temperature (light will fade some tablet colors but will not change their effect).

Keep the tablets in the container in which you received them. Most containers aid you in keeping track of your dosage schedule.

Side Effects of This Medicine

Along with their needed effects, birth control tablets sometimes cause some unwanted effects such as blood clots and problems of the breasts, gallbladder, liver, and uterus.

The following side effects may be caused by blood clots but rarely occur; however, if they do occur, they require immediate medical attention. If your doctor is not available, go to the nearest hospital emergency room.

Pains in chest, groin, or legs (especially in calves of legs)	Sudden loss of coordination
	Sudden loss of vision or change in vision
Severe, sudden headache	Sudden shortness of breath
Slurring of speech (sudden)	

Other side effects which may occur and require medical attention (but usually not on an emergency basis) are:

Less common or rare

Changes in vaginal bleeding (spotting, breakthrough bleeding, prolonged bleeding, or complete stoppage of bleeding)	Mental depression
	Pains in stomach or side
	Skin rash
	Vaginal discharge (thick, white, and curd-like)
Increased blood pressure	Yellowing of eyes and skin
Lumps in breasts	

Other side effects may occur which usually do not require medical attention. These side effects may go away during treatment as your body adjusts to the medicine. However, check with your doctor if any of the following side effects continue or are bothersome:

More common

Acne (usually less common after first 3 months)	Swelling of ankles and feet
Cramps of lower stomach	Swelling and increased tenderness of breasts
Loss of appetite	Unusual tiredness or weakness
Nausea	

Less common to rare

Brown, blotchy spots on exposed skin	Increased body and facial hair
Changes in sexual interest	Increased skin sensitivity to sun
Changes in weight	Irritability
Diarrhea (mild)	Some loss of scalp hair
Dizziness	Vomiting

Other side effects not listed above may also occur in some patients. If you notice any other effects, check with your doctor.

ETHACRYNIC ACID (Systemic)
A commonly used brand name is Edecrin.

Ethacrynic acid (eth-a-KRIN-ik AS-id) belongs to the general family of medicines called diuretics. It is given by mouth or injection to help reduce the amount of water in the body by increasing the flow of urine. Ethacrynic acid may also be used for other conditions as determined by your doctor. This medicine is available only with your doctor's prescription.

Before Using This Medicine

In order to decide on the best treatment for your medical problem, your doctor should be told:

—if you have ever had any unusual reaction to ethacrynic acid in the past. This medicine should not be taken if you are allergic to it.

—if you are pregnant or if you intend to become pregnant while using this medicine. Although ethacrynic acid has not been shown to cause birth defects or other problems in humans, the chance always exists.

—if you are breast-feeding an infant. Although ethacrynic acid has not been shown to cause problems, the chance always exists.

—if you have any of the following medical problems:

Diabetes	Liver disease
Gout	Pancreas disease
Hearing problems	Severe kidney
History of lupus	disease
erythematosus	

—if you are now taking any of the following medicines or types of medicine:

Anticoagulants (blood thinners)	Narcotics or prescription pain medicine
Corticosteroids (cortisone-like medicines)	Other diuretics (water pills) or antihyper-
Diabetes medicine	tensives (high
Digitalis glycosides (heart medicine)	blood pressure medicine)
Gout medicine	Sleeping medicine, such as bar-
Lithium	biturates

Proper Use of This Medicine

This medicine may cause you to have an unusual feeling of tiredness when you begin to take it.

You may also notice an increase in the amount of urine or in your frequency of urination. After taking the medicine for a while, these effects should lessen. In general, in order to keep the increase in urine from affecting your sleep:

• If you are to take a single dose a day, take it in the morning after breakfast.

• If you are to take more than one dose a day, take the last dose no later than 6 p.m., unless otherwise directed by your doctor.

However, it is best to plan your dose or doses according to a schedule that will least affect your personal activities and sleep. Ask your doctor, nurse, or pharmacist to help you plan the best time to take this medicine.

In order to help remember to take your medicine, try to get into the habit of taking it at the same time each day.

If this medicine upsets your stomach, it may be taken with meals or milk. If stomach upset (nausea, vomiting, or stomach pain) continues or gets worse, or if you suddenly get severe diarrhea, check with your doctor.

If you miss a dose of this medicine, take it as soon as possible. However, if it is almost time for your next dose, do not take the missed dose at all and do not double the next one. Instead, go back to your regular dosing schedule. If you have any questions about this, check with your doctor.

Precautions While Using This Medicine

It is important that your doctor check your progress at regular visits.

This medicine may cause a loss of potassium from your body. To help prevent this, your doctor may want you to:

—eat or drink foods that have a high potassium content (for example, orange or other citrus fruit juices), or

—take a potassium supplement, or

—take another medicine to help prevent the loss of the potassium in the first place.

It is very important to follow these directions. Also, it is important not to change your diet on your own. This is more important if you are already on a special diet (as for diabetes), or if you are taking a potassium supplement or a medicine to reduce potassium loss. Extra potassium may not be necessary and, in some cases, too much potassium could be harmful.

To prevent the loss of too much water and potassium, tell your doctor if you become sick, especially with severe or continuing nausea and vomiting or diarrhea.

Caution: Diabetics—Ethacrynic acid may affect blood sugar levels. While you are using this medicine, be especially careful in testing for sugar in your urine. If you have any questions about this, check with your doctor.

Before having any kind of surgery (including dental surgery), make sure the doctor or dentist in charge knows that you are taking this medicine.

Dizziness, lightheadedness, or fainting may occur, especially when you get up from a lying or sitting position. This is more likely to occur in the morning. *Getting up slowly may help* but if the problem continues or gets worse, check with your doctor.

The dizziness, lightheadedness, or fainting is also more likely to occur if you drink alcohol, stand for long periods of time, or exercise, or if the weather is hot. *While you are taking this medicine, be careful of the amount of alcohol you drink. Also, use extra care during exercise or hot weather or if you must stand for long periods of time.* Check with your doctor if you have any questions about this.

Side Effects of This Medicine

Along with its needed effects, a medicine may cause some unwanted effects. Although not all of these side effects appear very often, when they do occur they may require medical attention. Check with your doctor if any of the following side effects occur:

Signs of loss of too much potassium

Dryness of mouth	Muscle cramps or
Increased thirst	pain
Irregular heartbeats	Nausea or vomiting
Mood or mental	Unusual tiredness or
changes	weakness
	Weak pulse

Less common

Ringing, buzzing sound, or full feeling in ears or any loss of hearing

Rare

Black tarry stools	Skin rash or hives
Blood in urine	Unexplained sore
Joint, flank, or	throat and fever
stomach pain	Unusual bleeding or
Severe stomach pain	bruising
with nausea and	Yellowing of the
vomiting	eyes or skin

Other side effects may occur which usually do not require medical attention. These side effects may go away during treatment as your body adjusts to the medicine. However, check with your doctor if any of the following side effects continue or are bothersome:

More common

Diarrhea	Loss of appetite
Dizziness or light-	Upset stomach
headedness when	
getting up from	
a lying or sitting	
position	

Uncommon

Blurred vision	Nervousness
Headache	Redness or pain at
Mental confusion	the site of in-
	jection

Other side effects not listed above may also occur in some patients. If you notice any other effects, check with your doctor.

ETHAMBUTOL (Systemic)
Some commonly used brand names are Etibi* and Myambutol.

---

*Not available in the United States.

Ethambutol (e-THAM-byoo-tole) belongs to the general family of medicines called anti-infectives. It is used to help the body overcome tuberculosis (TB) and is given by mouth with one or more other medicines for TB. Ethambutol is available only with your doctor's prescription.

Before Using This Medicine

In order to decide on the best treatment for your medical problem, your doctor should be told:

—if you have ever had any unusual reaction to ethambutol. This medicine should not be taken if you are allergic to it.

—if you are pregnant, if you intend to become pregnant, or if you are breast-feeding an infant, although ethambutol has not been shown to cause problems in humans.

—if you have any of the following medical problems:

Gout	Optic neuritis
Kidney disease	(eye nerve
	damage)

Proper Use of This Medicine

Ethambutol may be taken with food if it upsets your stomach.

To help clear up your tuberculosis (TB) completely, *it is very important that you keep taking this medicine for the full time of treatment* even if you begin to feel better after a few weeks. You may have to take it every day for as long as 1 to 2 years or more. *It is important that you do not miss any doses.*

If you do miss a dose of this medicine, take it as soon as possible. However, if it is almost time for your next dose, do not take the missed dose or double your next dose. Instead, go back to your regular dosing schedule.

Precautions While Using This Medicine

If your symptoms do not improve within 2 to 3 weeks or if they become worse, check with your doctor.

It is very important that your doctor check your progress at regular visits. In addition, you should *check with your doctor immediately if blurred vision, eye pain, red-green color blindness, or any loss of vision occurs during treatment.* Your doctor may want you to have your eyes checked by an ophthalmologist (eye doctor).

Also, if this medicine causes chills; pain and swelling of joints (especially great toe, ankle, knee); or tense, hot skin over affected joints, check with your doctor immediately.

Side Effects of This Medicine

Along with its needed effects, a medicine may cause some unwanted effects. Although not all of these side effects appear very often, when they do occur they may require medical attention. Check with your doctor *immediately* if any of the following side effects occur:

Less common

Chills	Tense, hot skin
Pain and swelling of joints (especially great toe, ankle, knee)	over affected joints

Rare

Any loss of vision	Numbness, tingling,
Blurred vision	burning pain, or
Eye pain	weakness in the
	hands or feet
	Red-green color
	blindness

Other side effects may occur which usually do not require medical attention. These side effects may go away during treatment as your body adjusts to the medicine. However, check with your doctor if any of the following side effects continue or are bothersome:

Less common

Dizziness	Rash
Itching	Stomach upset

Other side effects not listed above may also occur in some patients. If you notice any other effects, check with your doctor.

ETHCHLORVYNOL (Systemic)
A commonly used brand name is Placidyl.

Ethchlorvynol (eth-klor-VI-nole) is used in the treatment of insomnia or sleeplessness. It helps patients to sleep. However, if used regularly (for example, every day) for insomnia or sleeplessness, it is usually not effective for more than 1 week. This medicine is available only with your doctor's prescription.

Before Using This Medicine

In order to decide on the best treatment for your medical problem, your doctor should be told:

—if you have ever had any unusual reaction to ethchlorvynol in the past. This medicine should not be taken if you are allergic to it.

—if you are pregnant or if you intend to become pregnant while using this medicine. Use of ethchlorvynol during pregnancy may cause unwanted effects in the baby.

—if you are breast-feeding an infant. Although ethchlorvynol has not been shown to cause problems, the chance always exists.

—if you have any of the following medical problems:

Kidney disease	Mental depression
Liver disease	Porphyria

—if you are now taking other central nervous system (CNS) depressants such as:

Antihistamines or medicine for hay fever, other allergies, or colds	Prescription pain medicine
	Seizure medicine
Barbiturates	Tricyclic anti-depressants
Narcotics	(medicine for
Other sedatives, tranquilizers, or sleeping medicine	depression)

—if you are now taking or have taken within the past 2 weeks monoamine oxidase (MAO) inhibitors such as:

Isocarboxazid	Phenelzine
Pargyline	Tranylcypromine

—if you are now taking anticoagulants (blood thinners).

Proper Use of This Medicine

Take this medicine only as directed by your doctor. Do not take more of it, do not take it more often, and do not take it for a longer period of time than your doctor ordered. If too much is taken, it may become habit-forming.

Keep this medicine out of the reach of children since overdose is especially dangerous in children.

This medicine is best taken with food or a glass of milk to lessen the possibility of dizziness, clumsiness, or unsteadiness which may occur shortly after you take this medicine.

Precautions While Using This Medicine

If you will be taking this medicine regularly for a long period of time:

—your doctor should check your progress at regular visits.

—do not stop taking it without first checking with your doctor. Your doctor may want you to reduce gradually the amount you are taking before stopping completely.

This medicine will add to the effects of alcohol and other medicines (CNS depressants) that slow down the nervous system. Some examples of CNS depressants are antihistamines or medicine for hay fever, other allergies, or colds; sedatives, tranquilizers, or sleeping medicine; prescription pain medicine or narcotics; barbiturates; medicine for seizures; tricyclic antidepressants (medicine for depression); or anesthetics, including some dental anesthetics. *Check with your doctor before taking any of the above while you are taking this medicine.*

If you think you may have taken an overdose, get emergency help at once. Taking an overdose of ethchlorvynol or taking alcohol or other CNS depressants with ethchlorvynol may lead to unconsciousness and possibly death. Some signs of an overdose are mental confusion, severe weakness, shortness of breath or troubled breathing, staggering, and unusually slow heartbeat.

This medicine may cause some people to become dizzy, lightheaded, drowsy, or less alert than they are normally. Even if taken at bedtime, it may cause some people to feel drowsy or less alert on arising. *Make sure you know how you react to this medicine before you drive, use machines, or do other jobs that require you to be alert.*

Side Effects of This Medicine

Along with its needed effects, a medicine may cause some unwanted effects. Although not all of these side effects appear very often, when they do occur they may require medical attention. Check with your doctor if any of the following side effects occur:

Less common

Skin rash or hives	Unusual excitement, nervousness, or
Unusual bleeding or bruising	restlessness

Rare

Darkening of urine	Unusually slow heartbeat, short-
Itching	ness of breath,
Pale stools	or troubled breathing
	Yellowing of eyes or skin

Other side effects may occur which usually do not require medical attention. These side effects may go away during treatment as your body adjusts to the medicine. However, check with your doctor if any of the following side effects continue or are bothersome:

More common

Blurred vision	Numbness of face
Dizziness or lightheadedness	Stomach pain
Indigestion	Unpleasant after- taste
Nausea or vomiting	Unusual tiredness or weakness

Less common

Clumsiness or unsteadiness	Mental confusion
Drowsiness (daytime)	Slurred speech

After you stop using this medicine, your body may need time to adjust. If you took this medicine in high doses or for a long time, this may take up to 2 weeks. During this period of time check with your doctor if you notice any of the following side effects:

Convulsions or seizures	Trembling
Hallucinations (see- ing, hearing, or feeling things that are not there)	Trouble in sleeping
	Unusual restlessness, nervousness, or irritability
Muscle twitching	Unusual sweating
Nausea or vomiting	Unusual weakness

Other side effects not listed above may also occur in some patients. If you notice any other effects, check with your doctor.

ETHINAMATE (Systemic)
A commonly used brand name is Valmid.

Ethinamate (e-THIN-a-mate) is used in the treatment of insomnia or sleeplessness. It helps patients to sleep. However, if used regularly (for example, every day) for insomnia or sleeplessness, it is usually not effective for more than 7 days. This medicine is available only with your doctor's prescription.

Before Using This Medicine
In order to decide on the best treatment for your medical problem, your doctor should be told:

—if you have ever had any unusual reaction to ethinamate in the past. This medicine should not be taken if you are allergic to it.

—if you are pregnant, if you intend to become pregnant, or if you are breast-feeding an infant. Although ethinamate has not been shown to cause problems, the chance always exists.

—if you have mental depression.

—if you are now taking other central nervous system (CNS) depressants such as:

Antihistamines or medicine for hay fever, other allergies, or colds	Prescription pain medicine
	Seizure medicine
Barbiturates	Tricyclic anti-
Narcotics	depressants
Other sedatives, tranquilizers, or sleeping medicine	(medicine for depression)

—if you are now taking or have taken within the past 2 weeks monoamine oxidase (MAO) inhibitors such as:

Isocarboxazid	Phenelzine
Pargyline	Tranylcypromine

Proper Use of This Medicine
Take this medicine only as directed by your doctor. Do not take more of it, do not take it more often, and do not take it for a longer period of time than your doctor ordered. If too much is taken, it may become habit-forming.

Keep this medicine out of the reach of children since overdose is especially dangerous in children.

Precautions While Using This Medicine
If you will be taking this medicine regularly for a long period of time:

—your doctor should check your progress at regular visits.

—do not stop taking it without first checking with your doctor. Your doctor may want you to reduce gradually the amount you are taking before stopping completely.

This medicine will add to the effects of alcohol and other medicines (CNS depressants) that slow down the nervous system. Some examples of CNS depressants are antihistamines or medicine for hay fever, other allergies, or colds; sedatives, tranquilizers, or sleeping medicine; prescription pain medicine or narcotics; barbiturates; medicine for seizures; tricyclic antidepressants (medicine for depression); or anesthetics, including some dental anesthetics. *Check with your doctor before taking any of the above while you are taking this medicine.*

If you think you may have taken an overdose, get emergency help at once. Taking an overdose of ethinamate or taking alcohol or other CNS depressants with ethinamate may lead to unconsciousness and possibly death. Some signs of an overdose are mental confusion, severe weakness, shortness of breath or troubled breathing, staggering, and unusually slow heartbeat.

This medicine may cause some people to become drowsy or less alert than they are normally. Even if taken at bedtime, it may cause some people to feel drowsy or less alert on arising. *Make sure you know how you react to this medicine before you drive, use machines, or do other jobs that require you to be alert.*

Side Effects of This Medicine
Along with its needed effects, a medicine may cause some unwanted effects. Although not all of these side effects appear very often, when they do occur they may require medical attention. Check with your doctor if any of the following side effects occur:

Less common

Skin rash	Unusual excitement (especially in children)

Rare

Unusual bleeding or bruising	Unusually slow heartbeat, shortness of breath, or troubled breathing

Other side effects may occur which usually do not require medical attention. These side effects may go away during treatment as your body adjusts to the medicine. However, check with your doctor if any of the following side effects continue or are bothersome:

Less common

| Indigestion | Stomach pain |
| Nausea | Vomiting |

Rare

Drowsiness
(daytime)

After you stop using this medicine, your body may need time to adjust. The length of time this takes depends on the amount of medicine you were using and how long you used it. During this period of time check with your doctor if you notice any of the following side effects:

| Convulsions or seizures | Mental confusion Trembling |
| Hallucinations (seeing, hearing, or feeling things that are not there) | Trouble in sleeping Unusual restlessness, nervousness, or irritability |

Other side effects not listed above may also occur in some patients. If you notice any other effects, check with your doctor.

ETHIONAMIDE (Systemic)
A commonly used brand name is Trecator-SC.

Ethionamide (e-thye-on-AM-ide) belongs to the general family of medicines called anti-infectives. It is used to help the body overcome tuberculosis (TB). It is given by mouth with one or more other medicines for TB. Ethionamide is available only with your doctor's prescription.

Before Using This Medicine

In order to decide on the best treatment for your medical problem, your doctor should be told:

—if you have had allergic reactions to isoniazid, pyrazinamide, or niacin (nicotinic acid).

—if you are pregnant or if you intend to become pregnant. Ethionamide may cause birth defects if it is taken during pregnancy.

—if you are breast-feeding an infant, although ethionamide has not been shown to cause problems.

—if you have either of the following medical problems:

Diabetes
Liver disease

—if you are now taking any of the following medicines:

Aminosalicylic acid (PAS)	Isoniazid Pyrazinamide
Capreomycin	Rifampin
Cycloserine	Streptomycin
Ethambutol	

Proper Use of This Medicine

Ethionamide may be taken with or after meals if it upsets your stomach.

To help clear up your tuberculosis (TB) completely, *it is very important that you keep taking this medicine for the full time of treatment* even if you begin to feel better after a few weeks. You may have to take it every day for as long as 1 to 2 years or more. *It is important that you do not miss any doses.*

Your doctor may also want you to take pyridoxine (vitamin B₆) every day to help prevent or lessen some of the side effects of ethionamide. If so, *it is very important to take pyridoxine every day along with this medicine; do not miss any doses.*

If you do miss a dose of either of these medicines, take it as soon as possible. However, if it is almost time for your next dose, do not take the missed dose or double your next dose. Instead, go back to your regular dosing schedule.

Precautions While Using This Medicine

If your symptoms do not improve within 2 to 3 weeks or if they become worse, check with your doctor.

It is very important that your doctor check your progress at regular visits. Also, *check with your doctor immediately if blurred vision or any loss of vision, with or without eye pain, occurs during treatment.* Your doctor may want you to have your eyes checked by an ophthalmologist (eye doctor).

If this medicine causes clumsiness; unsteadiness; or numbness, tingling, burning, or pain in the hands and feet, stop taking it and check with your doctor immediately. These may be early warning signs of more serious nerve problems that could develop later.

Side Effects of This Medicine

Along with its needed effects, a medicine may cause some unwanted effects. Although not all of these side effects appear very often, when they do occur they may require medical attention. Stop taking this medicine and check with your doctor *immediately* if any of the following side effects occur:

More common

Mental depression

Less common

Clumsiness or unsteadiness	Numbness, tingling, burning, or pain in hands and feet
Confusion	
Mood or other mental changes	Yellowing of eyes or skin

Rare

Blurred vision or any loss of vision, with or without eye pain	Decreased sexual ability (males)
	Dry, puffy skin
	Pain, stiffness, or swelling of joints
Changes in menstrual periods	Swelling of front part of neck
Coldness	Unusual weight gain

Other side effects may occur which usually do not require medical attention. These side effects may go away during treatment as your body adjusts to the medicine. However, check with your doctor if any of the following side effects continue or are bothersome:

More common

Diarrhea	Loss of appetite
Dizziness, including when arising from a horizontal or sitting position	Metallic taste
	Nausea
	Sore mouth
	Stomach pain or upset
Drowsiness	Vomiting
Increased amount of saliva or drooling	Weakness

Less common

Acne	Increased sensitivity to sunlight
Enlargement of the breasts (males)	Rash

Rare

Hair loss

Other side effects not listed above may also occur in some patients. If you notice any other effects, check with your doctor.

ETHYLNOREPINEPHRINE (Systemic)
A commonly used brand name is Bronkephrine.

Ethylnorepinephrine (ETH-il-nor-ep-i-NEF-rin) is given by injection to treat bronchial asthma. It relieves wheezing, shortness of breath, and troubled breathing. This medicine is available only with your doctor's prescription.

Before Using This Medicine

In order to decide on the best treatment for your medical problem, your doctor should be told:

—if you have ever had any unusual reaction to medicines like ethylnorepinephrine such as amphetamines, ephedrine, epinephrine, isoproterenol, metaproterenol, norepinephrine (levarterenol), phenylephrine, phenylpropanolamine, pseudoephedrine, or terbutaline.

—if you are pregnant, if you intend to become pregnant, or if you are breast-feeding an infant. Although ethylnorepinephrine has not been shown to cause problems, the chance always exists.

—if you have any of the following medical problems:

Heart or blood vessel disease	High blood pressure

—if you are now taking any of the following medicines or types of medicine:

Amphetamines	Propranolol
Other medicine for asthma or breathing problems	

Proper Use of This Medicine

Use this medicine only as directed. Do not use more of it and do not use it more often than your doctor ordered. To do so may increase the chance of side effects.

This medicine is for injection only. If you will be giving yourself the injections, make sure you understand exactly how to give them. If you have any questions about this, check with your doctor.

Side Effects of This Medicine

Along with its needed effects, a medicine may cause some unwanted effects. The following side effects may go away during treatment as your body adjusts to the medicine; however, check with your doctor if they continue or are bothersome:

Dizziness or lightheadedness	Unusually fast or pounding heartbeat
Headache	
Nausea	Weakness

Other side effects not listed above may also occur in some patients. If you notice any other effects, check with your doctor.

FENFLURAMINE (Systemic)
A commonly used brand name is Pondimin.

Fenfluramine (fen-FLURE-a-meen) belongs to the group of medicines called appetite suppressants. It is used in the short-term (a few weeks) treatment of obesity to help patients lose weight.

For a few weeks (6 to 12), fenfluramine in combination with dieting can help patients lose weight. However, since its appetite-reducing effect is only temporary, it is useful only for the first few weeks of dieting until new eating habits are established. It is not effective for continuous use in diet control.

This medicine is available only with your doctor's prescription.

Before Using This Medicine

In order to decide on the best treatment for your medical problem, your doctor should be told:

—if you have ever had any unusual reaction to amphetamine, dextroamphetamine, ephedrine, epinephrine, isoproterenol, metaproterenol, methamphetamine, norepinephrine (levarterenol), phenylephrine, phenylpropanolamine, pseudoephedrine, or terbutaline.

—if you are pregnant, if you intend to become pregnant, or if you are breast-feeding an infant. Although fenfluramine has not been shown to cause problems in humans, the chance always exists.

—if you have any of the following medical problems:

Alcoholism	High blood pressure
Diabetes	Mental depression
Glaucoma	(or history of)
Heart or blood vessel disease	Overactive thyroid

—if you are now taking any of the following medicines or types of medicine:

Guanethidine	Oral hypoglycemics
Insulin	(diabetes medicine
Methyldopa	you take by mouth)
	Reserpine

—if you are now taking central nervous system (CNS) depressants such as:

Antihistamines or medicine for hay fever, other allergies, or colds	Sedatives, tranquilizers, or sleeping medicine
Barbiturates	Seizure medicine
Narcotics	Tricyclic antidepressants
Prescription pain medicine	(medicine for depression)

—if you are now taking or have taken within the past 2 weeks monoamine oxidase (MAO) inhibitors such as:

Isocarboxazid	Phenelzine
Pargyline	Tranylcypromine

Proper Use of This Medicine

Take this medicine only as directed by your doctor. Do not take more of it, do not take it more often, and do not take it for a longer period of time than your doctor ordered. If too much is taken, it may become habit-forming.

If you think this medicine is not working as well after you have taken it for a few weeks, *do not increase the dose.* Instead, check with your doctor.

Precautions While Using This Medicine

Your doctor should check your progress at regular visits in order to make sure that this medicine does not cause unwanted effects.

If you will be taking this medicine in large doses for a long period of time, do not stop taking it without first checking with your doctor. Your doctor may want you to reduce gradually the amount you are taking before stopping completely.

Caution: Diabetics—This medicine may affect blood sugar levels. If you notice a change in the results of your urine sugar test or if you have any questions, check with your doctor.

Fenfluramine will add to the effects of alcohol and other medicines (CNS depressants) that slow down the nervous system. Some examples of CNS depressants are antihistamines or medicine for hay fever, other allergies, or colds; sedatives, tranquilizers, or sleeping medicine; prescription pain medicine or narcotics; barbiturates; medicine for seizures; tricyclic antidepressants (medicine for depression); or anesthetics, including some dental anesthetics. *Check with your doctor before taking any of the above while you are taking this medicine.*

Dryness of the mouth may occur while you are taking this medicine. Sucking on hard sugarless candy or ice chips or chewing sugarless gum may help to relieve the dry mouth.

This medicine may cause some people to become dizzy, lightheaded, drowsy, or less alert than they are normally. *Make sure you know how you react to this medicine before you drive, use machines, or do other jobs that require you to be alert.*

Side Effects of This Medicine

Along with its needed effects, a medicine may cause some unwanted effects. Although not all of these side effects appear very often, when they do occur they may require medical attention. Check with your doctor if any of the following side effects occur:

Less common

    Mental confusion or   Skin rash or hives
      depression

Other side effects may occur which usually do not require medical attention. These side effects may go away during treatment as your body adjusts to the medicine. However, check with your doctor if any of the following side effects continue or are bothersome:

More common

Diarrhea	Dryness of mouth
Drowsiness	

Less common

Blurred vision	Nausea or
Changes in	vomiting
sexual desire	Nervousness or
Clumsiness or	restlessness
unsteadiness	Stomach cramps
Constipation	or pain
Difficult or painful	Trouble in sleeping
urination	or nightmares
Difficulty in talking	Unpleasant taste
Dizziness or	Unusual pounding
lightheadedness	heartbeat
Frequent urge to	Unusual sweating
urinate	Unusual tiredness
Headache	or weakness

After you stop using this medicine, your body may need time to adjust. The length of time this takes depends on the amount of medicine you were using and how long you used it. During this period of time check with your doctor if you notice either of the following side effects:

Mental depression	Trouble in sleeping
	or nightmares

Other side effects not listed above may also occur in some patients. If you notice any other effects, check with your doctor.

FENOPROFEN (Systemic)
A commonly used brand name is Nalfon.

Fenoprofen (fen-oh-PROE-fen) is used to treat the symptoms of arthritis. It helps relieve inflammation, swelling, stiffness, and joint pain. Also, it is used as an analgesic to relieve pain. This medicine is available only with your doctor's prescription.

Before Using This Medicine

In order to decide on the best treatment for your medical problem, your doctor should be told:

—if you have ever had any unusual reaction to aspirin or other salicylates, ibuprofen, meclofenamate, naproxen, sulindac, or tolmetin.

—if you are pregnant, if you intend to become pregnant, or if you are breast-feeding an infant. Although fenoprofen has not been shown to cause problems in humans, the chance always exists.

—if you have any of the following medical problems:

Bleeding problems	Kidney disease
Heart disease	Stomach ulcer or
High blood pressure	other stomach
	problems

—if you are now taking any of the following medicines or types of medicine:

Anticoagulants	Inflammation
(blood thinners)	medicine (for
	example, aspirin
	or other arthritis
	medicine)

Proper Use of This Medicine

When used for arthritis, this medicine must be taken regularly as ordered by your doctor in order for it to help you. A few days may pass before you begin to feel better and up to 2 to 3 weeks may pass before you feel the full effects of this medicine.

It is best to take this medicine 30 minutes before meals or 2 hours after meals so that it will get into the blood more quickly. However, to lessen stomach upset, your doctor may want you to take the medicine with food, milk, or antacids. If stomach upset (indigestion, nausea, vomiting, stomach pain, or diarrhea) continues or if you have any questions about how you should be taking this medicine, check with your doctor.

If you are taking this medicine regularly (for example, every day) and you miss a dose, take it as soon as possible. Then go back to your regular dosing schedule. However, if it is almost time for your next dose, do not take the missed dose at all and do not double the next one. Instead, go back to your regular dosing schedule. If you have any questions about this, check with your doctor.

Precautions While Using This Medicine

Your doctor should check your progress at regular visits in order to make sure that this medicine does not cause unwanted effects.

Stomach problems may be more likely to occur if you take aspirin regularly (for example, every day) or drink alcoholic beverages while being treated with this medicine. Therefore, *do not take aspirin regularly or drink alcoholic beverages while taking this medicine,* unless otherwise directed by your doctor.

Before having any kind of surgery (including dental surgery), tell the doctor or dentist in charge that you are taking this medicine.

This medicine may cause some people to become dizzy, drowsy, or less alert than they are normally. *Make sure you know how you react to this medicine before you drive, use machines, or do other jobs that require you to be alert.*

Side Effects of This Medicine

Along with its needed effects, a medicine may cause some unwanted effects. Although not all of these side effects appear very often, when they do occur they may require medical attention. Check with your doctor if any of the following side effects occur:

More common

Ringing or buzzing in ears	Skin rash, hives, or itching

Less common

Bloody or black tarry stools	Decreased hearing
Blurred vision or any change in vision	Swelling of feet or lower legs
	Unusual weight gain

Rare

Bloody urine	Unexplained sore throat and fever
Difficult or painful urination	Unusual tiredness or weakness
Frequent urge to urinate	
Shortness of breath, troubled breathing, wheezing, or tightness in chest	

Other side effects may occur which usually do not require medical attention. These side effects may go away during treatment as your body adjusts to the medicine. However, check with your doctor if any of the following side effects continue or are bothersome:

More common

Constipation	Indigestion
Diarrhea	Loss of appetite
Drowsiness	Nausea or vomiting
Headache	Stomach pain or discomfort

Less common

Dizziness	Trouble in sleeping
Dry mouth	Unusual sweating
Mental confusion	Unusually fast or pounding heartbeat
Nervousness	
Trembling	

Other side effects not listed above may also occur in some patients. If you notice any other effects, check with your doctor.

FLOXURIDINE (Systemic)

Floxuridine is also commonly known as FUDR.

Floxuridine (flox-YOOR-i-deen) belongs to the group of medicines known as antimetabolites. It is used by injection to treat some kinds of cancer. Floxuridine is available only with a prescription and is to be administered only by or under the immediate supervision of your doctor.

Before Using This Medicine

Floxuridine is a very strong medicine. In addition to its helpful effects in treating your medical problem, it has side effects that could be very serious. Before you receive this medicine, be sure that you have discussed the use of it with your doctor.

In order to decide on the best treatment for your medical problem, your doctor should be told:

—if you have ever had any unusual reaction to floxuridine in the past.

—if you are pregnant or if you intend to have children. This medicine may cause birth defects if either the male or female is taking it at the time of conception or if it is taken during pregnancy. It may also cause permanent sterility after it has been taken for a while. Be sure that you have discussed this with your doctor before taking this medicine.

—if you are breast-feeding an infant. Although floxuridine has not been shown to cause problems, the chance always exists.

—if you have any of the following medical problems:

Infection	Liver disease
Kidney disease	

—if you have been treated with x-rays or cancer drugs by another doctor.

Proper Use of This Medicine

This medicine is sometimes given together with certain other medicines. If you are using a combination of drugs, make sure that you take each medicine at the right time and do not mix them. Ask your doctor, nurse, or pharmacist to help you plan a way to take your medicine at the right time.

Precautions While Using This Medicine

It is very important that your doctor check your progress at regular visits.

Side Effects of This Medicine

Along with its needed effects, a medicine may cause some unwanted effects. Although not all of these side effects appear very often, when they do occur they may require medical attention. Check with your doctor *immediately* if any of the following side effects occur:

More common

Diarrhea	Sores in the mouth
Nausea and	and on the lips
vomiting	Stomach pain or
Redness of skin at	cramps
injection site	

Less common

Black tarry stools	Unexplained sore
Fever and chills	throat
Heartburn	Unusual bleeding or
Swelling or soreness	bruising
of the tongue	

Other side effects may occur which usually do not require medical attention. These side effects may go away during treatment as your body adjusts to the medicine. However, check with your doctor if any of the following side effects continue or are bothersome:

Less common

Loss of appetite	Swelling of feet or
Skin rash or itching	lower legs
Sores on the skin	

Rare

Blurred vision	Hiccups
Difficulty in walk-	Loss of hair
ing	Tiredness or
Dizziness	weakness

Other side effects not listed above may also occur in some patients. If you notice any other effects, check with your doctor.

FLUCYTOSINE (Systemic)
Some commonly used brand names are Ancobon and Ancotil*.

---

*Not available in the United States.

Flucytosine (floo-SYE-toe-seen) belongs to the group of medicines called antifungals. It is used in the treatment of certain fungus infections. This medicine is available only with your doctor's prescription.

Before Using This Medicine

In order to decide on the best treatment for your medical problem, your doctor should be told:

—if you have ever had any unusual reaction to flucytosine in the past. This medicine should not be taken if you are allergic to it.

—if you are pregnant, if you intend to become pregnant, or if you are breast-feeding an infant. Although flucytosine has not been shown to cause problems in humans, the chance always exists.

—if you have any of the following medical problems:

Blood disease	Liver disease
Kidney disease	

—if you are taking medicines that affect the bone marrow such as:

Anticancer	Oxyphenbutazone
medicines	Penicillamine
Colchicine	Phenylbutazone
Gold salts	

Proper Use of This Medicine

To help clear up your infection completely, *keep taking this medicine for the full time of treatment* even if you begin to feel better after a few days; *do not miss any doses.*

If you do miss a dose of this medicine, take it as soon as possible. Then go back to your regular dosing schedule. If it is almost time for your next dose, do not take the missed dose at all and do not double the next one. Instead, go back to your regular dosing schedule. If you have any questions about this, check with your doctor.

In some patients this medicine may cause nausea or vomiting. If you are taking more than 1 capsule for each dose, you may space them out over a period of 15 minutes to help lessen the nausea or vomiting. If this does not help or if you have any questions, check with your doctor.

Precautions While Using This Medicine

Your doctor should check your progress at regular visits in order to make sure that this medicine does not cause unwanted effects.

Side Effects of This Medicine

Along with its needed effects, a medicine may cause some unwanted effects. Although not all of these side effects appear very often, when they do occur they may require medical attention. Check with your doctor if any of the following side effects occur:

More common

Skin rash	Unusual bleeding
Unexplained sore	or bruising
throat and fever	Unusual tiredness
	or weakness

Less common

Hallucinations (see-	Mental confusion
ing, hearing,	
or feeling	
things that are	
not there)	

Other side effects may occur which usually do not require medical attention. These side effects may go away during treatment as your body adjusts to the medicine. However, check with your doctor if any of the following side effects continue or are bothersome:

More common

Diarrhea	Vomiting
Nausea	

Less common

Dizziness or	Drowsiness
lightheadedness	Headache

Other side effects not listed above may also occur in some patients. If you notice any other effects, check with your doctor.

FLUOROURACIL (Systemic)

A commonly used brand name is Adrucil.

Fluorouracil (flure-oh-YOOR-a-sill) belongs to the group of medicines known as antimetabolites. It is used by injection to treat some kinds of cancer. Fluorouracil is available only on prescription and is to be administered only by or under the immediate supervision of your doctor.

Before Using This Medicine

Fluorouracil is a very strong medicine. In addition to its helpful effects in treating your medical problem, it has side effects that could be very serious. Before you receive this medicine, be sure that you have discussed the use of it with your doctor.

In order to decide on the best treatment for your medical problem, your doctor should be told:

—if you have ever had any unusual reaction to fluorouracil in the past.

—if you are pregnant or if you intend to have children. This medicine may cause birth defects if either the male or female is taking it at the time of conception or if it is taken during pregnancy. It may also cause permanent sterility after it has been taken for a while. Be sure that you have discussed this with your doctor before taking this medicine.

—if you are breast-feeding an infant. Although fluorouracil has not been shown to cause problems, the chance always exists.

—if you have any of the following medical problems:

Infection	Liver disease
Kidney disease	

—if you have been treated with x-rays or cancer drugs by another doctor.

Proper Use of This Medicine

This medicine is sometimes given together with certain other medicines. If you are using a combination of drugs, it is important that you receive each medicine at the proper time. If you are taking some of these medicines by mouth, ask your doctor, nurse, or pharmacist to help you plan a way to remember to take them at the right time.

Fluorouracil often causes nausea and vomiting. However, it is very important that you continue to receive the medicine, even if your stomach is upset. If you have any questions about this, check with your doctor.

Precautions While Using This Medicine

It is very important that your doctor check your progress at regular visits.

Side Effects of This Medicine

Along with its needed effects, a medicine may cause some unwanted effects. Although not all of these side effects appear very often, when they do occur they may require medical attention. Check with your doctor *immediately* if any of the following side effects occur:

More common

Diarrhea	Unexplained fever,
Heartburn	chills, or sore
Sores in the mouth	throat
and on the lips	

Less common

Black tarry stools	Stomach cramps
Severe nausea and vomiting	Unusual bleeding or bruising

Rare

Chest pain	Difficulty with balance
Cough	Shortness of breath

Other side effects may occur which usually do not require medical attention. These side effects may go away during treatment as your body adjusts to the medicine. However, check with your doctor if any of the following side effects continue or are bothersome:

More common

Loss of appetite	Skin rash and itching
Loss of hair	Weakness
Nausea and vomiting	

Rare

Changes in finger- nails and toenails	Increased sensitivity of the skin to sunlight
Darkening of the skin	Watery eyes
Dry, cracking skin	

This medicine often causes a temporary loss of hair. After treatment with fluorouracil has ended, normal hair growth should return.

After you stop using this medicine, it may still produce some side effects that need attention. During this period of time check with your doctor if you notice any of the following:

Unexplained fever, chills, or sore throat	Unusual bleeding or bruising

Other side effects not listed above may also occur in some patients. If you notice any other effects, check with your doctor.

FLUOROURACIL (Topical)

Some commonly used brand names are Efudex and Fluoroplex.

Fluorouracil (flure-oh-YOOR-a-sill) belongs to the group of medicines known as antimetabolites. When applied to the skin, it is used to treat certain skin problems, including cancer or conditions that could become cancerous if not treated. Fluorouracil is available only with your doctor's prescription.

Before Using This Medicine

In order to decide on the best treatment for your medical problem, your doctor should be told:

—if you have ever had any unusual reaction to fluorouracil in the past.

—if you are pregnant, if you intend to become pregnant, or if you are breast-feeding an infant. Although fluorouracil has not been shown to cause problems, the chance always exists.

Proper Use of This Medicine

Keep using this medicine for the full time of treatment. However, *do not use this medicine more often or for a longer period of time than your doctor ordered.* Apply enough medicine each time to cover the entire affected area with a thin layer.

This medicine may cause redness, scaling, blistering, and peeling of affected skin after 1 or 2 weeks of use. This effect may last for several weeks after you stop using the medicine and is to be expected. Do not stop using this medicine without first checking with your doctor.

Use a cotton-tipped applicator or your fingertips to apply the medicine in a thin layer to your skin.

If you apply this medicine with your fingertips, make sure you *wash your hands immediately afterwards,* to prevent any of the medicine from accidentally getting in your eyes or mouth.

Precautions While Using This Medicine

It is very important that your doctor check your progress at regular visits.

Apply this medicine very carefully when using it on your face. Avoid getting any in your eyes, nose, or mouth.

While using this medicine, and for 1 or 2 months after you stop using it, avoid too much sun or use of a sunlamp since your skin may become more sensitive to sunlight than usual and too much sunlight may increase the effect of the drug. In case of a severe burn, check with your doctor.

Side Effects of This Medicine

Along with its needed effects, a medicine may cause some unwanted effects. Although not all of these side effects appear very often, when

they do occur they may require medical attention. *Check with your doctor immediately* if the following side effect occurs:

Redness and swelling of normal skin

Other side effects may occur which usually do not require medical attention. These side effects may go away during treatment as your body adjusts to the medicine. However, check with your doctor if any of the following side effects continue, worsen, or are bothersome:

More common

Burning sensation where medicine is applied	Itching
	Oozing
	Skin rash
Increased sensitivity of skin to sunlight	Soreness or tenderness

Less common
Darkening of skin
Scaling

Rare
Watery eyes

Sometimes a pink, smooth scar is left when the area treated with this medicine heals. This scar will usually fade after 1 to 2 months. If you have any questions about this, check with your doctor.

Other side effects not listed above may also occur in some patients. If you notice any other effects, check with your doctor.

FUROSEMIDE (Systemic)

Some commonly used brand names are:

Furoside*	Novosemide*
Lasix	Uritol*
Neo-Renal*	

---

* Not available in the United States.

Furosemide (fur-OH-se-mide) belongs to the general family of medicines called diuretics. It is given by mouth or by injection to help reduce the amount of water in the body by increasing the flow of urine. It is also used to treat high blood pressure in those patients who are not helped by other medicines or in those patients who have kidney problems. Furosemide may also be used for other conditions as determined by your doctor. This medicine is available only with your doctor's prescription.

Before Using This Medicine

In order to decide on the best treatment for your medical problem, your doctor should be told:

—if you are allergic to sulfonamides (sulfa drugs) or thiazide diuretics.

—if you are pregnant or if you intend to become pregnant while using this medicine. Although furosemide has not been shown to cause birth defects in humans, the chance always exists.

—if you are breast-feeding an infant. Although furosemide has not been shown to cause problems, the chance always exists.

—if you have been told by another doctor that you have any of the following medical problems:

Diabetes	Liver disease
Gout	Pancreas disease
History of lupus erythematosus	Severe kidney disease

—if you are now taking any of the following medicines or types of medicine:

Aspirin or other salicylates in very large doses (such as for arthritis)	Gout medicine
	Lithium
	Narcotics or prescription pain medicine
Clofibrate	Other diuretics (water pills) or antihypertensives (high blood pressure medicine)
Corticosteroids (cortisone-like medicines)	
Diabetes medicine	
Digitalis glycosides (heart medicine)	Sleeping medicine, such as barbiturates

Proper Use of This Medicine

Furosemide may cause you to have an unusual feeling of tiredness when you begin to take it. You may also notice an increase in the amount of urine or in your frequency of urination. After taking the medicine for awhile, these effects should lessen. In order to keep the increase in urine from affecting your nighttime sleep:

—if you are to take a single dose a day, take it in the morning after breakfast.

—if you are to take more than one dose a day, take the last dose no later than 6 p.m., unless otherwise directed by your doctor.

However, it is best to plan your dose or doses according to a schedule that will least affect your personal activities and sleep. Ask your doctor, nurse, or pharmacist to help you plan the best time to take this medicine.

In order to help remember to take your medicine, try to get into the habit of taking it at the same time each day.

If you miss a dose of this medicine, take it as soon as possible. However, if it is almost time for your next dose, do not take the missed dose at all and do not double the next one. Instead, go back to your regular dosing schedule. If you have any questions about this, check with your doctor.

For patients taking this medicine for high blood pressure:

• Importance of Diet—In addition to prescribing medicine for your condition, your doctor may prescribe a personal diet for you. Such a diet may be low in sodium (salt). Medicine is more effective when this diet is properly followed.

Also, it may be very important for you to go on a reducing diet. However, check with your doctor before going on any diet.

• Many patients who have high blood pressure will not notice any signs of the problem. In fact, many may feel normal. It is very important that you take your medicine exactly as directed and that you keep your doctor's appointments even if you feel well.

• Remember that this medicine will not cure your high blood pressure but it does control it. Therefore, you must continue to take it as directed if you expect to keep your blood pressure down. *You may have to take medicine for the rest of your life.* If high blood pressure is not treated, it can cause serious problems such as heart failure, blood vessel disease, stroke, or kidney disease.

For patients taking the oral liquid form of this medicine:

• This medicine is to be taken by mouth even though it may come in a dropper bottle. If this medicine does not come in a dropper bottle, use a specially marked measuring spoon or other device to measure each dose accurately, since the average household teaspoon may not hold the right amount of liquid.

Precautions While Using This Medicine

It is important that your doctor check your progress at regular visits.

This medicine may cause a loss of potassium from your body.

• To help prevent this, your doctor may want you to:

—eat or drink foods that have a high potassium content (for example, orange or other citrus fruit juices), or

—take a potassium supplement, or

—take another medicine to help prevent the loss of the potassium in the first place.

• It is very important to follow these directions. Also, it is important not to change your diet on your own. This is more important if you are already on a special diet (as for diabetes), or if you are taking a potassium supplement or a medicine to reduce potassium loss. Extra potassium may not be necessary and, in some cases, too much potassium could be harmful.

To prevent the loss of too much water and potassium, tell your doctor if you become sick, especially with severe or continuing nausea and vomiting or diarrhea.

Caution: Diabetics—Furosemide may affect blood sugar levels. While you are using this medicine, be especially careful in testing for sugar in your urine. If you have any questions about this, check with your doctor.

Before having any kind of surgery (including dental surgery), make sure the doctor or dentist in charge knows that you are taking this medicine.

Dizziness, lightheadedness, or fainting may occur, especially when you get up from a lying or sitting position. This is more likely to occur in the morning. *Getting up slowly may help* but if the problem continues or gets worse, check with your doctor.

The dizziness, lightheadedness, or fainting is also more likely to occur if you drink alcohol, stand for long periods of time, exercise, or if the weather is hot. *While you are taking this medicine, be careful in the amount of alcohol you drink. Also, use extra care during exercise or hot weather or if you must stand for long periods of time.* Check with your doctor if you have any questions about this.

A few people who take this medicine may become more sensitive to sunlight than they are normally. When you begin to take this medicine, avoid too much sun or use of a sunlamp until you see how you react, especially if you tend to burn easily. If you have a severe reaction, check with your doctor.

For patients taking this medicine for high blood pressure:

• *Do not take other medicines unless they have been discussed with your doctor.* This especially includes over-the-counter (nonprescription) medicines for appetite control, asthma, colds, cough, hay fever, or sinus, since they may tend to increase your blood pressure.

Side Effects of This Medicine

Along with its needed effects, a medicine may cause some unwanted effects. Although not all of these side effects appear very often, when they do occur they may require medical attention. Check with your doctor if any of the following side effects occur:

Signs of loss of too much potassium

Dryness of mouth	Muscle cramps or
Increased thirst	pain
Irregular heartbeats	Nausea or vomiting
Mood or mental	Unusual tiredness or
changes	weakness
	Weak pulse

Rare

Flank or stomach	Skin rash or hives
pain	Unexplained sore
Joint pain	throat and fever
Ringing or buzzing	Unusual bleeding or
sound in ears or	bruising
any loss of hear-	Yellow vision
ing	Yellowing of eyes
Severe stomach pain	or skin
with nausea and	
vomiting	

Other side effects may occur which usually do not require medical attention. These side effects may go away during treatment as your body adjusts to the medicine. However, check with your doctor if any of the following side effects continue or are bothersome:

More common

Dizziness or light-
headedness when
getting up from
a lying or
sitting position

Less common

Diarrhea	Loss of appetite
Increased sensitivity	Upset stomach
of skin to	
sunlight	

Other side effects not listed above may also occur in some patients. If you notice any other effects, check with your doctor.

GENTAMICIN (Ophthalmic)
Some commonly used brand names are Garamycin and Genoptic.

Gentamicin (jen-ta-MYE-sin) belongs to the general family of medicines called antibiotics. Gentamicin ophthalmic preparations are used to help the body overcome infections of the eye. Gentamicin may also be used for other problems as determined by your doctor. They are available only with your doctor's prescription.

Before Using This Medicine

In order to decide on the best treatment for your medical problem, your doctor should be told:

—if you have had allergic reactions to any related antibiotics such as amikacin, gentamicin (by injection), kanamycin, neomycin, streptomycin, or tobramycin.

—if you are pregnant, if you intend to become pregnant, or if you are breast-feeding an infant, although gentamicin ophthalmic preparations have not been shown to cause problems.

Proper Use of This Medicine

If you are using the eye drop form of this medicine:

• Bottle is not full; this is to provide proper drop control.

• To prevent contamination of the eye drops, do not touch the applicator tip to any surface (including the eye), and keep the container tightly closed.

• How to apply this medicine: First, wash hands. Then tilt head back and pull lower eyelid away from eye to form a pouch. Drop medicine into the pouch and gently close eyes. Do not blink. Keep eyes closed for 1 or 2 minutes to allow medicine to come into contact with the infection.

• If you think you did not get the drop of medicine into your eye properly, use another drop.

If you are using the eye ointment form of this medicine:

• To prevent contamination of the eye ointment, do not touch the applicator tip to any surface (including the eye). After using, wipe the tip of the ointment tube with a clean tissue and keep the tube tightly closed.

• How to apply this medicine: First, wash hands. Then pull the lower eyelid away from eye to form a pouch. Squeeze a thin strip of ointment into the pouch. A 1-cm (approximately 1/3-inch) strip of ointment is usually enough unless otherwise directed by your doctor. Gently close eyes and keep them closed for 1 or 2 minutes to allow medicine to come into contact with the infection.

To help clear up your infection completely, *keep using this medicine for the full time of treatment,* even though your symptoms may have disappeared; *do not miss any doses.*

If you do miss a dose of this medicine, apply it as soon as possible. However, if it is almost time for your next application, skip the missed dose and go back to your regular dosing schedule.

Precautions While Using This Medicine

After application of this medicine to the eye, occasional stinging or burning may be expected.

After application, eye ointments usually cause your vision to blur for a few minutes.

If your symptoms do not improve within a few days or if they become worse, check with your doctor.

Side Effects of This Medicine

Along with its needed effects, a medicine may cause some unwanted effects. Although not all of these side effects appear very often, when they do occur they may require medical attention. Stop using this medicine and check with your doctor if any of the following side effects occur:

Itching, redness, swelling, or other sign of irritation not present before you started using this medicine

Other side effects not listed above may also occur in some patients. If you notice any other effects, check with your doctor.

GENTAMICIN (Topical)
A commonly used brand name is Garamycin.

Gentamicin (jen-ta-MYE-sin) belongs to the general family of medicines called antibiotics. Gentamicin topical preparations are used to help the body overcome infections of the skin. Gentamicin is available only with your doctor's prescription.

Before Using This Medicine

In order to decide on the best treatment for your medical problem, your doctor should be told:

—if you have had allergic reactions to any related antibiotics such as amikacin, gentamicin (by injection), kanamycin, neomycin, streptomycin, or tobramycin.

—if you are pregnant, if you intend to become pregnant, or if you are breast-feeding an infant, although gentamicin topical preparations have not been shown to cause problems.

—if you are now taking any of the following medicines:

Amikacin	Neomycin
Gentamicin (by injection)	Streptomycin
Kanamycin	Tobramycin

Proper Use of This Medicine

Before applying this medicine, wash the area to be treated with soap and water, and dry thoroughly. Apply a small amount to the affected area and rub in gently.

After this medicine is applied, the treated area may be covered with a gauze dressing if desired.

To help clear up your infection completely, *keep using this medicine for the full time of treatment,* even though your symptoms may have disappeared; *do not miss any doses.*

If you do miss a dose of this medicine, apply it as soon as possible. However, if it is almost time for your next application, skip the missed dose and go back to your regular dosing schedule.

Precautions While Using This Medicine

If there is no improvement in your skin problem after you have used this medicine for 1 week or if it becomes worse, check with your doctor.

Side Effects of This Medicine

Along with its needed effects, a medicine may cause some unwanted effects. Although not all of these side effects appear very often, when they do occur they may require medical attention. Stop using this medicine and check with your doctor if any of the following side effects occur:

Itching, redness, swelling, or other sign of irritation not present before you started using this medicine

Other side effects not listed above may also occur in some patients. If you notice any other effects, check with your doctor.

GENTIAN VIOLET (Topical)

Gentian violet (JEN-shun VYE-oh-let) belongs to the group of medicines called antifungals. Topical gentian violet is used to treat some types of fungal infections inside the mouth (thrush) and of the skin. This medicine is available without a prescription; however, your doctor may have special instructions on the proper use of gentian violet for your medical condition.

Before Using This Medicine

In order to decide on the best treatment for your medical problem, your doctor should be told:

—if you have ever had any unusual reaction to gentian violet in the past. This medicine should not be used if you are allergic to it.

—if you are pregnant, if you intend to become pregnant, or if you are breast-feeding an infant, although gentian violet has not been shown to cause problems.

Proper Use of This Medicine

To help clear up your infection completely, *keep using this medicine for the full time of treatment* even though your condition may have improved.

Using a cotton swab, apply enough gentian violet to cover only the affected area.

If you are applying this medicine to affected areas in the mouth, avoid swallowing any of the medicine.

If you are using this medicine in a child's mouth, make sure you understand exactly how to apply it so that it is not swallowed. If you have any questions about this, check with your doctor.

Do not apply an occlusive dressing or airtight covering (for example, kitchen plastic wrap) over this medicine, since it may cause irritation of the skin.

If you miss a dose of this medicine, apply it as soon as possible. Then go back to your regular dosing schedule. But if it is almost time for your next dose, do not apply the missed dose at all. Instead, go back to your regular dosing schedule. If you have any questions about this, check with your doctor.

Precautions While Using This Medicine

To help cure the infection and to help prevent reinfection, good health habits are required. These include the following:

• Wash all towels and bedding after each use.

• Use only freshly laundered clothes each time clothing is changed.

If you have any questions about this, check with your doctor, nurse, or pharmacist.

Gentian violet will stain the skin and clothing. Avoid getting the medicine on your clothes.

Side Effects of This Medicine

Along with its needed effects, a medicine may cause some unwanted effects. Although not all of these side effects appear very often, when they do occur they may require medical attention. Check with your doctor if the following side effect occurs:

Irritation of skin not present before using this medicine

Other side effects not listed above may also occur in some patients. If you notice any other effects, check with your doctor.

GENTIAN VIOLET (Vaginal)
Some commonly used brand names are Genapax and Hyva.

Gentian violet (JEN-shun VYE-oh-let) belongs to the group of medicines called antifungals. Vaginal gentian violet is used to treat fungal infections of the vagina. This medicine is available only with your doctor's prescription.

Before Using This Medicine

In order to decide on the best treatment for your medical problem, your doctor should be told:

—if you have ever had any unusual reaction to gentian violet in the past. This medicine should not be used if you are allergic to it.

—if you are pregnant, if you intend to become pregnant, or if you are breast-feeding an infant, although gentian violet has not been shown to cause problems.

Proper Use of This Medicine

To help clear up your infection completely, *keep using this medicine for the full time of treatment* even though your condition may have improved. Also, keep using this medicine even if you begin to menstruate during the time of treatment.

If you miss a dose of this medicine, insert it as soon as possible. Then go back to your regular dosing schedule. But if it is almost time for your next dose, do not insert the missed dose at all. Instead, go back to your regular dosing schedule. If you have any questions about this, check with your doctor.

Gentian violet usually comes with patient directions. Read them carefully before using this medicine.

If you are using the vaginal suppository or tablet form of this medicine:

• This medicine is usually inserted into the vagina using an applicator. However, if you are pregnant, check with your doctor before using the applicator to insert the vaginal suppository or tablet.

If you are using the vaginal tampon form of this medicine:

• After insertion, remove the tampon from the vagina after 3 to 4 hours unless otherwise directed by your doctor.

Precautions While Using This Medicine

To help cure the infection and to help prevent reinfection, good health habits are required. These include the following:

• Wear cotton panties (or panties or pantyhose with cotton crotches) instead of synthetic (for example, nylon, rayon) underclothes.

• Wear freshly laundered underclothes.

If you have any questions about this, check with your doctor, nurse, or pharmacist.

If you have intercourse during the time of treatment with this medicine, make sure your partner wears a condom (prophylactic). If you have any questions about this, check with your doctor or pharmacist.

If you have any questions about douching during the time of treatment with this medicine, check with your doctor.

Gentian violet will stain the skin and clothing. Avoid getting the medicine on your clothes.

Since there may be some vaginal drainage while you are using this medicine, a sanitary napkin may be worn to protect your clothing.

Side Effects of This Medicine

Along with its needed effects, a medicine may cause some unwanted effects. Although not all of these side effects appear very often, when they do occur they may require medical attention. Check with your doctor if any of the following side effects occur:

Vaginal burning, itching, pain, or other sign of irritation not present before using this medicine

Other side effects not listed above may also occur in some patients. If you notice any other effects, check with your doctor.

GLUCAGON (Systemic)

Glucagon (GLOO-ka-gon) belongs to the group of medicines called hormones. It is an emergency medicine used to treat severe hypoglycemia (low blood sugar) reactions of diabetic patients who are unconscious or unable to swallow food or liquids. It is also used during certain examination procedures to improve patient comfort and examination results. Glucagon is available only with your doctor's prescription.

Before Using This Medicine

In order to decide on the best treatment for your medical problem, your doctor should be told:

—if you have ever had any unusual reaction to glucagon in the past. This medicine should not be taken if you are allergic to it.

Proper Use of This Medicine

Glucagon is an emergency medicine and must be used only as directed by your doctor. Glucagon is used by injection if the patient becomes unconscious as a result of hypoglycemia (low blood sugar), or is unable to take some form of sugar by mouth. *Make sure that you and your family or a friend understand exactly when and how to use this medicine before it must be used.*

Glucagon is packaged in a kit containing two vials (one powder and one liquid) whose contents must be mixed before using. *Directions for mixing and injecting are in the package. Read them carefully* and ask your doctor, nurse, or pharmacist for additional explanation, if necessary.

Glucagon may be mixed when an emergency occurs. However, if glucagon is needed often, it may be mixed and kept ready for use ahead of time. The date of mixing should be noted on the package. When refrigerated, the mixed glucagon may be used within 3 months of that date. Mixed glucagon kept 3 months or more should be discarded and replaced by a fresh preparation.

Before mixing, glucagon may be stored at room temperature but should not be used after the expiration date printed on the kit and on one vial. This expiration date does not apply after mixing.

Precautions While Using This Medicine

Diabetic patients should be aware of the symptoms of hypoglycemia (low blood sugar) which may develop in a very short time. These symptoms may result from:

—using too much insulin ("insulin reaction").

—delaying or missing a scheduled snack or meal.

—sickness (especially with vomiting).

—exercising more than usual.

Such symptoms are:

Anxious feeling	Nervousness
Chills	Shakiness
Cool pale skin	Sweating
Headache	Unusual tiredness
Hunger	Weakness
Nausea	

Eating some form of sugar when these symptoms first appear will usually prevent them from getting worse, and will probably make the use of glucagon unnecessary.

However, if it becomes necessary to inject glucagon:

—*Turn the patient on one side.* Glucagon may cause some patients to vomit and this position will reduce the possibility of choking.

—*Call the patient's doctor at once.*

—The patient will often become conscious in 5 to 20 minutes, but if not, a second dose may be given. *Arrange to get the patient to a doctor or to hospital emergency care as soon as possible,* since being unconscious too long may be harmful.

—*When a patient has regained consciousness enough to swallow, give some form of sugar by mouth.* Orange juice, corn syrup, honey, sugar cubes, or table sugar all work more quickly when mixed with or dissolved in water. If a snack or meal is not scheduled for an hour or more, the patient should also eat some crackers

or half a sandwich. This will prevent hypoglycemia from occurring again soon.

—Glucagon is not effective for much longer than 1 1/2 hours and is *used only until the patient is able to swallow liquids.*

—*If nausea prevents a patient from swallowing some form of sugar for an hour after glucagon is given, medical help should be obtained.*

Diabetic patients should routinely check:

—glucagon expiration date.

—availability of sterile syringe and needles.

Keep your doctor informed of any hypoglycemic attacks or use of glucagon even if the symptoms are successfully controlled and there seem to be no continuing problems. Complete information is necessary to provide the best possible treatment of any condition.

GLUTETHIMIDE (Systemic)
Some commonly used brand names are Doriden and Dormtabs.

Glutethimide (gloo-TETH-i-mide) is used in the treatment of insomnia or sleeplessness. It helps patients to sleep. However, if used regularly (for example, every day), it is usually not effective for more than 7 days. This medicine is available only with your doctor's prescription.

Before Using This Medicine

In order to decide on the best treatment for your medical problem, your doctor should be told:

—if you have ever had any unusual reaction to glutethimide in the past. This medicine should not be taken if you are allergic to it.

—if you are pregnant or if you intend to become pregnant while using this medicine. Too much use of glutethimide during pregnancy may cause the baby to become dependent on the medicine. This may lead to withdrawal side effects after birth.

—if you are breast-feeding an infant. Glutethimide passes into the breast milk and may cause unwanted effects in infants of mothers taking this medicine.

—if you have any of the following medical problems:

Enlarged prostate	Kidney disease
Glaucoma	Porphyria
Intestinal blockage	Stomach ulcer
Irregular heartbeat	Urinary tract blockage

—if you are now taking other central nervous system (CNS) depressants such as:

Antihistamines or medicine for hay fever, other allergies, or colds	Prescription pain medicine
Barbiturates	Seizure medicine
Narcotics	Tricyclic antidepressants (medicine for depression)
Other sedatives, tranquilizers, or sleeping medicine	

—if you are now taking or have taken within the past 2 weeks monoamine oxidase (MAO) inhibitors such as:

| Isocarboxazid | Phenelzine |
| Pargyline | Tranylcypromine |

—if you are now taking coumarin-type anticoagulants (blood thinners).

Proper Use of This Medicine

Take this medicine only as directed by your doctor. Do not take more of it, do not take it more often, and do not take it for a longer period of time than your doctor ordered. If too much is taken, it may become habit-forming.

Keep this medicine out of the reach of children since overdose is especially dangerous in children.

Precautions While Using This Medicine

If you will be taking this medicine regularly for a long period of time:

—your doctor should check your progress at regular visits.

—do not stop taking it without first checking with your doctor. Your doctor may want you to reduce gradually the amount you are taking before stopping completely.

This medicine will add to the effects of alcohol and other medicines (CNS depressants) that slow down the nervous system. Some examples of CNS depressants are antihistamines or medicine for hay fever, other allergies, or colds; sedatives, tranquilizers, or sleeping medicine; prescription pain medicine or narcotics; barbiturates; medicine for seizures; tricyclic antidepressants (medicine for depression); or anesthetics, including some dental anesthetics. *Check with your doctor before taking any of the above while you are using this medicine.*

If you think you may have taken an overdose of this medicine, get emergency help at once. Taking an overdose of glutethimide or taking it with alcohol or other CNS depressants may lead to unconsciousness and possibly death. Some signs of an overdose are mental confusion, severe weakness, shortness of breath or troubled breathing, staggering, and unusually slow heartbeat.

This medicine may cause some people to become dizzy, drowsy, or less alert than they are normally. Even if taken at bedtime, it may cause some people to feel drowsy or less alert on arising. *Make sure you know how you react to this medicine before you drive, use machines, or do other jobs that require you to be alert.*

Side Effects of This Medicine

Along with its needed effects, a medicine may cause some unwanted effects. Although not all of these side effects appear very often, when they do occur they may require medical attention. Check with your doctor if any of the following side effects occur:

Less common
Skin rash

Rare

Unexplained sore throat and fever	Unusually slow heartbeat, shortness of breath, or troubled breathing
Unusual bleeding or bruising	
Unusual excitement	
Unusual tiredness or weakness	

Other side effects may occur which usually do not require medical attention. These side effects may go away during treatment as your body adjusts to the medicine. However, check with your doctor if any of the following side effects continue or are bothersome:

More common
Drowsiness (daytime)

Less common

Blurred vision	Headache
Clumsiness or unsteadiness	Mental confusion
	Nausea
Dizziness	Slurred speech
"Hangover" effect	Vomiting

After you stop using this medicine, your body may need time to adjust. The length of time this takes depends on the amount of medicine you were using and how long you used it. During this period of time check with your doctor if you notice any of the following side effects:

Convulsions or seizures	Nausea or vomiting
Hallucinations (seeing, hearing, or feeling things that are not there)	Nightmares
	Stomach cramps or pain
	Trembling
	Trouble in sleeping
Increased dreaming	Unusually fast heartbeat
Muscle cramps or spasms	

Other side effects not listed above may also occur in some patients. If you notice any other effects, check with your doctor.

GLYCERIN (Systemic)
Some commonly used brand names are Glyrol and Osmoglyn.

Glycerin (GLI-ser-in), when taken by mouth, is used to treat certain conditions in which there is increased eye pressure, such as glaucoma, or increased intracranial pressure. It may also be used before eye surgery to reduce pressure in the eye. This medicine is available only with your doctor's prescription.

Before Using This Medicine
In order to decide on the best treatment for your medical problem, your doctor should be told:

—if you have ever had any unusual reaction to glycerin in the past. This medicine should not be taken if you are allergic to it.

—if you are pregnant, if you intend to become pregnant, or if you are breast-feeding an infant. Although this medicine has not been shown to cause problems, the chance always exists.

—if you have any of the following medical problems:

Diabetes	Kidney disease
Heart disease	

Proper Use of This Medicine
It is very important that you take this medicine only as directed. Do not take more of it and do not take it more often than your doctor ordered.

To improve the taste of this medicine, mix with unsweetened lemon, lime, or orange juice, pour over cracked ice, and sip through a straw.

If you miss a dose of this medicine, take it as soon as possible. Then go back to your regular dosing schedule. But if it is almost time for your next dose, do not take the missed dose at all. Instead, take your next dose at the regularly scheduled time. Then continue with your regular dosing schedule. If you have any questions about this, check with your doctor.

Precautions While Using This Medicine
Your doctor should check your progress at regular visits.

In some patients, headaches may occur when this medicine is taken. To help prevent or relieve the headache, lie down while you are taking this medicine and for a short time after taking it. If headaches become severe or continue, check with your doctor.

Side Effects of This Medicine
Along with its needed effects, a medicine may cause some unwanted effects. Although not all of these side effects appear very often, when they do occur they may require medical attention. Check with your doctor if either of the following side effects occurs:

Less common
    Mental confusion

Rare
    Irregular heartbeat

Other side effects may occur which usually do not require medical attention. These side effects may go away during treatment as your body adjusts to the medicine. However, check with your doctor if any of the following side effects continue or are bothersome:

More common
    Headache
    Nausea or vomiting

Less common

Diarrhea	Unusual dryness of mouth or increased thirst
Dizziness	

Other side effects not listed above may also occur in some patients. If you notice any other effects, check with your doctor.

GOLD COMPOUNDS (Systemic)

This information applies to the following medicines:

Aurothioglucose (aur-oh-thye-oh-GLOO-kose)
Gold Sodium Thiomalate (gold SO-dee-um thye-oh-MAH-late)

Some commonly used brand names are:	Generic names:
Solganal	Aurothioglucose
Myochrysine	Gold Sodium Thiomalate

The gold compounds belong to the group of medicines called antirheumatics. They are used in the treatment of rheumatoid arthritis. These medicines are available only with your doctor's prescription.

Before Using This Medicine

In addition to the helpful effects of this medicine in treating your medical problem, it has side effects that could be very serious. Before you take this medicine, be sure that you have discussed the use of it with your doctor.

In order to decide on the best treatment for your medical problem, your doctor should be told:

—if you have ever had any unusual reaction to gold or other metals.

—if you are pregnant or if you intend to become pregnant while using this medicine. Although gold compounds have not been shown to cause birth defects or other problems in humans, the chance always exists.

—if you are breast-feeding an infant. Aurothioglucose, and possibly gold sodium thiomalate, passes into the breast milk and may cause unwanted effects in infants of mothers taking this medicine.

—if you have any of the following medical problems:

Blood disease	Kidney disease
Colitis	(or history of)
Diabetes	Liver disease (or
Heart or blood	history of)
vessel disease	Lupus
High blood pressure	erythematosus
	Sjogren's syndrome
	Skin disease

—if you have recently been treated with x-rays.

—if you are now taking any of the following medicines or types of medicine:

Amodiaquine	Oxyphenbutazone
Chlcroquine	Penicillamine
Hydroxychloroquine	Phenylbutazone

Precautions While Using This Medicine

Immediately following an injection of this medicine, side effects such as dizziness, feeling faint, flushing or redness of face, nausea or vomiting, unusual sweating, or unusual weakness may occur. These will usually go away after you lie down for a few minutes. If any of these effects continue or become worse, check with your doctor.

Joint pain may occur for 1 or 2 days after you receive an injection of this medicine and will usually disappear after the first few injections. If this continues or is bothersome, check with your doctor.

Side Effects of This Medicine

Along with its needed effects, a medicine may cause some unwanted effects. Although not all of these side effects appear very often, they may occur at any time during treatment with this medicine and up to many months after treatment has ended, and they may require medical attention. Check with your doctor if any of the following side effects occur:

More common

Irritation or soreness of tongue or gums	Skin rash or itching Ulcers, sores, or white spots in mouth or throat
Metallic taste in mouth	

Less common

Cloudy urine

Rare

Bloody urine	Unexplained sore throat and fever
Coughing or shortness of breath	Unusual bleeding or bruising
Diarrhea or stomach pain	Unusual tiredness or weakness

With long-term use

Eye problems	Numbness, tingling, pain, or weakness in hands or feet
Grayish-blue coloration of skin	Yellowing of eyes or skin

Other side effects may occur which usually do not require medical attention. These side effects may go away during treatment as your body

adjusts to the medicine. However, check with your doctor if the following side effect continues or is bothersome:

Less common

Joint pain

Other side effects not listed above may also occur in some patients. If you notice any other effects, check with your doctor.

GRISEOFULVIN (Systemic)

Some commonly used brand names are:

Fulvicin P/G	Grisactin
Fulvicin-U/F	Grisovin-FP*
Grifulvin V	grisOwen
	Gris-PEG

---

*Not available in the United States.

Griseofulvin (gri-see-oh-FUL-vin) belongs to the group of medicines called antifungals. It is used to treat fungus infections of the skin, hair, fingernails, and toenails. This medicine is available only with your doctor's prescription.

Before Using This Medicine

In order to decide on the best treatment for your medical problem, your doctor should be told:

—if you have ever had any unusual reaction to penicillin.

—if you are pregnant, if you intend to become pregnant, or if you are breast-feeding an infant. Although griseofulvin has not been shown to cause problems in humans, the chance always exists.

—if you have any of the following medical problems:

Liver disease	Porphyria
Lupus	
erythematosus	

—if you are now taking any of the following medicines or types of medicine:

Barbiturates	Coumarin-type
	anticoagulants
	(blood thinners)

Proper Use of This Medicine

To help clear up your infection completely, *keep taking this medicine for the full time of treatment* even if you begin to feel better after a few days; *do not miss any doses.*

If you do miss a dose of this medicine, take it as soon as possible. Then go back to your regular dosing schedule. But if it is almost time for your next dose, do not take the missed dose at all and do not double the next one. Instead, go back to your regular dosing schedule. If you have any questions about this, check with your doctor.

Take griseofulvin with or after meals to lessen possible stomach upset, unless otherwise directed by your doctor. In some cases, your doctor may want you to take this medicine with or after high-fat meals since the medicine may be absorbed faster. If you have any questions about this, check with your doctor.

Precautions While Using This Medicine

Your doctor should check your progress at regular visits in order to make sure that griseofulvin does not cause unwanted effects.

To help cure the infection and to help make sure it does not come back, good health habits are required. If you have any questions about this, check with your doctor or pharmacist.

Griseofulvin may increase the effects of alcohol. It may also cause unusually fast heartbeat or flushing or redness of the face if taken with alcohol. Therefore, *do not drink alcoholic beverages while you are taking this medicine,* unless you have first checked with your doctor.

A few people who take this medicine may become more sensitive to sunlight than they are normally. When you first begin taking this medicine, avoid too much sun or use of a sunlamp until you see how you react, especially if you tend to burn easily. If you have a severe reaction, check with your doctor.

Side Effects of This Medicine

Along with its needed effects, a medicine may cause some unwanted effects. Although not all of these side effects appear very often, when they do occur they may require medical attention. Check with your doctor if any of the following side effects occur:

Less common

Mental confusion	Soreness or irrita-
Skin rash, hives,	tion of mouth
or itching	or tongue

Rare

Numbness, tingling,	Unexplained sore
pain, or weakness	throat and fever
in hands or feet	

Other side effects may occur which usually do not require medical attention. These side effects may go away during treatment as your body adjusts to the medicine. However, check with your doctor if any of the following side effects continue or are bothersome:

More common

Headache

Less common

Diarrhea	Stomach pain
Dizziness	Trouble in sleeping
Nausea or vomiting	Unusual tiredness

Other side effects not listed above may also occur in some patients. If you notice any other effects, check with your doctor.

GUAIFENESIN (Systemic)
Some commonly used brand names are:

2/G	Hytuss
Anti-Tuss	Malotuss
Breonesin	Nortussin
Genetuss	Proco
Glycotuss	Robitussin
Glytuss	

Guaifenesin (gwye-FEN-e-sin) is used to relieve coughs due to colds, bronchitis, influenza, laryngitis, and certain other respiratory (lung) conditions. It loosens mucus or phlegm (pronounced flem) in the lungs.

This medicine is usually not used for the chronic cough that occurs with smoking, asthma, or emphysema or when there is an unusually large amount of mucus or phlegm with the cough.

Guaifenesin is available without a prescription; however, your doctor may have special instructions on the proper dose of this medicine for your medical condition.

Before Using This Medicine

In order to decide on the best treatment for your medical problem, your doctor should be told:

—if you have ever had any unusual reaction to guaifenesin in the past. This medicine should not be taken if you are allergic to it.

—if you are pregnant, if you intend to become pregnant, or if you are breast-feeding an infant. Although guaifenesin has not been shown to cause problems, the chance always exists.

Proper Use of This Medicine

To help loosen mucus or phlegm (flem) in the lungs, *drink a glass of water after each dose of this medicine,* unless otherwise directed by your doctor.

If you miss a dose of this medicine, take it as soon as possible. Then go back to your regular dosing schedule. But if it is almost time for your next dose, do not take the missed dose at all. Instead, take your next dose at the regularly scheduled time. Then continue with your regular dosing schedule. If you have any questions about this, check with your doctor or pharmacist.

Precautions While Using This Medicine

If your cough has not improved after 7 days or if you have a high fever, skin rash, continuing headache, or sore throat with the cough, check with your doctor. These signs may mean that you have other medical problems.

Side Effects of This Medicine

Along with its needed effects, a medicine may cause some unwanted effects. Although no serious side effects have been reported for guaifenesin, the following side effects may be noticed by some patients. Check with your doctor if any of these effects continue or are bothersome:

Less common or rare

Diarrhea	Nausea or vomiting
Drowsiness	Stomach pain

Other side effects not listed above may also occur in some patients. If you notice any other effects, check with your doctor.

GUAIFENESIN AND CODEINE (Systemic)
[Formerly called Glyceryl Guaiacolate and Codeine]
Some commonly used brand names are:

Cheracol	Robitussin A-C
Nortussin w/ Co-deine	Tolu-Sed

Guaifenesin (gwye-FEN-e-sin) and codeine (KOE-deen) combination is taken by mouth to relieve coughs due to colds, bronchitis, laryngitis, influenza, and other respiratory (lung) conditions. It is usually not used for chronic cough that occurs with smoking, asthma, or emphysema or when there is an unusually large amount of mucus or phlegm (pronounced flem) with the cough.

In some states, this medicine is available only with your doctor's prescription. In other states, it is available without a prescription; however, your doctor may have special instructions on the proper use of this medicine for your medical condition.

In the states where this medicine is available without a prescription, you must ask your pharmacist for it, show personal identification, and sign a record book showing that you bought the medicine, since codeine is a narcotic.

Before Using This Medicine

In order to decide on the best treatment for your medical problem, your doctor should be told:

—if you have ever had any unusual reaction to guaifenesin or codeine in the past. This medicine should not be taken if you are allergic to it.

—if you are pregnant or if you intend to become pregnant while using this medicine. Although guaifenesin and codeine have not been shown to cause birth defects or other problems, the chance always exists.

—if you are breast-feeding an infant. The codeine in this medicine passes into the breast milk. Although the amount of codeine in recommended doses of this medicine does not usually cause problems, the chance always exists.

—if you have any of the following medical problems:

Brain disease or injury	Kidney disease
Colitis	Liver disease
Emphysema, asthma, or chronic lung disease	Underactive adrenal gland (Addison's disease)
Enlarged prostate or problems with urination	Underactive thyroid Unusually slow or irregular heartbeat
Gallbladder disease or gallstones	

—if you are now taking central nervous system (CNS) depressants such as:

Antihistamines or medicine for hay fever, other allergies, or colds	Prescription pain medicine
	Sedatives, tranquilizers, or sleeping medicine
Barbiturates	Seizure medicine
Narcotics	Tricyclic antidepressants (medicine for depression)

—if you are now taking prescription medicine for stomach cramps or spasms.

—if you are now taking or have taken within the past 2 weeks monoamine oxidase (MAO) inhibitors such as:

Isocarboxazid	Phenelzine
Pargyline	Tranylcypromine

Proper Use of This Medicine

Take this medicine only as directed. Do not take more of it, do not take it more often, and do not take it for a longer period of time than recommended on the label, unless otherwise directed by your doctor. If too much is taken, the codeine in this medicine may become habit-forming.

Precautions While Using This Medicine

If your cough has not improved after 7 days or if you have a high fever, skin rash, or continuing headache with the cough, check with your doctor. These signs may mean that you have other medical problems.

The codeine in this medicine will add to the effects of alcohol and other medicines (CNS depressants) that slow down the nervous system. Some examples of CNS depressants are antihistamines or medicine for hay fever, other allergies, or colds; sedatives, tranquilizers, or sleeping medicine; prescription pain medicine or narcotics; barbiturates; medicine for seizures; tricyclic antidepressants (medicine for depression); or anesthetics, including some dental anesthetics. *Check with your doctor before taking any of the above while you are taking this medicine.*

This medicine may cause some people to become drowsy or less alert than they are normally. *Make sure you know how you react to this medicine before you drive, use machines, or do other jobs that require you to be alert.*

Dizziness, lightheadedness, or fainting may occur, especially when you get up from a lying or sitting position. Getting up slowly may help. If the problem continues or gets worse, check with your doctor.

Nausea may occur, especially after the first couple of doses. This effect usually goes away if you lie down for a while. However, if nausea continues, check with your doctor.

Side Effects of This Medicine

Along with its needed effects, a medicine may cause some unwanted effects. Although not all of these side effects appear very often, when

they do occur they may require medical attention. Check with your doctor if any of the following side effects occur:

Rare

Shortness of breath	Unusually slow
Troubled breathing	heartbeat
Unusual excitement	
(especially in	
children)	

Other side effects may occur which usually do not require medical attention. These side effects may go away during treatment as your body adjusts to the medicine. However, check with your doctor if any of the following side effects continue or are bothersome:

More common
Constipation
Drowsiness

Less common

Diarrhea	Nausea or vomiting
Difficult urination	Redness or flushing
Dizziness	of face
Feeling faint	Stomach pain
Frequent urge to	Unusual increase in
urinate	sweating
Lightheadedness	Unusual tiredness or
Loss of appetite	weakness

Other side effects not listed above may also occur in some patients. If you notice any other effects, check with your doctor.

GUAIFENESIN AND DEXTROMETHORPHAN
(Systemic)

[Formerly called Glyceryl Guaiacolate and Dextromethorphan]

Some commonly used brand names are:

Anti-Tuss	G-Tuss DM	Silexin
DM	Guaiadex	Tolu-Sed DM
Cheracol D	Neo-Vadrin	Trocal
Dextro-Tuss	Queltuss	Unproco
GG	Robitussin-	
2/G-DM	DM	

Guaifenesin (gwye-FEN-e-sin) and dextromethorphan (dex-troe-meth-OR-fan) combination is taken by mouth to relieve coughs due to colds, bronchitis, laryngitis, influenza, and other respiratory (lung) conditions. It is usually not used for chronic cough that occurs with smoking, asthma, or emphysema or when there is an unusually large amount of mucus or phlegm (pronounced flem) with the cough.

Some of these preparations are available only with your doctor's prescription. Others are available without a prescription; however, your doctor may have special instructions on the proper use of this medicine for your medical condition.

Before Using This Medicine

In order to decide on the best treatment for your medical problem, your doctor should be told:

—if you have ever had any unusual reaction to guaifenesin or dextromethorphan in the past. This medicine should not be taken if you are allergic to it.

—if you are pregnant, if you intend to become pregnant, or if you are breast-feeding an infant. Although guaifenesin and dextromethorphan have not been shown to cause problems, the chance always exists.

—if you have either of the following medical problems:
Asthma
Liver disease

—if you are now taking or have taken within the past 2 weeks monoamine oxidase (MAO) inhibitors such as:

| Isocarboxazid | Phenelzine |
| Pargyline | Tranylcypromine |

Precautions While Using This Medicine

If your cough has not improved after 7 days or if you have a high fever, skin rash, or continuing headache with the cough, check with your doctor. These signs may mean that you have other medical problems.

Side Effects of This Medicine

Along with its needed effects, a medicine may cause some unwanted effects. The following side effects may go away during treatment as your body adjusts to the medicine. However, check with your doctor if any of the following side effects continue or are bothersome:

Less common or rare

Diarrhea	Nausea or vomiting
Dizziness	Stomach pain
Drowsiness	

Other side effects not listed above may also occur in some patients. If you notice any other effects, check with your doctor.

GUANETHIDINE (Systemic)
A commonly used brand name is Ismelin.

Guanethidine (gwahn-ETH-i-deen) belongs to the general class of medicines called antihypertensives. It is used to treat high blood pressure. Guanethidine is available only with your doctor's prescription.

Before Using This Medicine
In order to decide on the best treatment for your medical problem, your doctor should be told:

—if you have ever had any unusual reaction to guanethidine in the past. This medicine should not be taken if you are allergic to it.

—if you are pregnant, if you intend to become pregnant, or if you are breast-feeding an infant. Although guanethidine has not been shown to cause problems, the chance always exists.

—if you have any of the following medical problems:

Asthma (history of)	Kidney disease
Diabetes	Liver disease
Diarrhea	Pheochromocytoma
Fever	Stomach ulcer
Heart or blood	(history of)
vessel disease	

—if you have recently had a heart attack or stroke.

—if you are now taking any of the following medicines or types of medicine:

Amphetamines	Other antihypertensives (high
Barbiturates	blood pressure
Diuretics (water	medicine)
pills)	Phenothiazines (for
Ephedrine	example, chlor-
Insulin or diabetes	promazine)
medicine you take	Phenylephrine
by mouth	Prescription pain
Medicine to help	medicine
you lose weight	Reserpine or
Methotrimeprazine	rauwolfia
Methylphenidate	Tricyclic an-
	tidepressants
	(medicine for
	depression)

—if you are now taking or have taken within the past 2 weeks monoamine oxidase (MAO) inhibitors such as:

Isocarboxazid	Phenelzine
Pargyline	Tranylcypromine

Proper Use of This Medicine
Importance of Diet—When prescribing medicine for your condition, your doctor may also prescribe a personal diet for you. Such a diet may be low in sodium (salt). Medicine is more effective when this diet is properly followed.

Also, it may be very important for you to go on a reducing diet. However, check with your doctor before going on any diet.

Many patients who have high blood pressure will not notice any signs of the problem. In fact, many may feel normal. It is very important that you take your medicine exactly as directed and that you keep your doctor's appointments even if you feel well.

Remember that guanethidine will not cure your high blood pressure but it does control it. Therefore, you must continue to take it as directed if you expect to keep your blood pressure down. *You may have to take medicine for the rest of your life.* If high blood pressure is not treated, it can cause serious problems such as heart failure, blood vessel disease, stroke, or kidney disease.

In order to help remember to take your medicine, try to get into the habit of taking it at the same time each day.

If you miss a dose of this medicine, take it as soon as possible. If it is almost time for your next dose, do not take the missed dose at all and do not double the next one. Instead, go back to your regular dosing schedule. If you have any questions about this, check with your doctor.

Precautions While Using This Medicine
It is important that your doctor check your progress at regular visits.

Dizziness, lightheadedness, or fainting may occur, especially when you get up from a lying or sitting position. This is more likely to occur in the morning. *Getting up slowly may help.* When you get up from lying down, sit on the edge of the bed with your feet dangling for 1 or 2 minutes. Then stand up slowly. If the problem continues or gets worse, check with your doctor.

The dizziness, lightheadedness, or fainting is also more likely to occur if you drink alcohol, stand for long periods of time, exercise, or if the weather is hot. *While you are taking this medicine, be careful in the amount of alcohol you drink. Also, use extra care during exercise or hot weather or if you must stand for long periods of time.* Check with your doctor if you have any questions about this.

Do not take other medicines unless they have been discussed with your doctor. This especially includes over-the-counter (nonprescription) medicines for appetite control, asthma, colds, cough, hay fever, or sinus, since they may tend to increase your blood pressure.

Before having any kind of surgery (including dental surgery) or emergency treatment, tell the doctor or dentist in charge that you are taking this medicine.

Tell your doctor if you get a fever since that may change the amount of medicine you have to take.

Side Effects of This Medicine

Along with its needed effects, a medicine may cause some unwanted effects. Although not all of these side effects appear very often, when they do occur they may require medical attention. Check with your doctor if any of the following side effects occur:

More common

    Swelling of feet or
      lower legs

Less common or rare

    Chest pains   Shortness of breath

Other side effects may occur which usually do not require medical attention. These side effects may go away during treatment as your body adjusts to the medicine. However, check with your doctor if any of the following side effects continue or are bothersome:

More common

Diarrhea or increase in bowel movements	Sexual problems in males
Dizziness, lightheadedness, or fainting, especially when getting up from a lying or sitting position	Stuffy nose
	Tiredness or weakness
	Unusually slow heartbeat

Less common or rare

Blurred vision	Muscle pain or tremors
Drooping eyelids	Nausea or vomiting
Dry mouth	Nighttime urination
Headache	Skin rash
Loss of hair on scalp	

Other side effects not listed above may also occur in some patients. If you notice any other effects, check with your doctor.

GUANETHIDINE AND HYDROCHLOROTHIAZIDE (Systemic)
A commonly used brand name is Esimil.

Guanethidine (gwahn-ETH-i-deen) and hydrochlorothiazide (hye-droe-klor-oh-THYE-a-zide) combination is used in the treatment of high blood pressure. It is available only with your doctor's prescription.

Before Using This Medicine

In order to decide on the best treatment for your medical problem, your doctor should be told:

—if you are allergic to sulfonamides (sulfa drugs) or other thiazide diuretics (water pills). This medicine should not be taken if you are allergic to it.

—if you are pregnant, or if you intend to become pregnant while using this medicine. When this medicine is used during pregnancy, it may cause side effects in the newborn infant. In addition, although this medicine has not been shown to cause birth defects, the chance always exists.

—if you are breast-feeding an infant. Although this medicine has not been shown to cause problems, the chance always exists.

—if you have any of the following medical problems:

Asthma (history of)	History of lupus erythematosus
Diabetes	Kidney disease
Diarrhea	Liver disease
Fever	Pancreas disease
Gout	Pheochromocytoma (PCC)
Heart or blood vessel disease	Stomach ulcer (history of)

—if you have recently had a heart attack or stroke.

—if you are now taking any of the following medicines or types of medicine:

Amphetamines	Diabetes medicine
Barbiturates	Digitalis glycosides (heart medicine)
Colestipol	
Corticosteroids (cortisone-like medicines)	Ephedrine
	Gout medicine
	Lithium
Corticotropin (ACTH)	Medicine to help you lose weight

Methenamine
Methotrimeprazine
Methylphenidate
Oral anticoagulants
(blood thinners
you take by
mouth)
Other diuretics
(water pills)
or antihyper-
tensives (high
blood pressure
medicine)

Phenothiazines
Phenylephrine
Prescription pain
medicine
Reserpine or
rauwolfia
Tricyclic an-
tidepressants
(medicine for
depression)

—if you are now taking or have taken within
the past 2 weeks monoamine oxidase (MAO)
inhibitors such as:

Isocarboxazid
Pargyline

Phenelzine
Tranylcypromine

Proper Use of This Medicine

This medicine may cause you to have an unusual
feeling of tiredness when you begin to take it.
You may also notice an increase in the amount
of urine or in your frequency of urination.
After taking the medicine for a while, these effects should lessen. In general, in order to keep
the increase in urine from affecting your sleep:

• If you are to take a single dose a day, take it
in the morning after breakfast.

• If you are to take more than one dose a day,
take the last dose no later than 6 p.m., unless
otherwise directed by your doctor.

• However, it is best to plan your dose or doses
according to a schedule that will least affect
your personal activities and sleep. Ask your
doctor, nurse, or pharmacist to help you plan
the best time to take this medicine.

Importance of Diet—When prescribing medicine
for your condition, your doctor may also
prescribe a personal diet for you. Such a diet
may be low in sodium (salt). Medicine is usually more effective when this diet is properly
followed.
Also, it may be very important for you to go on
a reducing diet. However, check with your doctor before going on any diet.

Many patients who have high blood pressure will
not notice any signs of the problem. In fact,
many may feel normal. It is very important
that you take your medicine exactly as directed
and that you keep your doctor's appointments
even if you feel well.

Remember that this medicine will not cure your
high blood pressure but it does control it.

Therefore, you must continue to take it as
directed if you expect to keep your blood
pressure down. *You may have to take medicine
for the rest of your life.* If high blood pressure
is not treated, it can cause serious problems
such as heart failure, blood vessel disease,
stroke, or kidney disease.

In order to help remember to take your medicine,
try to get into the habit of taking it at the same
time each day.

If you miss a dose of this medicine, take it as soon
as possible. If it is almost time for your next
dose, do not take the missed dose at all and do
not double the next one. Instead, go back to
your regular dosing schedule. If you have any
questions about this, check with your doctor.

Precautions While Using This Medicine

It is important that your doctor check your progress at regular visits.

This medicine may cause a loss of potassium from
your body.
• To help prevent this, your doctor may want
you to:

—eat or drink foods that have a high
potassium content (for example, orange or
other citrus fruit juices), or

—take a potassium supplement, or

—take another medicine to help prevent the
loss of the potassium in the first place.

• It is very important to follow these directions.
Also, it is important not to change your diet on
your own. This is more important if you are
already on a special diet (as for diabetes), or if
you are taking a potassium supplement or a
medicine to reduce potassium loss. Extra
potassium may not be necessary and, in some
cases, too much potassium could be harmful.

Check with your doctor if you become sick and
have severe or continuing vomiting or diarrhea.
These problems may cause you to lose additional water and potassium.

Caution: Diabetics—This medicine may raise
blood sugar levels. While you are using this
medicine, be especially careful in testing for
sugar in your urine. If you have any questions
about this, check with your doctor.

A few people who take this medicine may become
more sensitive to sunlight than they are normally. When you begin to take this medicine,
avoid too much sun or use of a sunlamp until
you see how you react, especially if you tend to

burn easily. If you have a severe reaction, check with your doctor.

Dizziness, lightheadedness, or fainting may occur, especially when you get up from a lying or sitting position. This is more likely to occur in the morning. *Getting up slowly may help.* When you get up from lying down, sit on the edge of the bed with your feet dangling for 1 or 2 minutes. Then stand up slowly. If the problem continues or gets worse, check with your doctor.

The dizziness, lightheadedness, or fainting is also more likely to occur if you drink alcohol, stand for long periods of time or exercise, or if the weather is hot. *While you are taking this medicine, be careful in the amount of alcohol you drink. Also, use extra care during exercise or hot weather or if you must stand for long periods of time.* Check with your doctor if you have any questions about this.

Do not take other medicines unless they have been discussed with your doctor. This especially includes over-the-counter (nonprescription) medicines for appetite control, asthma, colds, cough, hay fever, or sinus, since they may tend to increase your blood pressure.

Before having any kind of surgery (including dental surgery) or emergency treatment, tell the doctor or dentist in charge that you are taking this medicine.

Tell your doctor if you get a fever since that may change the amount of medicine you have to take.

Side Effects of This Medicine

Along with its needed effects, a medicine may cause some unwanted effects. Although not all of these side effects appear very often, when they do occur they may require medical attention. Check with your doctor if any of the following side effects occur *especially since some of them may mean that your body is losing too much potassium:*

Signs of too much potassium loss

Dryness of mouth	Muscle cramps or
Increased thirst	pain
Irregular heartbeats	Nausea or vomiting
Mood or mental	Unusual tiredness or
changes	weakness
	Weak pulse

Less common

Chest pains

Rare

Severe stomach pain	Unexplained sore
with nausea and	throat and fever
vomiting	Unusual bleeding or
Skin rash or hives	bruising
	Yellowing of eyes or
	skin

Other side effects may occur which usually do not require medical attention. These side effects may go away during treatment as your body adjusts to the medicine. However, check with your doctor if any of the following side effects continue or are bothersome:

More common

Diarrhea or increase	Sexual problems in
in bowel	males
movements	Stuffy nose
Dizziness,	Unusually slow
lightheaded-	heartbeat
ness, or fainting,	
especially when	
getting up from	
a lying or	
sitting position	

Less common or rare

Blurred vision	Loss of appetite
Drooping eyelids	Loss of hair
Headache	Nighttime urination
Increased sensitivity	
to sunlight	

Other side effects not listed above may also occur in some patients. If you notice any other effects, check with your doctor.

HALOPERIDOL (Systemic)
A commonly used brand name is Haldol.

Haloperidol (ha-loe-PER-i-dole) is used to treat nervous, mental, and emotional conditions. It is used also to control the effects of Gilles de la Tourette's disease and has been used in trial treatments of other conditions. Haloperidol is available only with your doctor's prescription.

Before Using This Medicine

In order to decide on the best treatment for your medical problem, your doctor should be told:

—if you have ever had any unusual reaction to haloperidol in the past. This medicine should not be taken if you are allergic to it.

—if you are pregnant, if you intend to become pregnant, or if you are breast-feeding an infant. Although haloperidol has not been shown to cause problems, the chance always exists.

—if you have any of the following medical problems:

Alcoholism	Lung disease
Blood disease	Overactive thyroid
Epilepsy	Parkinson's disease
Glaucoma	Prostate enlarge-
Heart or circulation	ment
disease	Severe mental
Kidney disease	depression
Liver disease	Stomach ulcers
	Urination problems

—if you are now taking any of the following medicines or types of medicine:

Amphetamines	Asthma medicine
Anticonvulsants	Epinephrine
(seizure medicine)	Lithium
Antihypertensives	Ulcer medicine
(high blood	
pressure	
medicine)	

—if you are now taking central nervous system (CNS) depressants such as:

Antihistamines or	Prescription pain
medicine for	medicine
hay fever,	Sedatives, tran-
other allergies, or	quilizers,
colds	or sleeping
Barbiturates	medicine
Narcotics	Tricyclic an-
	tidepressants
	(medicine for de-
	pression)

Proper Use of This Medicine

Use this medicine only as directed by your doctor. Do not use more of it, do not use it more often, and do not use it for a longer period of time than your doctor ordered.

If this medicine upsets your stomach, it may be taken with food or milk to lessen stomach irritation.

If you miss a dose of this medicine, take it as soon as possible unless it is within 6 hours of your next scheduled dose. Do not double doses. Instead, go back to your regular dosing schedule. If you have any questions about this, check with your doctor.

For patients taking the liquid form of this medicine:

• This medicine is to be taken by mouth even though it may come in a dropper bottle. Each dose is to be measured with the included, specially marked dropper. This medicine may be taken alone or mixed with food or beverages.

Precautions While Using This Medicine

Your doctor should check your progress at regular visits, especially for the first few months you take this medicine.

Sometimes haloperidol must be taken for several days to several weeks before its full effect is reached in the treatment of certain mental and emotional conditions.

Do not suddenly stop taking this medicine without first checking with your doctor. Your doctor may want you to reduce gradually the amount you are taking before stopping completely.

This medicine will add to the effects of alcohol and other medicines (CNS depressants) that slow down the nervous system. Some examples of CNS depressants are antihistamines or medicine for hay fever, other allergies, or colds; sedatives, tranquilizers, or sleeping medicine; prescription pain medicine or narcotics; barbiturates; medicine for seizures; tricyclic antidepressants (medicine for depression); or anesthetics, including some dental anesthetics. *Check with your doctor before taking any of the above while you are taking this medicine.*

This medicine may cause some people to become drowsy or less alert than they are normally, especially as the amount of medicine is increased. Even if you take this medicine at bedtime, you may feel drowsy or less alert on arising. *Make sure you know how you react to this medicine before you drive, use machines, or do other jobs that require you to be alert.*

Although not a problem for many patients, dizziness, lightheadedness, or fainting may occur, especially when you get up from a lying or sitting position. Getting up slowly may help. However, if the problem continues or gets worse, check with your doctor.

A few people who take this medicine may become more sensitive to sunlight than they are normally. When you first begin taking this medicine, use sun screen lotions, or avoid too much sun or too much use of a sunlamp until you see how you react. If you have a severe reaction, check with your doctor.

When using the liquid form of this medicine, try to avoid getting it on your skin or clothing because it may cause a skin rash or other irritation.

Side Effects of This Medicine

Along with its needed effects, a medicine may cause some unwanted effects. Although not all of these side effects appear very often, when they do occur they may require medical attention. Check with your doctor if any of the following side effects occur:

More common

Shuffling walk	Tic-like, jerky
Stiffness of arms	movements of
and legs	head, face,
	mouth, and neck
	Trembling and
	shaking of hands
	and fingers

Less common

Difficulty in urina-	Fine, worm-like
tion	movements of
Dizziness,	tongue
lightheadedness,	Skin rash
or fainting	

Rare

Unexplained sore	Yellowing of eyes
throat and fever	and skin

Other side effects may occur which usually do not require medical attention. These side effects may go away during treatment as your body adjusts to the medicine. However, check with your doctor if any of the following side effects continue or are bothersome:

More common

Blurred vision	Dry mouth
Constipation	

Less common

Decreased sexual	Increased sensitivity
ability	of skin to sun
Drowsiness	Nausea or vomiting

Other side effects not listed above may also occur in some patients. If you notice any other effects, check with your doctor.

HALOPROGIN (Topical)

A commonly used brand name is Halotex.

Haloprogin (ha-loe-PROE-jin) belongs to the group of medicines called antifungals. It is applied to the skin to treat some types of fungal infections. This medicine is available only with your doctor's prescription.

Before Using This Medicine

In order to decide on the best treatment for your medical problem, your doctor should be told:

—if you have ever had any unusual reaction to haloprogin in the past. This medicine should not be used if you are allergic to it.

—if you are pregnant, if you intend to become pregnant, or if you are breast-feeding an infant, although haloprogin has not been shown to cause problems.

Proper Use of This Medicine

To help clear up your infection completely, *keep using this medicine for the full time of treatment* even though your condition may have improved.

Apply enough haloprogin to cover the affected area, and rub in gently.

Keep this medicine away from the eyes.

If you miss a dose of this medicine, apply it as soon as possible. Then go back to your regular dosing schedule. But if it is almost time for your next dose, do not apply the missed dose at all. Instead, go back to your regular dosing schedule. If you have any questions about this, check with your doctor.

Precautions While Using This Medicine

If your skin problem has not improved after you have used haloprogin for 4 weeks, check with your doctor.

To help cure the infection and to help prevent reinfection, good health habits are required. These include the following:

• Wash all towels and bedding after each use.

• Use only freshly laundered clothes each time clothing is changed.

If you have any questions about this, check with your doctor, nurse, or pharmacist.

Side Effects of This Medicine

Along with its needed effects, a medicine may cause some unwanted effects. Although not all of these side effects appear very often, when they do occur they may require medical attention. Check with your doctor if any of the following side effects occur:

Blistering, burning, itching, or other sign of skin irritation not present before using this medicine

When you apply the solution form of this medicine, a mild temporary stinging may be expected.

Other side effects not listed above may also occur in some patients. If you notice any other effects, check with your doctor.

HEPARIN (Systemic)
Some commonly used brand names are:

Hepalean*	Lipo-Hepin
Heprinar	Liquaemin
	Panheprin

*Not available in the United States.

Heparin (HEP-a-rin) is an anticoagulant. It decreases the clotting ability of the blood and therefore helps prevent harmful clots from forming in the blood vessels. Anticoagulants are often used as treatment for certain blood vessel, heart, and lung conditions. This medicine is sometimes called a blood thinner, although it does not actually thin the blood. Heparin is used by injection and is available only with your doctor's prescription.

Before Using This Medicine
In order to decide on the best treatment for your medical problem, your doctor should be told:

—if you have ever had any unusual reaction to heparin in the past.

—if you have a history of allergies or asthma.

—if you are pregnant and within 3 months of your delivery date, or if you have delivered a baby within the past month. Although heparin has not been shown to cause birth defects or other problems in the baby, use during the last 3 months of pregnancy or during the month following the baby's delivery may cause bleeding problems in the mother.

—if you have any of the following medical problems:

Blood disease	Liver disease
High blood pressure	Problems with
Kidney disease	bleeding

—if you are now taking any of the following medicines or types of medicine:

Aspirin or other salicylates	Corticotropin
	Dipyridamole
Corticosteroids (cortisone-like medicines)	Ethacrynic acid

Inflammation medicine (for example, arthritis medicine)	Oral anticoagulants (blood thinners you take by mouth)
Mefenamic acid	Propylthiouracil
Methimazole	

—if you are now receiving any kind of medicine by intramuscular (IM) injection.

Proper Use of This Medicine
If you are using these injections at home, make sure your doctor has explained exactly how this medicine is to be given.

Use this medicine only as directed by your doctor. Do not use more of it, do not use it more often, and do not use it for a longer period of time than your doctor ordered.

Your doctor should check your progress at regular visits. A blood test must be taken regularly to see how fast your blood is clotting, so that your doctor can decide on the proper amount of anticoagulant you should be receiving each day.

If you miss a dose of this medicine, use it as soon as possible. Then go back to your regular dosing schedule. If it is almost time for your next dose, do not use the missed dose at all and do not double the next one. Instead, go back to your regular dosing schedule. Be sure to give your doctor a record of any doses you miss. If you have any questions about this, check with your doctor.

Precautions While Using This Medicine
Do not take aspirin while using this medicine. Many over-the-counter (OTC) or nonprescription medicines and some prescription medicines contain aspirin. Check the labels of all medicines you take. If you have any questions about this, check with your doctor or pharmacist.

Tell all doctors and dentists you visit that you are using this medicine.

Your doctor may want you to carry an identification card stating that you are using this medicine.

While you are using this medicine, it is very important that you avoid sports and other activities where you may be injured. Report to your doctor any falls, blows to the body or head, or other injuries since serious internal bleeding may occur without your knowing about it.

Side Effects of This Medicine

Along with its needed effects, a medicine may cause some unwanted effects. Although not all of these side effects appear very often, when they do occur they may require medical attention. Check with your doctor if any of the following side effects occur:

Signs of bleeding inside the body

Abdominal pain or swelling	Coughing up blood Dizziness
Back pain or backaches	Severe or continuing headaches
Bloody or black tarry stools	Vomiting blood or material that looks like coffee grounds
Bloody urine	
Constipation	

Other less common or rare side effects

Back or rib pain	Numbness or tingling in hands or feet
Chest pain	
Chills or fever	
Collection of blood under skin (blood blister) at place of injection	Pain or irritation at place of injection
	Pains in arms or legs
Decrease in height	Peeling of skin at place of injection
Frequent or persistent erection	Shortness of breath, wheezing, or tightness in chest
Itching, skin rash, or hives	Unusual hair loss

Since many things can affect the way your body reacts to this medicine, you should always watch for signs of unusual bleeding. Unusual bleeding may mean that your body is getting more medicine than it needs. Check with your doctor if any of the following signs of overdose occur:

Bleeding from gums when brushing teeth	Unexplained bruising or purplish areas on skin
Excessive bleeding or oozing from cuts or wounds	Unexplained nosebleeds
	Unusually heavy or unexpected menstrual bleeding

Other side effects not listed above may also occur in some patients. If you notice any other effects, check with your doctor.

HYDANTOIN-TYPE ANTICONVULSANTS
(Systemic)

This information applies to the following medicines:

Ethotoin (ETH-oh-toyn)
Mephenytoin (me-FEN-i-toyn)
Phenytoin (FEN-i-toyn)

Some commonly used brand names and other names are:	Generic names:
Peganone	Ethotoin
Mesantoin Methoin*	Mephenytoin
Dantoin* Dilantin Di-Phen Diphenylan Diphenylhydantoin	Phenytoin

*Not available in the United States.

These medicines belong to the general family of medicines called anticonvulsants and are used most often to control certain seizures in the treatment of epilepsy. Phenytoin may also be used for other conditions as determined by your doctor. These medicines are available only with your doctor's prescription.

Before Using This Medicine

In order to decide on the best treatment for your medical problem, your doctor should be told:

—if you have had any unusual reaction to any other anticonvulsant medicine in the past. This medicine should not be taken if you are allergic to it.

—if you are pregnant or if you intend to become pregnant while using this medicine. Although most mothers who take medicine for seizure control deliver normal babies, there are reports of increased birth defects when these medicines were used during pregnancy. It is not definitely known if any of these medicines are the cause of such problems.

—if you are breast-feeding an infant. Phenytoin is found to be present in breast milk in amounts large enough to cause unwanted effects in the baby. Although information concerning breast-feeding is not available for other medicines of this type, they may also produce similar unwanted effects.

—if you have any of the following medical problems:

Alcoholism	High blood sugar
Blood disease	Liver disease
Diabetes	

—if you are now taking any of the following medicines or types of medicine:

Barbiturates	Folic acid (con-
Birth control pills	tained in some
Chloramphenicol	vitamin formulas)
Coumarin-type	Isoniazid (INH)
anticoagulants	Levodopa
(blood thinners)	Medicine for mental
Dexamethasone or	illness
other cortisone-	Oxyphenbutazone
like medicines	Phenylbutazone
Diabetes medicine	Sulfonamides (sulfa
you take by	drugs)
mouth	Tricyclic an-
Disulfiram	tidepressants
(medicine for	(medicine for
alcoholism)	depression)
Doxycycline	

Proper Use of This Medicine

Take this medicine every day exactly as ordered by your doctor.

If this medicine upsets your stomach, take it with food or milk, unless otherwise directed by your doctor.

If you miss a dose of this medicine and your dosing schedule is one dose to be taken:

Once a day—
Take the missed dose as soon as possible. Then go back to your regular dosing schedule. But if you do not remember the missed dose until the next day, do not take it at all and do not double the next one. Instead, go back to your regular dosing schedule.

Several times a day—
Take the missed dose as soon as possible unless your next scheduled dose is within 4 hours. Then go back to your regular dosing schedule. Do not double doses.

If you have any questions about this, check with your doctor.

Precautions While Using This Medicine

Your doctor should check your progress at regular visits, especially during the first few months you take this medicine. During this time the amount of medicine you are taking may have to be changed often to meet your individual needs.

If you have been taking this medicine regularly for several weeks or more, do not suddenly stop taking it. Your doctor may want you to reduce gradually the amount you are taking before stopping completely.

Your doctor may want you to carry a medical identification card or bracelet stating that you are taking this medicine.

Caution: Diabetics—This medicine may affect blood sugar levels. If you notice a change in the results of your urine sugar tests or if you have any questions, check with your doctor.

Drinking alcohol may change the way this medicine works. Check with your doctor before drinking alcoholic beverages while you are taking this medicine.

Before having any kind of surgery (including dental surgery), or emergency treatment, tell the doctor or dentist in charge that you are using this medicine.

For patients taking phenytoin:

• In some patients (usually younger patients), tenderness, swelling, or bleeding of the gums may appear after 2 or 3 months of treatment with phenytoin. Brushing and flossing your teeth carefully and regularly and massaging your gums may help prevent this. *Check with your doctor or dentist if you have any questions about how to take care of your teeth and gums, or if you notice any tenderness, swelling, or bleeding of your gums.*

For patients taking ethotoin or mephenytoin:

• This medicine may cause some people to become dizzy, lightheaded, drowsy, or less alert than they are normally. After you have taken this medicine for a while, this effect may not be so bothersome. *Make sure you know how you react to this medicine before you drive, use machines, or do other jobs that require you to be alert.*

Side Effects of This Medicine

Along with its needed effects, a medicine may cause some unwanted effects. Although not all

of these side effects appear very often, when they do occur they may require medical attention. Check with your doctor if any of the following side effects occur:

More common

Bleeding, swollen, or tender gums (usually in pheny-toin patients only)	Continuous, uncontrolled back-and-forth or rolling eye movements
	Staggering walk

Less common

Skin rash
Slurred speech

Rare

Darkening of urine	Unusual bleeding or bruising
Enlarged lymph glands	Yellowing of skin or eyes
Unexplained sore throat and fever	

Other side effects may occur which usually do not require medical attention. These side effects may go away during treatment as your body adjusts to the medicine. However, check with your doctor if any of the following side effects continue or are bothersome:

More common

Constipation	Nausea and vomiting
Dizziness	
Drowsiness (usually in ethotoin and mephenytoin patients)	

Less common

Blurred vision	Excessive growth of body and facial hair
Diarrhea (has occurred with ethotoin)	Headache
Double vision	Mental confusion
	Muscle twitching
	Sleeplessness

This medicine may cause the urine to turn pinkish red to red or reddish brown; this is harmless and may be expected. If you have questions about this, ask your doctor or pharmacist.

Other side effects not listed above may also occur in some patients. If you notice any other effects, check with your doctor.

HYDRALAZINE (Systemic)

Some commonly used brand names are Apresoline and Rolazine.*

---

*Not available in the United States.

Hydralazine (hye-DRAL-a-zeen) belongs to the general class of medicines called antihypertensives. It is used to treat high blood pressure. Hydralazine is available only with your doctor's prescription.

Before Using This Medicine

In order to decide on the best treatment for your medical problem, your doctor should be told:

—if you have ever had any unusual reaction to hydralazine in the past. This medicine should not be taken if you are allergic to it.

—if you are pregnant or if you intend to become pregnant while using this medicine. Although hydralazine has not been shown to cause birth defects or other problems in humans, the chance always exists.

—if you are breast-feeding an infant. Although hydralazine has not been shown to cause problems, the chance always exists.

—if you have either of the following medical problems:

Heart disease
Kidney disease

—if you have recently had a stroke.

—if you are now taking any of the following medicines or types of medicine:

Diuretics (water pills)	Other antihypertensives (high blood pressure medicine)

Proper Use of This Medicine

Importance of Diet—In addition to prescribing medicine for your condition, your doctor may also prescribe a personal diet for you. Such a diet may be low in sodium (salt). Medicine is more effective when this diet is properly followed.

Also, it may be very important for you to go on a reducing diet. However, check with your doctor before going on any diet.

Many people who have high blood pressure will not notice any signs of the problem. In fact, many may feel normal. It is very important that you *take your medicine exactly as directed* and that you keep your doctor's appointments even if you feel well.

Remember that hydralazine will not cure your high blood pressure but it does control it. Therefore, you must continue to take it as directed if you expect to keep your blood pressure down. *You may have to take medicine for the rest of your life.* If high blood pressure is not treated, it can cause serious problems such as heart failure, blood vessel disease, stroke, or kidney disease.

In order to help remember to take your medicine, try to get into the habit of taking it at the same time each day.

If you miss a dose of this medicine, take it as soon as possible. If it is almost time for your next dose, do not take the missed dose at all and do not double the next one. Instead, go back to your regular dosing schedule. If you have any questions about this, check with your doctor.

Precautions While Using This Medicine

It is important that your doctor check your progress at regular visits.

Hydralazine may cause some people to have headaches or to feel dizzy. *Make sure you know how you react to this medicine before you drive, use machines, or do other jobs that require you to be alert.*

Dizziness, lightheadedness, or fainting may occur, especially when you get up from a lying or sitting position. Getting up slowly may help, but if the problem continues or gets worse, check with your doctor.

The dizziness, lightheadedness, or fainting is also more likely to occur if you drink alcohol, stand for long periods of time, exercise, or if the weather is hot. *While you are taking this medicine, be careful in the amount of alcohol you drink. Also, use extra care during exercise or hot weather or if you must stand for long periods of time.* Check with your doctor if you have any questions about this.

Do not take other medicines unless they have been discussed with your doctor. This especially includes over-the-counter (nonprescription) medicines for appetite control, asthma, colds, cough, hay fever, or sinus, since they may tend to increase your blood pressure.

Side Effects of This Medicine

Along with its needed effects, a medicine may cause some unwanted effects. Although not all of these side effects appear very often, when they do occur they may require medical attention. In general, side effects with hydralazine are rare at lower doses. However, check with your doctor if any of the following occur:

Less common

Chest pain	Skin rash or itching
General feeling of body discomfort or weakness	Swelling of feet or lower legs Swelling of the lymph glands
Joint pain	
Numbness, tingling, pain, or weakness in hands or feet	Unexplained sore throat and fever

Other side effects may occur which usually do not require medical attention. These side effects may go away during treatment as your body adjusts to the medicine. However, check with your doctor if any of the following side effects continue or are bothersome:

More common

Diarrhea	Nausea or vomiting
Headache	Rapid or irregular heartbeat
Loss of appetite	

Less common

Constipation	Redness or flushing of the face
Dizziness or lightheadedness, especially when getting up from a lying or sitting position	Shortness of breath with exercise or work
	Stuffy nose
	Watering or irritated eyes

Other side effects not listed above may also occur in some patients. If you notice any other effects, check with your doctor.

HYDROCODONE (Systemic)

Some commonly used brand names are:

Codone	Dicodid
*Corutol DH	*Robidone

---

*Not available in the United States.

Hydrocodone (hye-droe-KOE-done) is a medicine used to relieve pain. It is also used to relieve coughing. Hydrocodone is available only with your doctor's prescription. Since prescriptions for hydrocodone cannot be refilled, a new prescription must be obtained from your doctor each time you need this medicine.

Before Using This Medicine

In order to decide on the best treatment for your medical problem, your doctor should be told:

—if you have ever had any unusual reaction to hydrocodone in the past. This medicine should not be taken if you are allergic to it.

—if you are pregnant, if you intend to become pregnant, or if you are breast-feeding an infant. Although hydrocodone has not been shown to cause problems, the chance always exists.

—if you have any of the following medical problems:

Brain disease or injury

Colitis

Emphysema, asthma, or chronic lung disease

Enlarged prostate or problems with urination

Gallbladder disease or gallstones

Kidney disease

Liver disease

Underactive adrenal gland (Addison's disease)

Underactive thyroid

Unusually slow or irregular heart- beat

—if you are now taking other central nervous system (CNS) depressants such as:

Antihistamines or medicine for hay fever, other allergies, or colds

Barbiturates

Other prescription pain medicine

Sedatives, tran- quilizers, or sleeping medicine

Tricyclic an- tidepressants (medicine for depression)

—if you are now taking prescription medicine for stomach cramps or spasms.

—if you are now taking or have taken within the past 2 weeks monoamine oxidase (MAO) inhibitors such as:

Isocarboxazid

Pargyline

Phenelzine

Tranylcypromine

Proper Use of This Medicine

Take this medicine only as directed by your doctor. Do not take more of it, do not take it more often, and do not take it for a longer period of time than your doctor ordered. If too much is taken, it may become habit-forming.

Precautions While Using This Medicine

If you will be taking this medicine for a long period of time (for example, for several months at a time), your doctor should check your progress at regular visits.

This medicine will add to the effects of alcohol and other medicines (CNS depressants) that slow down the nervous system. Some examples of CNS depressants are antihistamines or medicine for hay fever, other allergies, or colds; sedatives, tranquilizers, or sleeping medicine; prescription pain medicine or narcotics; barbiturates; medicine for seizures; tricyclic antidepressants (medicine for depression); or anesthetics, including some dental anesthetics. *Check with your doctor before taking any of the above while you are using this medicine.*

This medicine may cause some people to become drowsy, dizzy, or lightheaded, or to feel a false sense of well-being. *Make sure you know how you react to this medicine before you drive, use machines, or do other jobs that require you to be alert and clear-headed.*

Dizziness, lightheadedness, or fainting may occur, especially when you get up from a lying or sitting position. Getting up slowly may help lessen this problem.

Nausea may occur, especially after the first couple of doses. This effect usually goes away if you lie down for a while.

Side Effects of This Medicine

Along with its needed effects, a medicine may cause some unwanted effects. Although not all of these side effects appear very often, when they do occur they may require medical attention. Check with your doctor if any of the following side effects occur:

Less common

Itching or skin rash

Shortness of breath

Troubled breathing

Unusually slow heartbeat

Other side effects may occur which usually do not require medical attention. These side effects may go away during treatment as your body adjusts to the medicine. However, check with your doctor if any of the following side effects continue or are bothersome:

More common

Dizziness

Drowsiness

Feeling faint

Lightheadedness

Nausea or vomiting

Less common

Constipation	Frequent urge to
Difficult urination	urinate
False sense of well-	Unusual tiredness or
being	weakness

Other side effects not listed above may also occur in some patients. If you notice any other effects, check with your doctor.

HYDROCODONE AND HOMATROPINE
(Systemic)
A commonly used brand name is Hycodan.

Hydrocodone (hye-droe-KOE-done) and homatropine (hoe-MA-troe-peen) is a combination used to relieve coughing. The combination is available only with your doctor's prescription.

Before Using This Medicine

In order to decide on the best treatment for your medical problem, your doctor should be told:

—if you have ever had an unusual reaction to hydrocodone, homatropine, or medicines like homatropine such as atropine or belladonna in the past. This medicine should not be taken if you are allergic to it.

—if you are pregnant, if you intend to become pregnant, or if you are breast-feeding an infant. Although this medicine has not been shown to cause problems, the chance always exists.

—if you have any of the following medical problems:

Brain disease or injury	Kidney disease
jury	Liver disease
Colitis	Underactive adrenal
Emphysema,	gland (Addison's
asthma, or	disease)
chronic lung	Underactive thyroid
disease	Unusually slow or
Enlarged prostate or	irregular heart-
problems with	beat
urination	
Gallbladder disease	
or gallstones	
Glaucoma	

—if you are now taking other central nervous system (CNS) depressants such as:

Antihistamines or	Barbiturates
medicine for hay	Other narcotics
fever, other	Prescription pain
allergies,	medicine
or colds	

Sedatives, tran-	Seizure medicine
quilizers,	Tricyclic an-
or sleeping	tidepressants
medicine	(medicine for
	depression)

—if you are now taking prescription medicine for stomach cramps or spasms.

—if you are now taking or have taken within the past 2 weeks monoamine oxidase (MAO) inhibitors such as:

Isocarboxazid	Phenelzine
Pargyline	Tranylcypromine

Proper Use of This Medicine

Take this medicine only as directed by your doctor. Do not take more of it, do not take it more often, and do not take it for a longer period of time than your doctor ordered. If too much is taken, it may become habit-forming.

Precautions While Using This Medicine

If you will be taking this medicine for a long period of time (for example, for several months at a time), your doctor should check your progress at regular visits.

This medicine will add to the effects of alcohol and other medicines (CNS depressants) that slow down the nervous system. Some examples of CNS depressants are antihistamines or medicine for hay fever, other allergies, or colds; sedatives, tranquilizers, or sleeping medicine; prescription pain medicine or narcotics; barbiturates; medicine for seizures; tricyclic antidepressants (medicine for depression); or anesthetics, including some dental anesthetics. *Check with your doctor before taking any of the above while you are using this medicine.*

This medicine may cause some people to become drowsy, dizzy, or lightheaded, or to feel a false sense of well-being. *Make sure you know how you react to this medicine before you drive, use machines, or do other jobs that require you to be alert and clear-headed.*

Also, dizziness, lightheadedness, or fainting may occur, especially when you get up from a lying or sitting position. Getting up slowly may help lessen this problem.

Nausea may occur, especially after the first couple of doses. This effect usually goes away if you lie down for a while. However, if nausea or vomiting continues, check with your doctor.

Side Effects of This Medicine

Along with its needed effects, a medicine may cause some unwanted effects. Although not all of these side effects appear very often, when they do occur they may require medical attention. Check with your doctor if any of the following side effects occur:

Less common

Itching or skin rash	Unusually slow
Shortness of breath	heartbeat
Troubled breathing	

Other side effects may occur which usually do not require medical attention. These side effects may go away during treatment as your body adjusts to the medicine. However, check with your doctor if any of the following side effects continue or are bothersome:

More common

Constipation	Feeling faint
Dizziness	Lightheadedness
Drowsiness	Nausea or vomiting

Less common

Difficult urination	Frequent urge to
False sense of well-	urinate
being	Unusual tiredness or
	weakness

Other side effects not listed above may also occur in some patients. If you notice any other effects, check with your doctor.

HYDROCODONE AND PHENYLTOLOX-AMINE RESIN COMPLEXES
(Systemic)
A commonly used brand name is Tussionex.

Hydrocodone (hye-droe-KOE-done) and phenyltoloxamine (fen-ill-tole-OX-a-meen) resin complexes combination is a medicine used to relieve coughing. It is available only with your doctor's prescription.

Before Using This Medicine

In order to decide on the best treatment for your medical problem, your doctor should be told:

—if you have ever had any unusual reaction to hydrocodone in the past. This medicine should not be taken if you are allergic to it.

—if you are pregnant, if you intend to become pregnant, or if you are breast-feeding an infant. Although hydrocodone and phenyltoloxamine have not been shown to cause problems, the chance always exists.

—if you have any of the following medical problems:

Brain disease or injury	Kidney disease
Colitis	Liver disease
Emphysema, asthma, or chronic lung disease	Underactive adrenal gland (Addison's disease)
Enlarged prostate or problems with urination	Underactive thyroid Unusually slow or irregular heartbeat
Gallbladder disease or gallstones	

—if you are now taking other central nervous system (CNS) depressants such as:

Antihistamines or medicine for hay fever, other allergies, or colds	Prescription pain medicine Sedatives, tranquilizers, or sleeping medicine
Barbiturates	
Other narcotics	Seizure medicine
	Tricyclic antidepressants (medicine for depression)

—if you are now taking prescription medicine for stomach cramps or spasms.

—if you are now taking or have taken within the past 2 weeks monoamine oxidase (MAO) inhibitors such as:

Isocarboxazid	Phenelzine
Pargyline	Tranylcypromine

Proper Use of This Medicine

Take this medicine only as directed by your doctor. Do not take more of it, do not take it more often, and do not take it for a longer period of time than your doctor ordered. If too much is taken, it may become habit-forming.

Precautions While Using This Medicine

If you will be taking this medicine for a long period of time (for example, for several months at a time), your doctor should check your progress at regular visits.

This medicine will add to the effects of alcohol and other medicines (CNS depressants) that slow down the nervous system. Some examples of CNS depressants are antihistamines or medicine for hay fever, other allergies, or colds; sedatives, tranquilizers, or sleeping medicine; prescription pain medicine or narcotics; barbiturates; medicine for seizures;

tricyclic antidepressants (medicine for depression); or anesthetics, including some dental anesthetics. *Check with your doctor before taking any of the above while you are using this medicine.*

This medicine may cause some people to become drowsy or less alert than they are normally. *Make sure you know how you react to this medicine before you drive, use machines, or do other jobs that require you to be alert.*

Nausea may occur, especially after the first couple of doses. This effect usually goes away if you lie down for a while.

Side Effects of This Medicine

Along with its needed effects, a medicine may cause some unwanted effects. Although not all of these side effects appear very often, when they do occur they may require medical attention. Check with your doctor if any of the following side effects occur:

Less common

Itching, especially on the face	Troubled breathing
Shortness of breath	Unusually slow heartbeat

Other side effects may occur which usually do not require medical attention. These side effects may go away during treatment as your body adjusts to the medicine. However, check with your doctor if any of the following side effects continue or are bothersome:

Less common

Constipation	Nausea
Drowsiness	

Other side effects not listed above may also occur in some patients. If you notice any other effects, check with your doctor.

HYDROCODONE AND PSEUDOEPHEDRINE
(Systemic)
A commonly used brand name is Tussend.

Hydrocodone (hye-droe-KOE-done) and pseudoephedrine (soo-doe-e-FED-rin) is a combination used to relieve coughing and nasal congestion caused by the common cold, influenza, bronchitis, sinusitis, and other upper respiratory tract infections or allergies. This combination medicine is available only with your doctor's prescription.

Before Using This Medicine

In order to decide on the best treatment for your medical problem, your doctor should be told:

—if you have ever had any unusual reaction to hydrocodone, pseudoephedrine, or medicines like pseudoephedrine such as amphetamines, ephedrine, epinephrine, isoproterenol, metaproterenol, norepinephrine (levarterenol), phenylephrine, phenylpropanolamine, or terbutaline.

—if you are pregnant or if you intend to become pregnant. Although hydrocodone and pseudoephedrine have not been shown to cause problems, the chance always exists.

—if you are breast-feeding an infant. Pseudoephedrine may cause unwanted side effects in infants.

—if you have any of the following medical problems:

Brain disease or injury	Heart or blood vessel disease
Colitis	High blood pressure
Diabetes	Kidney disease
Emphysema, asthma, or chronic lung disease	Liver disease
	Overactive or underactive thyroid
Enlarged prostate or problems with urination	Underactive adrenal gland (Addison's disease)
Gallbladder disease or gallstones	Unusually slow or irregular heartbeat
Glaucoma	

—if you are now taking any of the following medicines or types of medicine:

Alkavervir	Metoprolol
Amphetamines	Nadolol
Digitalis glycosides (heart medicine)	Prescription medicine for stomach cramps or spasms
Guanethidine	
Mecamylamine	
Medicine for asthma or breathing problems	Propranolol
Methyldopa	Protoveratrine A
	Reserpine
	Veratrum viride alkaloids

—if you are now taking other central nervous system (CNS) depressants such as:

Antihistamines or medicine for hay fever, other allergies, or colds	Barbiturates
	Other narcotics
	Prescription pain medicine

Sedatives, tran-   Tricyclic an-
    quilizers,   tidepressants
    or sleeping   (medicine for
    medicine   depression)
Seizure medicine

—if you are now taking or have taken within the past 2 weeks monoamine oxidase (MAO) inhibitors such as:

Isocarboxazid   Phenelzine
Pargyline   Tranylcypromine

Proper Use of This Medicine

Take this medicine only as directed by your doctor. Do not take more of it, do not take it more often, and do not take it for a longer period of time than your doctor ordered. If too much is taken, it may become habit-forming.

Precautions While Using This Medicine

If you will be taking this medicine for a long period of time (for example, for several months at a time), your doctor should check your progress at regular visits.

The hydrocodone in this medicine will add to the effects of alcohol and other medicines (CNS depressants) that slow down the nervous system. Some examples of CNS depressants are antihistamines or medicine for hay fever, other allergies, or colds; sedatives, tranquilizers, or sleeping medicine; prescription pain medicine or narcotics; barbiturates; medicine for seizures; tricyclic antidepressants (medicine for depression); or anesthetics, including some dental anesthetics. *Check with your doctor before taking any of the above while you are using this medicine.*

This medicine may cause some people to become drowsy, dizzy, or lightheaded, or to feel a false sense of well-being. *Make sure you know how you react to this medicine before you drive, use machines, or do other jobs that require you to be alert and clear-headed.*

Also, dizziness, lightheadedness, or fainting may occur when you get up from a lying or sitting position. Getting up slowly may help lessen this problem.

Nausea may occur, especially after the first couple of doses. This effect usually goes away if you lie down for a while. However, if nausea or vomiting continues, check with your doctor.

Side Effects of This Medicine

Along with its needed effects, a medicine may cause some unwanted effects. Although not all of these side effects appear very often, when they do occur they may require medical attention. Check with your doctor if any of the following side effects occur:

Less common

Itching or skin rash   Unusually slow
Shortness of breath   heartbeat
Troubled breathing

With high doses of pseudoephedrine

Hallucinations (see-   Irregular heartbeat
ing, hearing, or   Seizures
feeling things that
are not there)

Other side effects may occur which usually do not require medical attention. These side effects may go away during treatment as your body adjusts to the medicine. However, check with your doctor if any of the following side effects continue or are bothersome:

More common

Dizziness   Nausea or vomiting
Drowsiness   Nervousness
Feeling faint   Restlessness
Lightheadedness   Trouble in sleeping

Less common

Constipation   Trembling
Difficult or painful   Unusual increase in
urination   sweating
False sense of well-   Unusual paleness
being   Unusual tiredness or
Frequent urge to   weakness
urinate   Unusually fast or
Headache   pounding heart-
                         beat

Other side effects not listed above may also occur in some patients. If you notice any other effects, check with your doctor.

HYDROCODONE, PSEUDOEPHEDRINE, AND GUAIFENESIN (Systemic)

A commonly used brand name is Tussend Expectorant.

Hydrocodone (hye-droe-KOE-done), pseudoephedrine (soo-doe-e-FED-rin), and guaifenesin (gwye-FEN-e-sin) is a combination used to relieve coughing, reduce nasal congestion, and loosen mucus and phlegm in the lungs. This combination medicine is available only with your doctor's prescription.

Before Using This Medicine

In order to decide on the best treatment for your medical problem, your doctor should be told:

—if you have ever had any unusual reaction to guaifenesin or hydrocodone in the past.

—if you have ever had any unusual reaction to pseudoephedrine or to medicines like pseudoephedrine such as amphetamines, ephedrine, epinephrine, isoproterenol, metaproterenol, norepinephrine (levarterenol), phenylephrine, phenylpropanolamine, or terbutaline.

—if you are pregnant or if you intend to become pregnant. Although hydrocodone, pseudoephedrine, and guaifenesin have not been shown to cause problems, the chance always exists.

—if you are breast-feeding an infant. Pseudoephedrine may cause unwanted side effects in infants.

—if you have any of the following medical problems:

Brain disease or injury	Heart or blood vessel disease
Colitis	High blood pressure
Diabetes	Kidney disease
Emphysema, asthma, or chronic lung disease	Liver disease
	Overactive or underactive thyroid
Enlarged prostate or problems with urination	Underactive adrenal gland (Addison's disease)
Gallbladder disease or gallstones	Unusually slow or irregular heartbeat
Glaucoma	

—if you are now taking any of the following medicines or types of medicine:

Alkavervir	Metoprolol
Amphetamines	Nadolol
Digitalis glycosides (heart medicine)	Prescription medicine for stomach cramps or spasms
Guanethidine	
Mecamylamine	
Medicine for asthma or breathing problems	Propranolol
	Protoveratrine A
Methyldopa	Reserpine
	Veratrum viride alkaloids

—if you are now taking other central nervous system (CNS) depressants such as:

Antihistamines or medicine for hay fever, other allergies, or colds	Barbiturates
	Other narcotics
	Prescription pain medicine

Sedatives, tranquilizers, or sleeping medicine	Tricyclic antidepressants (medicine for depression)
Seizure medicine	

—if you are now taking or have taken within the past 2 weeks monoamine oxidase (MAO) inhibitors such as:

Isocarboxazid	Phenelzine
Pargyline	Tranylcypromine

Proper Use of This Medicine

Take this medicine only as directed by your doctor. Do not take more of it, do not take it more often, and do not take it for a longer period of time than your doctor ordered. If too much is taken, it may become habit-forming.

To help the guaifenesin in this medicine loosen the phlegm and mucus in the lungs, *drink a glass of water after each dose of this medicine,* unless otherwise directed by your doctor.

Precautions While Using This Medicine

If you will be taking this medicine for a long period of time (for example, for several months at a time), your doctor should check your progress at regular visits.

The hydrocodone in this medicine will add to the effects of alcohol and other medicines (CNS depressants) that slow down the nervous system. Some examples of CNS depressants are antihistamines or medicine for hay fever, other allergies, or colds; sedatives, tranquilizers, or sleeping medicine; prescription pain medicine or narcotics; barbiturates; medicine for seizures; tricyclic antidepressants (medicine for depression); or anesthetics, including some dental anesthetics. *Check with your doctor before taking any of the above while you are using this medicine.*

This medicine may cause some people to become drowsy, dizzy, or lightheaded, or to feel a false sense of well-being. *Make sure you know how you react to this medicine before you drive, use machines, or do other jobs that require you to be alert and clear-headed.*

Also, dizziness, lightheadedness, or fainting may occur when you get up from a lying or sitting position. Getting up slowly may help lessen this problem.

Nausea may occur, especially after the first couple of doses. This effect usually goes away if you lie down for a while. However, if nausea or vomiting continues, check with your doctor.

Side Effects of This Medicine

Along with its needed effects, a medicine may cause some unwanted effects. Although not all of these side effects appear very often, when they do occur they may require medical attention. Check with your doctor if any of the following side effects occur:

Less common

Itching or skin rash	Unusually slow
Shortness of breath	heartbeat
Troubled breathing	

With high doses of pseudoephedrine

Hallucinations (see-	Irregular heartbeat
ing, hearing,	Seizures
or feeling things	
that are not there)	

Other side effects may occur which usually do not require medical attention. These side effects may go away during treatment as your body adjusts to the medicine. However, check with your doctor if any of the following side effects continue or are bothersome:

More common

Dizziness	Nausea or vomiting
Drowsiness	Nervousness
Feeling faint	Restlessness
Lightheadedness	Trouble in sleeping

Less common

Constipation	Stomach pain
Diarrhea	Trembling
Difficult or painful	Unusual increase in
urination	sweating
False sense of well-	Unusual paleness
being	Unusual tiredness or
Frequent urge to	weakness
urinate	Unusually fast or
Headache	pounding heart-
	beat

Other side effects not listed above may also occur in some patients. If you notice any other effects, check with your doctor.

HYDROCORTISONE (Rectal)

Some commonly used brand names are Cortifoam, Cort-Dome, and Proctocort.

Hydrocortisone (hye-droe-KOR-ti-sone) is an adrenocorticoid (cortisone-like medicine). It belongs to the general family of medicines called steroids. Cortisone-like medicines are used in the rectum to help relieve swelling, itching, and discomfort of some rectal problems. Hydrocortisone is used in the form of a rectal cream, foam,

or suppository. Adrenocorticoids for rectal use are available only with your doctor's prescription.

Before Using This Medicine

In order to decide on the best treatment for your medical problem, your doctor should be told:

—if you have ever had any unusual reaction to hydrocortisone in the past. This medicine should not be taken if you are allergic to it.

—if you are pregnant, if you intend to become pregnant, or if you are breast-feeding an infant. Although rectal adrenocorticoids have not been shown to cause birth defects or other problems in humans, the chance always exists. In addition, use in large amounts or for prolonged periods of time is not recommended since the medicine may be absorbed through the skin.

—if you think you may have an infection at the site of treatment.

Proper Use of This Medicine

Do not use this medicine more often or for a longer period of time than your doctor ordered. To do so may increase the chance of absorption through the lining of the rectum and the chance of side effects.

Do not use any leftover medicine for future rectal problems without first checking with your doctor. The medicine should not be used on many kinds of bacterial, viral, or fungal infections.

If you miss a dose of this medicine, use it as soon as possible. Then go back to your regular dosing schedule. But if it is almost time for your next dose, do not use the missed dose at all. Instead, go back to your regular dosing schedule. If you have any questions about this, check with your doctor.

For patients using hydrocortisone rectal cream:

• This medicine usually comes with patient directions. Read them carefully before using this medicine.

For patients using hydrocortisone acetate suppositories:

• How to insert suppository: First remove the foil wrapper and moisten the suppository with water. Lie down on side and push the suppository well up into rectum with finger. If the suppository is too soft to insert because of storage in a warm place, chill the suppository in the refrigerator for 30 minutes or run cold water over it before removing the foil wrapper.

For patients using hydrocortisone acetate rectal foam aerosol:

- This medicine usually comes with patient directions. Read them carefully before using this medicine.

- This medicine is used with a special applicator. Do not insert any part of the aerosol container into the rectum.

- Container provides about 24 applications of foam.

- Store away from heat and direct sunlight. Do not puncture, break, or burn the container.

Precautions While Using This Medicine

This medicine may be absorbed through the lining of the rectum and can affect growth. *Children who must use this medicine should be followed closely by their doctor.*

Side Effects of This Medicine

Along with its needed effects, a medicine may cause some unwanted effects. Although not all of these side effects appear very often, when they do occur they may require medical attention. Check with your doctor if any of the following side effects occur:

Signs of irritation or infection such as rectal bleeding, pain, burning, itching, or blistering not present before using this medicine

Other side effects not listed above may also occur in some patients. If you notice any other effects, check with your doctor.

HYDROCORTISONE AND ACETIC ACID
(Otic)
A commonly used brand name is VōSol HC.

Hydrocortisone (hye-droe-KOR-ti-sone) and acetic acid (a-SEE-tik AS-id) combination is used to treat certain infections of the ear canal. It also helps relieve the redness, itching, and swelling that may accompany these infections. Hydrocortisone is an adrenocorticoid (cortisone-like medicine) and belongs to the general family of medicines called steroids. Hydrocortisone and acetic acid combination is available only with your doctor's prescription.

Before Using This Medicine

In order to decide on the best treatment for your medical problem, your doctor should be told:

—if you have ever had any unusual reaction to steroids in the past. This medicine should not be used if you are allergic to it.

—if you have any of the following medical problems:

Any other ear infec-   Punctured ear drum
tion or condition

Proper Use of This Medicine

Do not use any leftover medicine for future ear problems without first checking with your doctor. This medicine should not be used on many kinds of bacterial, viral, or fungal infections.

Before applying this medicine, wash the area to be treated (including the ear canal) with soap and water, and dry thoroughly. The ear canal should be dried with a sterile cotton applicator.

To prevent contamination of the ear drops, do not touch the dropper to any surface (including the ear).

How to apply this medicine: Lie down or tilt the head so that the infected ear faces up. For adults, gently pull the ear lobe up and back to straighten the ear canal. (For children, gently pull the ear lobe down and back to straighten the ear canal.) Drop medicine into the ear canal. Keep ear facing up for several minutes to allow medicine to run to the bottom of the ear canal. A clean, soft cotton plug may be gently inserted into the ear opening to prevent the medicine from leaking out.

Do not rinse dropper after use. Wipe the tip of the dropper with a clean tissue and keep the container tightly closed.

If you miss a dose of this medicine, apply it as soon as possible. Then go back to your regular dosing schedule. But if it is almost time for your next dose, do not apply the missed dose at all. Instead, go back to your regular dosing schedule. If you have any questions about this, check with your doctor.

Precautions While Using This Medicine

If your symptoms have not improved after 5 to 7 days, of if your ear problem becomes worse, check with your doctor.

Side Effects of This Medicine

After this medicine is applied to the ear, some stinging, itching, or burning may be expected. If this continues or is bothersome, check with your doctor.

There have not been any other common or important side effects reported with this medicine. However, if you notice any other effects, check with your doctor.

HYDROCORTISONE, BELLADONNA, EPHEDRINE, ZINC OXIDE, BORIC ACID, BISMUTH, AND PERUVIAN BALSAM
(Rectal)
A commonly used brand name is Wyanoids HC.

Hydrocortisone (hye-droe-KOR-ti-sone), belladonna (bell-a-DON-a), ephedrine (e-FED-rin), zinc oxide (ZINK OX-ide), boric acid (BOR-ik AS-id), bismuth (BIZ-muth), and Peruvian balsam (pe-ROO-vee-an BAL-sam) combination is used to relieve the swelling, itching, and discomfort caused by certain rectal problems. This medicine is used as a rectal suppository and is available only with your doctor's prescription.

Before Using This Medicine

In order to decide on the best treatment for your medical problem, your doctor should be told:

—if you have ever had any unusual reaction to hydrocortisone, ephedrine, belladonna, or to hemorrhoid or other rectal medicines.

—if you are pregnant or if you intend to become pregnant while using this medicine. Although this medicine has not been shown to cause birth defects or other problems, the chance always exists, especially if it is used in large amounts or for a long period of time.

—if you are breast-feeding an infant. Although this medicine has not been shown to cause problems, the chance always exists.

—if you have any of the following medical problems:

Brain damage (children)	Infection at the place of treatment
Difficult urination	Pyloric stenosis
Down's syndrome (mongolism)	(intestinal blockage)
Enlarged prostate	Spastic paralysis (children)
Glaucoma	

—if you are now taking any of the following medicines or types of medicine:

Amantadine	Medicine for Parkinson's disease
Antihistamines or medicine for hay fever, other allergies, or colds	Phenothiazines
Haloperidol	Tricyclic antidepressants (medicine for depression)
Medicine for intestinal or stomach cramping	

—if you are now taking or have taken within the past 2 weeks monoamine oxidase (MAO) inhibitors such as:

Isocarboxazid	Phenelzine
Pargyline	Tranylcypromine

Proper Use of This Medicine

How to insert suppository: First remove the foil wrapper and moisten the suppository with water. Lie down on side and push the suppository well up into rectum with finger. If the suppository is too soft to insert because of storage in a warm place, chill the suppository in the refrigerator for 30 minutes or run cold water over it before removing the foil wrapper.

Do not use this medicine more often or for a longer period of time than your doctor ordered. To do so may increase the chance of absorption through the lining of the rectum and the chance of side effects.

Do not use any leftover medicine for future rectal problems without first checking with your doctor. The hydrocortisone in this medicine should not be used on many kinds of bacterial, viral, or fungal infections.

If you miss a dose of this medicine, use it as soon as possible. Then go back to your regular dosing schedule. But if it is almost time for your next dose, do not use the missed dose at all. Instead, go back to your regular dosing schedule. If you have any questions about this, check with your doctor.

Precautions While Using This Medicine

The hydrocortisone in this medicine may be absorbed through the lining of the rectum and can affect growth. *Children who must use this medicine should be followed closely by their doctor.*

If this medicine stains your clothing, the stain may be removed by hand- or machine-washing with laundry detergent.

The belladonna in this medicine may make you sweat less, causing your body temperature to increase. *Use extra care not to become overheated during exercise or hot weather while you are using this medicine,* as overheating could possibly result in heat stroke.

Side Effects of This Medicine

Along with its needed effects, a medicine may cause some unwanted effects. Although not all of these side effects appear very often, when they do occur they may require medical attention. Check with your doctor if any of the following side effects occur:

Rare

    Eye pain
    Signs of irritation or infection such as rectal bleeding, pain, burning, itching, or blistering not present before using this medicine

Possible signs of too much medicine being absorbed into the body

Blurred vision	Dryness of mouth
Dizziness	Rapid heartbeat

Other side effects not listed above may also occur in some patients. If you notice any other effects, check with your doctor.

HYDROCORTISONE, BISMUTH, BENZYL BENZOATE, PERUVIAN BALSAM, AND ZINC OXIDE (Rectal)
A commonly used brand name is Anusol-HC.

Hydrocortisone (hye-droe-KOR-ti-sone), bismuth (BIZ-muth), benzyl benzoate (BEN-zill BENZ-oh-ate), Peruvian balsam (pe-ROO-vee-an BAL-sam) and zinc oxide (ZINK OX-ide) combination is used to relieve the swelling, itching, and discomfort of hemorrhoids and certain other rectal problems. This medicine is used as a rectal cream or suppository and is available only with your doctor's prescription.

Before Using This Medicine

In order to decide on the best treatment for your medical problem, your doctor should be told:

—if you have ever had any unusual reaction to hydrocortisone or to hemorrhoid or other rectal medicines.

—if you are pregnant or if you intend to become pregnant while using this medicine. Although this medicine has not been shown to cause birth defects or other problems, the chance always exists, especially if it is used in large amounts or for a long period of time.

—if you are breast-feeding an infant. Although this medicine has not been shown to cause problems, the chance always exists.

—if you have an infection at the place of treatment.

Proper Use of This Medicine

Do not use this medicine more often or for a longer period of time than your doctor ordered. To do so may increase the chance of absorption through the lining of the rectum and the chance of side effects.

Do not use any leftover medicine for future rectal problems without first checking with your doctor. The hydrocortisone in this medicine should not be used on many kinds of bacterial, viral, or fungal infections.

If you miss a dose of this medicine, use it as soon as possible. Then go back to your regular dosing schedule. But if it is almost time for your next dose, do not use the missed dose at all. Instead, go back to your regular dosing schedule. If you have any questions about this, check with your doctor.

For patients using the rectal cream:

• Bathe and dry the rectal area. Apply a small amount of cream and gently rub in.

• If your doctor wants you to insert the cream into the rectum: First attach the plastic applicator tip onto the opened tube. Insert the applicator tip into the rectum and gently squeeze the tube to deliver the cream. Remove the applicator tip from the tube and wash with hot, soapy water. Replace the cap of the tube after use.

For patients using the suppositories:

• How to insert suppository: First remove the foil wrapper and moisten the suppository with water. Lie down on side and push the suppository well up into rectum with finger. If the suppository is too soft to insert because of storage in a warm place, chill the suppository in the refrigerator for 30 minutes or run cold water over it before removing the foil wrapper.

Precautions While Using This Medicine

The hydrocortisone in this medicine may be absorbed through the lining of the rectum and can affect growth. *Children who must use this medicine should be followed closely by their doctor.*

If this medicine stains your clothing, the stain may be removed by hand- or machine-washing with laundry detergent.

Side Effects of This Medicine

Along with its needed effects, a medicine may cause some unwanted effects. Although not all of these side effects appear very often, when they do occur they may require medical attention. Check with your doctor if any of the following side effects occur:

Rare

Signs of irritation or infection such as rectal bleeding, pain, burning, itching, or blistering not present before using this medicine

Other side effects not listed above may also occur in some patients. If you notice any other effects, check with your doctor.

HYDROXYSTILBAMIDINE (Systemic)

Hydroxystilbamidine (hye-drox-ee-stil-BAM-i-deen) belongs to the group of medicines called antifungals. It is given by injection to treat certain fungal infections. This medicine is available only with your doctor's prescription.

Before Using This Medicine

In order to decide on the best treatment for your medical problem, your doctor should be told:

—if you have ever had any unusual reaction to hydroxystilbamidine in the past. This medicine should not be used if you are allergic to it.

—if you are pregnant, if you intend to become pregnant, or if you are breast-feeding an infant. Although hydroxystilbamidine has not been shown to cause problems, the chance always exists.

—if you have either of the following medical problems:
    Kidney disease
    Liver disease

Side Effects of This Medicine

Along with its needed effects, a medicine may cause some unwanted effects. Although not all of these side effects appear very often, when they do occur they may require medical attention. Check with your doctor if any of the following side effects occur:

Less common

Chills and fever	Troubled breathing
Redness, swelling, or pain at place of injection	Unexplained sore throat and fever
Skin rash or itching	Unusual tiredness or weakness
Swelling of face or eyelids	Unusually fast heartbeat

Rare

Numbness, tingling, pain, or weakness in hands or feet	Yellowing of eyes or skin

Other side effects may occur which usually do not require medical attention. These side effects may go away during treatment as your body adjusts to the medicine. However, check with your doctor if any of the following side effects continue or are bothersome:

More common

Diarrhea	Nausea
Loss of appetite	Vomiting

Less common

Dizziness or lightheadedness	Headache
Drowsiness	Joint pain

Other side effects not listed above may also occur in some patients. If you notice any other effects, check with your doctor.

HYDROXYUREA (Systemic)
A commonly used brand name is Hydrea.

Hydroxyurea (hye-DROX-ee-yoo-REE-ah) belongs to the group of medicines called antimetabolites. It is used to treat some kinds of cancer as well as some noncancerous conditions such as psoriasis. It is used also in some situations to reduce the body's natural immunity. Hydroxyurea is available only with your doctor's prescription.

Before Using This Medicine

Hydroxyurea is a very strong medicine. In addition to its helpful effects in treating your medical problem, it has side effects that could be very serious. Before you take this medicine, be sure that you have discussed the use of it with your doctor.

In order to decide on the best treatment for your medical problem, your doctor should be told:

—if you have ever had any unusual reaction to hydroxyurea in the past.

—if you are pregnant or if you intend to have children. This medicine may cause birth defects if either the male or female is taking it at the time of conception or if it is taken during pregnancy. It may also cause permanent sterility after it has been taken for a while. Be sure that you have discussed this with your doctor before taking this medicine.

—if you are breast-feeding an infant. Although hydroxyurea has not been shown to cause problems, the chance always exists.

—if you have any of the following medical problems:

Anemia	Kidney disease
Blood disease	Kidney stones
Gout	Liver disease
Infection	

—if you are taking gout medicine.

—if you have been treated with x-rays or cancer drugs by another doctor.

Proper Use of This Medicine

Take this medicine only as directed by your doctor. Do not use more or less of it, and do not use it more often than your doctor ordered.

This medicine is sometimes given together with certain other medicines. If you are using a combination of drugs, make sure that you take each medicine at the right time and do not mix them. Ask your doctor, nurse, or pharmacist to help you plan a way to take your medicine at the right time.

Do not stop taking this medicine without first checking with your doctor.

If you miss a dose of this medicine, do not take the missed dose at all and do not double the next one. Instead, go back to your regular dosing schedule and check with your doctor.

Precautions While Using This Medicine

It is very important that your doctor check your progress at regular visits.

While you are using this medicine, your doctor may want you to drink plenty of fluids and urinate often. This will help prevent kidney problems and keep your kidneys working well. If you have any questions about this, check with your doctor.

Side Effects of This Medicine

Along with its needed effects, a medicine may cause some unwanted effects. Although not all of these side effects appear very often, when they do occur they may require medical attention. Check with your doctor if any of the following side effects occur:

More common
Unexplained fever, chills, or sore throat	Unusual bleeding or bruising

Less common
Diarrhea	Sores in the mouth and on the lips
Loss of appetite	
Nausea	Vomiting

Rare
Dizziness	Headache
Flank or stomach pain	Joint pain
Hallucinations (seeing, hearing, or feeling things that are not there)	Mental confusion
	Swelling of feet or lower legs

Other side effects may occur which usually do not require medical attention. These side effects may go away during treatment as your body adjusts to the medicine. However, check with your doctor if any of the following side effects continue or are bothersome:

More common
Drowsiness

Less common
Constipation	Skin rash and itching
Redness of the face	

Rare
Loss of hair

After you stop using this medicine, your body may need time to adjust. The length of time this takes depends on the amount of medicine you were using and how long you used it. During this period of time check with your doctor if you notice any of the following side effects:

Unexplained fever, chills, or sore throat	Unusual bleeding or bruising

Other side effects not listed above may also occur in some patients. If you notice any other effects, check with your doctor.

HYDROXYZINE (Systemic)
Some commonly used brand names are Atarax and Vistaril.

Hydroxyzine (hye-DROX-i-zeen) is a medicine used in the treatment of nervous and emotional conditions. It can also be used to help control anxiety.

Because hydroxyzine has antihistamine action, it can be used to relieve or prevent the symptoms of hay fever and other types of allergy. It also can be used to prevent motion sickness, nausea, and vomiting.

Hydroxyzine is available only with your doctor's prescription.

Before Using This Medicine
In order to decide on the best treatment for your medical problem, your doctor should be told:

—if you have ever had any unusual reaction to hydroxyzine in the past. This medicine should not be taken if you are allergic to it.

—if you are pregnant, if you intend to become pregnant, or if you are breast-feeding an infant. Although hydroxyzine has not been shown to cause problems in humans, the chance always exists.

—if you are now taking any central nervous system (CNS) depressants such as:

Antihistamines or medicine for hay fever, other allergies, or colds	Prescription pain medicine
	Sedatives, tranquilizers, or sleeping medicine
Barbiturates	
Medicine for seizures	Tricyclic antidepressants (medicine for depression)
Narcotics	

Proper Use of This Medicine
Take hydroxyzine only as directed by your doctor. Do not take more of it and do not take it more often than your doctor ordered.

If you are taking this medicine regularly and you miss a dose, take it as soon as possible. However, if it is almost time for your next dose, do not take the missed dose at all and do not double the next one. Instead, go back to your regular dosing schedule. If you have any questions about this, check with your doctor.

Precautions While Using This Medicine
Hydroxyzine will add to the effects of alcohol and other medicines (CNS depressants) that slow down the nervous system. Some examples of CNS depressants are antihistamines or medicine for hay fever, other allergies, or colds; sedatives, tranquilizers, or sleeping medicine; prescription pain medicine or narcotics; barbiturates; medicine for seizures; tricyclic antidepressants (medicine for depression); or anesthetics, including some dental anesthetics. *Check with your doctor before taking any of the above while you are using this medicine.*

This medicine may cause some people to become drowsy or less alert than they are normally. Even if taken at bedtime, it may cause some people to feel drowsy or less alert on arising. *Make sure you know how you react to this medicine before you drive, use machines, or do other jobs that require you to be alert.*

Your mouth may feel very dry while you are taking hydroxyzine. To help relieve this feeling, chew sugarless gum or dissolve bits of ice in your mouth.

Side Effects of This Medicine
Along with its needed effects, a medicine may cause some unwanted effects. Although not all of these side effects appear very often, when they do occur they may require medical attention. Check with your doctor if either of the following side effects occurs:

Rare
 Skin rash
 Tremors or
  shakiness

Other side effects may occur which usually do not require medical attention. These side effects may go away during treatment as your body adjusts to the medicine. However, check with your doctor if either of the following side effects is bothersome:

More common
 Drowsiness
Less common
 Dryness of the
  mouth

Other side effects not listed above may also occur in some patients. If you notice any other effects, check with your doctor.

IBUPROFEN (Systemic)
A commonly used brand name is Motrin.

Ibuprofen (eye-BYOO-proe-fen) is used to treat the symptoms of arthritis. It helps relieve inflammation, swelling, stiffness, and joint pain. Also, it is used as an analgesic to relieve pain. This medicine is available only with your doctor's prescription.

Before Using This Medicine
In order to decide on the best treatment for your medical problem, your doctor should be told:

—if you have ever had any unusual reaction to aspirin or other salicylates, fenoprofen, meclofenamate, naproxen, sulindac, or tolmetin.

—if you are pregnant, if you intend to become pregnant, or if you are breast-feeding an infant. Although ibuprofen has not been shown to cause problems in humans, the chance always exists.

—if you have any of the following medical problems:

Bleeding problems	Kidney disease
Heart disease	Stomach ulcer or
High blood pressure	other stomach
	problems

—if you are now taking any of the following medicines or types of medicine:

Anticoagulants	Inflammation
(blood thinners)	medicine (for
	example, aspirin
	or other arthritis
	medicine)

Proper Use of This Medicine
When used for arthritis, this medicine must be taken regularly as ordered by your doctor in order for it to help you. One to 2 weeks may pass before you feel its full effects.

It is best to take this medicine 30 minutes before meals or 2 hours after meals so that it will get into the blood more quickly. However, to lessen stomach upset, your doctor may want you to take the medicine with food, milk, or antacids. If stomach upset (indigestion, nausea, vomiting, stomach pain, or diarrhea) continues or if you have any questions about how you should be taking this medicine, check with your doctor.

If you are taking this medicine regularly (for example, every day) and you miss a dose, take it as soon as possible. Then go back to your regular dosing schedule. However, if it is almost time for your next dose, do not take the missed dose at all and do not double the next one. Instead, go back to your regular dosing schedule. If you have any questions about this, check with your doctor.

Precautions While Using This Medicine
Your doctor should check your progress at regular visits in order to make sure that this medicine does not cause unwanted effects.

Stomach problems may be more likely to occur if you take aspirin regularly (for example, every day) or drink alcoholic beverages while being treated with this medicine. Therefore, *do not take aspirin regularly or drink alcoholic beverages while taking this medicine,* unless otherwise directed by your doctor.

Before having any kind of surgery (including dental surgery), tell the doctor or dentist in charge that you are taking this medicine.

This medicine may cause some people to become dizzy. *Make sure you know how you react to this medicine before you drive, use machines, or do other jobs that require you to be alert.*

Side Effects of This Medicine
Along with its needed effects, a medicine may cause some unwanted effects. Although not all of these side effects appear very often, when they do occur they may require medical attention. Check with your doctor if any of the following side effects occur:

More common
    Skin rash
Less common

Itching of skin	Swelling of feet or
Ringing or buzzing	lower legs
in ears	Unusual weight gain

Rare

Bloody or black	Hives
tarry stools	Mental depression
Bloody urine	Shortness of breath,
Blurred vision or	troubled
any change in	breathing,
vision	wheezing, or
Difficult or painful	tightness
urination	in chest
Frequent urge to	Unexplained sore
urinate	throat and fever

Other side effects may occur which usually do not require medical attention. These side effects may go away during treatment as your body adjusts to the medicine. However, check with your doctor if any of the following side effects continue or are bothersome:

More common

Bloated feeling or gas	Heartburn or indigestion
Constipation	Nausea or vomiting
Diarrhea	Stomach pain or discomfort
Dizziness	

Less common

Decreased appetite	Nervousness
Headache	

Other side effects not listed above may also occur in some patients. If you notice any other effects, check with your doctor.

IDOXURIDINE (Ophthalmic)
Some commonly used brand names are Dendrid, Herplex, and Stoxil.

Idoxuridine (eye-dox-YOOR-i-deen) belongs to the general family of medicines called antivirals. Idoxuridine ophthalmic preparations are used to help the body overcome virus infections of the eye. They are available only with your doctor's prescription.

Before Using This Medicine

In order to decide on the best treatment for your medical problem, your doctor should be told:

—if you have had allergic reactions to iodine or iodine-containing preparations.

—if you are pregnant, if you intend to become pregnant, or if you are breast-feeding an infant, although idoxuridine ophthalmic preparations have not been shown to cause problems in humans.

—if you are now using boric acid in the eyes.

Proper Use of This Medicine

For patients using the eye drop form of this medicine:

• Bottle is not full; this is to provide proper drop control.

• To prevent contamination of the eye drops, do not touch the applicator tip to any surface (including the eye), and keep the container tightly closed.

• How to apply this medicine: First, wash hands. Then tilt head back and pull lower eyelid away from eye to form a pouch. Drop medicine into the pouch and gently close eyes. Do not blink. Keep eyes closed for 1 or 2 minutes to allow medicine to come into contact with the infection.

• If you think you did not get the drop of medicine into your eye properly, use another drop.

For patients using the eye ointment form of this medicine:

• To prevent contamination of the eye ointment, do not touch the applicator tip to any surface (including the eye). After using, wipe the tip of the ointment tube with a clean tissue and keep the tube tightly closed.

• How to apply this medicine: First, wash hands. Then pull the lower eyelid away from eye to form a pouch. Squeeze a thin strip of ointment into the pouch. A 1-cm (approximately 1/3-inch) strip of ointment is usually enough unless otherwise directed by your doctor. Gently close eyes and keep them closed for 1 or 2 minutes to allow medicine to come into contact with the infection.

Do not use this medicine more often or for a longer time than your doctor ordered. To do so may cause problems in the eyes. If you have any questions about this, check with your doctor.

To help clear up your infection completely, *keep using this medicine for the full time of treatment,* even though your symptoms may have disappeared; *do not miss any doses.*

If you do miss a dose of this medicine, apply it as soon as possible. However, if it is almost time for your next application, skip the missed dose and go back to your regular dosing schedule.

Precautions While Using This Medicine

After application, eye ointments usually cause your vision to blur for a few minutes.

It is very important that your doctor check your progress at regular visits.

If your symptoms do not improve within a week or if they become worse, check with your doctor.

Side Effects of This Medicine

Along with its needed effects, a medicine may cause some unwanted effects. Although not all of these side effects appear very often, when they do occur they may require medical attention. Check with your doctor if any of the following side effects occur:

Less common

Increased sensitivity of eyes to light
Itching, redness, swelling, pain, or other sign of irritation not present before you started using this medicine

Rare
>Blurring, dimming, or haziness of vision

Other side effects may occur which usually do not require medical attention. These side effects may go away during treatment as your body adjusts to the medicine. However, check with your doctor if the following side effect continues or is bothersome:

Less common
>Excess flow of tears

Other side effects not listed above may also occur in some patients. If you notice any other effects, check with your doctor.

INDOMETHACIN (Systemic)

Some commonly used brand names are Indocid* and Indocin.

---

*Not available in the United States.

Indomethacin (in-doe-METH-a-sin) is used to treat the symptoms of many medical problems, including certain types of arthritis. It helps relieve inflammation, swelling, stiffness, joint pain, and fever. This medicine is available only with your doctor's prescription.

Before Using This Medicine

In order to decide on the best treatment for your medical problem, your doctor should be told:

—if you have ever had any unusual reaction to aspirin or other salicylates, fenoprofen, ibuprofen, meclofenamate, naproxen, oxyphenbutazone, phenylbutazone, sulindac, or tolmetin.

—if you are pregnant, if you intend to become pregnant, or if you are breast-feeding an infant. Although indomethacin has not been shown to cause problems in humans, the chance always exists.

—if you have any of the following medical problems:

Bleeding problems	Mental illness
Colitis	Parkinsonism
Epilepsy	Stomach ulcer or
Kidney disease	other stomach
Liver disease	problems

—if you are now taking any of the following medicines or types of medicine:

Anticoagulants (blood thinners)	Inflammation medicine (for example, aspirin or other arthritis medicine)
Furosemide	
	Lithium
	Probenecid

Proper Use of This Medicine

Take this medicine only as directed by your doctor. Do not take more of it, do not take it more often, and do not take it for a longer period of time than your doctor ordered.

If you are taking this medicine to relieve arthritis, you must take it regularly as ordered by your doctor. In some types of arthritis, up to 2 weeks may pass before you begin to feel better and up to 1 month may pass before you feel the full effects of this medicine.

Take this medicine immediately after meals or with food or milk to lessen stomach upset. If this does not work, ask your doctor if you may use antacids. If stomach upset (indigestion, heartburn, nausea, vomiting, stomach pain, or diarrhea) continues, check with your doctor.

If you miss a dose of this medicine and remember within an hour or so of the missed dose, take it right away. Then go back to your regular dosing schedule. But if you do not remember until later, do not take the missed dose at all and do not double the next one. Instead, go back to your regular dosing schedule. If you have any questions about this, check with your doctor.

Precautions While Using This Medicine

If you will be taking this medicine for a long period of time:

—your doctor should check your progress at regular visits.

—your doctor may want you to have your eyes examined by an ophthalmologist.

Before having any kind of surgery (including dental surgery), tell the doctor or dentist in charge that you are taking this medicine.

Stomach problems may be more likely to occur if you take aspirin regularly (for example, every day) or drink alcoholic beverages while being treated with this medicine. Therefore, *do not take aspirin regularly or drink alcoholic beverages while taking this medicine,* unless otherwise directed by your doctor.

This medicine may cause some people to become dizzy, light-headed, drowsy, or less alert than they are normally. *Make sure you know how you react to this medicine before you drive, use machines, or do other jobs that require you to be alert.*

Side Effects of This Medicine

Along with its needed effects, a medicine may cause some unwanted effects. Although not all of these side effects appear very often, when they do occur they may require medical attention. Check with your doctor if any of the following side effects occur:

Less common

    Ringing or buzzing in ears

Rare

Bloody or black tarry stools	Skin rash, hives, or itching
Blurred vision (with prolonged use)	Swelling of feet or lower legs
Hearing problems	Unexplained sore throat and fever
Mental confusion or depression	Unusual bleeding or bruising
Shortness of breath, troubled breathing, wheezing, or tightness in chest	Unusual weight gain
	Yellowing of eyes or skin

Other side effects may occur which usually do not require medical attention. These side effects may go away during treatment as your body adjusts to the medicine. However, check with your doctor if any of the following side effects continue or are bothersome:

More common

Dizziness or lightheadedness	Heartburn or indigestion
Headache	Nausea
	Stomach pain

Less common

Constipation	Unusual tiredness or weakness
Diarrhea	
Unusual drowsiness	Vomiting

Other side effects not listed above may also occur in some patients. If you notice any other effects, check with your doctor.

INSULIN (Systemic)

This information applies to the following medicines:

Insulin (IN-su-lin)
Globin Zinc Insulin
Isophane Insulin Suspension
Isophane Insulin Suspension and Insulin Injection
Insulin Zinc Suspension
Extended Insulin Zinc Suspension
Prompt Insulin Zinc Suspension
Protamine Zinc Insulin Suspension

Some commonly used brand names and other names are:	Generic names:
Actrapid Regular Insulin Regular Iletin II (new) Velosulin	Insulin Injection
Globin Insulin	Globin Zinc Insulin Injection
Insulatard NPH NPH Iletin II	Isophane Insulin Suspension
Mixtard	Isophane Insulin Suspension and Insulin Injection
Lentard Lente Insulin Lente Iletin II Monotard	Insulin Zinc Suspension
Ultralente Ultralente Iletin Ultratard	Extended Insulin Zinc Suspension
Semilente Semilente Iletin Semitard	Prompt Insulin Zinc Suspension
Protamine Zinc & Iletin II PZI	Protamine Zinc Insulin Suspension

Insulin (IN-su-lin) belongs to the group of medicines called hormones. It is made naturally by the body to help produce energy from the carbohydrates and sugars in food.

If the body does not make enough insulin to meet its needs, a condition known as diabetes mellitus (sugar diabetes) may develop. Eating the right foods along with proper exercise may control this condition. If not, your doctor may prescribe insulin along with diet and exercise to help keep your health in balance.

Insulin is made from beef or pork sources and many insulin preparations contain a mixture of both, although one-source preparations are available. Insulin must be injected under the skin because when taken by mouth, it is destroyed by stomach acids.

Although a prescription is not necessary to purchase most insulin, your doctor must first determine your personal insulin needs and provide you with special instructions for control of your diabetic condition.

Before Using This Medicine

Importance of Diet

Before prescribing medicine for your diabetes, your doctor will probably try to control your condition by prescribing a personal diet for you. Such a diet is low in refined carbohydrates (foods such as sugar and candy used for quick energy). The daily number of calories in this diet should be adjusted to help you reach and maintain your ideal body weight. In addition, meals and snacks are arranged to meet the energy needs of your body at different times of the day.

Many diabetics are able to control their condition by carefully following their doctor's orders for proper diet and exercise. *Medicine is prescribed only when additional help is needed.*

In order to decide on the best treatment for your medical problem, your doctor should be told:

—if you are allergic to beef or pork insulins.

—if you are pregnant.

—if you have any of the following medical problems:

Infection	Liver disease
Kidney disease	Thyroid disease

—if you are now taking any of the following medicines or types of medicine:

Anabolic steroids	Oral contraceptives
Aspirin or other	(birth control
salicylates (in	pills)
large doses)	Phenytoin
Cortisone-like	Propranolol
medicine	Sinus or
Diabetes medicine	asthma medicine
you take by	Thyroid medicine
mouth	Water pills (such
Disopyramide	as chlorthalidone,
Epinephrine	ethacrynic acid,
Guanethidine	furosemide,
Monoamine oxidase	thiazides)
(MAO) inhibitors	
(medicine for	
depression)	

Proper Use of This Medicine

Make sure you have the correct type and strength of insulin as ordered for you by your doctor. You may find that keeping an insulin label with you is helpful when buying insulin supplies.

It is very important to use insulin only as directed. Do not change the strength or the type unless told to do so by your doctor. Some insulin products have recently been changed and may require a different dosage for some users. If your insulin package has a red number beginning with "CP"—, in the upper right corner, discuss its use with your doctor or pharmacist if you have not already done so.

The strength (concentration) of insulin is measured by Units and is sometimes expressed in terms such as U-100 insulin instead of insulin 100 Units.

Insulin doses are measured and given with specially marked insulin syringes. For patients using only a few units of U-100 insulin per dose, a special low-dose syringe is available to make dose measurement easier and more accurate. The syringes are marked with a scale in Units which match the Unit strength of insulin being used. To help you quickly check for the strength, insulin syringes, packages, and bottles are color-coded as follows according to the strength of insulin: red for U-40, and orange or black for U-100.

A prescription from your doctor may be required to purchase insulin syringes in some states.

Each package of insulin contains a patient instruction sheet. Read this sheet carefully for information concerning your syringe and needle and steps to follow when injecting a dose of insulin. You may prefer to use disposable insulin syringes and needles which are presterilized and designed to be used one time only, and then discarded. A glass insulin syringe and metal needles may be used repeatedly if they are sterilized each time. The patient instruction sheet included in each insulin package will explain how to sterilize the syringe and needle. For more information or for explanation of instructions you do not understand, ask your doctor, nurse, or pharmacist.

It is very important to follow carefully any instructions from your doctor such as these for:

• Alcohol. Drinking alcohol may cause severe hypoglycemia (low blood sugar). Discuss the use of alcoholic beverages with your doctor.

• Diabetic diet. The success of your treatment depends on closely following the diet your doctor prescribed for you.

• Exercise. Your doctor will tell you what kind of exercise and how much you should do daily.

• Foot care. Special care of your feet will prevent possible future trouble.

• Urine tests. These tests are used to guide you in the control of your condition and must be done properly. Two urine tests for sugar are widely used: the tablet urine test and the paper-strip urine test. In addition, your doctor may instruct you to test your urine for acetone.

Precautions While Using This Medicine

It is very important that your doctor check your progress at regular visits, especially during the first few weeks of insulin treatment.

Do not take other medicines unless they have been discussed with your doctor. This especially includes over-the-counter (nonprescription) medicines such as aspirin, and those for appetite control, asthma, colds, cough, hay fever, or sinus.

In case of emergency:

• Carry a diabetic identification card.

• A medical I.D. bracelet may be helpful.

• Keep handy an extra supply of insulin and a syringe with needles.

• Keep handy a glucagon kit and syringe with needle and know how it is used; also, members of your household should know how it is used.

• Make sure a source of sugar such as orange juice, non-diet cola or soda, honey, table sugar, corn syrup, sugar cubes, or candy is always available to correct an insulin reaction (hypoglycemia).

• Have on hand several phone numbers you can call for help, such as those of your doctor, the emergency room, your pharmacy, friends, and neighbors.

Storage and expiration date:

• When buying insulin always check the package expiration date to make sure the insulin will be used before it expires. This expiration date applies only when the insulin has been stored under refrigeration.

• Do not use insulin after the expiration date stated on the label even if the bottle has never been opened. Check with your pharmacist about the possibility of exchanging an outdated bottle not yet opened.

• Insulin should be refrigerated without freezing until it is to be used. Insulin you are now using regularly may be kept out of the refrigerator at room temperature if it will be used up within a month. Insulin stored at room temperature which has not been used for a month or more should be discarded. Insulin which is used only occasionally is best kept refrigerated.

Do not expose insulin to extremely hot temperatures. Do not leave insulin in the hot summer sun or in a hot, closed automobile. Extreme heat will cause it to spoil more quickly.

Do not shake the insulin bottle hard before using. Frothing or bubbles can cause an incorrect dose. Mix contents well by rolling the bottle slowly between the palms of the hands or by tipping the bottle end-to-end a few times. Do not use if contents look lumpy or grainy, or stick to the bottle.

Your doctor may want you to mix two types of insulin in the same syringe to match your needs more closely with one injection. Although it is not critical which type of insulin of a mixture is drawn into the syringe first, patients should always mix insulins in the same order.

Check with your doctor immediately if these symptoms of low blood sugar (hypoglycemia) insulin reaction appear:

Anxiety	Nausea
Chills	Nervousness
Cold sweats	Rapid pulse
Cool pale skin	Shakiness
Drowsiness	Unusual tiredness
Excessive hunger	or weakness
Headache	

Such symptoms may occur suddenly if you use too much insulin, delay or skip a meal, become sick (especially with nausea or vomiting), or exercise more than usual. Eating some type of sugar when these symptoms first appear will usually prevent them from getting worse. Orange juice, corn syrup, honey, sugar cubes, or table sugar will work faster if first dissolved in water. Also, you should eat some crackers or half a sandwich if you will not be having a snack or a meal for an hour or more.

If you become sick, especially with nausea and vomiting, or are not able to eat for other reasons, you may still need some insulin. Before you become sick, check with your doctor for instructions regarding sick days. Even if you control the symptoms of low blood sugar and have no continuing problems, you should keep your doctor informed.

Check with your doctor right away if the symptoms of high blood sugar (hyperglycemia) occur. These symptoms appear more slowly than those of hypoglycemia, and usually include:

Drowsiness	Increased urination
Flushed, dry skin	Loss of appetite
Fruit-like breath odor	Unusual thirst

These symptoms may occur if you do not take enough insulin, if you skip a dose, if you do not follow a proper diet or if you overeat, or if you have a fever or infection.

Symptoms of both low blood sugar and high blood sugar must be corrected before they progress to a more serious condition. In either situation, you should check with your doctor immediately.

When traveling:

• Carry a recent prescription from your doctor for your diabetes medicine, and also for the correct syringe and needles, since state and city laws and regulations may vary.

• Do not change your diet or medicine schedule. Before you leave, discuss your trip with your doctor.

• Consider the use of disposable syringes since they are presterilized.

• Carry your diabetic supplies on your person or in a purse or briefcase to reduce the possibility of loss.

• Remember time zone changes and changes in meal times. Such changes may affect your diabetic schedule unless you allow for them.

• In hot climates, consider the use of a vacuum container to help maintain the temperature of your insulin. These can be obtained at most pharmacies.

• In foreign countries, it is advisable to carry enough diabetic supplies to last until you return home, although most countries have some form of insulin available.

• When carrying a large quantity of diabetic supplies, divide your insulin supplies equally throughout your pieces of luggage. This will reduce the amount of loss if any of your luggage is lost or delayed.

IODOCHLORHYDROXYQUIN (Topical)
A commonly used brand name is Vioform.

Iodochlorhydroxyquin (eye-oh-doe-klor-hye-DROX-ee-kwin) belongs to the general family of medicines called anti-infectives. Iodochlorhydroxyquin topical preparations are used to help the body overcome infections of the skin. Iodochlorhydroxyquin is available without a prescription; however, your doctor may have special instructions on the proper use of this medicine for your medical problem.

Before Using This Medicine
In order to decide on the best treatment for your medical problem, your doctor should be told:

—if you have had allergic reactions to iodine or iodine-containing preparations.

—if you are pregnant, if you intend to become pregnant, or if you are breast-feeding an infant, although iodochlorhydroxyquin topical preparations have not been shown to cause problems.

Proper Use of This Medicine
This medicine may stain clothing, skin, hair, and nails yellow. Avoid getting this medicine on your clothing since bleaching may not remove the stain.

Do not use this medicine in or around the eyes.

Before applying this medicine, wash the area to be treated with soap and water, and dry thoroughly.

If you are using the cream form of this medicine:

• Apply a thin layer of cream to the affected area and rub in gently until cream disappears. Do not apply a thick layer; this only wastes medicine and does no more good than a thin layer.

If you are using the ointment form of this medicine:

• Apply a thin layer of ointment to the affected area and rub in gently. Do not apply a thick layer; this only wastes medicine and does no more good than a thin layer.

To help clear up your infection completely, *keep using this medicine for the full time of treatment,* even though your symptoms may have disappeared; *do not miss any doses.*

If you do miss a dose of this medicine, apply it as soon as possible. However, if it is almost time for your next application, skip the missed dose and go back to your regular dosing schedule.

Precautions While Using This Medicine

To help make sure your infection does not return, good health habits are required. If you have any questions about this, check with your doctor or pharmacist.

If there is no improvement in your skin problem after you have used this medicine for 1 to 2 weeks or if it becomes worse, check with your doctor or pharmacist.

Side Effects of This Medicine

Along with its needed effects, a medicine may cause some unwanted effects. Although not all of these side effects appear very often, when they do occur they may require medical attention. Stop using this medicine and check with your doctor if any of the following side effects occur:

Rare

Itching, rash, redness, swelling, or other sign of irritation not present before you started using this medicine

Other side effects not listed above may also occur in some patients. If you notice any other effects, check with your doctor.

IODOCHLORHYDROXYQUIN AND HYDROCORTISONE (Topical)

Some commonly used brand names are:

Dek-Quin	Mity-Quin
Domeform-HC	Racet
HCV	Vioform-HC

Iodochlorhydroxyquin (eye-oh-doe-klor-hye-DROX-ee-kwin) and hydrocortisone (hye-droe-KOR-ti-sone) is a combined anti-infective and cortisone-like medicine. Iodochlorhydroxyquin and hydrocortisone topical preparations are used to help the body overcome infections of the skin and to help provide relief from the redness, itching, and discomfort of many skin problems. They are available only with your doctor's prescription.

Before Using This Medicine

In order to decide on the best treatment for your medical problem, your doctor should be told:

—if you have had allergic reactions to iodine or iodine-containing preparations.

—if you are pregnant, if you intend to become pregnant, or if you are breast-feeding an infant, although iodochlorhydroxyquin and hydrocortisone topical preparations have not been shown to cause problems. However, use of large amounts on the skin or use for a long time is not recommended during pregnancy.

—if you have any other skin infection.

Proper Use of This Medicine

This medicine may stain clothing, skin, hair, and nails yellow. Avoid getting this medicine on your clothing since bleaching may not remove the stain.

Do not use this medicine in or around the eyes.

Check with your doctor before using this medicine on any other skin problems, since it should not be used on certain kinds of bacterial, viral, or fungal skin infections.

Before applying this medicine, wash the area to be treated with soap and water, and dry thoroughly.

If you are using the cream form of this medicine:

• Apply a thin layer of cream to the affected area and rub in gently until cream disappears. Do not apply a thick layer; this only wastes medicine and does no more good than a thin layer.

If you are using the lotion form of this medicine:

• Gently squeeze bottle and apply a few drops of lotion to the affected area. Rub in gently until lotion disappears. Do not use more than is necessary to cover the area; using more only wastes medicine and does no more good.

If you are using the ointment form of this medicine:

• Apply a thin layer of ointment to the affected area and rub in gently. Do not apply a thick layer; this only wastes medicine and does no more good than a thin layer.

Do not bandage or otherwise wrap the area of the skin being treated unless directed to do so by your doctor.

To help clear up your infection completely, *keep using this medicine for the full time of treatment,* even though your symptoms may have disappeared; *do not miss any doses.* However, *do not use this medicine more often or for a longer period of time than your doctor ordered.* To do so may increase the chance of absorption through your skin and the chance of side effects. In addition, too much use, especially on thin skin areas (for example, face, armpits, groin), may result in thinning of the skin and stretch marks.

If you do miss a dose of this medicine, apply it as soon as possible. However, if it is almost time for your next application, skip the missed dose and go back to your regular dosing schedule.

Precautions While Using This Medicine

To help make sure your infection does not return, good health habits are required. If you have any questions about this, check with your doctor or pharmacist.

If there is no improvement in your skin problem after you have used this medicine for 1 to 2 weeks or if it becomes worse, check with your doctor.

This medicine may be absorbed through the skin and too much use can affect growth. *Children who must use this medicine should be followed closely by their doctor.*

Side Effects of This Medicine

Along with its needed effects, a medicine may cause some unwanted effects. Although not all of these side effects appear very often, when they do occur they may require medical attention. Stop using this medicine and check with your doctor if any of the following side effects occur:

Rare

Blistering, burning, itching, peeling, rash, redness, swelling, or other sign of irritation not present before you started using this medicine

Other side effects not listed above may also occur in some patients. If you notice any other effects, check with your doctor.

IODOQUINOL (Systemic)

Some commonly used brand names are Moebiquin and Yodoxin.

Iodoquinol (eye-oh-doe-KWIN-ole) belongs to the group of medicines called antiprotozoals. Although sometimes used to treat other types of infection, it is used most often in the treatment of intestinal infections. This medicine is available only with your doctor's prescription.

Before Using This Medicine

In order to decide on the best treatment for your medical problem, your doctor should be told:

—if you have ever had any unusual reaction to clioquinol (iodochlorhydroxyquin), iodine, primaquine, seafood, or shellfish.

—if you are pregnant, if you intend to become pregnant, or if you are breast-feeding an infant. Although iodoquinol has not been shown to cause problems, the chance always exists.

—if you have any of the following medical problems:

Eye disease	Liver disease
Kidney disease	Thyroid disease

Proper Use of This Medicine

To help clear up your infection completely, *keep taking this medicine for the full time of treatment* even if you begin to feel better after a few days; *do not miss any doses.*

If you do miss a dose of this medicine, take it as soon as possible. Then go back to your regular dosing schedule.

Take this medicine after meals to lessen possible stomach upset, unless otherwise directed by your doctor.

If these tablets are too large to swallow whole, they may be crushed and mixed with a small amount of applesauce or chocolate syrup.

Precautions While Using This Medicine

If you must have thyroid function tests, make sure the doctor knows that you are taking this medicine or have taken it within the past 6 months.

Side Effects of This Medicine

Along with its needed effects, a medicine may cause some unwanted effects. Although not all of these side effects appear very often, when they do occur they may require medical attention. Check with your doctor if any of the following side effects occur:

Less common

Fever or chills	Swelling of neck
Skin rash, hives, or itching	

With long-term use of high doses

Blurred vision or any change in vision (especially in children)	Muscle pain
	Numbness, tingling, pain, or weakness in hands or feet (especially in children)
Clumsiness or unsteadiness	
Eye pain (especially in children)	Unusual weakness

Other side effects may occur which usually do not require medical attention. These side effects may go away during treatment as your body

adjusts to the medicine. However, check with your doctor if any of the following side effects continue or are bothersome:

More common

| Diarrhea | Stomach pain |
| Nausea | Vomiting |

Less common

Dizziness or	Itching around rec-
lightheadedness	tum
Headache	

Other side effects not listed above may also occur in some patients. If you notice any other effects, check with your doctor.

IPECAC (Systemic)

Ipecac (IP-e-kak) is used in the emergency treatment of certain kinds of poisoning. Only the syrup form of ipecac should be used. It is taken by mouth to cause vomiting of the poison.

Ordinarily, this medicine should not be used if strychnine, corrosives such as alkalies (lye) and strong acids, or petroleum distillates such as kerosene, gasoline, coal oil, fuel oil, paint thinner, or cleaning fluid have been swallowed, since it may cause seizures, additional injury to the throat, or pneumonia.

This medicine in amounts of more than 1 ounce is available only with your doctor's prescription. It is available in 1 ounce bottles without a prescription; however, before using ipecac syrup, call your doctor, a poison control center, or an emergency room for advice.

Before Using This Medicine

In order to decide on the best treatment for your medical problem, your doctor should be told:

—if you are pregnant, if you intend to become pregnant, or if you are breast-feeding an infant. Although ipecac has not been shown to cause problems, the chance always exists.

—if you have heart disease.

Proper Use of This Medicine

It is very important that you take this medicine only as directed. Do not take more of it and do not take it more often than recommended on the label, unless otherwise directed.

Keep this medicine out of the reach of children, since overdose is very dangerous in children.

Before using this medicine to cause vomiting in poisoning, call your doctor, a poison control

center, or an emergency room for advice. It is a good idea to have these telephone numbers readily available.

Do not give this medicine to unconscious or very drowsy persons, since the vomited material may enter the lungs and cause pneumonia.

To help this medicine cause vomiting of the poison, adults should drink 1 to 2 full glasses (8 to 16 ounces) of water and children should drink 1/2 to 1 full glass (4 to 8 ounces) of water immediately after taking this medicine.

Do not take this medicine with milk, milk products, or with carbonated beverages. Milk or milk products may prevent this medicine from working properly and carbonated beverages may cause swelling of the stomach.

If vomiting does not occur within 20 minutes after you have taken the first dose of this medicine, take a second dose. If vomiting does not occur after you have taken the second dose, you must immediately see your doctor or go to an emergency room.

If you have been told to take both this medicine and activated charcoal to treat the poisoning, *do not take the activated charcoal until after you have taken this medicine to cause vomiting and the vomiting has stopped. This is usually about 30 minutes.* Taking the activated charcoal before or with this medicine may prevent this medicine from causing vomiting of the poison.

Side Effects of This Medicine

Along with its needed effects, a medicine may cause some unwanted effects. Although side effects usually do not occur with recommended doses of ipecac, when they do occur they may require medical attention. Check with your doctor if any of the following side effects occur:

Possible signs of overdose

Diarrhea	Unusual tiredness or
Nausea or vomiting	weakness
(continuing more	Unusually fast or
than 30 minutes)	irregular heart-
Stomach cramps or	beat
pain	Weakness, aching,
Troubled breathing	and stiffness
	of muscles,
	especially those of
	the neck, arms,
	and legs

Other side effects not listed above may also occur in some patients. If you notice any other effects, check with your doctor.

ISOETHARINE (Systemic)

Some commonly used brand names are Bronkometer and Bronkosol.

Isoetharine (eye-soe-ETH-a-reen) is used in the treatment of bronchial asthma, bronchitis, and emphysema. It relieves wheezing, shortness of breath, and troubled breathing. This medicine is available only with your doctor's prescription.

Before Using This Medicine

In order to decide on the best treatment for your medical problem, your doctor should be told:

—if you have ever had any unusual reaction to medicines like isoetharine such as amphetamines, ephedrine, epinephrine, isoproterenol, metaproterenol, norepinephrine (levarterenol), phenylephrine, phenylpropanolamine, pseudoephedrine, or terbutaline.

—if you are pregnant, if you intend to become pregnant, or if you are breast-feeding an infant. Although isoetharine has not been shown to cause problems, the chance always exists.

—if you have any of the following medical problems:

Heart or blood vessel disease	High blood pressure
	Overactive thyroid

—if you are now taking any of the following medicines or types of medicine:

Amphetamines	Propranolol
Other medicine for asthma or breathing problems	

Proper Use of This Medicine

Do not use if the solution turns brownish in color or if it becomes cloudy.

Use this medicine only as directed. Do not use more of it and do not use it more often than your doctor ordered. To do so may increase the chance of side effects.

If you are using this medicine in a nebulizer, make sure you understand exactly how to use it. If you have any questions about this, check with your doctor.

If you are using the aerosol form of this medicine:

• This medicine usually comes with patient directions. Read them carefully before using.

• Keep spray away from the eyes.

• *Do not take more than 2 inhalations of this medicine at any one time,* unless otherwise

directed by your doctor. Allow 1 to 2 minutes after the first inhalation to make certain that a second inhalation is necessary.

• Save your applicator. Refill units of this medicine may be available.

• Store away from heat and direct sunlight. Do not puncture, break, or burn container.

Precautions While Using This Medicine

If you still have trouble breathing after using this medicine, or if your condition gets worse, *check with your doctor at once.*

Side Effects of This Medicine

Along with its needed effects, a medicine may cause some unwanted effects. The following side effects may go away during treatment as your body adjusts to the medicine. However, check with your doctor if they continue or are bothersome:

Dizziness or lightheadedness	Restlessness
	Trouble in sleeping
Headache	Unusually fast or
Nausea	pounding heart-
Nervousness	beat
	Weakness

Other side effects not listed above may also occur in some patients. If you notice any other effects, check with your doctor.

ISOMETHEPTENE, DICHLORALPHENAZONE, AND ACETAMINOPHEN (Systemic)

A commonly used brand name is Midrin.

Isometheptene (eye-soe-meth-EP-teen), dichloralphenazone (dye-klor-al-FEN-a-zone), and acetaminophen (a-set-a-MEE-noe-fen) is a combination medicine used to treat migraine headaches and some kinds of throbbing headaches. It is not used to prevent headaches, but is used to treat an attack once it has started. This medicine is available only with your doctor's prescription.

Before Using This Medicine

In order to decide on the best treatment for your medical problem, your doctor should be told:

—if you have ever had any unusual reaction to isometheptene, dichloralphenazone, or acetaminophen in the past. This medicine should not be taken if you are allergic to it.

—if you are pregnant, if you intend to become pregnant, or if you are breast-feeding an infant. Although this medicine has not been shown to cause problems, the chance always exists.

—if you have any of the following medical problems:

Blood vessel disease	High blood pressure
Glaucoma	Kidney disease
Heart disease	Liver disease

—if you have recently had a heart attack or stroke.

—if you are now taking or have taken within the past 2 weeks monoamine oxidase (MAO) inhibitors such as:

Isocarboxazid	Phenelzine
Pargyline	Tranylcypromine

Proper Use of This Medicine

This medicine works best if you:

• *Take it at the first sign of headache.*

• *Lie down in a quiet, dark room for at least 2 hours after taking it.*

Take this medicine only as directed by your doctor. Do not take more of it, do not take it more often, and do not take it for a longer period of time than your doctor ordered. If too much acetaminophen is taken, liver damage may occur.

Precautions While Using This Medicine

If you will be taking this medicine regularly for a long period of time, your doctor should check your progress at regular visits.

Check the labels of all over-the-counter (OTC), nonprescription, and prescription medicines you now take. If any contain acetaminophen be especially careful, since taking them while taking this medicine may lead to overdose. If you have any questions about this, check with your doctor or pharmacist.

Side Effects of This Medicine

Along with its needed effects, a medicine may cause some unwanted effects. Although not all of these side effects appear very often, when they do occur they may require medical attention. Check with your doctor if any of the following side effects occur:

Rare

Itching or skin rash	Unusual tiredness or
Unexplained sore	weakness
throat and fever	Yellowing of eyes or
Unusual bleeding or	skin
bruising	

Possible signs of acetaminophen overdose

Diarrhea	Stomach cramps or
Nausea or vomiting	pain

Other side effects may occur which usually do not require medical attention. These side effects may go away during treatment as your body adjusts to the medicine. However, check with your doctor if any of the following side effects continue or are bothersome:

Rare

Dizziness	Rapid or irregular
Drowsiness	heartbeat

Other side effects not listed above may also occur in some patients. If you notice any other effects, check with your doctor.

ISONIAZID (Systemic)

Some commonly used brand names and other names are:

INH	Nydrazid
Isotamine*	Rimifon*

*Not available in the United States.

Isoniazid (eye-soe-NYE-a-zid) belongs to the general family of medicines called anti-infectives. It is used to prevent or help the body overcome tuberculosis (TB). It is given by mouth or by injection and may be given alone or with one or more other medicines for TB. Isoniazid is available only with your doctor's prescription.

Before Using This Medicine

In order to decide on the best treatment for your medical problem, your doctor should be told:

—if you have had allergic reactions to ethionamide, pyrazinamide, or niacin (nicotinic acid).

—if you are pregnant, if you intend to become pregnant, or if you are breast-feeding an infant, although isoniazid has not been shown to cause problems.

—if you have any of the following medical problems:

Alcoholism	Liver disease
Convulsive	Severe kidney
disorders such	disease
as seizures or	
epilepsy	

—if you are taking aluminum- or magnesium-containing antacids and you are to take this medicine by mouth.

—if you are now also taking any of the following medicines:

Cycloserine   Phenytoin
Disulfiram   Rifampin

—if you have had any problems with this medicine in the past.

Proper Use of This Medicine

If you are taking isoniazid by mouth and it upsets your stomach, you may take it with food. Antacids may also help. However, do not take aluminum- or magnesium-containing antacids within 1 hour of the time you take isoniazid since they may keep this medicine from working as well.

To help clear up your tuberculosis (TB) completely, *it is very important that you keep taking this medicine for the full time of treatment* even if you begin to feel better after a few weeks. You may have to take it every day for as long as 1 to 2 years or more. *It is important that you do not miss any doses.*

Your doctor may also want you to take pyridoxine (vitamin B$_6$) every day to help prevent or lessen some of the side effects of isoniazid. If so, *it is very important to take pyridoxine every day along with this medicine; do not miss any doses.*

If you do miss a dose of either of these medicines, take it as soon as possible. However, if it is almost time for your next dose, do not take the missed dose or double your next dose. Instead, go back to your regular dosing schedule.

Precautions While Using This Medicine

Certain foods such as fish (tuna, skipjack, or Sardinella) or cheese (Swiss or Cheshire) may rarely cause reactions in some patients taking isoniazid. Check with your doctor if redness or itching of the skin, hot feeling, rapid or pounding heartbeat, sweating, chills or clammy feeling, headache, or lightheadedness occurs while you are taking this medicine.

If your symptoms do not improve within 2 to 3 weeks or if they become worse, check with your doctor.

It is very important that your doctor check your progress at regular visits. Also, *check with your doctor immediately if blurred vision or any loss of vision, with or without eye pain, occurs during treatment.* Your doctor may want you to have your eyes checked by an ophthalmologist (eye doctor).

If this medicine causes you to feel very tired or very weak; or causes clumsiness; unsteadiness; a loss of appetite; nausea; numbness, tingling, burning, or pain in the hands and feet; or vomiting, stop taking it and check with your doctor immediately. These may be early warning signs of more serious liver or nerve problems that could develop later.

Caution: Diabetics—This medicine may cause false test results with some urine sugar tests. Check with your doctor before changing your diet or the dosage of your diabetes medicine.

Liver problems may be more likely to occur if you drink alcoholic beverages regularly while you are taking this medicine. Also, the regular use of alcohol may keep this medicine from working as well. Therefore, *you should not drink alcoholic beverages while you are taking this medicine.*

Side Effects of This Medicine

Along with its needed effects, a medicine may cause some unwanted effects. Although not all of these side effects appear very often, when they do occur they may require medical attention. Stop taking this medicine and check with your doctor immediately if any of the following side effects occur:

More common

Clumsiness or unsteadiness	Unusual tiredness or weakness
Dark urine	Vomiting
Loss of appetite	Yellowing of eyes or skin
Nausea	
Numbness, tingling, burning, or pain in hands and feet	

Rare
Blurred vision or any loss of vision, with or without eye pain

Other side effects may occur which usually do not require medical attention. These side effects may go away during treatment as your body adjusts to the medicine. However, check with your doctor if any of the following side effects continue or are bothersome:

More common
Dizziness
Stomach upset

Less common
Enlargement of the breasts (males)

For injection form
Irritation at the place of injection

Other side effects not listed above may also occur in some patients. If you notice any other effects, check with your doctor.

ISOPROTERENOL (Systemic)
Some commonly used brand names are:

Aerolone	Norisodrine
Iprenol	Aerotrol
Isuprel	Proternol
Medihaler-Iso	Vapo-Iso

Isoproterenol (eye-soe-proe-TER-e-nole) is given by injection or taken by mouth or oral inhalation to treat bronchial asthma, chronic bronchitis, emphysema, and other lung diseases. It relieves wheezing, shortness of breath, and troubled breathing. Also, some forms of isoproterenol are used in the treatment of certain heart disorders. This medicine is available only with your doctor's prescription.

Before Using This Medicine

In order to decide on the best treatment for your medical problem, your doctor should be told:

—if you have ever had any unusual reaction to medicines like isoproterenol such as amphetamines, ephedrine, epinephrine, metaproterenol, norepinephrine (levarterenol), phenylephrine, phenylpropanolamine, pseudoephedrine, or terbutaline.

—if you are pregnant, if you intend to become pregnant, or if you are breast-feeding an infant. Although isoproterenol has not been shown to cause problems, the chance always exists.

—if you have any of the following medical problems:

Diabetes	High blood pressure
Heart or blood vessel disease	Overactive thyroid

—if you are now taking any of the following medicines or types of medicine:

Amphetamines	Propranolol
Other medicine for asthma or breathing problems	

Proper Use of This Medicine

Use this medicine only as directed. Do not use more of it and do not use it more often than your doctor ordered. To do so may increase the chance of side effects.

If you are using the inhalation form of this medicine:

• Do not use if the solution turns pinkish to brownish in color or becomes cloudy.

• Some of these preparations may come with patient directions. Read them carefully before using this medicine.

• If you are using this medicine in a nebulizer, make sure you understand exactly how to use it. Using the dropper provided, place in the nebulizer only that amount of solution needed for 1 day's treatment. If you have any questions about this, check with your doctor.

• If you are using the aerosol form of this medicine:

—Keep spray away from the eyes.

—*Do not take more than 2 inhalations of this medicine at any one time,* unless otherwise directed by your doctor. Allow 1 to 5 minutes after the first inhalation to make certain that a second inhalation is necessary.

—Save your applicator. Refill units of this medicine may be available.

—Store away from heat and direct sunlight. Do not puncture, break, or burn the container.

If you are taking the tablet form of this medicine:

• If you are taking the sublingual tablet form of this medicine (isoproterenol hydrochloride tablets), do not chew or swallow the tablet. This medicine is meant to be absorbed through the lining of the mouth. Place the tablet under your tongue (sublingual) and let it slowly dissolve there. Do not swallow until the tablet has dissolved completely.

• If you are taking isoproterenol hydrochloride extended-release tablets, swallow the tablets whole. Do not chew, break, or crush the tablets.

Precautions While Using This Medicine

If after using this medicine for asthma or other breathing problems you still have trouble breathing, or if your condition gets worse, *check with your doctor at once.*

If you are using the inhalation form of this medicine:

• Dryness of the mouth and throat may occur after using this medicine. Rinsing the mouth with water after each dose may help prevent the dryness.

Side Effects of This Medicine

Along with its needed effects, a medicine may cause some unwanted effects. Although not all of these side effects appear very often, when they do occur they may require medical attention. Check with your doctor if either of the following side effects occurs:

>Chest pain
>Irregular heartbeat

Other side effects may occur which usually do not require medical attention. These side effects may go away during treatment as your body adjusts to the medicine. However, check with your doctor if any of the following side effects continue or are bothersome:

More common

Dryness of mouth and throat (for inhalation dosage forms only)	Nervousness Restlessness Trouble in sleeping

Less common

Dizziness or lightheadedness	Trembling Unusual increase in
Flushing or redness of face or skin	sweating Unusually fast or
Headache	pounding heart-
Nausea or vomiting	beat Weakness

Isoproterenol may cause the saliva to turn pinkish to red. This is to be expected while you are using the inhalation or sublingual (under-the-tongue) forms of this medicine.

Other side effects not listed above may also occur in some patients. If you notice any other effects, check with your doctor.

ISOPROTERENOL AND PHENYLEPHRINE
(Systemic)
A commonly used brand name is Duo-Medihaler.

Isoproterenol and phenylephrine (eye-soe-proe-TER-e-nole and fen-ill-EF-rin) is a combination medicine taken by oral inhalation to treat bronchial asthma, bronchitis, emphysema, and other lung diseases. It relieves wheezing, shortness of breath, and troubled breathing. This medicine is available only with your doctor's prescription.

Before Using This Medicine

In order to decide on the best treatment for your medical problem, your doctor should be told:

—if you have ever had any unusual reaction to medicines like isoproterenol and phenylephrine such as amphetamines, ephedrine, epinephrine, metaproterenol, norepinephrine (levarterenol), phenylpropanolamine, pseudoephedrine, or terbutaline.

—if you are pregnant, if you intend to become pregnant, or if you are breast-feeding an infant. Although isoproterenol and phenylephrine have not been shown to cause problems, the chance always exists.

—if you have any of the following medical problems:

Diabetes	High blood pressure
Heart or blood vessel disease	Overactive thyroid

—if you are now taking any of the following medicines or types of medicine:

Amphetamines	Propranolol
Guanethidine	Tricyclic an-
Other medicine for asthma or breathing prob- lems	tidepressants (medicine for depression)

—if you are now taking or have taken within the past 2 weeks monoamine oxidase (MAO) inhibitors such as:

Isocarboxazid	Phenelzine
Pargyline	Tranylcypromine

Proper Use of This Medicine

Use this medicine only as directed. Do not use more of it and do not use it more often than your doctor ordered. To do so may increase the chance of side effects.

This medicine usually comes with patient directions. Read them carefully before using this medicine.

Keep spray away from the eyes.

Do not take more than 2 inhalations of this medicine at any one time, unless otherwise directed by your doctor. Allow 2 to 5 minutes after the first inhalation to make certain that a second inhalation is necessary.

Save your applicator. Refill units of this medicine may be available.

Store away from heat and direct sunlight. Do not puncture, break, or burn container.

Precautions While Using This Medicine

If you still have trouble breathing after using this medicine, or if your condition gets worse, *check with your doctor at once.*

Side Effects of This Medicine

Along with its needed effects, a medicine may cause some unwanted effects. Although not all of these side effects appear very often, when they do occur they may require medical attention. Check with your doctor if either of the following side effects occurs:

>Chest pain
>Irregular heartbeat

Other side effects may occur which usually do not require medical attention. These side effects may go away during treatment as your body adjusts to the medicine. However, check with your doctor if any of the following side effects continue or are bothersome:

More common

Nervousness	Trouble in sleeping
Restlessness	

Less common

Dizziness or	Trembling
lightheadedness	Unusual increase in
Flushing or redness	sweating
of face or skin	Unusually fast or
Headache	pounding heart-
Nausea or	beat
vomiting	Weakness

This medicine may cause the saliva to turn pinkish to red in color. This is to be expected while you are using this medicine.

Other side effects not listed above may also occur in some patients. If you notice any other effects, check with your doctor.

ISOXSUPRINE (Systemic)
Some commonly used brand names are Vasodilan and Vasoprine.

Isoxsuprine (eye-SOX-syoo-preen) belongs to the group of medicines called vasodilators. Vasodilators increase the size of blood vessels. Isoxsuprine is used to treat problems resulting from poor blood circulation. It may also be used for other conditions as determined by your doctor. Isoxsuprine is available only with your doctor's prescription.

Before Using This Medicine

In order to decide on the best treatment for your medical problem, your doctor should be told:

—if you have ever had any unusual reaction to isoxsuprine in the past. This medicine should not be taken if you are allergic to it.

—if you are pregnant, if you intend to become pregnant, or if you are breast-feeding an infant. Although isoxsuprine has not been shown to cause problems, the chance always exists.

—if you have any of the following medical problems:

Angina (chest pain)	Glaucoma
Bleeding problems	Hardening of the
	arteries

—if you have recently had a heart attack or stroke.

—if you are to receive this medicine by injection and you have low blood pressure or an unusually rapid heart rate.

—if you smoke.

Proper Use of This Medicine

If this medicine upsets your stomach, it may be taken with meals, milk, or antacids.

If you miss a dose of this medicine, take it as soon as you remember. If it is almost time for your next dose, do not take the missed dose at all and do not double the next one. Instead, go back to your regular dosing schedule. If you have any questions about this, check with your doctor.

Precautions While Using This Medicine

It may take some time for this medicine to work. If you feel that the medicine is not working, do not stop taking it on your own. Instead, check with your doctor.

The helpful effects of this medicine may be decreased if you smoke. If you have any questions about this, check with your doctor.

Dizziness may occur, especially when you get up from a lying or sitting position or climb stairs. Getting up slowly may help. If this problem continues or gets worse, check with your doctor.

Side Effects of This Medicine

Along with its needed effects, a medicine may cause some unwanted effects. Although not all of these side effects appear very often, when they do occur they may require medical attention. Check with your doctor if the following side effects occur:

Rare

Dizziness or faint-	Skin rash
ness	
Rapid or irregular	
heartbeat	

Other side effects not listed above may also occur in some patients. If you notice any other effects, check with your doctor.

KANAMYCIN (Oral)
A commonly used brand name is Kantrex.

Oral kanamycin (kan-a-MYE-sin) belongs to the general family of medicines called antibiotics. Oral kanamycin is given by mouth to help lessen the symptoms of hepatic coma, a complication of liver disease. It may also be used before any surgery affecting the bowels to help prevent infection during surgery. In addition, oral kanamycin may be given for other problems as determined by your doctor. Kanamycin is available only with your doctor's prescription.

Before Using This Medicine
In order to decide on the best treatment for your medical problem, your doctor should be told:

—if you have had allergic reactions to any related antibiotics such as amikacin, gentamicin, kanamycin (by injection), neomycin, streptomycin, or tobramycin.

—if you are pregnant, if you intend to become pregnant, or if you are breast-feeding an infant, although oral kanamycin has not been shown to cause problems.

—if you have any of the following medical problems:

Blockage of the bowel	Kidney disease
Eighth-cranial-nerve disease (loss of hearing and/or balance)	Ulcers of the bowel

Proper Use of This Medicine
This medicine may be taken without regard to meals.

Keep taking this medicine for the full time of treatment; do not miss any doses.

If you are taking this medicine for hepatic coma and you miss a dose, take it as soon as possible. However, if it is almost time for your next dose, do not take the missed dose or double your next dose. Instead, go back to your regular dosing schedule.

If you are taking this medicine before any surgery affecting the bowels and you miss a dose, take it as soon as possible. However, if it is almost time for your next dose and your dosing schedule is:

• 1 dose every hour (for 4 hours)—Space the missed dose and the next dose 1/2 hour apart.

• 3 or more doses a day—Space the missed dose and the next dose 2 to 4 hours apart or double your next dose.

Then go back to your regular dosing schedule.

Precautions While Using This Medicine
If this medicine causes any loss of hearing, a ringing or buzzing sound or a feeling of fullness in the ears, clumsiness, unsteadiness, dizziness, excessive thirst, or greatly decreased frequency of urination or amount of urine, stop taking it and check with your doctor as soon as possible.

Side Effects of This Medicine
Along with its needed effects, a medicine may cause some unwanted effects. Although not all of these side effects appear very often, when they do occur they may require medical attention. Stop taking this medicine and check with your doctor as soon as possible if any of the following side effects occur:

Rare

Any loss of hearing	Ringing or buzzing sound or a feeling of fullness in the ears
Clumsiness	
Dizziness	
Excessive thirst	
Greatly decreased frequency of urination or amount of urine	Unsteadiness

Other side effects may occur which usually do not require medical attention. These side effects may go away during treatment as your body adjusts to the medicine. However, check with your doctor if any of the following side effects continue or are bothersome:

More common

Irritation or soreness of the mouth or rectal area	Nausea Vomiting

Rare

Diarrhea	Light-colored, frothy, fatty-appearing stools
Excessive gas	Rash

Other side effects not listed above may also occur in some patients. If you notice any other effects, check with your doctor.

KAOLIN AND PECTIN (Oral)
Some commonly used brand names are Kaomead, Kaopectate, and Pargel.

Kaolin (KAY-oh-lin) and pectin (PEK-tin) is a combination medicine used to treat diarrhea. This medicine is available without a prescription; however, the product's directions and warnings should be carefully followed. In addition, your doctor may have special instructions on the proper dose or use of kaolin and pectin for your medical condition.

Before Using This Medicine

Whether you are taking this medicine on your own or on your doctor's orders, your doctor should be told:

—if you are pregnant, if you intend to become pregnant, or if you are breast-feeding an infant. Although this medicine is not absorbed into the body and is not likely to cause problems, the chance always exists.

—if you have a chronic medical problem such as asthma, heart disease, stomach ulcer, or other problem.

—if you are taking any other medicine, especially digoxin or lincomycin, since this medicine may interfere with its effects.

Proper Use of This Medicine

Do not give this medicine to children less than 3 years of age without first checking with your doctor. Patients over 60 years of age should also check with their doctor before taking this medicine.

Take this medicine after each loose bowel movement until the diarrhea is controlled, unless otherwise directed by your doctor.

Precautions While Using This Medicine

Check with your doctor if your diarrhea does not stop after 1 or 2 days or if you develop a fever.

Side Effects of This Medicine

Along with its needed effects, a medicine may cause some unwanted effects. No serious side effects have been reported for this medicine. However, constipation may occur in some patients, especially if they take a lot of it. Check with your doctor if constipation continues or is bothersome.

Other side effects not listed above may also occur in some patients. If you notice any other effects, check with your doctor.

KAOLIN, PECTIN, BELLADONNA ALKALOIDS, AND OPIUM (Systemic)
A commonly used brand name is Donnagel-PG.

Kaolin (KAY-oh-lin), pectin (PEK-tin), belladonna alkaloids (bell-a-DON-a AL-ka-loyds), and opium (OH-pee-um) is a combination medicine used to treat diarrhea. In some states, this medicine is available without a prescription; however, the product's directions and warnings should be carefully followed. In addition, your doctor may have special instructions on the proper dose or use of this medicine for your medical condition.

Before Using This Medicine

Whether you are taking this medicine on your own or on your doctor's orders, your doctor should be told:

—if you have ever had an unusual reaction to atropine, belladonna, or medicines like morphine, codeine, or papaverine. This medicine should not be taken if you are allergic to it.

—if you are pregnant, if you intend to become pregnant, or if you are breast-feeding an infant. Although this medicine has not been shown to cause problems, the chance always exists.

—if you have any of the following medical problems:

Alcoholism	
Brain damage	Heart disease
(children)	Hiatal hernia
Colitis or other	Irregular heartbeat
intestinal disease	Kidney disease
Difficult urination	Liver disease
Emphysema,	Spastic paralysis
asthma, bron-	(children)
chitis, or	Underactive adrenal
other chronic	gland (Addison's
lung disease	disease)
Enlarged prostate	Underactive thyroid
Gallbladder disease	
or gallstones	
Glaucoma	

—if you are now taking any of the following medicines or types of medicine:

Amantadine	Medicine for
Digoxin	intestinal or
Lincomycin	stomach cramping
	Ulcer medicine
	Any other medicine

—if you are now taking other central nervous system (CNS) depressants such as:

Antihistamines or medicine for hay fever, other allergies, or colds	Sedatives, tranquilizers, or sleeping medicine
Barbiturates	Seizure medicine
Other narcotics	Tricyclic antidepressants (medicine for depression)
Prescription pain medicine	

—if you are now taking or have taken within the past 2 weeks monoamine oxidase (MAO) inhibitors such as:

Isocarboxazid	Phenelzine
Pargyline	Tranylcypromine

Proper Use of This Medicine

Do not give this medicine to children less than 3 years of age without first checking with your doctor. Patients over 60 years of age should also check with their doctor before taking this medicine.

Take this medicine only as directed on the label. Do not take more of it, do not take it more often, and do not take it for a long period of time. If too much is taken, it may become habit-forming.

Keep this medicine out of the reach of children since overdose is especially dangerous in children.

If this medicine upsets your stomach, you may take it with food.

Precautions While Using This Medicine

Check with your doctor if your diarrhea does not stop after 1 or 2 days or if you develop a fever.

This medicine will add to the effects of alcohol and other medicines (CNS depressants) that slow down the nervous system. Some examples of CNS depressants are antihistamines or medicine for hay fever, other allergies, or colds; sedatives, tranquilizers, or sleeping medicine; prescription pain medicine or narcotics; barbiturates; medicine for seizures; tricyclic antidepressants (medicine for depression); or anesthetics, including some dental anesthetics. *Check with your doctor before taking any of the above while you are taking this medicine.*

This medicine may cause some people to become dizzy, drowsy, or less alert than they are normally. Even if taken at bedtime, it may cause some people to feel drowsy or less alert on arising. *Make sure you know how you react to this medicine before you drive, use machines, or do other jobs that require you to be alert.*

This medicine may cause your eyes to become more sensitive to light than they are normally. Wearing sunglasses may help lessen the discomfort from bright light.

This medicine may make you sweat less, causing your body temperature to increase. *Use extra care not to become overheated during exercise or hot weather while you are taking this medicine,* as overheating could possibly result in heat stroke.

Your mouth, nose, and throat may feel very dry while you are taking this medicine. To help relieve mouth dryness, chew sugarless gum or dissolve bits of ice in your mouth.

Side Effects of This Medicine

Along with its needed effects, a medicine may cause some unwanted effects. Although not all of these side effects appear very often, when they do occur they may require medical attention. Check with your doctor *immediately* if any of the following side effects are severe and occur suddenly since they may indicate a more severe and dangerous problem with your bowels:

Rare

Bloating	Nausea and vomiting
	Stomach pain

Check with your doctor also if the following effects occur:

Rare

Eye pain	Shortness of breath
Hallucinations (seeing, hearing, or feeling things that are not there)	Skin rash or itching
	Troubled breathing
	Unusually slow heartbeat

Other side effects may occur which usually do not require medical attention. These side effects may go away during treatment as your body adjusts to the medicine. However, check with your doctor if any of the following side effects continue or are bothersome:

More common with large doses

Constipation
Difficult urination
  or frequent urge
  to urinate
Dizziness
Drowsiness
Dryness of mouth,
  nose, throat,
  and skin
Faintness
Headache

Lightheadedness
Mental confusion
Rapid heartbeat
Redness or flushing
  of face
Reduced sweating
Unusual increase in
  sweating
Unusual tiredness or
  weakness

Less common

Blurred vision
Decreased sexual
  ability

Increased sensitivity
  of eyes to
  sunlight
Nervousness
Reduced sense of
  taste

Other side effects not listed above may also occur in some patients. If you notice any other effects, check with your doctor.

KAOLIN, PECTIN, AND PAREGORIC
(Systemic)
A commonly used brand name is Parepectolin.

Kaolin (KAY-oh-lin), pectin (PEK-tin), and paregoric (par-e-GOR-ik) is a combination medicine used to treat diarrhea. In some states, this medicine is available without a prescription; however, the product's directions and warnings should be carefully followed. In addition, your doctor may have special instructions on the proper dose or use of this medicine for your medical condition.

Before Using This Medicine

Whether you are taking this medicine on your own or on your doctor's orders, your doctor should be told:

—if you have ever used a medicine like morphine, codeine, or papaverine and had an unusual reaction to it. This medicine should not be taken if you are allergic to it.

—if you are pregnant, if you intend to become pregnant, or if you are breast-feeding an infant. Although this medicine has not been shown to cause problems, the chance always exists.

—if you have any of the following medical problems:

Alcoholism
Colitis
Difficult urination
Emphysema,
  asthma, bron-
  chitis, or other
  chronic lung
  disease
Enlarged prostate
Gallbladder disease
  or gallstones

Heart disease
Hiatal hernia
Kidney disease
Liver disease
Underactive adrenal
  gland (Addison's
  disease)
Underactive thyroid

—if you are now taking any of the following medicines or types of medicine:

Digoxin
Lincomycin

Ulcer medicine
Any other medicine

—if you are now taking other central nervous system (CNS) depressants such as:

Antihistamines or
  medicine for
  hay fever,
  other allergies, or
  colds
Barbiturates
Other narcotics
Prescription pain
  medicine

Sedatives, tran-
  quilizers,
  or sleeping
  medicine
Seizure medicine
Tricyclic an-
  tidepressants
  (medicine for
  depression)

—if you are now taking or have taken within the past 2 weeks monoamine oxidase (MAO) inhibitors such as:

Isocarboxazid
Pargyline

Phenelzine
Tranylcypromine

Proper Use of This Medicine

Do not give this medicine to children less than 3 years of age without first checking with your doctor. Patients over 60 years of age should also check with their doctor before taking this medicine.

Take this medicine only as directed on the label or by your doctor. Do not take more of it, do not take it more often, and do not take it for a long period of time. If too much is taken, it may become habit-forming.

Keep this medicine out of the reach of children since overdose is especially dangerous in children.

Keep the container for this medicine tightly closed to prevent the alcohol from evaporating and the medicine from becoming stronger. Do not store this medicine in the refrigerator. If it does get cold and you notice any solid particles in it, throw it away.

If this medicine upsets your stomach, you may take it with food.

Precautions While Using This Medicine

Check with your doctor if your diarrhea does not stop after 1 or 2 days or if you develop a fever.

This medicine will add to the effects of alcohol and other medicines (CNS depressants) that slow down the nervous system. Some examples of CNS depressants are antihistamines or medicine for hay fever, other allergies, or colds; sedatives, tranquilizers, or sleeping medicine; prescription pain medicine or narcotics; barbiturates; medicine for seizures; tricyclic antidepressants (medicine for depression); or anesthetics, including some dental anesthetics. *Check with your doctor before taking any of the above while you are taking this medicine.*

This medicine may cause some people to become dizzy, drowsy, or less alert than they are normally. Even if taken at bedtime, it may cause some people to feel drowsy or less alert on arising. *Make sure you know how you react to this medicine before you drive, use machines, or do other jobs that require you to be alert.*

Side Effects of This Medicine

Along with its needed effects, a medicine may cause some unwanted effects. Although not all of these side effects appear very often, when they do occur they may require medical attention. Check with your doctor *immediately* if any of the following side effects are severe and occur suddenly since they may indicate a more severe and dangerous problem with your bowels:

Rare

Bloating	Severe stomach pain with nausea and vomiting

Check with your doctor also if the following effects occur:

Rare

Shortness of breath	Troubled breathing
Skin rash or itching	Unusually slow heartbeat

Other side effects may occur which usually do not require medical attention. These side effects may go away during treatment as your body adjusts to the medicine. However, check with your doctor if any of the following side effects continue or are bothersome:

More common with large doses

Constipation	Lightheadedness
Difficult urination or frequent urge to urinate	Redness or flushing of face
Dizziness	Unusual increase in sweating
Drowsiness	Unusual tiredness or weakness
Faintness	

Other side effects not listed above may also occur in some patients. If you notice any other effects, check with your doctor.

LAXATIVES, BULK-FORMING (Oral)

This information applies to the following medicines:

Malt Soup Extract
Methylcellulose (meth-ill-SELL-yoo-lose)
Polycarbophil (pol-i-KAR-boe-fil)
Psyllium (SILL-i-yum)

Some commonly used brand names are:	Generic names:
Maltsupex	Malt Soup Extract
Cellothyl Cologel Hydrolose	Methylcellulose
	Polycarbophil
Mitrolan	Polycarbophil Calcium
Effersyllium Konsyl L.A. Formula Metamucil Modane Bulk Mucilose Plova Serutan Siblin	Psyllium Mucilloid Psyllium Seed Psyllium

Note: Many laxative formulas include two or more laxative substances. Only those formulas containing one primary laxative are listed above.

Bulk-forming laxatives are medicines taken by mouth to encourage bowel movements to relieve constipation and to prevent straining. This type of laxative is not digested but absorbs liquid in the intestines and swells to form a soft, bulky stool. The bowel is then stimulated normally by the presence of the bulky mass. To allow bulk-forming laxatives to work properly and to prevent intestinal blockage, it is necessary to drink plenty of fluids during their use. Most bulk-forming laxatives are available without a prescription; however, your doctor may have special instructions for the proper use and dose for your medical condition.

When indicated, bulk-forming laxatives may provide relief in a number of situations such as:

—during pregnancy.

—for a few days after giving birth.

—constipation caused by other medicines.

—to aid in developing normal bowel function following a period of poor eating habits or a lack of physical exercise.

—following surgery when straining should be avoided.

—with some medical conditions that may be made worse by straining, for example:

Heart disease	High blood pressure
Hemorrhoids	History of stroke
Hernia (rupture)	

Before Using This Medicine

Importance of diet, fluids, and exercise—Laxatives are to be used to provide short-term relief only, unless otherwise directed by a doctor. A proper diet containing roughage (whole grain breads and cereals, bran, fruit, and green, leafy vegetables), with 6 to 8 full glasses (8 ounces each) of liquids each day, and daily exercise are most important in maintaining a healthy bowel function.

In order to decide on the best treatment for your medical problem, the following should be kept in mind and/or your doctor should be told:

—if you have ever had any unusual reaction to laxatives in the past. This medicine should not be taken if you are allergic to it.

—if you are pregnant. Some bulk-forming laxatives contain a large amount of sodium or sugars which may have possible unwanted effects such as increasing blood pressure or causing water to be held in the tissues.

—if you have any of the following medical problems:

Appendicitis (or signs of)	Intestinal blockage
	Kidney disease
Colostomy	Laxative habit
Diabetes	Rectal bleeding of
Heart disease	unknown cause
High blood pressure	Swallowing difficulty
Ileostomy	

—if you are now taking any of the following medicines or types of medicine:

Antibiotics	Digitalis preparations (heart medicine)
Anticoagulants (blood thinners)	
Aspirin	Laxatives (other)
Contraceptives, oral (birth control pills)	Sodium salicylate

Proper Use of This Medicine

Each dose should be taken in or with a full glass (8 ounces) or more of cold water or fruit juice. This will provide enough liquid for the laxative to work properly. A second glass of water or juice by itself is often recommended with each dose for best effect.

Results often may be obtained in 12 to 24 hours but may not occur for some individuals until after 2 or 3 days.

For safe and effective use of bulk-forming laxatives:

• Follow your doctor's orders if this laxative was prescribed.

• Follow the manufacturer's package directions if you are treating yourself.

• Drink at least 6 to 8 full glasses (8 ounces each) of liquid each day.

• Do not try to swallow in the dry form. Take with liquid.

Precautions While Using This Medicine

Do not take any type of laxative:

—*if you have signs of appendicitis or inflamed bowel* (such as stomach or lower abdominal pain, cramping, bloating, soreness, nausea, or vomiting).

—*for more than 1 week* unless your doctor has prescribed or ordered a special schedule for you. This is true even when you have had no results from the laxative.

—*within 2 hours of taking other medicine* because the desired effect of the other medicine may be reduced.

—*if you do not need it,* as for the common cold, "to clean out your system," or as a "tonic to make you feel better."

—*if you miss a bowel movement for a day or two.*

—*if you develop a skin rash* while taking a laxative or if you had a rash the last time you took it.

If you notice a sudden change in bowel habits or function that lasts longer than 2 weeks, or that keeps returning off and on, check with your doctor before using a laxative. This will allow the cause of your problem to be determined before it becomes more serious.

The "laxative habit"—Laxative products are overused by many people. Such a practice often leads to dependence on the laxative action to produce a bowel movement. In severe cases, overuse of some laxatives has caused damage to the nerves, muscles, and tissues of the intestines and bowel. If you have any questions about the use of laxatives, check with your doctor, nurse, or pharmacist.

Caution: Bulk-forming laxatives often contain large amounts of sugars, carbohydrates, and sodium. If you are on a low-sugar, low-caloric, or low-salt diet, check with your doctor, nurse, or pharmacist before using this type of laxative.

Side Effects of This Medicine

Along with its needed effects, a medicine may cause some unwanted effects. Although not all of these side effects appear very often, when they do occur they may require medical attention. Check with your doctor if any of the following side effects occur:

Rare

Asthma	Swallowing difficul-
Itching	ty (feeling of
Intestinal blockage	lump in throat)
Skin rash	

Other side effects not listed above may also occur in some patients. If you notice any other effects, check with your doctor.

LAXATIVES, EMOLLIENT (Oral)

This information applies to the following medicines:

Docusate (DOK-yoo-sate)
Poloxamer 188 (pol-OX-a-mer)

Some commonly used brand names and other names are:	Generic names:
Surfak	Docusate Calcium
Kasof	Docusate Potassium

Afko-Lube	
Colace	
Colax	Docusate Sodium
Comfolax	
Dioctyl Sodium Sulfosuccinate	

Alaxin	Poloxamer 188
Magcyl	

Note: Many laxative formulas include two or more laxative substances. Only those formulas containing one primary laxative are listed above.

Emollient laxatives (stool softeners) are medicines taken by mouth to encourage bowel movements by helping liquids mix into the stool and prevent dry, hard stool masses. This type of laxative has been said not to *cause* a bowel movement but instead *allows* the patient to have a bowel movement without straining. Emollient laxatives are available without a prescription; however, your doctor may have special instructions for the proper use and dose for your medical condition.

When indicated, emollient laxatives may provide relief when constipation is associated with hard, dry stools such as:

—during pregnancy.

—a few days after giving birth.

—constipation caused by other medicines.

—following surgery when straining should be avoided.

—with some medical conditions that may be made worse by straining, for example:

Heart disease	High blood pressure
Hemorrhoids	History of stroke
Hernia (rupture)	

Before Using This Medicine

Importance of diet, fluids, and exercise—Laxatives are to be used to provide short-term relief only, unless otherwise directed by a doctor. A proper diet containing roughage (whole grain breads and cereals, bran, fruit, and green, leafy vegetables), with 6 to 8 full glasses (8 ounces each) of liquids each day, and daily exercise are most important in maintaining a healthy bowel function.

In order to decide on the best treatment for your medical problem, the following should be kept in mind and/or your doctor should be told:

—if you have ever had any unusual reaction to laxatives in the past. This medicine should not be taken if you are allergic to it.

—if you have any of the following medical problems:

Appendicitis (or signs of)	Intestinal blockage
	Laxative habit
Congestive heart failure	Rectal bleeding of unknown cause
Diabetes	
High blood pressure	

—if you are now taking any medicines, especially other laxatives, or mineral oil.

Proper Use of This Medicine

For safe and effective use of your laxative carefully follow,

—your doctor's instructions if this laxative was prescribed.

—the manufacturer's package directions if you are treating yourself.

Results may not occur until 1 to 3 days after the first dose.

Liquid forms may be taken in milk or fruit juice to improve flavor.

Moisture is necessary to produce a soft bowel movement. A person using any type of laxative should drink at least 6 to 8 full glasses (8 ounces each) of liquid each day.

Precautions While Using This Medicine

Do not take any type of laxative:
—*if you have signs of appendicitis or inflamed bowel* (such as stomach or lower abdominal pain, cramping, bloating, soreness, nausea, or vomiting).

—*for more than 1 week* unless your doctor has prescribed or ordered a special schedule for you. This is true even when you have had no results from the laxative.

—*within 2 hours of taking other medicine* because the desired effect of the other medicine may be reduced.

—*if you do not need it*, as for the common cold, "to clean out your system," or as a "tonic to make you feel better."

—*if you miss a bowel movement for a day or two.*

—*if you develop a skin rash* while taking a laxative or if you had a rash the last time you took it.

If you notice a sudden change in bowel habits or function that lasts longer than 2 weeks, or that keeps returning off and on, check with your doctor before using a laxative. This will allow the cause of your problem to be determined before it may become more serious.

The "laxative habit"—Laxative products are overused by many people. Such a practice often leads to dependence on the laxative action to produce a bowel movement. In severe cases, overuse of some laxatives has caused damage to the nerves, muscles, and tissues of the intestines and bowel. If you have any questions about the use of laxatives, check with your doctor, nurse, or pharmacist.

You should check with your doctor before using stool softeners:

—when taking mineral oil in the same period of time. An increased amount of mineral oil may be absorbed into the body tissues where it can cause problems.

—when taking other laxative products because their absorption may be increased.

Side Effects of This Medicine

Along with its needed effects, a medicine may cause some unwanted effects. Although not all of these side effects appear very often, when they do occur they may require medical attention. Check with your doctor if any of the following side effects occur:

Rare
 Skin rash

Other side effects may occur which usually do not require medical attention. These side effects may go away during treatment as your body adjusts to the medicine. However, check with your doctor if any of the following side effects continue or are bothersome:

Less common

Stomach and/or intestinal cramping	Throat irritation (liquid forms only)

Other side effects not listed above may also occur in some patients. If you notice any other effects, check with your doctor.

LAXATIVES, HYPEROSMOTIC— LACTULOSE AND SALINE (Oral)

This information applies to the following medicines:

Lactulose
Saline
    Magnesium Citrate (mag-NEE-zhum SI-trate)
    Magnesium Sulfate (mag-NEE-zhum SUL-fate)
    Sodium Phosphate (SOE-dee-um FOS-fate)

Some commonly used brand names and other names are:	Generic names:
Chronulac	Lactulose
Citrate of Magnesia	Magnesium Citrate
Adlerika Epsom Salts	Magnesium Sulfate
Phospho-Soda Sal Hepatica	Sodium Phosphate (or phosphates) Effervescent Sodium Phosphate

Note: Many laxative formulas include two or more laxative substances. Only those formulas containing one primary laxative are listed above.

This information does not apply to milk of magnesia or sodium phosphate, when used for purposes other than laxative.

Hyperosmotic laxatives are medicines taken by mouth to encourage bowel movements by drawing water into the bowel from surrounding body tissues. This provides a soft stool mass and increased bowel action.

There are two types of hyperosmotic laxatives taken by mouth—the saline and the lactulose types. The saline type is often called "salts." They are used for rapid emptying of the lower intestine and bowel. They are not used for long-term or repeated correction of constipation. This type of laxative is available without a prescription; however, your doctor may have special instructions for the proper use and dose for your medical condition.

The lactulose type is a special sugar-like laxative that works the same way as the saline type. However, it produces results much more slowly and is often used for long-term treatment of chronic constipation. This type of laxative may sometimes be used in the treatment of medical conditions other than constipation and is available only with your doctor's prescription.

When indicated, saline laxatives may provide rapid results in situations such as:

—preparation for examination or surgery.

—elimination of food or drugs from the body in cases of poisoning or overdose.

—simple constipation that happens on occasion (although another type of laxative may be preferred).

—to supply fresh stool sample for diagnosis.

Before Using This Medicine

Importance of diet, fluids, and exercise—Laxatives are to be used to provide short-term relief only, unless otherwise directed by a doctor. A proper diet containing roughage (whole grain breads and cereals, bran, fruit, and green, leafy vegetables), with 6 to 8 full glasses (8 ounces each) of liquids each day, and daily exercise are most important in maintaining a healthy bowel function.

In order to decide on the best treatment for your medical problem, the following should be kept in mind and/or your doctor should be told:

—if you have ever had any unusual reaction to laxatives in the past. This medicine should not be taken if you are allergic to it.

—if you are pregnant. Saline laxatives containing magnesium or potassium may have to be avoided if your kidney function is not normal. Saline laxatives containing sodium (salt) are usually avoided if you tend to retain (keep) body water.

—if you have any of the following medical problems:

Appendicitis (or signs of)	Ileostomy
Colostomy	Intestinal blockage
Congestive heart disease	Kidney disease
Diabetes	Laxative habit
Diverticulitis	Rectal bleeding of unknown cause
High blood pressure	Ulcerative colitis

—if you are now taking any of the following medicines or types of medicine:

Anticoagulants (blood thinners)	Isoniazid
Contraceptives, oral (birth control pills)	Laxatives (other)
	Medicine for nervousness or emotional condition
Digitalis preparations (heart medicine)	Tetracycline antibiotics
Insulin or other medicine for diabetes	

Proper Use of This Medicine

For safe and effective use of your laxative carefully follow,

—your doctor's instructions if this laxative was prescribed.

—the manufacturer's package directions if you are treating yourself.

The unpleasant taste produced by some hyperosmotic laxatives may be improved by following each dose with citrus fruit juice or citrus-flavored carbonated beverage.

Lactulose may not produce laxative results for 24 to 28 hours.

Saline laxatives usually produce results within 2 to 8 hours following a dose. When a larger dose is taken on an empty stomach, the results are quicker. When a smaller dose is taken with food, the results are delayed. Therefore, large doses of saline laxatives are usually not taken late in the day on an empty stomach.

Each dose should be taken in or with a full glass (8 ounces) or more of cold water or fruit juice. This will provide enough liquid for the laxative to work properly. A second glass of water or juice by itself is often recommended with each dose for best effect.

Moisture is necessary to produce a soft bowel movement. A person using any type of laxative should drink at least 6 to 8 full glasses (8 ounces each) of liquid each day.

You should not use saline laxatives until you have checked with your doctor if:

—you have kidney disease.

—you are on a low-salt (sodium restricted) diet, since many of these products contain large amounts of sodium.

—if you have diabetes. Some preparations contain sugar.

—you are taking any tetracycline antibiotics, since their effect may be reduced by the salts of the laxative.

Young children (up to 6 years of age) should not take saline laxatives unless prescribed by their doctor.

Precautions While Using This Medicine

Do not take any type of laxative:

—*if you have signs of appendicitis or inflamed bowel* (such as stomach or lower abdominal pain, cramping, bloating, soreness, nausea, or vomiting).

—*for more than 1 week* unless your doctor has prescribed or ordered a special schedule for you. This is true even when you have had no results from the laxative.

—*within 2 hours of taking other medicine* because the desired effect of the other medicine may be reduced.

—*if you do not need it,* as for the common cold, "to clean out your system," or as a "tonic to make you feel better."

—*if you miss a bowel movement for a day or two.*

—*if you develop a skin rash* while taking a laxative or if you had a rash the last time you took it.

If you notice a sudden change in bowel habits or function that lasts longer than 2 weeks, or that keeps returning off and on, check with your doctor before using a laxative. This will allow the cause of your problem to be determined before it may become more serious.

The "laxative habit"—Laxative products are overused by many people. Such a practice often leads to dependence on the laxative action to produce a bowel movement. In severe cases, overuse of some laxatives has caused damage to the nerves, muscles, and tissues of the intestines and bowel. If you have any questions about the use of laxatives, check with your doctor, nurse, or pharmacist.

Side Effects of This Medicine

Along with its needed effects, a medicine may cause some unwanted effects. Although not all of these side effects appear very often, when they do occur they may require medical attention. Check with your doctor if any of the following side effects occur:

Rare

Dizziness or lightheadedness	Muscle cramps
Irregular heartbeat	Unusual tiredness or weakness
Mental confusion	

Other side effects may occur which usually do not require medical attention. These side effects may go away during treatment as your body adjusts to the medicine. However, check with your doctor if any of the following side effects continue or are bothersome:

Less common

Cramping	Increased thirst
Diarrhea	Nausea
Gas	

Other side effects not listed above may also occur in some patients. If you notice any other effects, check with your doctor.

LAXATIVES, LUBRICANT (Oral)
This information applies to Mineral Oil.

Some commonly used brand names or other names are:	Generic names:
Liquid petrolatum Nujol	Mineral Oil
Neo-Cultol	Mineral Oil (Jellied)

Note: Many laxative formulas include two or more laxative substances. Only those formulas containing one primary laxative are listed above.

Lubricant laxatives are today mostly products containing mineral oil, although some vegetable oils have been used. Mineral oil taken by mouth encourages bowel movements by coating the bowel and the stool mass with a waterproof film. This keeps moisture in the stool. The stool remains soft and its passage is made easier. Mineral oil is available without a prescription; however, your doctor may have special instructions for the proper use and dose for your medical condition.

When indicated, lubricant laxatives may provide relief in situations such as:

—following surgery when straining should be avoided.

—with some medical conditions that may be made worse by straining, for example:

Heart disease	High blood pressure
Hemorrhoids	History of stroke
Hernia (rupture)	

Before Using This Medicine

Importance of diet, fluids, and exercise—Laxatives are to be used to provide short-term relief only, unless otherwise directed by a doctor. A proper diet containing roughage (whole grain breads and cereals, bran, fruit, and green, leafy vegetables), with 6 to 8 full glasses (8 ounces each) of liquids each day, and daily exercise are most important in maintaining a healthy bowel function.

In order to decide on the best treatment for your medical problem, the following should be kept in mind and/or your doctor should be told:

—if you have ever had any unusual reaction to laxatives in the past. This medicine should not be taken if you are allergic to it.

—if you are pregnant. Laxative preparations containing mineral oil, castor oil, or sodium are usually not used during pregnancy because of possible unwanted effects on the mother or baby.

—if you have any of the following medical problems:

Appendicitis (or signs of)	Ileostomy
	Intestinal blockage
Colostomy	Laxative habit
Congestive heart disease	Rectal bleeding of unknown cause
Diabetes	

—if you are now taking any of the following medicines or types of medicine:

Antibiotics	Digitalis preparations (heart medicine)
Anticoagulants (blood thinners)	
Contraceptives, oral (birth control pills)	Laxatives (other)
	Vitamins A, D, E, or K

Proper Use of This Medicine

Moisture is necessary to produce a soft bowel movement. A person using any type of laxative should drink at least 6 to 8 full glasses (8 ounces each) of liquid each day.

For safe and effective use of your laxative carefully follow,

—your doctor's instructions if this laxative was prescribed.

—the manufacturer's package directions if you are treating yourself.

Lubricant laxatives are usually taken at bedtime for convenience and because they require about 8 hours to produce results.

This type of laxative should not be taken within 2 hours of meals because of possible interference with food digestion and absorption of nutrients and vitamins.

Precautions While Using This Medicine

Do not take any type of laxative:

—*if you have signs of appendicitis or inflamed bowel* (such as stomach or lower abdominal pain, cramping, bloating, soreness, nausea, or vomiting).

—*for more than 1 week* unless your doctor has prescribed or ordered a special schedule for you. This is true even when you have had no results from the laxative.

—*within 2 hours of taking other medicine* because the desired effect of the other medicine may be reduced.

—*if you do not need it,* as for the common cold, "to clean out your system," or as a "tonic to make you feel better."

—*if you miss a bowel movement for a day or two.*

—*if you develop a skin rash* while taking a laxative or if you had a rash the last time you took it.

If you notice a sudden change in bowel habits or function that lasts longer than 2 weeks, or that keeps returning off and on, check with your doctor before using a laxative. This will allow the cause of your problem to be determined before it may become more serious.

The "laxative habit"—Laxative products are overused by many people. Such a practice often leads to dependence on the laxative action to produce a bowel movement. In severe cases, overuse of some laxatives has caused damage to the nerves, muscles, and tissues of the intestines and bowel. If you have any questions about the use of laxatives, check with your doctor, nurse, or pharmacist.

Lubricant laxatives should not be taken often or for long periods of time because:

—gradual build-up in body tissues may create additional problems.

—a form of pneumonia may be caused by the inhalation of oil droplets into the lungs. Young children (up to 6 years of age) and elderly patients seem more likely to suffer from this effect, and use by such patients is discouraged.

—the use of mineral oil may interfere with the body's ability to absorb certain food nutrients and vitamins A, D, E, and K.

Lubricant laxatives should not be taken within 1 or 2 hours of other medicines, especially oral anticoagulants (blood-thinners) or oral contraceptives (birth control pills). The effect of the other medicine may be reduced.

Large doses of lubricant laxatives may cause some leakage from the rectum. The use of absorbant pads or a decrease in dose may be necessary to prevent the soiling of clothing.

Side Effects of This Medicine

Side effects from mineral oil are actually the result of improper use and are referred to under *Precautions While Using This Medicine.*

Other side effects not listed above may also occur in some patients. If you notice any other effects, check with your doctor.

LAXATIVES, STIMULANT (Oral)

This information applies to the following medicines:

Bisacodyl (bis-a-KOE-dill)
Cascara (kas-KAR-a) Sagrada
Castor (KAS-tor) Oil
Danthron (DAN-thron)
Dehydrocholic (dee-hye-droe-KOE-lik) Acid
Phenolphthalein (fee-nole-THAY-leen)
Senna
Sennosides A and B (SEN-oh-sides)

Some commonly used brand names and other names are:	Generic names:
Cenalax Codylax Dulcolax Theralax	Bisacodyl
Cascara Sagrada Cas-Evac	Cascara
Alphamul Neoloid	Castor Oil
Dorbane Modane	Danthron
Cholan-DH Decholin Neocholan	Dehydrocholic Acid
Alophen Espotabs Evac-U-Gen Evac-U-Lax Ex-Lax Feen-A-Mint Phenolax Prulet	Phenolphthalein
Black Draught Casa Fru Dr. Caldwell's Senna Laxative Fletcher's Castoria Senokot Swiss Kriss X-Prep	Senna
Glysennid Senokot X-Prep	Sennosides A and B

Note: Many laxative formulas include two or more laxative substances. Only those formulas containing one primary laxative are listed above.

Stimulant laxatives, also known as contact laxatives, encourage bowel movements by acting on the intestinal wall. They increase the muscle contractions that move along the stool mass. Stimulant laxatives are available in many brand names, package designs, and dosage forms. They are a popular type of laxative for self-treatment. However, they also are more likely to cause side effects. Most stimulant laxatives are available without a prescription; however, your doctor may have special instructions for the proper use and dose for your medical condition.

When indicated, stimulant laxatives may provide relief in situations such as:

—constipation caused by other medicines.

—preparation for examination or surgery (castor oil and bisacodyl).

—constipation of bedfast patients.

Before Using This Medicine

Importance of diet, fluids, and exercise—Laxatives are to be used to provide short-term relief only, unless otherwise directed by a doctor. A proper diet containing roughage (whole grain breads and cereals, bran, fruit, and green, leafy vegetables), with 6 to 8 full glasses (8 ounces each) of liquids each day, and daily exercise are most important in maintaining a healthy bowel function.

In order to decide on the best treatment for your medical problem, the following should be kept in mind and/or your doctor should be told:

—if you have ever had any unusual reaction to laxatives in the past. This medicine should not be taken if you are allergic to it.

—if you are pregnant. Stimulant laxatives may cause unwanted effects in the expectant mother if improperly used. Castor oil in particular should not to be used as it may cause contractions of the womb.

—if you are breast-feeding an infant. Laxatives containing cascara, danthron, and phenolphthalein may be excreted in breast milk. Although the amount of laxative in the milk is generally thought to be too small to cause problems in the child, your doctor should be told that you plan to use such laxatives. Some reports claim that diarrhea has been caused in the infants.

—if you have any of the following medical problems:

Appendicitis (or signs of)
Colostomy
Congestive heart disease
Diabetes
Diverticulitis
High blood pressure
Ileostomy
Intestinal blockage
Kidney disease
Laxative habit
Rectal bleeding of unknown cause
Ulcerative colitis

—if you are now taking any of the following medicines or types of medicine:

Antacids
Antibiotics
Anticoagulants (blood thinners)
Contraceptives, oral (birth control pills)
Digitalis preparations
Laxatives (other)

Proper Use of This Medicine

For safe and effective use of your laxative carefully follow,

—your doctor's instructions if this laxative was prescribed.

—the manufacturer's package directions if you are treating yourself.

Stimulant laxatives are usually taken on an empty stomach for rapid effect. Results are slowed if taken with food.

Many stimulant laxatives (but not castor oil) are often taken at bedtime to produce results the next morning (although some may require up to 24 hours or more).

If you are taking castor oil:

• Castor oil is not usually taken late in the day because its results occur within 2 to 6 hours.

• The unpleasant taste may be improved by chilling in the refrigerator for at least an hour and then stirring the dose into a full glass of cold orange juice just before it is taken. Also, flavored preparations of castor oil are available.

If you are taking bisacodyl:

• Bisacodyl tablets are specially coated to allow them to work properly without causing irritation and/or nausea. To protect this coating, do not chew, crush, or take the tablets within an hour of milk or antacids.

Moisture is necessary to produce a soft bowel movement. A person using any type of laxative should drink at least 6 to 8 full glasses (8 ounces each) of liquid each day.

Precautions While Using This Medicine

Do not take any type of laxative:

—*if you have signs of appendicitis or inflamed bowel* (such as stomach or lower abdominal pain, cramping, bloating, soreness, nausea, or vomiting).

—*for more than 1 week* unless your doctor has prescribed or ordered a special schedule for you. This is true even when you have had no results from the laxative.

—*within 2 hours of taking other medicine* because the desired effect of the other medicine may be reduced.

—*if you do not need it,* as for the common cold, "to clean out your system," or as a "tonic to make you feel better."

—*if you miss a bowel movement for a day or two.*

—*if you develop a skin rash* while taking a laxative or if you had a rash the last time you took it.

If you notice a sudden change in bowel habits or function that lasts longer than 2 weeks, or that keeps returning off and on, check with your doctor before using a laxative. This will allow the cause of your problem to be determined before it may become more serious.

The "laxative habit"—Laxative products are overused by many people. Such a practice often leads to dependence on the laxative action to produce a bowel movement. In severe cases, overuse of some laxatives has caused damage to the nerves, muscles, and tissues of the intestines and bowel. If you have any questions about the use of laxatives, check with your doctor, nurse, or pharmacist.

Stimulant laxatives are most often associated with:

—occasional coloration of urine or stool (pink to red most common).

—overuse and the laxative habit.

—skin rashes.

—intestinal cramping after dosing.

—potassium loss.

If you are taking laxative products containing phenolphthalein:
• Because of the way this ingredient works in the body, a single dose may cause a laxative effect in some people for up to 3 days.

Side Effects of This Medicine

Along with its needed effects, a medicine may cause some unwanted effects. Although not all of these side effects appear very often, when they do occur they may require medical attention. Check with your doctor if any of the following side effects occur:

Rare

Breathing difficulty	Skin rash
Burning on urina-	Unusual tiredness or
tion	weakness
Irregular heartbeat	
Mental confusion	

Other side effects may occur which usually do not require medical attention. These side effects may go away during treatment as your body adjusts to the medicine. However, check with your doctor if any of the following side effects continue or are bothersome:

Less common

Belching	Irritation of tissues
Cramping	around the rectal
Diarrhea	area
	Nausea

Other side effects not listed above may also occur in some patients. If you notice any other effects, check with your doctor.

LEVODOPA (Systemic)

This information applies to the following medicines:

Carbidopa and Levodopa
Levodopa

Some commonly used brand names are:	Generic names:
Sinemet	Carbidopa and Levodopa
Bendopa Dopar Larodopa Levopa*	Levodopa

*Not available in the United States.

Levodopa (lee-voe-DOE-pa) is a medicine used alone or in combination with carbidopa (kar-bi-DOE-pa) to treat Parkinson's disease, also referred to as shaking palsy or paralysis agitans. Some patients require the combination of medicine while others benefit from levodopa alone. By improving muscle control, this medicine allows body movements to become more normal. Levodopa alone or in combination is available only with your doctor's prescription.

Before Using This Medicine

In order to decide on the best treatment for your medical problem, your doctor should be told:

—if you have ever had any unusual reaction to levodopa in the past. This medicine should not be taken if you are allergic to it.

—if you are pregnant, if you intend to become pregnant, or if you are breast-feeding an infant. Although this medicine has not been shown to cause problems in humans, animal studies have indicated possible unwanted effects on the baby's growth.

—if you have any of the following medical problems:

Convulsive disorders like epilepsy	Heart or blood vessel disease
Diabetes	Hormone problems
Emphysema, asthma, bronchitis, or other chronic lung disease	Kidney disease
	Liver disease
	Mental illness
	Skin cancer
Glaucoma	Stomach ulcer

—if you are now taking any of the following medicines or types of medicine:

Asthma or bronchitis medicine; for example, epinephrine, ephedrine, or isoproterenol	Medicine for high blood pressure
Haloperidol	Methyldopa
Medicine for appetite control (for example phenylpropanolamine)	Papaverine
	Phenytoin
	Pyridoxine (vitamin B6) (present in some foods and vitamin formulas)
	Reserpine

—if you are now taking phenothiazine medicines such as:

Chlorpromazine	Prochlorperazine
Fluphenazine	Trifluoperazine
Perphenazine	Triflupromazine

—if you are now taking or have taken within the past 2 weeks monoamine oxidase (MAO) inhibitors such as:

Isocarboxazid	Phenelzine
Pargyline	Tranylcypromine

Proper Use of This Medicine

Take this medicine only as directed. Do not take more or less of it, do not take it more often, and do not stop taking it unless ordered to by your doctor.

Pyridoxine (vitamin B6) has been found to reduce the effects of levodopa. Do not take vitamin products containing vitamin B6 unless prescribed by your doctor. High concentrations of pyridoxine are also contained in some common foods such as avocado, bacon, beans, beef liver, dry skim milk, oatmeal, peas, pork, sweet potato, tuna, and certain health foods. Check with your doctor about how much of these foods you may have in your diet while you are taking levodopa. Also, ask your doctor or pharmacist for help when selecting vitamin products.

Some people must take this medicine for several weeks before full benefit is received.

Take this medicine with solid food to lessen possible stomach upset. If upset continues, check with your doctor.

If you miss a dose of this medicine, take it as soon as possible. If your next scheduled dose is within 2 hours, do not take the missed dose at all and do not double the next one. Instead, go back to your regular dosing schedule. If you have any questions about this, check with your doctor.

Precautions While Using This Medicine

Before having any kind of surgery (including dental surgery) or emergency treatment, tell the doctor or dentist in charge that you are taking this medicine.

This medicine may cause some people to become drowsy or less alert than they are normally. *Make sure you know how you react to this medicine before you drive, use machines, or do other jobs that require you to be alert.*

Dizziness, lightheadedness, or fainting may occur especially when you get up from a lying or sitting position. Getting up slowly may help. If the problem continues or gets worse, check with your doctor.

Diabetics—This medicine may cause test results for urine sugar or ketones to be wrong. Check with your doctor before depending on home tests using the paper-strip or tablet method.

As your condition improves and your body movements become easier, *be careful not to overdo physical activities since injuries resulting from falls may occur.* Such activities must be gradually increased to allow your body to adjust to changing balance, circulation, and coordination.

Side Effects of This Medicine

Along with its needed effects, a medicine may cause some unwanted effects. Although not all of these side effects appear very often, when they do occur they may require medical attention. Check with your doctor if any of the following side effects occur:

More common

Mental depression	Unusual and uncontrolled movements of the body (such as the face, tongue, arms, hands, head, and upper body)
Mood or mental changes (such as aggressive behavior)	

Less common

Difficult urination	Irregular heart beats (skipping, fluttering, pounding, racing)
Fainting or severe dizziness	
	Nausea and vomiting (severe or continuing)

Rare

Anemia	High blood pressure
Duodenal ulcer	

Other side effects may occur which usually do not require medical attention. These side effects may go away during treatment as your body adjusts to the medicine. However, check with your doctor if any of the following side effects continue or are bothersome:

More common

Anxiety	Dry mouth
Diarrhea	

Less common

Constipation	Sleeping difficulty
Flushing of skin	Tiredness
Headache	Urine discoloration or darkening
Muscle twitching	
Nightmares	

After taking this medicine for long periods of time, such as 1 to several years, some patients suddenly lose the ability to move because their muscles seem not to work. This loss of movement may last from a few minutes to hours. The patient is then able to move as before until the condition unexpectedly occurs again. If you should have this problem, sometimes called the "on-off" phenomenon, check with your doctor.

This medicine may sometimes cause the urine and sweat to be darker than usual. The urine may at first be reddish, then turn to nearly black after being exposed to air. Some bathroom cleaning products will produce a similar darkening when in contact with urine containing this medicine. This effect is not important and is to be expected during treatment with this medicine.

Other side effects not listed above may also occur in some patients. If you notice any other effects, check with your doctor.

LIME, SULFURATED (Topical)
Some commonly used brand names or other names are Vlem-Dome and Vleminckx's solution.

Sulfurated (SUL-fur-ay-ted) lime solution is applied to the skin to treat acne, scabies, and other skin disorders. This medicine is available without a prescription; however, your doctor may have special instructions on the proper use of this medicine for your medical problem.

Before Using This Medicine

In order to decide on the best treatment for your medical problem, your doctor should be told:

—if you have ever had any unusual reaction to sulfurated lime in the past. This medicine should not be used if you are allergic to it.

—if you are pregnant, if you intend to become pregnant, or if you are breast-feeding an infant, although sulfurated lime has not been shown to cause problems.

—if you are now using any topical acne preparation or preparation containing a peeling agent such as benzoyl peroxide, resorcinol, salicylic acid, sulfur, or tretinoin.

—if you are now using any topical preparation containing mercury, such as ammoniated mercury ointment.

Proper Use of This Medicine

Use this medicine only as directed. Do not use more of it, do not use it more often, and do not use it for a longer period of time than recommended on the label, unless otherwise directed by your doctor.

Sulfurated lime solution must be diluted before you use it on your skin. Make sure you understand exactly how you should use this solution since it may be used for wet dressings, as a soak, or in a bath. If you have any questions about this, check with your doctor or pharmacist.

Before diluting and applying this solution, remove all jewelry and metallic ornaments since the solution may discolor metals. Also, avoid getting this solution on metal spoons or bath fixtures.

Keep this medicine away from the eyes. If you should accidentally get some in your eyes, flush them thoroughly with water.

If you miss a dose of this medicine, apply it as soon as possible. Then go back to your regular dosing schedule. But if it is almost time for your next dose, do not apply the missed dose at all. Instead, go back to your regular dosing schedule. If you have any questions about this, check with your doctor or pharmacist.

Precautions While Using This Medicine

Do not use any acne preparation or preparation containing a peeling agent (for example, benzoyl peroxide, resorcinol, salicylic acid, sulfur, or tretinoin) *on the same affected area as this medicine,* unless otherwise directed by your doctor. To do so may cause severe irritation of the skin.

Do not use any topical mercury-containing preparation such as ammoniated mercury ointment on the same affected area as this medicine. To do so may cause a foul odor, be irritating to the skin, and stain the skin black. If you have any questions about this, check with your doctor.

Side Effects of This Medicine

Along with its needed effects, a medicine may cause some unwanted effects. Although not all of these side effects appear very often, when they do occur they may require medical attention. Check with your doctor or pharmacist if the following side effect occurs:

Irritation of skin not present before using this medicine

Other side effects may occur which usually do not require medical attention. However, check with your doctor or pharmacist if the following side effect continues or is bothersome:

Unusual dryness of skin

After you use this medicine for a few days, some redness and peeling of the skin may be expected.

Other side effects not listed above may also occur in some patients. If you notice any other effects, check with your doctor or pharmacist.

LINCOMYCINS (Systemic)

This information applies to the following medicines:

Clindamycin (klin-da-MYE-sin)
Lincomycin (lin-koe-MYE-sin)

Some commonly used brand names are:	Generic names:
Cleocin Dalacin C*	Clindamycin
Lincocin	Lincomycin

*Not available in the United States.

Lincomycins belong to the general family of medicines called antibiotics. They are given by mouth or by injection to help the body overcome infections. Lincomycins are available only with your doctor's prescription.

Before Using This Medicine

In order to decide on the best treatment for your medical problem, your doctor should be told:

—if you have had allergic reactions to any of the lincomycins.

—if you are pregnant, if you intend to become pregnant, or if you are breast-feeding an infant, although lincomycins have not been shown to cause problems.

—if you have any of the following medical problems:

| Kidney disease | Stomach or |
| Liver disease | intestinal disease, especially colitis |

—if you are now taking any of the following medicines or types of medicine:

| Chloramphenicol | Erythromycins |
| Diarrhea medicine | |

—if you have had any problems with this medicine in the past.

Proper Use of This Medicine

If you are taking the capsule form of clindamycin, it should be taken with a full glass (8 ounces) of water or with meals to prevent irritation of the esophagus (tube between the throat and stomach).

Lincomycin is best taken with a full glass (8 ounces) of water on an empty stomach (either 1 hour before or 2 hours after meals), unless otherwise directed by your doctor.

If you are taking the oral liquid form of this medicine:

• Use a specially marked measuring spoon or other device to measure each dose accurately since the average household teaspoon may not hold the right amount of liquid.

• Do not refrigerate the oral liquid form of clindamycin. If chilled, the liquid may thicken and be difficult to pour.

To help clear up your infection completely, *keep taking this medicine for the full time of treatment* even if you begin to feel better after a few days; *do not miss any doses.* This is especially important if you have a "strep" infection since serious heart problems could develop later if your infection is not completely cleared up.

If you do miss a dose of this medicine, take it as soon as possible. However, if it is almost time for your next dose and your dosing schedule is:

• 3 or more doses a day—Space the missed dose and the next dose 2 to 4 hours apart or double your next dose.

Then go back to your regular dosing schedule.

Precautions While Using This Medicine

If your symptoms do not improve within a few days or if they become worse, check with your doctor.

It is important that your doctor check your progress at regular visits.

Before having surgery (including dental surgery) with a general anesthetic, tell the doctor or dentist in charge that you are taking a lincomycin.

If this medicine causes severe stomach cramps, pain, and bloating; severe, watery diarrhea, which may be accompanied by blood, mucus, pus, or pieces of intestinal lining in the stool; or unexplained fever, stop taking this medicine and check with your doctor immediately. These side effects may also occur up to several weeks after you stop taking this medicine.

If diarrhea occurs, do not take any diarrhea medicine without first checking with your doctor or pharmacist. These medicines may make your diarrhea worse or make it last longer.

Side Effects of This Medicine

Along with its needed effects, a medicine may cause some unwanted effects. Although not all of these side effects appear very often, when they do occur they may require medical attention. Stop taking this medicine and check with your doctor *immediately* if any of the follow-

ing side effects occur (these side effects may also occur up to several weeks after you stop taking this medicine):

More common

Severe stomach cramps, pain, and bloating	Severe, watery diarrhea, which may be accompanied by blood, mucus, pus, or pieces of intestinal lining in the stool
	Unexplained fever

Other side effects may occur which usually do not require medical attention. These side effects may go away during treatment as your body adjusts to the medicine. However, check with your doctor if any of the following side effects continue or are bothersome:

More common

Mild diarrhea	Rash
Nausea	Vomiting

Less common

Itching of skin, rectal, or genital areas

Other side effects not listed above may also occur in some patients. If you notice any other effects, check with your doctor.

LINDANE (Topical)
Some commonly used brand names are GBH*, Kwell, and Kwellada*.

---

*Not available in the United States.

Lindane (LIN-dane), formerly known as gamma benzene hexachloride, is applied to the skin or scalp to treat scabies and lice infections. It is available only with your doctor's prescription.

Before Using This Medicine

In order to decide on the best treatment for your medical problem, your doctor should be told:

—if you have ever had any unusual reaction to lindane in the past. This medicine should not be used if you are allergic to it.

—if you are pregnant or if you intend to become pregnant while using this medicine. Use of too much lindane may cause unwanted effects in both the mother and baby, since it may be absorbed through the skin.

—if you are breast-feeding an infant. Although lindane has not been shown to cause problems, the chance always exists.

—if you are now using any other skin preparations such as lotions, ointments, or oils.

Proper Use of This Medicine

Use this medicine only as directed by your doctor. Do not use more of it, do not use it more often, and do not use it for a longer period of time than your doctor ordered. To do so may increase the chance of absorption through the skin and the chance of lindane poisoning.

Keep this medicine away from the eyes. If you should accidentally get some in your eyes, flush them thoroughly with water at once.

This medicine usually comes with patient directions. Read them carefully before using this medicine.

If you are using the cream or lotion form of this medicine:

For scabies
• If you take a warm bath before using this medicine, dry the skin well before applying this medicine.

• Apply enough medicine to cover the entire skin surface from the neck down, and rub in well.

• Leave the medicine on for 8 to 12 hours, then remove by washing thoroughly.

• Put on freshly washed or dry-cleaned clothing in order to prevent reinfection.

For lice
• Apply enough medicine to cover only the affected areas, and rub well into the hair and skin or scalp.

• Leave the medicine on for 12 hours, then remove by washing thoroughly.

• Put on freshly washed or dry-cleaned clothing in order to prevent reinfection.

If you are using the shampoo form of this medicine:

• Apply enough shampoo to thoroughly wet the hair and skin or scalp of the affected and surrounding hairy areas. Then use enough water to work up a lather while rubbing into the hair and skin or scalp.

• Continue rubbing the lather into the hair and skin or scalp for 4 minutes. Then rinse thoroughly and dry with a clean towel.

• When the hair is dry, comb with a fine-tooth comb.

• This shampoo may also be used to wash combs and brushes to prevent spread of the infection.

• Do not use as a regular shampoo.

If you are using this medicine for pubic (crab) lice, your sexual partner should also be treated since the lice may spread to persons in close contact. If your partner is not being treated or if you have any questions about this, check with your doctor.

Precautions While Using This Medicine

To prevent reinfection or spreading of the infection to other people, all clothing, bed linen, and towels should be washed in very hot water or dry-cleaned.

Side Effects of This Medicine

Along with its needed effects, a medicine may cause some unwanted effects. Although not all of these side effects appear very often, when they do occur they may require medical attention. Check with your doctor if any of the following side effects occur:

Irritation of skin not present before using this medicine	Skin rash

Possible signs of lindane poisoning

Clumsiness or unsteadiness	Unusual nervousness, restlessness, or irritability
Convulsions or seizures	
Muscle cramps	Unusually fast heartbeat
	Vomiting

Other side effects may occur which usually do not require medical attention. These side effects may go away during treatment as your body adjusts to the medicine. However, check with your doctor if the following side effect continues or is bothersome:

Itching of skin

After you stop using this medicine, itching may occur and continue for 1 to several weeks. If this continues longer or is bothersome, check with your doctor.

Other side effects not listed above may also occur in some patients. If you notice any other effects, check with your doctor.

LITHIUM (Systemic)
Some commonly used brand names are:

Eskalith   Lithonate-S
Lithonate   Lithane
Lithobid

Lithium (LI-thee-um) is a medicine used in the treatment of certain mental and emotional conditions. Lithium is available only with your doctor's prescription.

Before Using This Medicine

In order to decide on the best treatment for your medical problem, your doctor should be told:

—if you have ever had any unusual reaction to lithium in the past. This medicine should not be taken if you are allergic to it.

—if you are pregnant or if you intend to become pregnant while using this medicine. Lithium may cause unwanted effects in the baby and may produce other problems for both mother and baby before and during delivery. Be sure you have discussed this with your doctor before taking lithium.

—if you are breast-feeding an infant. Lithium passes into the breast milk and may cause unwanted effects in the infant. Be sure you have discussed this with your doctor before taking this medicine.

—if you have any of the following medical problems:

Diabetes   Low blood pressure
Difficult urination   Parkinson's disease
Epilepsy   Severe infection
Heart disease   Thyroid disease
Kidney disease

—if you drink large amounts of coffee, tea, or colas.

—if you are on a low-salt diet.

—if you are now taking any of the following medicines or types of medicine:

Asthma medicine   Methyldopa
Caffeine   Potassium iodide or
Chlorpromazine   other iodide
Diuretic tablets   medicines
  (water pills,   Sodium bicarbonate
  especially   (baking soda)
  thiazide-type)   Sodium chloride
Haloperidol   (salt)
Indomethacin   Tetracycline

Proper Use of This Medicine

Take this medicine exactly as directed. Do not take more of it, do not take it more often, and do not take it for a longer period of time than your doctor ordered.

Sometimes this medicine must be taken for 1 to several weeks before you begin to feel better.

While taking this medicine, drink 2 or 3 quarts of water or other fluids each day, and use a normal amount of table salt in your food, unless otherwise directed by your doctor.

Take this medicine immediately after meals or with food or milk to lessen stomach upset, unless otherwise directed by your doctor.

If you miss a dose of this medicine, take it as soon as possible unless it is 2 hours or less until your next scheduled dose. Do not double doses. Instead, go back to your regular dosing schedule. If you have any questions about this, check with your doctor.

Precautions While Using This Medicine

Your doctor should check your progress at regular visits to make sure that the medicine is working properly and that possible side effects are avoided. Laboratory tests may be necessary.

This medicine may cause some people to become drowsy or less alert than they are normally. *Make sure you know how you react to this medicine before you drive, use machines, or do other jobs that require you to be alert.*

Use extra care in hot weather and during activities that cause you to sweat heavily, such as hot baths, saunas, or exercising. The loss of too much water and salt from your body may lead to serious side effects from this medicine.

Drinking large amounts of coffee, tea, or colas may cause this medicine to build up in your body to serious levels. Check with your doctor before using large amounts of these beverages.

Side Effects of This Medicine

Along with its needed effects, a medicine may cause some unwanted effects. Although not all of these side effects appear very often, when they do occur they may require medical attention. Check with your doctor if any of the following side effects occur:

More common

Nausea and   Shakiness and
  vomiting   tremor

Less common

Drowsiness	Swelling of hands
Mental confusion	and feet
Pains in lower	Weakness
stomach	
Slurred speech	

Rare

Blurred vision	Jerking of arms
	and legs

Other side effects may occur which usually do not require medical attention. These side effects may go away during treatment as your body adjusts to the medicine. However, check with your doctor if any of the following side effects continue or are bothersome:

More common

Decreased sexual	Dry mouth
ability	Increased thirst
Diarrhea	Increased urination
	Dizziness

Less common

Skin eruption
or rash

Signs of possible low thyroid function such as:

Coldness of fingers	Menstrual changes
and toes	Muscle aches
Constipation	Sleepiness
Dry, puffy skin	Tiredness
Headaches	Unusual weight gain

LOMUSTINE (Systemic)
A commonly used brand name is CeeNU.

Lomustine (loe-MUS-teen) belongs to the group of medicines known as alkylating agents. It is used to treat some kinds of cancer. Lomustine is available only with your doctor's prescription.

Before Using This Medicine

Lomustine is a very strong medicine. In addition to its helpful effects in treating your medical problem, it has side effects that could be very serious. Before you take this medicine, be sure that you have discussed the use of it with your doctor.

In order to decide on the best treatment for your medical problem, your doctor should be told:

—if you have ever had any unusual reaction to lomustine in the past.

—if you are pregnant or if you intend to have children. This medicine may cause birth defects if either the male or female is taking it at the time of conception or if it is taken during pregnancy. It may also cause permanent sterility after it has been taken for a while. Be sure that you have discussed this with your doctor before taking this medicine.

—if you are breast-feeding an infant. Although lomustine has not been shown to cause problems, the chance always exists.

—if you have any of the following medical problems:

Anemia	Infection
Blood disease	Kidney disease

—if you have been treated with x-rays or cancer drugs by another doctor.

Proper Use of This Medicine

Take this medicine only as directed by your doctor.

In order that you receive the proper dose of this medicine, there may be two or more different types of capsules in the container. This is not an error. It is important that you take all of the capsules in the container as one dose so that you receive the right dose of the medicine.

This medicine is sometimes given together with certain other medicines. If you are using a combination of drugs, make sure that you take each medicine at the right time and do not mix them. Ask your doctor, nurse, or pharmacist to help you plan a way to remember to take your medicines at the right time.

Nausea and vomiting occur often after taking this drug, but usually last less than 24 hours. Loss of appetite may last for several days. This medicine is best taken on an empty stomach at bedtime so that it will cause less stomach upset. To help prevent nausea, your doctor may also prescribe a drug that you may take before you take this medicine.

Do not stop using this medicine without first checking with your doctor.

Precautions While Using This Medicine

It is important that your doctor check your progress at regular visits.

Side Effects of This Medicine

Along with its needed effects, a medicine may cause some unwanted effects. Although not all of these side effects appear very often, when they do occur they may require medical attention. Check with your doctor if any of the following side effects occur:

More common

Unexplained fever, chills, or sore throat	Unusual bleeding or bruising

Less common

Awkwardness	Swelling of feet
Mental confusion	or lower legs
Slurred speech	Unusual tiredness or
Sores in the mouth and on the lips	weakness

Rare

Yellowing of eyes
and skin

Other side effects may occur which usually do not require medical attention. These side effects may go away during treatment as your body adjusts to the medicine. However, check with your doctor if any of the following side effects continue or are bothersome:

More common

Loss of appetite
Nausea and
vomiting

Less common

Darkening of skin	Skin rash and
Loss of hair	itching

After you stop using this medicine, it may still produce some side effects that need attention. During this period of time check with your doctor if you notice any of the following side effects:

Unexplained fever, chills, or sore throat	Unusual bleeding or bruising

Other side effects not listed above may also occur in some patients. If you notice any other effects, check with your doctor.

LOPERAMIDE (Systemic)

A commonly used brand name is Imodium.

Loperamide (loe-PER-a-mide) is a medicine used along with other measures to treat severe diarrhea. This medicine is available only with your doctor's prescription.

Before Using This Medicine

In order to decide on the best treatment for your medical problem, your doctor should be told:

—if you have ever had any unusual reaction to loperamide in the past. This medicine should not be used if you are allergic to it.

—if you are pregnant, if you intend to become pregnant, or if you are breast-feeding an infant. Although loperamide has not been shown to cause problems, the chance always exists.

—if you have either of the following medical problems:

Colitis
Liver disease

Proper Use of This Medicine

Take this medicine only as directed by your doctor. Do not take more of it, do not take it more often, and do not take it for a longer period of time than your doctor ordered.

If you must take loperamide regularly and if you miss a dose, do not take the missed dose at all and do not double the next one. Instead, go back to your regular dosing schedule. If you have any questions about this, check with your doctor.

Precautions While Using This Medicine

If you will be taking this medicine regularly for a long period of time, your doctor should check your progress at regular visits.

Check with your doctor if your diarrhea doesn't stop after a few days or if you develop a fever.

Side Effects of This Medicine

Along with its needed effects, a medicine may cause some unwanted effects. *When this medicine is used for short periods of time at low doses, side effects usually are rare* and they may go away during treatment as your body adjusts to the medicine. However, check with your doctor if any of the following side effects continue, worsen, or are bothersome:

Rare

Bloating	Fever
Constipation	Loss of appetite
Dizziness	Nausea and
Drowsiness	vomiting
Dry mouth	Skin rash
	Stomach pain

Other side effects not listed above may also occur in some patients. If you notice any other effects, check with your doctor.

LOXAPINE (Systemic)

Some commonly used brand names are Daxolin and Loxitane.

Loxapine (LOX-a-peen) is used to treat nervous, mental, and emotional conditions. Loxapine is taken by mouth as a capsule or a liquid and sometimes is given by injection. Loxapine is available only with your doctor's prescription.

Before Using This Medicine

In order to decide on the best treatment for your medical problem, your doctor should be told:

—if you have ever had any unusual reaction to loxapine in the past. This medicine should not be taken if you are allergic to it.

—if you are pregnant, if you intend to become pregnant, or if you are breast-feeding an infant. Although loxapine has not been shown to cause problems, the chance always exists.

—if you have any of the following medical problems:

Alcoholism	Liver disease
Epilepsy	Parkinson's disease
Glaucoma	Prostate enlarge-
Heart or circulation	ment
disease	Urination problems

—if you are now taking any of the following medicines or types of medicine:

Amphetamines	Epinephrine
Antacids	Guanethidine (high
Antibiotics	blood pressure
Anticonvulsants	medicine)
(seizure medicine)	Levodopa
Asthma medicine	Ulcer medicine
Diarrhea medicine	

—if you are now taking central nervous system (CNS) depressants such as:

Antihistamines or	Prescription pain
medicine for	medicine
hay fever, other	Sedatives, tran-
allergies, or	quilizers,
colds	or sleeping
Barbiturates	medicine
Narcotics	Tricyclic an-
	tidepressants
	(medicine for
	depression)

—if you are now taking or have taken within the past 2 weeks monoamine oxidase (MAO) inhibitors such as:

Isocarboxazid	Phenelzine
Pargyline	Tranylcypromine

Proper Use of This Medicine

Do not take more of this medicine or take it more often than your doctor ordered.

Do not stop taking this medicine without first checking with your doctor. Your doctor may want you to reduce gradually the amount you are taking before stopping completely to prevent side effects or making your condition worse.

If you miss a dose of this medicine and you remember within an hour or so of the missed dose, take it right away. Then go back to your regular dosing schedule. But if you do not remember until later, do not take the missed dose at all and do not double the next one. Instead, go back to your regular dosing schedule. If you have any questions about this, check with your doctor.

This medicine may be taken with food or a full glass (8 ounces) of water or milk to reduce stomach irritation.

Precautions While Using This Medicine

Your doctor should check your progress at regular visits, especially for the first few weeks you take this medicine. This will allow your dosage to be changed if necessary to meet your needs.

This medicine will add to the effects of alcohol and other medicines (CNS depressants) that slow down the nervous system. Some examples of CNS depressants are antihistamines or medicine for hay fever, other allergies, or colds; sedatives, tranquilizers, or sleeping medicine; prescription pain medicine or narcotics; barbiturates; medicine for seizures; tricyclic antidepressants (medicine for depression); or anesthetics, including some dental anesthetics. *Check with your doctor before taking any of the above while you are taking this medicine.*

Dizziness, lightheadedness, or fainting may occur, especially when you get up from a lying or sitting position. Getting up slowly may help. If the problem continues or gets worse, check with your doctor.

This medicine may cause some people to become drowsy or less alert than they are normally, especially during the first few days the medicine is being taken or when the dosage is increased. Even if you take this medicine only at bedtime, you may feel drowsy or less alert on arising. *Make sure you know how you react to this medicine before you drive, use machines, or do other jobs that require you to be alert.*

Do not take this medicine within an hour of taking antacids or medicine for diarrhea. Taking them too close together may make this medicine less effective.

A few people who take this medicine may become more sensitive to sunlight than they are normally. When you first begin taking this medicine, use sun screen lotions, or avoid too much sun or too much use of a sunlamp until you see how you react. If you have a severe reaction, check with your doctor.

Side Effects of This Medicine

Along with its needed effects, a medicine may cause some unwanted effects. Although not all of these side effects appear very often, when they do occur they may require medical attention. Check with your doctor if any of the following side effects occur:

More common (occurring with increase of dosage)

Muscle spasms, especially of neck and back	Tic-like (jerky) movements of head, face, mouth, and neck
Restlessness	Trembling and
Shuffling walk	shaking of hands and fingers

Less common

Difficult urination	Fine, worm-like movements of tongue
Fainting	Skin rash

Other side effects may occur which usually do not require medical attention. These side effects may go away during treatment as your body adjusts to the medicine. However, check with your doctor if any of the following side effects continue or are bothersome:

More common

Blurred vision	Dizziness
Constipation	Drowsiness
	Dry mouth

Less common

Headache	Nausea
Increased sensitivity of skin to sun	Unusually fast heartbeat

Other side effects not listed above may also occur in some patients. If you notice any other effects, check with your doctor.

MAGNESIA, MILK OF (Oral)

Some other commonly used names are magnesia and magnesium hydroxide.

Milk of magnesia is used to relieve heartburn or acid stomach by neutralizing excess stomach acid. When used for this purpose, it is said to belong to the group of medicines called antacids. With larger doses than those used for antacid, milk of magnesia produces a laxative effect. Milk of magnesia is available without a prescription; however, your doctor may have special instructions on the proper use for your medical condition.

Before Using This Medicine

For laxative effect

Importance of diet, fluids, and exercise—Laxatives are to be used to provide short-term relief only, unless otherwise directed by a doctor. A proper diet containing roughage (whole-grain breads and cereals, bran, fruit, and green, leafy vegetables), with 6 to 8 full glasses (8 ounces each) of liquids each day, and daily exercise are most important in maintaining a healthy bowel function.

For antacid or laxative effect

In order to decide on the best treatment for your medical problem, the following should be kept in mind and/or your doctor should be told:

—if you have ever had any unusual reaction to milk of magnesia in the past. This medicine should not be taken if you are allergic to it.

—if you are pregnant. Milk of magnesia contains magnesium and may be more likely to cause serious side effects if your kidneys are not working well.

—if you have any of the following medical problems:

Appendicitis (or signs of)	Kidney disease
Colostomy	Laxative habit
Diverticulitis	Rectal bleeding (of unknown cause)
Ileostomy	Ulcerative colitis
Intestinal blockage	

—if you are now taking any of the following medicines or types of medicine:

Anticoagulants (blood thinners)	Isoniazid
Digitalis preparations (heart medicine)	Laxatives (other)
	Medicine for nerves
	Tetracycline

Proper Use of This Medicine

For safe and effective use of milk of magnesia:

• Follow your doctor's instructions if this was prescribed.

• Follow the manufacturer's package directions if you are treating yourself.

For antacid use:

Milk of magnesia provides relief from hyperacidity (over-acid stomach) within minutes of a dose. Although it is used when needed, it is often taken 1 to 3 hours after meals when the stomach acid is usually highest.

The tablets must be chewed or crushed well before being taken to allow the medicine to work more quickly and effectively. Both tablet and liquid doses should be followed with a full glass (8 ounces) of water to increase their effect.

For laxative use:

Results are usually obtained within 2 to 8 hours. Milk of magnesia should not be taken late in the day unless at bedtime with food for morning results. When taken on an empty stomach with a full glass of liquid, results are obtained in a shorter time.

Moisture is necessary to produce a soft bowel movement. A person using any type of laxative should drink at least 6 to 8 full glasses (8 ounces each) of liquid each day.

Precautions While Using This Medicine

For antacid use:

Using milk of magnesia as an antacid too often during the day, or in high doses, may produce a laxative effect. This happens fairly often and depends on the individual's sensitivity to the medicine.

Do not continue to rely on antacids if your stomach problem continues more than 2 weeks or if the problem comes back often. Instead, check with your doctor. Antacids should be used only for occasional relief.

For laxative use:

Do not take milk of magnesia for its laxative effect:

—*if you have symptoms of appendicitis or inflamed bowel* (such as stomach or lower abdominal pain, cramping, bloating, or soreness, nausea, and/or vomiting)

—*for more than 1 week* unless your doctor has prescribed or ordered a special schedule for you. This is true even when you have had no results from the laxative.

—*within 2 hours of taking other medicine* because the desired effect of the other medicine may be reduced.

—*if you do not need it,* as for the common cold, "to clean out your system," or as a "tonic to make you feel better."

—*if you have kidney disease.* This medicine may cause serious side effects if your kidneys do not work well.

—*if you miss a bowel movement for a day or two.*

If you notice a sudden change in bowel habits or function that lasts longer than 2 weeks, or that keeps returning off and on, check with your doctor before using a laxative. This will allow the cause of your problem to be determined before it becomes more serious.

The "laxative habit"—Laxative products are overused by many people. Such a practice often leads to dependence on the laxative action to produce a bowel movement. In severe cases, overuse of some laxatives has caused damage to the nerves, muscles, and tissues of the intestines and bowel. If you have any questions about the use of laxatives, check with your doctor, nurse, or pharmacist.

Side Effects of This Medicine

Along with its needed effects, a medicine may cause some unwanted effects. Although not all of these side effects appear very often, when they do occur they may require medical attention. Check with your doctor if any of the following side effects occur:

Signs of overuse

Dizziness or lightheadedness	Mental confusion
Irregular heartbeat	Unusual tiredness or weakness

Other side effects may occur which usually do not require medical attention. These side effects may go away during treatment as your body adjusts to the medicine. However, check with your doctor if any of the following side effects continue or are bothersome:

More common

Diarrhea (when used for antacid effect)

Less common

Cramping	Nausea
Increased thirst	

Other side effects not listed above may also occur in some patients. If you notice any other effects, check with your doctor.

MANNITOL (Systemic)
A commonly used brand name is Osmitrol.

Mannitol (MAN-i-tole) is given by injection to treat certain medical conditions in which there is an increased pressure in the eye, such as glaucoma, or increased pressure on the brain. It may be used before eye surgery to reduce pressure in the eye. It may also be used to help reduce the amount of water in the body by increasing the flow of urine. Sometimes it may be used as a test to determine how well your kidneys are working. This medicine is available only with your doctor's prescription.

Before Using This Medicine

In order to decide on the best treatment for your medical problem, your doctor should be told:

—if you have ever had any unusual reaction to mannitol in the past. This medicine should not be used if you are allergic to it.

—if you are pregnant, if you intend to become pregnant, or if you are breast-feeding an infant. Although mannitol has not been shown to cause problems, the chance always exists.

—if you have any of the following medical problems:

Heart disease	Lung disease
Kidney disease	

Side Effects of This Medicine

Along with its needed effects, a medicine may cause some unwanted effects. Although not all of these side effects appear very often, when they do occur they may require medical attention. Check with your doctor if any of the following side effects occur:

Rare

Chest pain or unusually fast or irregular heartbeat	Redness, swelling, or pain at the place of injection
Chills or fever	Seizures
Coughing, troubled breathing, or wheezing	Swelling of feet or lower legs
Difficult urination	Trembling
Mental confusion	Unusual tiredness or weakness
Muscle cramps or pain	Weakness and heaviness of legs
Numbness, tingling, pain, or weakness in hands or feet	

Other side effects may occur which usually do not require medical attention. These side effects may go away during treatment as your body adjusts to the medicine. However, check with your doctor if any of the following side effects continue or are bothersome:

More common

Headache	Nausea or vomiting
Increased urination	Unusual dryness of mouth or increased thirst

Less common

Blurred vision	Skin rash or hives
Dizziness	

Other side effects not listed above may also occur in some patients. If you notice any other effects, check with your doctor.

MECAMYLAMINE (Systemic)
A commonly used brand name is Inversine.

Mecamylamine (mek-a-MILL-a-meen) belongs to the general class of medicines called antihypertensives. It is used to treat high blood pressure. Mecamylamine is available only with your doctor's prescription.

Before Using This Medicine

In order to decide on the best treatment for your medical problem, your doctor should be told:

—if you have ever had any unusual reaction to mecamylamine in the past. This medicine should not be taken if you are allergic to it.

—if you are pregnant or if you intend to become pregnant while using this medicine. Too much use of it during pregnancy may cause unwanted effects in the baby. Be sure that you have discussed this with your doctor before taking this medicine. In addition, although this medicine has not been shown to cause birth defects, the chance always exists.

—if you are breast-feeding an infant. Although this medicine has not been shown to cause problems, the chance always exists.

—if you have any of the following medical problems:

Bladder or prostate problems	Glaucoma
Bowel problems	Heart or blood vessel disease
Diarrhea	Kidney disease
Fever or infection	Nausea or vomiting

—if you have recently had a heart attack or stroke.

—if you are now taking any of the following medicines or types of medicine:

Acetazolamide	Diuretics (water
Antibiotics	pills) or other
	antihyperten-
	sives (medicine
	for high blood
	pressure)
	Sulfa drugs

Proper Use of This Medicine

Importance of Diet—When prescribing medicine for your condition, your doctor may also prescribe a personal diet for you. Such a diet may be low in sodium (salt). Medicine is usually more effective when this diet is properly followed.

Also, it may be very important for you to go on a reducing diet. However, check with your doctor before going on any diet.

Many patients who have high blood pressure will not notice any signs of the problem. In fact, many may feel normal. *It is very important that you take your medicine exactly as directed and that you keep your doctor's appointments* even if you feel well.

Remember that this medicine will not cure your high blood pressure but it does control it. Therefore, you must continue to take it as directed if you expect to keep your blood pressure down. *You may have to take medicine for the rest of your life.* If high blood pressure is not treated, it can cause serious problems such as heart failure, blood vessel disease, stroke, or kidney disease.

In order to help remember to take your medicine, try to get into the habit of taking it at the same time each day.

If you do miss a dose of this medicine, take it as soon as possible. Then go back to your regular dosing schedule. *If you miss more than one dose in a row check with your doctor right away.* If your body goes without this medicine for too long, your blood pressure may go up to a dangerously high level.

Precautions While Using This Medicine

It is important that your doctor check your progress at regular visits.

Dizziness, lightheadedness, or fainting may occur, especially when you get up from a lying or sitting position. This is more likely to occur in the morning. *Getting up slowly may help.* When you get up from lying down, sit on the edge of the bed with your feet dangling for one or two minutes. Then stand up slowly. If the problem continues or gets worse, check with your doctor.

The dizziness, lightheadedness, or fainting is also more likely to occur if you drink alcohol, stand for long periods of time, exercise, or if the weather is hot. *While you are taking this medicine, be careful in the amount of alcohol you drink. Also, use extra care during exercise or hot weather or if you must stand for long periods of time.* Check with your doctor if you have any questions about this.

Do not take other medicines unless they have been discussed with your doctor. This especially includes over-the-counter (nonprescription) medicines for appetite control, asthma, colds, cough, hay fever, or sinus, since they may tend to increase your blood pressure.

Sodium bicarbonate (commonly known as baking soda) may cause you to get a greater effect from this medicine than normal. To prevent problems, check with your doctor or pharmacist before using an antacid or medicine for heartburn since some of these contain sodium bicarbonate.

Before having any kind of surgery (including dental surgery) or emergency treatment, tell the doctor or dentist in charge that you are taking this medicine.

Tell your doctor if you get a fever or infection since that may change the amount of medicine you have to take.

Check with your doctor before you stop taking this medicine. Your doctor may want you to reduce gradually the amount you are taking before stopping completely.

Make sure that you have enough medicine on hand to last through weekends, holidays, or vacations. You should not miss taking any doses. You may want to ask your doctor for another prescription for mecamylamine to carry in your wallet or purse. You could then have it filled if you run out when you are away from home.

Your mouth, nose, and throat may feel very dry while you are taking this medicine. To help relieve mouth dryness, chew sugarless gum or dissolve bits of ice in your mouth.

Check with your doctor if you become sick and have severe or continuing vomiting or diarrhea. These problems may cause you to lose water and salt, which could be harmful.

Side Effects of This Medicine

Along with its needed effects, a medicine may cause some unwanted effects. Although not all of these side effects appear very often, when they do occur they may require medical attention. Check with your doctor if any of the following side effects occur:

More common

Dizziness or lightheadedness, especially when getting up from a lying or sitting position

Less common

Difficult urination

Rare

Confusion or unusual excitement
Mental depression

Shortness of breath
Trembling

Other side effects may occur which usually do not require medical attention. These side effects may go away during treatment as your body adjusts to the medicine. However, check with your doctor if any of the following side effects continue or are bothersome:

More common

Constipation

Drowsiness
Tiredness

Less common or rare

Blurred vision
Decreased sexual ability
Dry mouth

Enlarged pupils
Loss of appetite
Nausea and vomiting
Weakness

Other side effects not listed above may also occur in some patients. If you notice any other effects, check with your doctor.

MECHLORETHAMINE (Systemic)
A commonly used brand name is Mustargen.

Mechlorethamine (me-klor-ETH-a-meen) belongs to the group of medicines called alkylating agents. It is used by injection to treat some kinds of cancer as well as some noncancerous conditions. It is also applied to the skin sometimes to treat certain conditions that could turn to cancer if left untreated. Mechlorethamine is available only on prescription and is to be administered only by or under the immediate supervision of your doctor.

Before Using This Medicine

Mechlorethamine is a very strong medicine. In addition to its helpful effects in treating your medical problem, it has side effects that could be very serious. Before you receive this medicine, be sure that you have discussed the use of it with your doctor.

In order to decide on the best treatment for your medical problem, your doctor should be told:

—if you have ever had any unusual reaction to mechlorethamine in the past.

—if you are pregnant or if you intend to have children. This medicine may cause birth defects if either the male or female is taking it at the time of conception or if it is taken during pregnancy. It may also cause permanent sterility after it has been taken for a while. Be sure that you have discussed this with your doctor before receiving this medicine.

—if you are breast-feeding an infant. Although mechlorethamine has not been shown to cause problems, the chance always exists.

—if you have any of the following medical problems:

Blood disease
Gout

Infection
Kidney stones

—if you are taking gout medicine.

—if you have been treated with x-rays or cancer drugs by another doctor.

Proper Use of This Medicine

This medicine is sometimes given together with certain other medicines. If you are using a combination of drugs, it is important that you receive each medicine at the proper time. If you are taking some of these medicines by mouth, ask your doctor, nurse, or pharmacist to help you plan a way to take them at the right time.

This medicine often causes nausea and vomiting, which usually last only 8 to 24 hours. It is very important that you continue to receive the medicine, even if you begin to feel ill. Your doctor may prescribe a medicine to relieve stomach upset. If you have any questions about this, check with your doctor.

Precautions While Using This Medicine

It is very important that your doctor check your progress at regular visits.

While you are using this medicine, your doctor may want you to drink plenty of fluids and urinate often. This will help prevent kidney problems and keep your kidneys working well. If you have any questions about this, check with your doctor.

Side Effects of This Medicine

Along with its needed effects, a medicine may cause some unwanted effects. Although not all of these side effects appear very often, when they do occur they may require medical attention. Check with your doctor if any of the following side effects occur:

More common

Missing menstrual periods	Unexplained fever, chills, or sore throat
Painful rash	Unusual bleeding or bruising

Less common

Dizziness	Pain or redness at the place of injection
Flank and stomach pain	
Joint pain	Ringing in the ears
Loss of hearing	Swelling of feet or lower legs

Rare

Black tarry stools	Shortness of breath
Itching	Wheezing
Numbness, tingling, or burning of fingers, toes, or face	Yellowing of eyes and skin

Other side effects may occur which usually do not require medical attention. These side effects may go away during treatment as your body adjusts to the medicine. However, check with your doctor if any of the following side effects continue or are bothersome:

More common

Nausea and vomiting

Less common

Diarrhea	Loss of appetite
Drowsiness	Loss of hair
Headache	Weakness

Rare

Skin rash or itching

This medicine may cause a temporary loss of hair in some people. After treatment with mechlorethamine has ended, normal hair growth should return.

If mechlorethamine accidentally seeps out of the vein into which it is injected, it may damage some tissues and cause scarring. Tell the doctor right away if you notice redness, pain, or swelling at the site of injection.

After you stop receiving this medicine, it may still produce some side effects that need attention. During this period of time check with your doctor if you notice any of the following side effects:

Unexplained fever, chills, or sore throat	Unusual bleeding or bruising

Other side effects not listed above may also occur in some patients. If you notice any other effects, check with your doctor.

MECLIZINE (Systemic)

This information applies to the following medicines:

Buclizine (BYOO-kli-zeen)
Cyclizine (SYE-kli-zeen)
Meclizine (MEK-li-zeen)

Some commonly used brand names are:	Generic names:
Bucladin-S	Buclizine
Marezine	Cyclizine
Antivert Bonine	Meclizine

Buclizine, cyclizine, and meclizine are used to prevent motion sickness, nausea, vomiting, and dizziness. These medicines may also be used for other conditions as determined by your doctor. Some of these preparations are available only with your doctor's prescription. Others are available without a prescription; however, your doctor may have special instructions on the proper dose of the medicine for your medical condition.

Before Using This Medicine

In order to decide on the best treatment for your medical problem, the following should be kept in mind and/or your doctor should be told:

—if you have ever had any unusual reaction to buclizine, cyclizine, or meclizine in the past. This medicine should not be taken if you are allergic to it.

—if you are pregnant or if you intend to become pregnant. Although this medicine has not been shown to cause problems in humans, the chance always exists.

—if you are breast-feeding an infant. This medicine may pass into the breast milk and cause unwanted effects in the infant.

—if you have any of the following medical problems:

Enlarged prostate   Stomach ulcer
Glaucoma   Urinary tract
                             blockage

—if you are now taking any central nervous system (CNS) depressants such as:

Antihistamines or   Narcotics
  medicine for hay   Prescription pain
  fever, other   medicine
  allergies,   Sedatives, tran-
  or colds   quilizers,
Barbiturates   or sleeping
Medicine for   medicine
  seizures

Proper Use of This Medicine

This medicine is used to relieve or prevent the symptoms of your medical problem. Take it only as directed. Do not take more of it or take it more often than as stated on the label or ordered by your doctor.

If necessary, take this medicine with food or a glass of water or milk to lessen stomach irritation.

If you are taking this medicine for motion sickness, take it at least 30 minutes to 1 hour before you begin to travel.

If you must take this medicine regularly and you miss a dose, take the missed dose as soon as possible. However, if it is almost time for your next dose, do not take the missed dose at all and do not double the next one. Instead, go back to your regular dosing schedule. If you have any questions about this, check with your doctor.

Precautions While Using This Medicine

Buclizine, cyclizine, or meclizine will add to the effects of alcohol and other medicines (CNS depressants) that slow down the nervous system. Some examples of CNS depressants are antihistamines or medicine for hay fever, other allergies, or colds; sedatives, tranquilizers, or sleeping medicine; prescription pain medicine or narcotics; barbiturates; medicine for

seizures; tricyclic antidepressants (medicine for depression); or anesthetics, including some dental anesthetics. *Check with your doctor before taking any of the above while you are using this medicine.*

This medicine may cause some people to become drowsy or less alert than they are normally. *Make sure you know how you react to this medicine before you drive, use machines, or do other jobs that require you to be alert.*

Your mouth may feel very dry while you are taking buclizine, cyclizine, or meclizine. To help relieve this feeling, chew sugarless gum or dissolve bits of ice in your mouth.

When taking this medicine on a regular basis, make sure your doctor knows if you are taking large amounts of aspirin at the same time (as in arthritis). Effects of too much aspirin, such as ringing in the ears, may be covered up by this medicine.

Side Effects of This Medicine

Along with its needed effects, a medicine may cause some unwanted effects. The following side effects may go away during treatment as your body adjusts to the medicine; however, check with your doctor if they continue or are bothersome:

More common
  Drowsiness

Less common or rare

Blurred vision   Nervousness,
Difficult or painful   restlessness,
  urination   or trouble in
Dizziness   sleeping
Dryness of mouth,   Skin rash
  nose, and throat   Unusually fast
Headache   heartbeat
Loss of appetite   Upset stomach

Although not all of the side effects listed above have been reported for all of these medicines, they have been reported for at least one of them. However, since buclizine, cyclizine, and meclizine are very similar, any of the above side effects may occur with any of these medicines.

Other side effects not listed above may also occur in some patients. If you notice any other effects, check with your doctor.

MECLOFENAMATE (Systemic)
A commonly used brand name is Meclomen.

Meclofenamate (me-kloe-fen-AM-ate) is used to treat the symptoms of certain types of arthritis. It helps relieve inflammation, swelling, stiffness, and joint pain. This medicine is available only with your doctor's prescription.

Before Using This Medicine
In order to decide on the best treatment for your medical problem, your doctor should be told:

—if you have ever had any unusual reaction to aspirin or other salicylates, fenoprofen, ibuprofen, naproxen, sulindac, or tolmetin.

—if you are pregnant, if you intend to become pregnant, or if you are breast-feeding an infant. Although meclofenamate has not been shown to cause problems in humans, the chance always exists.

—if you have a stomach ulcer or other stomach problems.

—if you are now taking either of the following medicines or types of medicine:

Inflammation medicine (for example, aspirin or other arthritis medicine)	Warfarin

Proper Use of This Medicine
In order for meclofenamate to help you, it must be taken regularly as ordered by your doctor. A few days may pass before you begin to feel better and up to 2 to 3 weeks may pass before you feel its full effects.

If this medicine upsets your stomach, it may be taken with meals, milk, or antacids. If stomach upset (nausea, vomiting, stomach pain, or diarrhea) continues, check with your doctor.

If you miss a dose of meclofenamate, take it as soon as possible. Then go back to your regular dosing schedule. However, if it is almost time for your next dose, do not take the missed dose at all and do not double the next one. Instead, go back to your regular dosing schedule. If you have any questions about this, check with your doctor.

Precautions While Using This Medicine
Your doctor should check your progress at regular visits, in order to make sure that this medicine does not cause unwanted effects.

Stomach problems may be more likely to occur if you take aspirin regularly (for example, every day) or drink alcoholic beverages while being treated with this medicine. Also, aspirin may lessen the effects of meclofenamate. Therefore, *do not take aspirin regularly or drink alcoholic beverages while taking this medicine,* unless otherwise directed by your doctor.

This medicine may cause some people to become dizzy. *Make sure you know how you react to this medicine before you drive, use machines, or do other jobs that require you to be alert.*

Side Effects of This Medicine
Along with its needed effects, a medicine may cause some unwanted effects. Although not all of these side effects appear very often, when they do occur they may require medical attention. Check with your doctor if any of the following side effects occur:

More common
  Hives
Less common

Ringing or buzzing in ears	Swelling of feet or lower legs
Skin rash or itching	Unusual weight gain

Rare

Bloody or black tarry stools	Unexplained sore throat and fever
Blurred vision or any change in vision	Unusual tiredness and weakness (with long-term use)

Other side effects may occur which usually do not require medical attention. These side effects may go away during treatment as your body adjusts to the medicine. However, check with your doctor if any of the following side effects continue or are bothersome:

More common

Diarrhea	Vomiting
Nausea	

Less common

Bloated feeling or gas	Irritation or soreness of mouth
Constipation	Loss of appetite
Dizziness	Stomach pain or burning in stomach
Headache	
Heartburn	

Other side effects not listed above may also occur in some patients. If you notice any other effects, check with your doctor.

MELPHALAN (Systemic)
A commonly used brand name is Alkeran.

Melphalan (MEL-fa-lan) belongs to the group of medicines called alkylating agents. It is used to treat some kinds of cancer as well as some noncancerous conditions. It is used also in some situations to reduce the body's natural immunity. Melphalan is available only with your doctor's prescription.

Before Using This Medicine
Melphalan is a very strong medicine. In addition to its helpful effects in treating your medical problem, it has side effects that could be very serious. Before you take this medicine, be sure that you have discussed the use of it with your doctor.

In order to decide on the best treatment for your medical problem, your doctor should be told:

—if you have ever had any unusual reaction to melphalan in the past.

—if you are pregnant or if you intend to have children. This medicine may cause birth defects if either the male or female is taking it at the time of conception or if it is taken during pregnancy. It may also cause permanent sterility after it has been taken for a while. Be sure that you have discussed this with your doctor before taking this medicine.

—if you are breast-feeding an infant. Although melphalan has not been shown to cause problems, the chance always exists.

—if you have any of the following medical problems:

Blood disease	Infection
Gout	Kidney disease
	Kidney stones

—if you are taking gout medicine.

—if you have been treated with x-rays or cancer drugs by another doctor.

Proper Use of This Medicine
Use this medicine only as directed by your doctor. Do not use more or less of it, do not use it more often, and do not use it for a longer period of time than your doctor ordered.

This medicine is sometimes given together with certain other medicines. If you are using a combination of drugs, make sure that you take each medicine at the proper time and do not mix them. Ask your doctor, nurse, or pharmacist to help you plan a way to remember to take your medicine at the right time.

This medicine may cause nausea, vomiting, and loss of appetite. However, it may have to be taken for several months to be effective. Even if you begin to feel ill, *do not stop using this medicine without first checking with your doctor.*

If you miss a dose of this medicine, do not take the missed dose at all and do not double the next one. Instead, go back to your regular dosing schedule and check with your doctor.

Precautions While Using This Medicine
It is very important that your doctor check your progress at regular visits.

While you are using this medicine, your doctor may want you to drink plenty of fluids and urinate often. This will help prevent kidney problems and keep your kidneys working well. If you have any questions about this, check with your doctor.

Side Effects of This Medicine
Along with its needed effects, a medicine may cause some unwanted effects. Although not all of these side effects appear very often, when they do occur they may require medical attention. Check with your doctor *immediately* if any of the following side effects occur:

More common

Black tarry stools	Unusual bleeding or
Unexplained fever, chills, or sore throat	bruising

Less common

Flank or stomach pain	Sores in the mouth and on the lips
Joint pain	Swelling of feet or lower legs

Other side effects may occur which usually do not require medical attention. These side effects may go away during treatment as your body adjusts to the medicine. However, check with your doctor if any of the following side effects continue or are bothersome:

More common

Nausea and
vomiting

Less common

Loss of hair

This medicine may cause a temporary loss of hair in some people. After treatment with melphalan has ended, normal hair growth should return.

After you stop using this medicine, it may still produce some side effects that need attention. During this period of time check with your doctor if you notice any of the following side effects:

Unexplained fever,   Unusual bleeding or
chills, or sore   bruising
throat

Other side effects not listed above may also occur in some patients. If you notice any other effects, check with your doctor.

MEPERIDINE (Systemic)
Some commonly used brand names are Demerol, Demer-Idine*, and Pethadol.

---

*Not available in the United States.

Meperidine (me-PER-i-deen) is a medicine used to relieve pain. Meperidine is available only with your doctor's prescription. Since prescriptions cannot be refilled, a new prescription must be obtained from your doctor each time you need this medicine.

Before Using This Medicine

In order to decide on the best treatment for your medical problem, your doctor should be told:

—if you have ever had any unusual reaction to meperidine in the past. This medicine should not be taken if you are allergic to it.

—if you are pregnant or if you intend to become pregnant while using this medicine. Although meperidine has not been shown to cause birth defects, the chance always exists.

—if you are breast-feeding an infant. Although meperidine has not been shown to cause problems, it passes into the breast milk and may cause unwanted side effects.

—if you have any of the following medical problems:

Brain disease or   Kidney disease
injury   Liver disease
Emphysema,   Underactive adrenal
asthma, or   gland (Addison's
chronic lung   disease)
disease   Underactive thyroid
Enlarged prostate or   Unusually slow or
problems with   irregular heart-
urination   beat
Gallbladder disease
or gallstones

—if you are now taking other central nervous system (CNS) depressants such as:

Antihistamines or   Sedatives, tran-
medicine for hay   quilizers,
fever, other   or sleeping
allergies,   medicine
or colds   Seizure medicine
Barbiturates   Tricyclic an-
Other narcotics   tidepressants
Other prescription   (medicine for
pain medicine   depression)

—if you are now taking prescription medicine for stomach cramps or spasms.

—if you are now taking or have taken within the past 2 weeks monoamine oxidase (MAO) inhibitors such as:

Isocarboxazid   Phenelzine
Pargyline   Tranylcypromine

Proper Use of This Medicine

Take this medicine only as directed by your doctor. Do not take more of it, do not take it more often, and do not take it for a longer period of time than your doctor ordered. If too much is taken, it may become habit-forming.

For patients taking the oral liquid form of this medicine:

• Unless otherwise directed by your doctor, take this medicine mixed with a half glass of water to lessen the numbing effect of the medicine on your mouth and throat.

Precautions While Using This Medicine

If you will be taking this medicine for a long period of time (for example, for several months at a time), your doctor should check your progress at regular visits.

This medicine will add to the effects of alcohol and other medicines (CNS depressants) that slow down the nervous system. Some examples of CNS depressants are antihistamines or medicine for hay fever, other allergies, or colds; sedatives, tranquilizers, or sleeping medicine; prescription pain medicine or narcotics; barbiturates; medicine for seizures; tricyclic antidepressants (medicine for depression); or anesthetics, including some dental anesthetics. *Check with your doctor before taking any of the above while you are using this medicine.*

This medicine may cause some people to become drowsy or less alert than they are normally. *Make sure you know how you react to this medicine before you drive, use machines, or do other jobs that require you to be alert.*

Dizziness, lightheadedness, or fainting may occur, especially when you get up from a lying or sitting position. Getting up slowly may help lessen this problem.

Nausea or vomiting may occur, especially after the first couple of doses. This effect usually goes away if you lie down for a while. However, if nausea or vomiting continues, check with your doctor.

Side Effects of This Medicine

Along with its needed effects, a medicine may cause some unwanted effects. Although not all of these side effects appear very often, when they do occur they may require medical attention. Check with your doctor if any of the following side effects occur:

Less common

Shortness of breath	Unusually slow
Troubled breathing	heartbeat

Other side effects may occur which usually do not require medical attention. These side effects may go away during treatment as your body adjusts to the medicine. However, check with your doctor if any of the following side effects continue or are bothersome:

More common

Dizziness	Redness or flushing
Drowsiness	of face
Feeling faint	Unusual increase in
Lightheadedness	sweating
Nausea or vomiting	

Less common

Blurred vision	Dry mouth
Constipation	Unusual tiredness or
Difficult urination	weakness
or frequent urge	Unusually fast or
to urinate	pounding heart-
	beat

Other side effects not listed above may also occur in some patients. If you notice any other effects, check with your doctor.

MEPROBAMATE (Systemic)

Some commonly used brand names are:

Equanil	Miltown
Lan-Dol*	Neo-Tran*
Medi-Tran*	Novo-Mepro*
Mep-E*	Quietal*
Meprospan	SK-Bamate
	Tranmap

*Not available in the United States.

Meprobamate (me-proe-BA-mate) is used to relieve nervousness or tension. It is available only with your doctor's prescription.

Before Using This Medicine

In order to decide on the best treatment for your medical problem, your doctor should be told:

—if you have ever had any unusual reaction to medicines like meprobamate such as carbromal, carisoprodol, mebutamate, or tybamate.

—if you are pregnant or if you intend to become pregnant while using this medicine. Meprobamate may cause birth defects if taken during the first 3 months of pregnancy.

—if you are breast-feeding an infant. Meprobamate passes into the breast milk and may cause drowsiness in infants of mothers taking this medicine.

—if you have any of the following medical problems:

Epilepsy	Liver disease
Kidney disease	Porphyria

—if you are now taking other central nervous system (CNS) depressants such as:

Antihistamines or	Other sedatives,
medicine for hay	tranquilizers, or
fever, other	sleeping medicine
allergies, or colds	Prescription pain
Barbiturates	medicine
Narcotics	Seizure medicine
	Tricyclic an-
	tidepressants
	(medicine for
	depression)

—if you are now taking or have taken within the past 2 weeks monoamine oxidase (MAO) inhibitors such as:

Isocarboxazid   Phenelzine
Pargyline   Tranylcypromine

Proper Use of This Medicine

Take this medicine only as directed by your doctor. Do not take more of it, do not take it more often, and do not take it for a longer period of time than your doctor ordered. If too much is taken, it may become habit-forming.

If you miss a dose of this medicine, and remember within an hour or so of the missed dose, take it right away. Then go back to your regular dosing schedule. But if you do not remember until later, do not take the missed dose at all and do not double the next one. Instead, go back to your regular dosing schedule. If you have any questions about this, check with your doctor.

Precautions While Using This Medicine

If you will be taking this medicine regularly for a long period of time:

• Your doctor should check your progress at regular visits.

• Check with your doctor at least every 4 months to make sure you need to continue taking this medicine.

If you will be taking this medicine in large doses or for a long period of time, do not stop taking it without first checking with your doctor. Your doctor may want you to reduce gradually the amount you are taking before stopping completely.

This medicine will add to the effects of alcohol and other medicines (CNS depressants) that slow down the nervous system. Some examples of CNS depressants are antihistamines or medicine for hay fever, other allergies, or colds; sedatives, tranquilizers, or sleeping medicine; prescription pain medicine or narcotics; barbiturates; medicine for seizures; tricyclic antidepressants (medicine for depression); or anesthetics, including some dental anesthetics. *Check with your doctor before taking any of the above while you are taking this medicine.*

If you think you may have taken an overdose, get emergency help at once. Taking an overdose of meprobamate or taking alcohol or other CNS depressants with meprobamate may lead to unconsciousness and possibly death. Some signs of an overdose are mental confusion, severe weakness, shortness of breath or troubled breathing, staggering, and unusually slow heartbeat.

This medicine may cause some people to become dizzy, lightheaded, drowsy, or less alert than they are normally. Even if taken at bedtime, it may cause some people to feel drowsy or less alert on arising. *Make sure you know how you react to this medicine before you drive, use machines, or do other jobs that require you to be alert.*

Side Effects of This Medicine

Along with its needed effects, a medicine may cause some unwanted effects. Although not all of these side effects appear very often, when they do occur they may require medical attention. Check with your doctor if any of the following side effects occur:

Less common

Skin rash, hives, or itching

Rare

Mental confusion	Unusually slow
Unexplained sore	heartbeat
throat and fever	Wheezing, shortness
Unusual bleeding or	of breath, or
bruising	troubled
Unusual excitement	breathing
Unusually fast,	
pounding, or	
irregular	
heartbeat	

Other side effects may occur which usually do not require medical attention. These side effects may go away during treatment as your body adjusts to the medicine. However, check with your doctor if any of the following side effects continue or are bothersome:

More common

Clumsiness or	Drowsiness
unsteadiness	

Less common

Blurred vision or	False sense of well-
change in near or	being
distant vision	Headache
Diarrhea	Nausea or vomiting
Dizziness or light-	Slurred speech
headedness	Unusual tiredness or
	weakness

After you stop using this medicine, your body may need time to adjust. If you took this medicine in high doses or for a long time, this may take about 2 days. During this period of time check with your doctor if you notice any of the following side effects:

Clumsiness or unsteadiness	Mental confusion
Convulsions or seizures	Muscle twitching
	Nausea or vomiting
Hallucinations (seeing, hearing, or feeling things that are not there)	Nightmares
	Trembling
	Trouble in sleeping
	Unusual nervousness or restlessness
Increased dreaming	

Other side effects not listed above may also occur in some patients. If you notice any other effects, check with your doctor.

MEPROBAMATE, ETHOHEPTAZINE, AND ASPIRIN (Systemic)

Some commonly used brand names are:

Equagesic	Mepro Compound
Heptogesic	Meprogesic

Meprobamate (me-proe-BA-mate), ethoheptazine (eth-oh-HEP-ta-zeen), and aspirin (AS-pir-in) combination is used to relieve pain, anxiety, and tension in certain disorders or diseases. This medicine is available only with your doctor's prescription.

Before Using This Medicine

In order to decide on the best treatment for your medical problem, your doctor should be told:

—if you have ever had any unusual reaction to aspirin or other salicylates including methyl salicylate (oil of wintergreen) or nonsteroidal anti-inflammatory agents (such as fenoprofen, ibuprofen, indomethacin, meclofenamate, naproxen, oxyphenbutazone, phenylbutazone, sulindac, or tolmetin); or to carbromal, carisoprodol, mebutamate, meprobamate, or tybamate.

—if you are pregnant or if you intend to become pregnant while using this medicine. Meprobamate (contained in this combination medicine) may cause birth defects if taken during the first 3 months of pregnancy. Too much use of aspirin (contained in this combination medicine) during the last 3 months of pregnancy may increase the length of pregnancy, prolong labor, and increase bleeding. Also, aspirin may cause the baby to have bleeding problems at birth if taken during the last 2 weeks of pregnancy. Although ethoheptazine (contained in this medicine) has not been shown to cause problems, the chance always exists.

—if you are breast-feeding an infant. Meprobamate (contained in this combination medicine) passes into the breast milk and may cause drowsiness in infants of mothers taking this medicine. Although aspirin and ethoheptazine (contained in this medicine) have not been shown to cause problems, the chance always exists.

—if you have any of the following medical problems:

Anemia	Hodgkin's disease
Asthma, allergies, and nasal polyps (history of)	Kidney disease
	Liver disease
	Porphyria
Epilepsy	Stomach ulcer or other stomach problems
Gout	
Hemophilia or other bleeding problems	

—if you are now taking other central nervous system (CNS) depressants such as:

Antihistamines or medicine for hay fever, other allergies, or colds	Sedatives, tranquilizers, or sleeping medicine
Barbiturates	Seizure medicine
Narcotics	Tricyclic antidepressants (medicine for depression)
Prescription pain medicine	

—if you are now taking or have taken within the past 2 weeks monoamine oxidase (MAO) inhibitors such as:

Isocarboxazid	Phenelzine
Pargyline	Tranylcypromine

—if you are now taking any of the following medicines or types of medicine:

Anticoagulants (blood thinners)	Oral hypoglycemics (diabetes medicine you take by mouth)
Inflammation medicine (for example, arthritis medicine)	Probenecid
	Spironolactone
Insulin	Sulfinpyrazone
Methotrexate	

Proper Use of This Medicine

Take this medicine only as directed by your doctor. Do not take more of it, do not take it more often, and do not take it for a longer period of time than your doctor ordered. If too much is taken, it may become habit-forming.

Keep this medicine out of the reach of children since overdose is very dangerous in children.

Do not use this medicine if it has a strong vinegar-like odor, since this means the aspirin is breaking down. If you have any questions about this, check with your doctor or pharmacist.

Precautions While Using This Medicine

If you will be taking this medicine regularly for a long period of time:

• Your doctor should check your progress at regular visits.

• Check with your doctor at least every 4 months to make sure you need to continue taking this medicine.

If you will be taking this medicine in large doses or for a long period of time, do not stop taking it without first checking with your doctor. Your doctor may want you to reduce gradually the amount you are taking before stopping completely.

Check the labels of all over-the-counter (OTC), nonprescription, and prescription medicines you now take. If any contain aspirin be especially careful, since taking them while taking this medicine may lead to overdose. If you have any questions about this, check with your doctor or pharmacist.

Stomach problems may be more likely to occur if you drink alcoholic beverages while being treated with this medicine, especially if you are taking it in high doses or for a long time. Check with your doctor if you have any questions about this.

This medicine will add to the effects of alcohol and other medicines (CNS depressants) that slow down the nervous system. Some examples of CNS depressants are antihistamines or medicine for hay fever, other allergies, or colds; sedatives, tranquilizers, or sleeping medicine; prescription pain medicine or narcotics; barbiturates; medicine for seizures; tricyclic antidepressants (medicine for depression); or anesthetics, including some dental anesthetics. *Check with your doctor before taking any of the above while you are taking this medicine.*

If you think you may have taken an overdose, get emergency help at once. Taking an overdose of meprobamate (contained in this combination medicine) or taking alcohol or other CNS depressants with the meprobamate may lead to unconsciousness and possibly death. Some signs of an overdose of meprobamate are mental confusion, severe weakness, shortness of breath or troubled breathing, staggering, and unusually slow heartbeat.

If you plan to have surgery, including dental surgery, do not take aspirin (contained in this combination medicine) for 5 days before the surgery, unless otherwise directed by your doctor. Taking aspirin during this time may cause bleeding problems.

This medicine may cause some people to become dizzy, drowsy, or less alert than they are normally. *Make sure you know how you react to this medicine before you drive, use machines, or do other jobs that require you to be alert.*

Side Effects of This Medicine

Along with its needed effects, a medicine may cause some unwanted effects. Although not all of these side effects appear very often, when they do occur they may require medical attention. Check with your doctor if any of the following side effects occur:

Rare

Skin rash, hives, or itching	Wheezing, shortness of breath,
Unexplained sore throat and fever	or tightness in chest
Unusual bleeding or bruising	

Possible signs of overdose

Blurred vision or change in near or distant vision	Ringing or buzzing in ears (continuing)
Clumsiness or unsteadiness	Severe or continuing headache
Mental confusion	Unusually slow heartbeat or troubled breathing
Rapid breathing	

Other side effects may occur which usually do not require medical attention. These side effects may go away during treatment as your body adjusts to the medicine. However, check with your doctor if any of the following side effects continue or are bothersome:

More common

Drowsiness	Stomach pain
Nausea or vomiting	

Less common

Dizziness

After you stop using this medicine, your body may need time to adjust. The length of time this takes depends on the amount of medicine you were using and how long you used it. During this period of time check with your doctor if you notice any of the following side effects:

Clumsiness or unsteadiness	Mental confusion
Convulsions or seizures	Muscle twitching
	Nausea or vomiting
Hallucinations (seeing, hearing, or feeling things that are not there)	Nightmares
	Trembling
	Trouble in sleeping
Increased dreaming	Unusual nervousness or restlessness

Other side effects not listed above may also occur in some patients. If you notice any other effects, check with your doctor.

MERCAPTOPURINE (Systemic)
A commonly used brand name is Purinethol.

Mercaptopurine (mer-kap-toe-PYOOR-een) belongs to the group of medicines known as antimetabolites. It is used to treat some kinds of cancer as well as some noncancerous conditions. It is used also in some situations to reduce the body's natural immunity. Mercaptopurine is available only with your doctor's prescription.

Before Using This Medicine
Mercaptopurine is a very strong medicine. In addition to its helpful effects in treating your medical problem, it has side effects that could be very serious. Before you take this medicine, be sure that you have discussed the use of it with your doctor.

In order to decide on the best treatment for your medical problem, your doctor should be told:

—if you have ever had any unusual reaction to mercaptopurine in the past.

—if you are pregnant or if you intend to have children. This medicine may cause birth defects if either the male or female is taking it at the time of conception or if it is taken during pregnancy. It may also cause permanent sterility after it has been taken for a while. Be sure that you have discussed this with your doctor before taking this medicine.

—if you are breast-feeding an infant. Although mercaptopurine has not been shown to cause problems, the chance always exists.

—if you have any of the following medical problems:

Alcoholism	Kidney disease
Blood disease	Kidney stones
Gout	Liver disease
Infection	

—if you are taking any of the following medicines or types of medicine:

Anticoagulants (blood thinners)	Gout medicine

—if you have been treated with x-rays or cancer drugs by another doctor.

Proper Use of This Medicine
Use this medicine only as directed by your doctor. Do not use more or less of it, and do not use it more often than your doctor ordered.

This medicine is often given together with certain other medicines. If you are using a combination of drugs, make sure that you take each medicine at the right time and do not mix them. Ask your doctor, nurse, or pharmacist to help you plan a way to remember to take your medicines at the right time.

Do not stop using this medicine without first checking with your doctor.

If you miss a dose of this medicine, do not take the missed dose at all and do not double the next one. Instead, go back to your regular dosing schedule and check with your doctor.

Precautions While Using This Medicine
It is very important that your doctor check your progress at regular visits.

While you are using this medicine, your doctor may want you to drink plenty of fluids and urinate often. This will help prevent kidney problems and keep your kidneys working well. If you have any questions about this, check with your doctor.

Avoid alcoholic beverages until you have discussed their use with your doctor. Alcohol may increase the harmful effects of this medicine.

Side Effects of This Medicine
Along with its needed effects, a medicine may cause some unwanted effects. Although not all of these side effects appear very often, when they do occur they may require medical attention. Check with your doctor *immediately* if any of the following side effects occur:

More common

Unexplained fever, chills, or sore throat	Yellowing of eyes and skin
Unusual bleeding or bruising	

Less common

Loss of appetite	Nausea and vomiting
Flank or stomach pain	Swelling of feet or lower legs
Joint pain	

Rare

Black tarry stools	Sores in the mouth and on the lips

Other side effects may occur which usually do not require medical attention. These side effects may go away during treatment as your body adjusts to the medicine. However, check with your doctor if any of the following side effects continue or are bothersome:

Less common

Darkening of skin	Headache
Diarrhea	Skin rash and
Fever	itching
	Weakness

Rare

Loss of hair

After you stop using this medicine, it may still produce some side effects that need attention. During this period of time check with your doctor if you notice any of the following side effects:

Unexplained fever, chills, or sore throat	Yellowing of eyes and skin
Unusual bleeding or bruising	

Other side effects not listed above may also occur in some patients. If you notice any other effects, check with your doctor.

MERCURY, AMMONIATED (Topical)

Ammoniated mercury (a-MOE-nee-ay-ted MER-kyoo-ree) is applied to the skin to treat psoriasis, minor skin infections, and other skin disorders. Some of these preparations are available only with your doctor's prescription. Others are available without a prescription; however, your doctor may have special instructions on the proper use of this medicine for your medical condition.

Before Using This Medicine

In order to decide on the best treatment for your medical problem, your doctor should be told:

—if you have ever had any unusual reaction to ammoniated mercury in the past. This medicine should not be used if you are allergic to it.

—if you are pregnant, if you intend to become pregnant, or if you are breast-feeding an infant, although ammoniated mercury has not been shown to cause problems.

—if you are now using any topical iodine-containing or sulfur-containing preparations.

Proper Use of This Medicine

It is very important that you use this medicine only as directed. Do not use more of it and do not use it more often than recommended on the label, unless otherwise directed by your doctor. To do so may increase the chance of absorption through the skin and the chance of mercury poisoning.

Apply enough ointment to cover the affected area, and rub in gently.

Do not use this medicine on deep or open wounds or serious burns.

Keep this medicine away from the eyes.

If you miss a dose of this medicine, apply it as soon as possible. Then go back to your regular dosing schedule. But if it is almost time for your next dose, do not apply the missed dose at all. Instead, go back to your regular dosing schedule. If you have any questions about this, check with your doctor or pharmacist.

Precautions While Using This Medicine

Do not use any topical iodine-containing preparations (for example, iodine solution, iodine tincture, or povidone-iodine) *on the same affected area as this medicine.* To do so may increase the possibility of side effects. If you have any questions about this, check with your doctor or pharmacist.

Do not use any sulfur-containing preparations on the same affected area as this medicine. To do so may cause a foul odor, be irritating to the skin, and stain the skin black. If you have any questions about this, check with your doctor or pharmacist.

Side Effects of This Medicine

Along with its needed effects, a medicine may cause some unwanted effects. Although not all of these side effects appear very often, when they do occur they may require medical attention. Check with your doctor or pharmacist if any of the following side effects occur:

Infection or irritation of skin not present before using this medicine

Possible signs of mercury poisoning

Cloudy urine	Irritation, soreness,
Continuing or	or swelling of
severe headache	gums
Dizziness	Nausea
	Skin rash or
	unusual redness
	of skin

Other side effects not listed above may also occur in some patients. If you notice any other effects, check with your doctor or pharmacist.

METAPROTERENOL (Systemic)

Some commonly used brand names are Alupent and Metaprel.

Metaproterenol (met-a-proe-TER-e-nole) is used in the treatment of bronchial asthma, bronchitis, and emphysema. It relieves wheezing, shortness of breath, and troubled breathing. This medicine is available only with your doctor's prescription.

Before Using This Medicine

In order to decide on the best treatment for your medical problem, your doctor should be told:

—if you have ever had any unusual reaction to medicines like metaproterenol such as amphetamines, ephedrine, epinephrine, isoproterenol, norepinephrine (levarterenol), phenylephrine, phenylpropanolamine, pseudoephedrine, or terbutaline.

—if you are pregnant, if you intend to become pregnant, or if you are breast-feeding an infant. Although metaproterenol has not been shown to cause problems in humans, the chance always exists.

—if you have any of the following medical problems:

Diabetes	High blood pressure
Heart or blood	Overactive thyroid
vessel disease	

—if you are now taking any of the following medicines or types of medicine:

Amphetamines	Propranolol
Other medicine	
for asthma or	
breathing prob-	
lems	

Proper Use of This Medicine

Use this medicine only as directed. Do not use more of it and do not use it more often than your doctor ordered. To do so may increase the chance of side effects.

If you are taking this medicine regularly (for example, every day) and you miss a dose, take it right away if you remember within an hour or so of the missed dose. Then go back to your regular dosing schedule. But if you do not remember until later, do not take the missed dose at all and do not double the next one. Instead, go back to your regular dosing schedule. If you have any questions about this, check with your doctor.

If you are using the inhalation form of this medicine:

• Some of these preparations may come with patient instructions. Read them carefully before using this medicine.

• If you are using this medicine in a nebulizer, make sure you understand exactly how to use it. If you have any questions about this, check with your doctor.

• If you are using the aerosol form of this medicine:

—save your applicator. Refill units of this medicine may be available.

—store away from heat and direct sunlight. Do not puncture, break, or burn container.

Precautions While Using This Medicine

If you still have trouble breathing after using this medicine, or if your condition gets worse, *check with your doctor at once.*

Side Effects of This Medicine

Along with its needed effects, a medicine may cause some unwanted effects. Although not all of these side effects appear very often, when they do occur they may require medical attention. Check with your doctor if either of the following side effects occurs:

Signs of overdose

Chest pain
Irregular heartbeat

Other side effects may occur which usually do not require medical attention. These side effects may go away during treatment as your body adjusts to the medicine. However, check with your doctor if any of the following side effects continue or are bothersome:

More common

Nervousness
Restlessness

Less common

Bad taste in mouth	Trembling
Dizziness or lightheadedness	Unusual increase in sweating
Headache	Unusually fast or pounding heart- beat
Muscle cramps in arms, hands, or legs	
Nausea or vomiting	Weakness

While using this medicine, you may notice a bad taste in your mouth. This may be expected and will go away when you stop using this medicine.

Other side effects not listed above may also occur in some patients. If you notice any other effects, check with your doctor.

METHADONE (Systemic)
Some commonly used brand names are Dolophine and Westadone.

Methadone (METH-a-done) is a medicine used to relieve pain. It is also used to help some people control their dependence on heroin or other narcotics. Methadone is available only with your doctor's prescription. Since prescriptions cannot be refilled, a new prescription must be obtained from your doctor each time you need this medicine. In addition, other rules and regulations may apply if methadone is being used to treat narcotic dependence.

Before Using This Medicine

In order to decide on the best treatment for your medical problem, your doctor should be told:

—if you have ever had any unusual reaction to methadone in the past. This medicine should not be taken if you are allergic to it.

—if you are pregnant or if you intend to become pregnant while using this medicine. Methadone may cause the unborn baby to become addicted to it. Also, it may cause breathing problems in the newborn infant.

—if you are breast-feeding an infant. Methadone passes into the breast milk and may cause dependence in the infant.

—if you have any of the following medical problems:

Brain disease or in- jury	Emphysema, asthma, or chronic lung disease
Colitis	

Enlarged prostate or problems with urination	Underactive adrenal gland (Addison's disease)
Gallbladder disease or gallstones	Underactive thyroid
Kidney disease	Unusually slow or irregular heart- beat
Liver disease	

—if you are now taking any of the following medicines or types of medicine:

Pentazocine	Rifampin
Phenytoin	Urine acidifiers (medicine to make your urine more acid)
Prescription medicine for stomach cramps or spasms	

—if you are now taking other central nervous system (CNS) depressants such as:

Antihistamines or medicine for hay fever, other aller- gies, or colds	Sedatives, tranqui- lizers, or sleeping medicine
Barbiturates	Seizure medicine
Other narcotics	Tricyclic antidepres- sants (medicine for depression)
Other prescription pain medicine	

—if you are now taking or have taken within the past 2 weeks monoamine oxidase (MAO) inhibitors such as:

Isocarboxazid	Phenelzine
Pargyline	Tranylcypromine

Proper Use of This Medicine

Keep this medicine out of the reach of children since overdose is especially dangerous in young children.

Take this medicine only as directed by your doctor. Do not take more of it, do not take it more often, and do not take it for a longer period of time than your doctor ordered. If too much is taken, it may become habit-forming.

For patients taking the oral liquid form of this medicine:

• *This medicine may have to be mixed with water before taking. Read the label carefully for directions.* If you have any questions, check with your pharmacist.

For patients taking the tablets for oral solution form of this medicine:

• *These tablets must be dissolved in water or fruit juice before taking. Read the label carefully for directions.* If you have any questions, check with your pharmacist.

Precautions While Using This Medicine

If you will be taking this medicine for a long period of time (for example, for several months at a time), your doctor should check your progress at regular visits.

This medicine will add to the effects of alcohol and other medicines (CNS depressants) that slow down the nervous system. Some examples of CNS depressants are antihistamines or medicine for hay fever, other allergies, or colds; sedatives, tranquilizers, or sleeping medicine; prescription pain medicine or narcotics; barbiturates; medicine for seizures; tricyclic antidepressants (medicine for depression); or anesthetics, including some dental anesthetics. *Check with your doctor before taking any of the above while you are using this medicine.*

This medicine may cause some people to become drowsy or less alert than they are normally. *Make sure you know how you react to this medicine before you drive, use machines, or do other jobs that require you to be alert.*

Dizziness, lightheadedness, or fainting may occur, especially when you get up from a lying or sitting position. Getting up slowly may help lessen this problem.

Nausea may occur, especially after the first couple of doses. This effect usually goes away if you lie down for a while. However, if nausea or vomiting continues, check with your doctor.

Side Effects of This Medicine

Along with its needed effects, a medicine may cause some unwanted effects. Although not all of these side effects appear very often, when they do occur they may require medical attention. Check with your doctor if any of the following side effects occur:

Shortness of breath	Unusually slow
Troubled breathing	heartbeat

Other side effects may occur which usually do not require medical attention. These side effects may go away during treatment as your body adjusts to the medicine. However, check with your doctor if any of the following side effects continue or are bothersome:

More common

Dizziness	Redness or flushing
Drowsiness	of face
Feeling faint	Unusual increase in
Lightheadedness	sweating
Nausea or	
vomiting	

Less common

Blurred vision	Loss of appetite
Constipation	Unusual tiredness or
Difficult urina-	weakness
tion or frequent	Unusually fast or
urge to urinate	pounding heart-
Dry mouth	beat

Other side effects not listed above may also occur in some patients. If you notice any other effects, check with your doctor.

METHAQUALONE (Systemic)

Some commonly used brand names are:

Mequelon*	Sedalone*
Mequin	Sopor
Parest	Triador*
Quaalude	Tualone*

*Not available in the United States.

Methaqualone (meth-A-kwa-lone) is used in the treatment of insomnia or sleeplessness. It helps patients fall asleep and stay asleep through the night. Also, it is used to help calm or relax patients who are nervous or tense. If used regularly (for example, every day) for insomnia, methaqualone is usually not effective for more than 2 weeks. This medicine is available only with your doctor's prescription. Since prescriptions cannot be refilled, a new prescription must be obtained from your doctor each time you need this medicine.

Before Using This Medicine

In order to decide on the best treatment for your medical problem, your doctor should be told:

—if you have ever had any unusual reaction to methaqulone in the past. This medicine should not be taken if you are allergic to it.

—if you are pregnant, if you intend to become pregnant, or if you are breast-feeding an infant. Although methaqualone has not been shown to cause problems in humans, the chance always exists.

—if you have liver disease.

—if you are now taking other central nervous system (CNS) depressants such as:

Antihistamines or	Barbiturates
medicine for hay	Narcotics
fever, other aller-	
gies, or colds	

Other sedatives, tranquilizers, or sleeping medicine	Seizure medicine Tricyclic antidepressants (medicine for depression)
Prescription pain medicine	

—if you are now taking or have taken within the past 2 weeks monoamine oxidase (MAO) inhibitors such as:

Isocarboxazid	Phenelzine
Pargyline	Tranylcypromine

Proper Use of This Medicine

Take this medicine only as directed by your doctor. Do not take more of it, do not take it more often, and do not take it for a longer period of time than your doctor ordered. If too much is taken, it may become habit-forming.

Keep this medicine out of the reach of children since overdose is especially dangerous in children.

If you miss a dose of this medicine, do not take the missed dose at all and do not double the next one. Instead, go back to your regular dosing schedule. If you have any questions about this, check with your doctor.

Precautions While Using This Medicine

If you will be taking this medicine regularly for a long period of time:

—your doctor should check your progress at regular visits.

—do not stop taking it without first checking with your doctor. Your doctor may want you to reduce gradually the amount you are taking before stopping completely.

This medicine will add to the effects of alcohol and other medicines (CNS depressants) that slow down the nervous system. Some examples of CNS depressants are antihistamines or medicine for hay fever, other allergies, or colds; sedatives, tranquilizers, or sleeping medicine; prescription pain medicine or narcotics; barbiturates; medicine for seizures; tricyclic antidepressants (medicine for depression); or anesthetics, including some dental anesthetics. *Check with your doctor before taking any of the above while you are taking this medicine.*

If you think you may have taken an overdose, get emergency help at once. Taking an overdose of methaqualone or taking alcohol or other CNS depressants with methaqualone may lead to unconsciousness and possibly death. Some signs of an overdose are mental confusion; severe weakness; shortness of breath or troubled breathing; staggering; unusually slow heartbeat, unusual excitement, nervousness, or restlessness; trembling; and seizures.

This medicine may cause some people to become dizzy, drowsy, or less alert than they are normally. Even if taken at bedtime, it may cause some people to feel drowsy or less alert on arising. *Make sure you know how you react to this medicine before you drive, use machines, or do other jobs that require you to be alert.*

Side Effects of This Medicine

Along with its needed effects, a medicine may cause some unwanted effects. Although not all of these side effects appear very often, when they do occur they may require medical attention. Check with your doctor if any of the following side effects occur:

Less common

Skin rash or hives	Unusual excitement, nervousness, or restlessness

Rare

Unusually slow heartbeat, shortness of breath, or troubled breathing

Other side effects may occur which usually do not require medical attention. These side effects may go away during treatment as your body adjusts to the medicine. However, check with your doctor if any of the following side effects continue or are bothersome:

More common

Diarrhea	Nausea
Dizziness	Stomach pain
Drowsiness (daytime)	Unusual tiredness or weakness
"Hangover" effect	Vomiting
Headache	

Less common

Numbness, tingling, pain, or weakness in hands or feet	Unusual sweating

After you stop using this medicine, your body may need time to adjust. The length of time this takes depends on the amount of medicine you were using and how long you used it. During this period of time check with your doctor if you notice any of the following side effects:

Convulsions or seizures	Nightmares
Hallucinations (seeing, hearing, or feeling things that are not there)	Stomach cramps
	Trembling
	Trouble in sleeping
	Unusual restlessness or nervousness
Increased dreaming	Unusual weakness
Mental confusion	
Nausea or vomiting	

Other side effects not listed above may also occur in some patients. If you notice any other effects, check with your doctor.

METHENAMINE (Systemic)

Some commonly used brand names are:	Generic names:
Hiprex	Methenamine Hippurate
Urex	
Mandelamine	Methenamine Mandelate
Methandine*	
Prov-U-Sep	
Sterine*	

*Not available in the United States.

Methenamine (meth-EN-a-meen) belongs to the general family of medicines called anti-infectives. It is given by mouth to help the body overcome infections of the urinary tract. Methenamine tablets are available without a prescription; however, your doctor may have special instructions on the proper use of this medicine for your medical problem. Methenamine hippurate (HIP-yoo-rate) and methenamine mandelate (MAN-de-late) are available only with your doctor's prescription.

Before Using This Medicine

In order to decide on the best treatment for your medical problem, your doctor should be told:

—if you have ever had any unusual reaction to methenamine. This medicine should not be taken if you are allergic to it.

—if you are pregnant, if you intend to become pregnant, or if you are breast-feeding an infant, although methenamine has not been shown to cause problems.

—if you have either of the following medical problems:
Kidney disease
Liver disease

—if you are now taking any of the following medicines or types of medicine:

Antacids	Sulfonamides (sulfa drugs)
Glaucoma medicine you take by mouth	Thiazide diuretics (water pills)

—if you are taking medicine to make your urine more alkaline such as:

Acetazolamide	Sodium citrate
Dichlorphenamide	Sodium citrate and citric acid
Ethoxzolamide	
Methazolamide	Sodium citrate, potassium citrate, and citric acid
Sodium bicarbonate (baking soda)	

Proper Use of This Medicine

If this medicine causes nausea or upset stomach, it may be taken after meals and at bedtime.

In order for this medicine to work well, your urine must be acid (pH 5.5 or below).

Before you start taking this medicine, check your urine with phenaphthazine paper or another test to see if it is acid. If you have any questions about this, check with your doctor or pharmacist.

The following changes in your diet may help make your urine more acid; however, check with your doctor first if you are on a special diet (for example, for diabetes). Avoid most fruits (especially citrus fruits and juices), milk and other dairy products, and other foods which make the urine more alkaline. Also, avoid antacids unless otherwise directed by your doctor. Eating more protein and foods such as cranberries (especially cranberry juice with vitamin C added), plums, or prunes may also help. If your urine is still not acid enough, check with your doctor.

If you are taking the dry granule form of this medicine:

• Dissolve the contents of each packet in 2 to 4 ounces of water immediately before taking. Stir well. Be sure to drink all the liquid in order to get the full dose of medicine.

If you are taking the oral liquid form of this medicine:

• Use a specially marked measuring spoon or other device to measure each dose accurately since the average household teaspoon may not hold the right amount of liquid.

If you are taking the enteric-coated tablet form of this medicine:

• Swallow tablets whole. Do not break, crush, or take if chipped.

To help clear up your infection completely, *keep taking this medicine for the full time of treatment* even if you begin to feel better after a few days; *do not miss any doses.*

If you do miss a dose of this medicine, take it as soon as possible. However, if it is almost time for your next dose and your dosing schedule is:

• 2 doses a day—Space the missed dose and the next dose 5 to 6 hours apart.

• 3 or more doses a day—Space the missed dose and the next dose 2 to 4 hours apart or double your next dose.

Then go back to your regular dosing schedule.

Precautions While Using This Medicine

If your symptoms do not improve within a few days or if they become worse, check with your doctor.

Side Effects of This Medicine

Along with its needed effects, a medicine may cause some unwanted effects. Although not all of these side effects appear very often, when they do occur they may require medical attention. Stop taking this medicine and check with your doctor if any of the following side effects occur:

Blood in urine	Pain or burning
Lower-back pain	while urinating

Other side effects may occur which usually do not require medical attention. These side effects may go away during treatment as your body adjusts to the medicine. However, check with your doctor if any of the following side effects continue or are bothersome:

Nausea	Rash
Painful or difficult urination	Stomach upset

Other side effects not listed above may also occur in some patients. If you notice any other effects, check with your doctor.

METHOCARBAMOL (Systemic)

Some commonly used brand names are:

Delaxin	Robamol
Forbaxin	Robaxin
Marbaxin-750	Spinaxin
Metho-500	Tumol

Methocarbamol (meth-oh-KAR-ba-mole) is a medicine that is used to help relax certain muscles in your body and relieve the pain and discomfort caused by strains, sprains, or other injury to your muscles. This medicine is available only with your doctor's prescription.

Before Using This Medicine

In order to decide on the best treatment for your medical problem, your doctor should be told:

—if you have ever had any unusual reaction to methocarbamol in the past. This medicine should not be taken if you are allergic to it.

—if you are pregnant, if you intend to become pregnant, or if you are breast-feeding an infant. Although methocarbamol has not been shown to cause problems, the chance always exists.

—if you are now taking other central nervous system (CNS) depressants such as:

Antihistamines or medicine for hay fever, other allergies, or colds	Sedatives, tranquilizers, or sleeping medicine
Barbiturates	Seizure medicine
Narcotics	Tricyclic antidepressants
Prescription pain medicine	(medicine for depression)

—if you are now taking or have taken within the past 2 weeks monoamine oxidase (MAO) inhibitors such as:

Isocarboxazid	Phenelzine
Pargyline	Tranylcypromine

Proper Use of This Medicine

If you miss a dose of this medicine and remember within an hour or so of the missed dose, take it right away. Then go back to your regular dosing schedule. But if you do not remember until later, do not take the missed dose at all and do not double the next one. Instead, go back to your regular dosing schedule. If you have any questions about this, check with your doctor.

Precautions While Using This Medicine

This medicine will add to the effects of alcohol and other medicines (CNS depressants) that slow down the nervous system. Some examples of CNS depressants are antihistamines or medicine for hay fever, other allergies, or colds; sedatives, tranquilizers, or sleeping medicine; prescription pain medicine or narcotics; barbiturates; medicine for seizures; tricyclic antidepressants (medicine for depression); or anesthetics, including some dental anesthetics. *Check with your doctor before taking any of the above while you are using this medicine.*

This medicine may cause some people to become drowsy, dizzy, lightheaded, or less alert than they are normally. *Make sure you know how you react to this medicine before you drive, use machines, or do other jobs that require you to be alert.*

Side Effects of This Medicine

Along with its needed effects, a medicine may cause some unwanted effects. Although not all of these side effects appear very often, when they do occur they may require medical attention. Check with your doctor if any of the following side effects occur:

Less common

Itching or skin rash	Stuffy nose and red or bloodshot eyes

Other side effects may occur which usually do not require medical attention. These side effects may go away during treatment as your body adjusts to the medicine. However, check with your doctor if any of the following side effects continue or are bothersome:

More common

Blurred or double vision	Drowsiness
Dizziness	Lightheadedness

Less common

Fever	Nausea
Headache	

Other side effects not listed above may also occur in some patients. If you notice any other effects, check with your doctor.

METHOTREXATE (Systemic)
A commonly used brand name is Mexate.

Methotrexate (meth-o-TREX-ate) belongs to the group of medicines known as antimetabolites. It is used to treat some kinds of cancer. It is also used to treat some medical conditions that are not cancerous, such as psoriasis. Methotrexate is available only with your doctor's prescription.

Before Using This Medicine

Methotrexate is a very strong medicine. In addition to its helpful effects in treating your medical problem, it has side effects that could be very serious. Before you take this medicine, be sure that you have discussed the use of it with your doctor.

In order to decide on the best treatment for your medical problem, your doctor should be told:

—if you have ever had any unusual reaction to methotrexate in the past. This medicine should not be taken if you are allergic to it.

—if you are pregnant or if you intend to have children. This medicine may cause birth defects if either the male or female is taking it at the time of conception or if it is taken during pregnancy. It may also cause permanent sterility after it has been taken for a while. Be sure that you have discussed this with your doctor before taking this medicine.

—if you are breast-feeding an infant. Although methotrexate has not been shown to cause problems, the chance always exists.

—if you have any of the following medical problems:

Alcoholism	Kidney disease
Blood disease	Kidney stones
Colitis	Liver disease
Gout	Stomach ulcer
Infection	

—if you are now taking any of the following medicines or types of medicine:

Aspirin or other salicylates	Probenecid
Gout medicine	Pyrimethamine
Phenylbutazone	Sulfonamides (sulfa drugs)

—if you have been treated with x-rays or cancer drugs by another doctor.

Proper Use of This Medicine

Use this medicine only as directed by your doctor. Do not use more or less of it, and do not use it more often than your doctor ordered.

This medicine is often given together with certain other medicines. If you are using a combination of drugs, make sure that you take each medicine at the proper time and do not mix them. Ask your doctor, nurse, or pharmacist to help you plan a way to remember to take your medicines at the right time.

This medicine commonly causes nausea, vomiting, and loss of appetite. Even if you begin to feel ill, *do not stop using this medicine without first checking with your doctor.*

If you miss a dose of this medicine, do not take the missed dose at all and do not double the next one. Instead, go back to your regular dosing schedule and check with your doctor.

Precautions While Using This Medicine

It is very important that your doctor check your progress at regular visits.

While you are using this medicine, your doctor may want you to drink plenty of fluids and urinate often. This will help prevent kidney problems and keep your kidneys working well. If you have any questions about this, check with your doctor.

Do not drink alcohol while using this medicine. Alcohol can increase the risk of liver problems. If you have any questions about this, check with your doctor.

When you begin to take this medicine, avoid too much sun or use of a sunlamp since you may become more sensitive to sunlight than usual. In case of a severe burn, check with your doctor. This is especially important if you are taking this medicine for psoriasis because sunlight can make the psoriasis worse.

Do not take aspirin (ASA) or any other preparations containing aspirin or salicylate compounds without first checking with your doctor. These medicines may increase the effects of methotrexate on your body.

Side Effects of This Medicine

Along with its needed effects, a medicine may cause some unwanted effects. Although not all of these side effects appear very often, when they do occur they may require medical attention. Check with your doctor if any of the following side effects occur:

More common

Black tarry stools	Stomach pain
Bloody vomit	Unexplained fever,
Diarrhea	chills, or sore
Sores in the mouth	throat
and on the lips	Unusual bleeding or
	bruising

Less common

Blood in urine	Mental confusion
Blurred vision	Shortness of breath
Convulsions or	Swelling of feet
seizures	or lower legs
Cough	Unusual tiredness or
Dark urine	weakness
Dizziness	Yellowing of eyes
Drowsiness	and skin
Headache	
Joint pain	

Other side effects may occur which usually do not require medical attention. These side effects may go away during treatment as your body adjusts to the medicine. However, check with your doctor if any of the following side effects continue or are bothersome:

More common

Loss of appetite
Nausea and
vomiting

Less common

Acne	Pale skin
Boils	Reddening of skin
Loss of hair	Skin rash or itching

Rare

Bone pain

This medicine may cause a temporary loss of hair in some people. After treatment with methotrexate has ended, normal hair growth should return.

After you stop using this medicine, it may still produce some side effects that need attention. During this period of time check with your doctor if you notice any of the following side effects:

Blurred vision	Headache
Convulsions or	Mental confusion
seizures	Unusual tiredness or
Dizziness	weakness
Drowsiness	

Other side effects not listed above may also occur in some patients. If you notice any other effects, check with your doctor.

METHOXSALEN (Systemic)
A commonly used brand name is Oxsoralen.

Methoxsalen (meth-OX-a-len) belongs to the group of medicines called psoralens. It is used along with ultraviolet light (found in sunlight and some special lamps) in a treatment called PUVA to treat vitiligo, a disease in which skin color is lost. Methoxsalen may also be used for other conditions as determined by your doctor. It is available only with your doctor's prescription.

Before Using This Medicine

Methoxsalen is a very strong medicine. In addition to causing serious sunburns if not properly used, in animals it has been reported to increase the chance of skin cancer and cataracts. Therefore, methoxsalen should be used only as directed and it should *not* be used simply for suntanning. Before using this medicine, be sure that you have discussed the use of it with your doctor.

In order to decide on the best treatment for your medical problem, your doctor should be told:

—if you have ever had any unusual reaction to methoxsalen in the past. This medicine should not be taken if you are allergic to it.

—if you are pregnant, if you intend to become pregnant, or if you are breast-feeding an infant. Although methoxsalen has not been shown to cause problems, the chance always exists.

—if you have any of the following medical problems:

Acute lupus   Liver disease
   erythematosus   Other skin condi-
Allergy to sunlight   tions
Infection   Stomach problems

—if you are now using any other medicine that increases the sensitivity of your skin to sunlight (check with your doctor or pharmacist to see if any of the medicines you are using can cause this effect).

—if you have recently had x-ray treatment.

Proper Use of This Medicine

Do not increase the amount of methoxsalen you are taking or spend extra time in the sunlight or under an ultraviolet lamp. This will not make the medicine act any more quickly and may result in a serious burn.

If this medicine upsets your stomach, it may be taken with meals or milk.

If you are late in taking or miss taking a dose of this medicine, take it as soon as you remember. However, remember that exposure to sunlight or ultraviolet light must take place 2 to 4 hours *after* taking the medicine or it won't work. If you don't remember until the next day, do not take the missed dose at all and do not double the next one. Instead, go back to your regular dosing schedule. If you have any questions about this, check with your doctor.

Precautions While Using This Medicine

Your doctor should check your progress at regular visits.

This medicine increases the sensitivity of your skin to sunlight; too much exposure could cause a serious burn. If you must go out in the sunlight, *cover your skin for at least 24 hours before and 8 hours following treatment.* A special sunscreening lotion may also help.

During and after treatment with sunlight or an ultraviolet lamp, *your eyes should be protected with special sunglasses;* your doctor will tell you what kind to use. *Protect your lips with a special lipstick to block sunlight.*

When taken with certain foods, methoxsalen may cause a serious reaction. To prevent such reactions, avoid eating limes, figs, parsley, parsnips, mustard, carrots, and celery while you are being treated with this medicine.

Side Effects of This Medicine

Along with its needed effects, a medicine may cause some unwanted effects. Although not all of these side effects appear very often, when they do occur they may require medical attention. Check with your doctor *immediately* if any of the following side effects occur since they may indicate a serious burn:

Blistering and peel-   Swelling, especially
   ing of skin   in feet or lower
Reddened, sore skin   legs

Other side effects may occur which usually do not require medical attention. These side effects may go away during treatment as your body adjusts to the medicine. However, check with your doctor if any of the following side effects continue or are bothersome:

More common

Dizziness   Mental depression
Headache   Nausea
Inability to sleep   Nervousness
Itching of skin

Other side effects not listed above may also occur in some patients. If you notice any other effects, check with your doctor.

METHOXSALEN (Topical)

Methoxsalen (meth-OX-a-len) belongs to the group of medicines called psoralens. It is used on the skin along with ultraviolet light (found in sunlight and some special lamps) in a treatment called PUVA to treat vitiligo, a disease in which skin color is lost. Methoxsalen may also be used for other conditions as determined by your doctor. It is available only with a prescription and is to be administered by or under the direct supervision of your doctor.

Before Using This Medicine

Methoxsalen is a very strong medicine. In addition to causing serious sunburns if not properly used, in animals it has been reported to increase the chance of skin cancer and cataracts. Therefore, methoxsalen should be used only as directed and it should *not* be used simply for suntanning. Before using this medicine, be sure that you have discussed the use of it with your doctor.

In order to decide on the best treatment for your medical problem, your doctor should be told:

—if you have ever had any unusual reaction to methoxsalen in the past. This medicine should not be used if you are allergic to it.

—if you are pregnant, if you intend to become pregnant, or if you are breast-feeding an infant. Although methoxsalen has not been shown to cause problems, the chance always exists.

—if you have any of the following medical problems:

Acute lupus erythematosus	Infection Other skin condi-
Allergy to sunlight	tions
	Stomach problems

—if you are now using any other medicine that increases the sensitivity of your skin to sunlight (check with your doctor or pharmacist to see if any of the medicines you are using can cause this effect).

—if you have recently had x-ray treatment.

Precautions While Using This Medicine

It is important that you visit your doctor as directed for treatments and so that your progress can be checked.

This medicine increases the sensitivity of your skin to sunlight; too much exposure could cause a serious burn. If you must go out in the sunlight, *cover the treated areas of your skin for at least 12 to 48 hours following treatment.* A special sunscreening lotion may also help.

During and after treatment with sunlight or an ultraviolet lamp, *your eyes should be protected with special sunglasses;* your doctor will tell you what kind to use. *Protect your lips with a special lipstick to block sunlight.*

When used with certain foods, methoxsalen may cause a serious reaction. To prevent such reactions, avoid eating limes, figs, parsley, parsnips, mustard, carrots, and celery while you are being treated with this medicine.

Side Effects of This Medicine

Along with its needed effects, a medicine may cause some unwanted effects. Although not all of these side effects appear very often, when they do occur they may require medical atten-

tion. Check with your doctor *immediately* if any of the following side effects occur since they may indicate a serious burn:

Blistering and peeling of skin	Swelling, especially in the feet or
Reddened, sore skin	lower legs

Other side effects not listed above may also occur in some patients. If you notice any other effects, check with your doctor.

METHYLDOPA (Systemic)
Some commonly used brand names are:

Aldomet	Medimet-250*
Dopamet*	Novomedopa*

*Not available in the United States.

Methyldopa (meth-ill-DOE-pa) belongs to the general class of medicines called antihypertensives. It is used to treat high blood pressure. Methyldopa is available only with your doctor's prescription.

Before Using This Medicine

In order to decide on the best treatment for your medical problem, your doctor should be told:

—if you have ever had any unusual reaction to methyldopa in the past. This medicine should not be taken if you are allergic to it.

—if you are pregnant, if you intend to become pregnant, or if you are breast-feeding an infant. Although methyldopa has not been shown to cause problems, the chance always exists.

—if you have any of the following medical problems:

Angina (chest pain)	Liver disease
Heart disease	Mental depression
Kidney disease	(history of)
	Pheochromocytoma
	(PCC)

—if you have taken methyldopa in the past and developed liver problems.

—if you are now taking any of the following medicines or types of medicine:

Levodopa	Other antihyperten-
Methotrimeprazine	sives (high blood
	pressure
	medicine)

—if you are now taking or have taken within the past 2 weeks monoamine oxidase (MAO) inhibitors such as:

Isocarboxazid	Phenelzine
Pargyline	Tranylcypromine

Proper Use of This Medicine

Importance of Diet—When prescribing medicine for your condition, your doctor may also prescribe a personal diet for you. Such a diet may be low in sodium (salt). Medicine is usually more effective when this diet is properly followed.

Also, it may be very important for you to go on a reducing diet. However, check with your doctor before going on any diet.

Many patients who have high blood pressure will not notice any signs of the problem. In fact, many may feel normal. It is very important that you take your medicine exactly as directed and that you keep your doctor's appointments even if you feel well.

Remember that methyldopa will not cure your high blood pressure but it does control it. Therefore, you must continue to take it as directed if you expect to keep your blood pressure down. *You may have to take medicine for the rest of your life.* If high blood pressure is not treated, it can cause serious problems such as heart failure, blood vessel disease, stroke, or kidney disease.

In order to help remember to take your medicine, try to get into the habit of taking it at the same time each day.

If you miss a dose of this medicine, take it as soon as possible. If it is almost time for your next dose, do not take the missed dose at all and do not double the next one. Instead, go back to your regular dosing schedule. If you have any questions about this, check with your doctor.

Precautions While Using This Medicine

It is important that your doctor check your progress at regular visits.

If you have a fever and there seems to be no reason for it, check with your doctor. This is especially important during the first few weeks you take methyldopa.

Before having any kind of surgery (including dental surgery), make sure the doctor or dentist in charge knows that you are taking this medicine.

Methyldopa may cause some people to become drowsy or less alert than they are normally.

This is more likely to happen when you begin to take it or when you increase the amount of medicine you are taking. *Make sure you know how you react to this medicine before you drive, use machines, or do other jobs that require you to be alert.*

Dizziness, lightheadedness, or fainting may occur, especially when you get up from a lying or sitting position. Getting up slowly may help but if the problem continues or gets worse, check with your doctor.

Do not take other medicines unless they have been discussed with your doctor. This especially includes over-the-counter (nonprescription) medicines for appetite control, asthma, colds, cough, hay fever, or sinus, since they may tend to increase your blood pressure.

Side Effects of This Medicine

Along with its needed effects, a medicine may cause some unwanted effects. Although not all of these side effects appear very often, when they do occur they may require medical attention. Check with your doctor if any of the following side effects occur:

More common

Swelling of feet
or lower legs

Less common

Inability to sleep	Unexplained fever
Mental depression	shortly after start-
or anxiety	ing to take this
Nightmares or	medicine
unusually vivid	
dreams	

Rare

Continuing tiredness	Severe stomach pain
or weakness	with nausea and
after having	vomiting
taken this	Shakiness or
medicine for	unusual
several weeks	body movements
Dark or amber	Unexplained sore
urine	throat and fever
Fever, chills,	Unusual bleeding or
troubled breath-	bruising
ing, and unusual-	Yellowing of eyes
ly fast heartbeat	and skin
Pale stools	
Severe or continuing	
diarrhea or	
stomach cramps	

Other side effects may occur which usually do not require medical attention. These side effects may go away during treatment as your body

adjusts to the medicine. However, check with your doctor if any of the following side effects continue or are bothersome:

More common

Drowsiness	Headache
Dry mouth	

Less common

Decreased sexual	Numbness, tingling,
ability	pain, or weakness
Diarrhea	in hands or feet
Dizziness or light-	Skin rash
headedness when	Stuffy nose
getting up from	Swelling of the
a lying or	breasts
sitting position	Unusually slow
Fainting	heartbeat
Nausea or vomiting	

Other side effects not listed above may also occur in some patients. If you notice any other effects, check with your doctor.

METHYLDOPA AND THIAZIDE DIURETICS
(Systemic)

This information applies to the following medicines:

Methyldopa (meth-ill-DOE-pa) and Chlorothiazide (klor-oh-THYE-a-zide)
Methyldopa and Hydrochlorothiazide (hye-droe-klor-oh-THYE-a-zide)

Some commonly used brand names are:	Generic names:
Aldoclor	Methyldopa and Chlorothiazide
Aldoril	Methyldopa and Hydrochlorothiazide

This medicine is a combination which is used in the treatment of high blood pressure. It is available only with your doctor's prescription.

Before Using This Medicine

In order to decide on the best treatment for your medical problem, your doctor should be told:

—if you are allergic to sulfonamides (sulfa drugs) or other thiazide diuretics (water pills). This medicine should not be taken if you are allergic to it.

—if you are pregnant or if you intend to become pregnant while using this medicine. When this medicine is used during pregnancy,

it may cause side effects in the newborn infant. In addition, although this medicine has not been shown to cause birth defects, the chance always exists.

—if you are breast-feeding an infant. Although this medicine has not been shown to cause problems, the chance always exists.

—if you have any of the following medical problems:

Diabetes	Mental depression
Gout	(history of)
History of lupus	Pancreas disease
erythematosus	Pheochromocytoma
Kidney disease	(PCC)
Liver disease	

—if you have taken methyldopa in the past and developed liver problems.

—if you are now taking any of the following medicines or types of medicine:

Colestipol	Gout medicine
Corticosteroids	Levodopa
(cortisone-like	Lithium
medicines)	Methenamine
Corticotropin	Methotrimeprazine
(ACTH)	Oral anticoagulants
Diabetes medicine	(blood thinners
Digitalis glycosides	you take by
(heart medicine)	mouth)
Diuretics (water	
pills) or other	
antihypertensives	
(high blood	
pressure	
medicine)	

—if you are now taking or have taken within the past 2 weeks monoamine oxidase (MAO) inhibitors such as:

Isocarboxazid	Phenelzine
Pargyline	Tranylcypromine

Proper Use of This Medicine

Importance of Diet—When prescribing medicine for your condition, your doctor may also prescribe a personal diet for you. Such a diet may be low in sodium (salt). Medicine is usually more effective when this diet is properly followed.

Also, it may be very important for you to go on a reducing diet. However, check with your doctor before going on any diet.

Many patients who have high blood pressure will not notice any signs of the problem. In fact, many may feel normal. It is very important that you take your medicine exactly as directed and that you keep your doctor's appointments even if you feel well.

Remember that this medicine will not cure your high blood pressure but it does control it. Therefore, you must continue to take it as directed if you expect to keep your blood pressure down. *You may have to take medicine for the rest of your life.* If high blood pressure is not treated, it can cause serious problems such as heart failure, blood vessel disease, stroke, or kidney disease.

This medicine may cause you to have an unusual feeling of tiredness when you begin to take it. You may also notice an increase in the amount of urine or in your frequency of urination. After taking the medicine for a while, these effects should lessen. In general, in order to keep the increase in urine from affecting your sleep:

• If you are to take a single dose a day, take it in the morning after breakfast.

• If you are to take more than one dose a day, take the last dose no later than 6 p.m., unless otherwise directed by your doctor.

• However, it is best to plan your dose or doses according to a schedule that will least affect your personal activities and sleep. Ask your doctor, nurse, or pharmacist to help you plan the best time to take this medicine.

In order to help remember to take your medicine, try to get into the habit of taking it at the same time each day.

If you miss a dose of this medicine, take it as soon as possible. If it is almost time for your next dose, do not take the missed dose at all and do not double the next one. Instead, go back to your regular dosing schedule. If you have any questions about this, check with your doctor.

Precautions While Using This Medicine

It is important that your doctor check your progress at regular visits.

This medicine may cause a loss of potassium from your body:

• To help prevent this, your doctor may want you to:

—eat or drink foods that have a high potassium content (for example, orange or other citrus fruit juices), or

—take a potassium supplement, or

—take another medicine to help prevent the loss of the potassium in the first place.

• It is very important to follow these directions. Also, it is important not to change your diet on your own. This is more important if you are already on a special diet (as for diabetes), or if you are taking a potassium supplement or a medicine to reduce potassium loss. Extra potassium may not be necessary and, in some cases, too much potassium could be harmful.

Check with your doctor if you become sick and have severe or continuing vomiting or diarrhea. These problems may cause you to lose additional water and potassium.

Caution: Diabetics—This medicine may raise blood sugar levels. While you are using this medicine, be especially careful in testing for sugar in your urine. If you have any questions about this, check with your doctor.

A few people who take this medicine may become more sensitive to sunlight than they are normally. When you begin to take this medicine, avoid too much sun or use of a sunlamp until you see how you react, especially if you tend to burn easily. If you have a severe reaction, check with your doctor.

If you have a fever and there seems to be no reason for it, check with your doctor. This is especially important during the first few weeks you take methyldopa.

Do not take other medicines unless they have been discussed with your doctor. This especially includes over-the-counter (nonprescription) medicines for appetite control, asthma, colds, cough, hay fever, or sinus, since they may tend to increase your blood pressure.

Before having any kind of surgery (including dental surgery), make sure the doctor or dentist in charge knows that you are taking this medicine.

This medicine may cause some people to become drowsy or less alert than they are normally. This is more likely to happen when you begin to take it or when you increase the amount of medicine you are taking. *Make sure you know how you react to this medicine before you drive, use machines, or do other jobs that require you to be alert.*

Dizziness, lightheadedness, or fainting may occur, especially when you get up from a lying or sitting position. Getting up slowly may help but if the problem continues or gets worse, check with your doctor.

The dizziness, lightheadedness, or fainting is also more likely to occur if you drink alcohol, stand for long periods of time, exercise, or if the weather is hot. Drinking alcoholic beverages may also make the drowsiness worse. *While* you are taking this medicine, be careful in the amount of alcohol you drink. Also, use extra care during exercise or hot weather or if you must stand for long periods of time. Check with your doctor if you have any questions about this.

Side Effects of This Medicine

Along with its needed effects, a medicine may cause some unwanted effects. Although not all of these side effects appear very often, when they do occur they may require medical attention. *Check with your doctor if any of the following side effects occur especially since some of them may mean that your body is losing too much potassium:*

Signs of too much potassium loss

Dryness of mouth	Nausea or vomiting
Increased thirst	Unusual tiredness or
Irregular heartbeats	weakness
Muscle cramps or	Weak pulse
pain	

Less common

Inability to sleep	Nightmares or
Mental depression	unusually vivid
or anxiety	dreams

Rare

Continuing tiredness	Shakiness or
or weakness after	unusual body
having taken	movements
this medicine	Skin rash or hives
for several weeks	Unexplained sore
Fever, chills, troub-	throat and fever
led breathing, and	Unexplained fever
unusually fast	shortly after start-
heartbeat	ing to take
Joint pain	this medicine
Severe or continuing	Unusual bleeding or
diarrhea or	bruising
stomach cramps	Yellowing of eyes
Severe stomach pain	and skin
with nausea and	
vomiting	

Other side effects may occur which usually do not require medical attention. These side effects may go away during treatment as your body adjusts to the medicine. However, check with your doctor if any of the following side effects continue or are bothersome:

More common

Dizziness or light-	Drowsiness
headedness when	Headache
getting up from	Stuffy nose
a lying or	
sitting position	

Less common

Decreased sexual	Numbness, tingling,
ability	pain, or weakness
Diarrhea	in hands or feet
Fainting	Skin rash
Increased sensitivity	Swelling of the
to sunlight	breasts
Loss of appetite	Unusually slow
	heartbeat

Other side effects not listed above may also occur in some patients. If you notice any other effects, check with your doctor.

METHYLPHENIDATE (Systemic)

Some commonly used brand names are Methidate* and Ritalin.

---

*Not available in the United States.

Methylphenidate (meth-ill-FEN-i-date) belongs to the group of medicines called central stimulants. It is used to treat behavior problems in children. Also, it is used in the treatment of narcolepsy (uncontrolled desire for sleep or sudden attacks of sleep at irregular intervals). Sometimes it is used in the treatment of mild mental depression. This medicine is available only with your doctor's prescription. Since prescriptions cannot be refilled, a new prescription must be obtained from your doctor each time you need this medicine.

Before Using This Medicine

In order to decide on the best treatment for your medical problem, your doctor should be told:

—if you have ever had any unusual reaction to methylphenidate in the past. This medicine should not be taken if you are allergic to it.

—if you are pregnant, if you intend to become pregnant, or if you are breast-feeding an infant. Although methylphenidate has not been shown to cause problems, the chance always exists.

—if you have any of the following medical problems:

Epilepsy	High blood pressure
Glaucoma	Severe anxiety, ten-
	sion, or depres-
	sion

—if you are now taking any of the following medicines or types of medicine:

Coumarin-type anti-coagulants (blood thinners)	Medicine for seizures
Guanethidine	Phenylbutazone
Medicine for asthma or breathing problems (for example, ephedrine, epinephrine, isoproterenol, phenylephrine)	Tricyclic antidepressants (medicine for depression)

—if you are now taking or have taken within the past 2 weeks monoamine oxidase (MAO) inhibitors such as:

Isocarboxazid	Phenelzine
Pargyline	Tranylcypromine

Proper Use of This Medicine

Take this medicine only as directed by your doctor. Do not take more of it, do not take it more often, and do not take it for a longer period of time than your doctor ordered. If too much is taken, it may become habit-forming.

To help prevent trouble in sleeping, take the last dose of this medicine for each day before 6 p.m. unless otherwise directed by your doctor.

If you miss a dose of this medicine and remember within an hour or so of the missed dose, take it right away. Then go back to your regular dosing schedule. But if you do not remember until later, do not take the missed dose at all and do not double the next one. Instead, go back to your regular dosing schedule. If you have any questions about this, check with your doctor.

Precautions While Using This Medicine

Your doctor should check your progress at regular visits in order to make sure that this medicine does not cause unwanted effects.

If you will be taking this medicine in large doses for a long period of time, do not stop taking it without first checking with your doctor. Your doctor may want you to reduce gradually the amount you are taking before stopping completely.

This medicine may cause some people to become dizzy or less alert than they are normally. *Make sure you know how you react to this medicine*

before you drive, use machines, or do other jobs that require you to be alert.

Side Effects of This Medicine

Along with its needed effects, a medicine may cause some unwanted effects. Although not all of these side effects appear very often, when they do occur they may require medical attention. Check with your doctor if any of the following side effects occur:

Less common

Chest pain	Unexplained fever
Joint pain	Unusual bruising
Skin rash or hives	Unusually fast, pounding, or irregular heart-beat
Uncontrolled movements of the body	

Rare

Blurred vision or any change in vision	Unexplained sore throat and fever
Convulsions or seizures	Unusual tiredness or weakness
Mood or mental changes	

Other side effects may occur which usually do not require medical attention. These side effects may go away during treatment as your body adjusts to the medicine. However, check with your doctor if any of the following side effects continue or are bothersome:

More common

Loss of appetite	Trouble in sleeping
Nervousness	

Less common

Dizziness	Nausea
Drowsiness	Stomach pain
Headache	Unusual weight loss (with long-term use)

After you stop using this medicine, your body may need time to adjust. The length of time this takes depends on the amount of medicine you were using and how long you used it. During this period of time check with your doctor if you notice any of the following side effects:

Mental depression	Unusual tiredness or weakness
Unusual behavior	

Other side effects not listed above may also occur in some patients. If you notice any other effects, check with your doctor.

METHYPRYLON (Systemic)
A commonly used brand name is Noludar.

Methyprylon (meth-i-PRYE-lon) is used in the treatment of insomnia or sleeplessness. It helps patients fall asleep and stay asleep through the night. However, if used regularly (for example, every day), methyprylon may not be effective for more than 1 week. This medicine is available only with your doctor's prescription.

Before Using This Medicine
In order to decide on the best treatment for your medical problem, your doctor should be told:

—if you have ever had any unusual reaction to methyprylon in the past. This medicine should not be taken if you are allergic to it.

—if you are pregnant or if you intend to become pregnant while using this medicine. Although methyprylon has not been shown to cause problems, the chance always exists.

—if you are breast-feeding an infant. Methyprylon passes into the breast milk and may cause unwanted effects in infants of mothers taking this medicine.

—if you have any of the following medical problems:

| Kidney disease | Porphyria |
| Liver disease | |

—if you are now taking other central nervous system (CNS) depressants such as:

Antihistamines or medicine for hay fever, other allergies, or colds	Other sedatives, tranquilizers, or sleeping medicine
Barbiturates	Prescription pain medicine
Narcotics	Seizure medicine
	Tricyclic antidepressants (medicine for depression)

—if you are now taking or have taken within the past 2 weeks monoamine oxidase (MAO) inhibitors such as:

| Isocarboxazid | Phenelzine |
| Pargyline | Tranylcypromine |

Proper Use of This Medicine
Take this medicine only as directed by your doctor. Do not take more of it, do not take it more often, and do not take it for a longer period of time than your doctor ordered. If too much is taken, it may become habit-forming.

Keep this medicine out of the reach of children since overdose is especially dangerous in children.

Precautions While Using This Medicine
If you will be taking this medicine regularly for a long period of time:

—your doctor should check your progress at regular visits.

—do not stop taking it without first checking with your doctor. Your doctor may want you to reduce gradually the amount you are taking before stopping completely.

This medicine will add to the effects of alcohol and other medicines (CNS depressants) that slow down the nervous system. Some examples of CNS depressants are antihistamines or medicine for hay fever, other allergies, or colds; sedatives, tranquilizers, or sleeping medicine; prescription pain medicine or narcotics; barbiturates; medicine for seizures; tricyclic antidepressants (medicine for depression); or anesthetics, including some dental anesthetics. *Check with your doctor before taking any of the above while you are using this medicine.*

If you think you may have taken an overdose, get emergency help at once. Taking an overdose of methyprylon or taking alcohol or other CNS depressants with methyprylon may lead to unconsciousness and possibly death. Some signs of an overdose are mental confusion, severe weakness, shortness of breath or troubled breathing, staggering, and unusually slow heartbeat.

This medicine may cause some people to become dizzy, drowsy, or less alert than they are normally. Even if taken at bedtime, it may cause some people to feel drowsy or less alert on arising. *Make sure you know how you react to this medicine before you drive, use machines, or do other jobs that require you to be alert.*

Side Effects of This Medicine
Along with its needed effects, a medicine may cause some unwanted effects. Although not all of these side effects appear very often, when they do occur they may require medical attention. Check with your doctor if any of the following side effects occur:

Less common

Skin rash
Unusual excitement

Rare

Ulcers or sores in mouth or throat (continuing)	Unusually slow heartbeat, short-ness of breath,
Unusual bleeding or bruising	or troubled breathing

Other side effects may occur which usually do not require medical attention. These side effects may go away during treatment as your body adjusts to the medicine. However, check with your doctor if any of the following side effects continue or are bothersome:

More common

Dizziness	Headache
Drowsiness (daytime)	

Less common

Diarrhea	Vomiting
Nausea	

After you stop using this medicine, your body may need time to adjust. The length of time this takes depends on the amount of medicine you were using and how long you used it. During this period of time check with your doctor if you notice any of the following side effects:

Convulsions or seizures	Nightmares
	Stomach cramps
Hallucinations (see-ing, hearing, or feeling things that are not there)	Trembling
	Trouble in sleeping
	Unusual restlessness or nervousness
Increased dreaming	Unusual sweating
Mental confusion	Unusual weakness
Nausea or vomiting	

Other side effects not listed above may also occur in some patients. If you notice any other ef-fects, check with your doctor.

METHYSERGIDE (Systemic)
A commonly used brand name is Sansert.

Methysergide (meth-i-SER-jide) is a medicine used to prevent migraine headaches and some kinds of throbbing headaches. It is not used to treat an attack once it has started. This medicine is available only with your doctor's prescription.

Before Using This Medicine

In order to decide on the best treatment for your medical problem, your doctor should be told:

—if you have ever had any unusual reaction to methysergide or other ergot medicines in the past. This medicine should not be taken if you are allergic to it.

—if you are pregnant or if you intend to become pregnant while using this medicine. Too much use of it during pregnancy may cause unwanted effects in the baby. Be sure that you have discussed this with your doctor before taking this medicine. In addition, although this medicine has not been shown to cause birth defects, the chance always exists.

—if you are breast-feeding an infant. This medicine passes into the breast milk and may cause unwanted effects in infants of mothers taking large doses of it. Be sure you have discussed this with your doctor before taking this medicine.

—if you have any of the following medical problems:

Angina	Kidney disease
Arthritis	Liver disease
Hardening of the arteries	Lung disease
	Problems with veins
Heart disease	Severe itching
High blood pressure	Stomach ulcer
Infection	

—if you ever take ergotamine or a medicine containing ergotamine for your migraine at-tacks.

Proper Use of This Medicine

Take this medicine only as directed by your doctor. If the amount you are to take does not relieve your headache, do not take more than your doctor ordered. Instead, check with your doctor. Taking too much of this medicine or taking it too frequently may cause serious ef-fects such as nausea and vomiting; cold, pain-ful hands or feet; or even gangrene.

If this medicine upsets your stomach, it may be taken with meals or milk. If stomach upset continues or is severe, check with your doctor.

If you miss a dose of this medicine, do not take the missed dose at all and do not double the next one. Instead, go back to your regular dosing schedule. If you have any questions about this, check with your doctor.

Precautions While Using This Medicine

If you have been taking this medicine regularly, *do not stop taking it without first checking with your doctor.* Your doctor may want you to reduce gradually the amount you are using before stopping completely. If you stop taking it suddenly, your headaches may return or worsen.

This medicine may cause some people to become dizzy, lightheaded, drowsy, or less alert than they are normally. Even if taken at bedtime, it may cause some people to feel drowsy or less alert on arising. *Make sure you know how you react to this medicine before you drive, use machines, or do other jobs that require you to be alert.*

If dizziness occurs, get up slowly after lying or sitting down. If the problem continues or gets worse, check with your doctor.

Since drinking alcoholic beverages may make headaches worse, it is best to avoid alcohol while you are suffering from them. If you have any questions about this, check with your doctor.

Since smoking may increase some of the harmful effects of this medicine, it is best to avoid smoking while you are using it. If you have any questions about this, check with your doctor.

Avoid prolonged exposure to very cold temperatures while you are using this medicine, since cold may increase the harmful effects of the medicine.

If you have an infection or illness of any kind, check with your doctor before taking this medicine, since you may be more sensitive to the effects of it.

Your doctor will tell you how long you should take this medicine. Usually it is not taken for longer than 6 months at a time. *If the doctor tells you to stop taking the medicine for a while, do not continue to take it.* If your body does not get a rest from the medicine, it can have harmful effects.

Side Effects of This Medicine
Along with its needed effects, a medicine may cause some unwanted effects. Although not all of these side effects appear very often, when they do occur they may require medical attention. Check with your doctor *immediately* if any of the following side effects occur:

Chest pain	Loss of appetite or
Difficult or painful	weight loss
urination	Pale or cold hands
Extreme thirst	or feet
Fever	Shortness of breath
Flank or groin pain	Swelling of hands
Leg cramps or	or ankles
lower back pain	

Check with your doctor also if the following side effects occur:

More common

Itching	Weakness in the
Numbness and	legs
tingling of	
fingers, toes, or	
face	

Less common or rare

Anxiety or ner-	Hallucinations (see-
vousness	ing, hearing, or
Changes in vision	feeling things that
Clumsiness	are not there)
Excitement or dif-	Nightmares
ficulty in	Unusually rapid or
thinking	slow heartbeat
Feeling of being	
outside the body	

Other side effects may occur which usually do not require medical attention. These side effects may go away during treatment as your body adjusts to the medicine. However, check with your doctor if any of the following side effects continue or are bothersome:

More common

Diarrhea	Drowsiness
Dizziness or	Nausea and
lighthead-	vomiting
edness, especially	
when getting up	
from a lying or	
sitting position	

Rare

Loss of hair
Weight gain

After you stop using this medicine, your body may need time to adjust. The length of time this takes depends on the amount of medicine you were using and how long you used it. During this period of time check with your doctor if your headaches begin again or worsen.

Other side effects not listed above may also occur in some patients. If you notice any other effects, check with your doctor.

METRONIDAZOLE (Systemic)
Some commonly used brand names are:

Flagyl	Novonidazole*
Neo-Tric*	Trikacide*

*Not available in the United States.

Metronidazole (me-troe-NI-da-zole) belongs to the group of medicines called antiprotozoals. Although sometimes used to treat other types of infection, it is probably used most often to treat infections of the genital-urinary tract. This medicine is available only with your doctor's prescription.

Before Using This Medicine

Metronidazole has been shown to cause tumors (some possibly cancerous) in animals. Before you take this medicine, be sure that you have discussed the use of it with your doctor.

In order to decide on the best treatment for your medical problem, your doctor should be told:

—if you have ever had any unusual reaction to metronidazole in the past. This medicine should not be taken if you are allergic to it.

—if you are pregnant, if you intend to become pregnant, or if you are breast-feeding an infant. Although metronidazole has not been shown to cause problems in humans, the chance always exists.

—if you have either of the following medical problems:

Blood disease or
 a history of
 blood disease

Central nervous
 system (CNS)
 disease

—if you are now taking any of the following medicines or types of medicine:

Anticoagulants
 (blood thinners)

Disulfiram

Proper Use of This Medicine

To help clear up your infection completely, *keep taking this medicine for the full time of treatment* even if you begin to feel better after a few days; *do not miss any doses.*

If you do miss a dose of this medicine, take it as soon as possible. Then go back to your regular dosing schedule. If you do not remember the missed dose until it is almost time for your next one, do not take the missed dose at all and do not double the next one. Instead, go back to your regular dosing schedule. If you have any questions about this, check with your doctor.

If this medicine upsets your stomach, it may be taken with meals or food. If stomach upset (nausea, vomiting, stomach pain, or diarrhea) continues, check with your doctor.

If you are taking this medicine for a genital infection, your sexual partner should also be treated since the infection may be spread to another person during intercourse. If your partner is not being treated or if you have any questions about this, check with your doctor.

Precautions While Using This Medicine

Your doctor should check your progress at regular visits.

If your symptoms do not improve within a few days or if they become worse, check with your doctor.

Drinking alcoholic beverages while taking this medicine may cause stomach pain, nausea, vomiting, headache, or flushing or redness of the face. *When you begin taking this medicine, be especially careful in the amount of alcohol you drink until you see how you react.* If you have any questions about this, check with your doctor.

Side Effects of This Medicine

Along with its needed effects, a medicine may cause some unwanted effects. Although not all of these side effects appear very often, when they do occur they may require medical attention. Check with your doctor if any of the following side effects occur:

Less common

Any irritation, dis-
 charge, or dryness
 of vagina not
 present before
 using this
 medicine
Irritation or sore-
 ness of mouth
 or tongue

Skin rash, hives,
 or itching
Unexplained sore
 throat and
 fever
White furry growth
 on tongue

Rare

Clumsiness or
 unsteadiness
Mood or
 mental changes

Numbness, tingling,
 pain, or weakness
 in hands or feet
 (with high doses)
Seizures (with
 high doses)

Other side effects may occur which usually do not require medical attention. These side effects may go away during treatment as your body adjusts to the medicine. However, check with your doctor if any of the following side effects continue or are bothersome:

More common

Diarrhea
Loss of appetite
Nausea

Stomach pain or
 cramps
Vomiting

Less common

Constipation
Dizziness or
 lightheadedness
Dryness of mouth

Headache
Unpleasant or sharp
 metallic taste
 in mouth
Unusual tiredness
 or weakness

Rare

Darkening of urine

Metronidazole may cause darkening of the urine. This is only temporary and will go away when you stop taking this medicine.

Other side effects not listed above may also occur in some patients. If you notice any other effects, check with your doctor.

METYROSINE (Systemic)
A commonly used brand name is Demser.

Metyrosine (me-TYE-roe-seen) belongs to the general class of medicines called antihypertensives. It is used to treat high blood pressure due to a disease called pheochromocytoma. It is also sometimes used to treat certain other medical problems. Metyrosine is available only with your doctor's prescription.

Before Using This Medicine

In order to decide on the best treatment for your medical problem, your doctor should be told:

—if you have ever had any unusual reaction to metyrosine in the past.

—if you are pregnant, if you intend to become pregnant, or if you are breast-feeding an infant. Although metyrosine has not been shown to cause problems, the chance always exists.

—if you have any of the following medical problems:

Kidney disease	Mental depression
Liver disease	(or history of)
	Parkinson's disease

—if you are now taking any of the following medicines or types of medicine:

Haloperidol	Phenothiazines
Levodopa	

—if you are now taking central nervous system (CNS) depressants such as:

Antihistamines or medicine for hay fever, other allergies, or colds	Prescription pain medicine
	Sedatives, tranquilizers, or sleeping medicine
Barbiturates	Seizure medicine
Narcotics	Tricyclic antidepressants (medicine for depression)

Proper Use of This Medicine

Take this medicine only as directed by your doctor. Do not take more or less of it than your doctor ordered.

In order to help remember to take your medicine, try to get into the habit of taking it at the same times each day.

If you miss a dose of this medicine, take it as soon as possible. If it is almost time for your next dose, do not take the missed dose at all and do not double the next one. Instead, go back to your regular dosing schedule. If you have any questions about this, check with your doctor.

Precautions While Using This Medicine

It is important that your doctor check your progress at regular visits.

While using this medicine, it is important that you drink plenty of fluids and urinate often. This will help prevent kidney problems and keep your kidneys working well. If you have any questions about how much you should drink, check with your doctor.

This medicine will add to the effects of alcohol and other medicines (CNS depressants) that slow down the nervous system. Some examples of CNS depressants are antihistamines or medicine for hay fever, other allergies, or colds; sedatives, tranquilizers, or sleeping medicine; prescription pain medicine or narcotics; barbiturates; medicine for seizures; tricyclic antidepressants (medicine for depression); or anesthetics, including some dental anesthetics. *Check with your doctor before taking any of the above while you are using this medicine.*

This medicine may cause most people to become drowsy or less alert than they are normally. *Make sure you know how you react to this medicine before you drive, use machines, or do other jobs that require you to be alert.*

Before having any kind of surgery (including dental surgery), make sure that the doctor or dentist in charge knows that you are using this medicine.

Side Effects of This Medicine

Along with its needed effects, a medicine may cause some unwanted effects. Although not all of these side effects appear very often, when they do occur they may require medical attention. Check with your doctor if any of the following side effects occur:

More common

Diarrhea	Drooling
Difficulty in speaking	Trembling and shaking of hands and fingers

Less common

Anxiety	Mental confusion
Hallucinations (see-	Mental depression
ing, hearing, or	
feeling things that	
are not there)	

Rare

Blood in urine	Skin rash and
Muscle spasms,	itching
especially of	Swelling of feet
neck and back	or lower legs
Painful urination	Tic-like (jerky)
Restlessness	movements of
Shortness of breath	head, face,
Shuffling walk	mouth, and neck
	Unusual decrease in
	urination

Other side effects may occur which usually do not require medical attention. These side effects may go away during treatment as your body adjusts to the medicine. However, check with your doctor if the following side effect continues or is bothersome:

More common

Drowsiness

After you stop using this medicine, it may still produce some side effects that need attention. During this period of time check with your doctor if you notice the following side effect:

Diarrhea

Also, after you stop using this medicine, you may have feelings of increased energy or you may have trouble in sleeping. However, these effects should last only for two or three days.

Other side effects not listed above may also occur in some patients. If you notice any other effects, check with your doctor.

MICONAZOLE (Systemic)
A commonly used brand name is Monistat.

Miconazole (mi-KON-a-zole) belongs to the group of medicines called antifungals. It is given by injection to treat certain fungal infections. This medicine is available only with your doctor's prescription.

Before Using This Medicine

In order to decide on the best treatment for your medical problem, your doctor should be told:

—if you have ever had any unusual reaction to miconazole in the past. This medicine should not be used if you are allergic to it.

—if you are pregnant, if you intend to become pregnant, or if you are breast-feeding an infant. Although miconazole has not been shown to cause problems, the chance always exists.

—if you are now taking coumarin-type anticoagulants (blood thinners).

Side Effects of This Medicine

Along with its needed effects, a medicine may cause some unwanted effects. Although not all of these side effects appear very often, when they do occur they may require medical attention. Check with your doctor if any of the following side effects occur:

More common

Fever and chills	Skin rash or itching
Redness, swelling,	
or pain at place	
of injection	

Less common or rare

Unusual bleeding or	Wheezing or trou-
bruising	bled breathing
Unusual tiredness or	
weakness	

Other side effects may occur which usually do not require medical attention. These side effects may go away during treatment as your body adjusts to the medicine. However, check with your doctor if any of the following side effects continue or are bothersome:

More common

Nausea
Vomiting

Less common

Diarrhea	Flushing or redness
Drowsiness	of face or skin
	Loss of appetite

Other side effects not listed above may also occur in some patients. If you notice any other effects, check with your doctor.

MICONAZOLE (Topical)
A commonly used brand name is Micatin.

Miconazole (mi-KON-a-zole) belongs to the group of medicines called antifungals. Topical miconazole is applied to the skin to treat some types of fungal infections. This medicine is available only with your doctor's prescription.

Before Using This Medicine

In order to decide on the best treatment for your medical problem, your doctor should be told:

—if you have ever had any unusual reaction to miconazole in the past. This medicine should not be used if you are allergic to it.

—if you are pregnant, if you intend to become pregnant, or if you are breast-feeding an infant, although miconazole is not absorbed into the body and has not been shown to cause problems.

Proper Use of This Medicine

To help clear up your infection completely, *keep using this medicine for the full time of treatment* even though your condition may have improved.

Apply enough miconazole to cover the affected area, and rub in gently.

Keep this medicine away from the eyes.

When miconazole is used to treat certain types of fungal infections of the skin, an occlusive dressing or airtight covering (for example, kitchen plastic wrap) should *not* be applied over this medicine. To do so may cause irritation of the skin. *Do not apply an occlusive dressing over this medicine unless you have been directed to do so by your doctor.*

If you miss a dose of this medicine, apply it as soon as possible. Then go back to your regular dosing schedule. But if it is almost time for your next dose, do not apply the missed dose at all. Instead, go back to your regular dosing schedule. If you have any questions about this, check with your doctor.

Precautions While Using This Medicine

If your skin problem has not improved after you have used miconazole for 4 weeks, check with your doctor.

To help cure the infection and to help prevent reinfection, good health habits are required. These include the following:

• Wash all towels and bedding after each use.

• Use only freshly laundered clothes each time clothing is changed.

If you have any questions about this, check with your doctor, nurse, or pharmacist.

Side Effects of This Medicine

Along with its needed effects, a medicine may cause some unwanted effects. Although not all of these side effects appear very often, when they do occur they may require medical attention. Check with your doctor if any of the following side effects occur:

Skin rash, blistering, burning, redness, or other sign of skin irritation not present before using this medicine

Other side effects not listed above may also occur in some patients. If you notice any other effects, check with your doctor.

MICONAZOLE (Vaginal)
A commonly used brand name is Monistat.

Miconazole (mi-KON-a-zole) belongs to the group of medicines called antifungals. Vaginal miconazole is used to treat fungal infections of the vagina. This medicine is available only with your doctor's prescription.

Before Using This Medicine

In order to decide on the best treatment for your medical problem, your doctor should be told:

—if you have ever had any unusual reaction to miconazole in the past. This medicine should not be used if you are allergic to it.

—if you are pregnant, if you intend to become pregnant, or if you are breast-feeding an infant. Although only a small amount of miconazole is absorbed into the body and has not been shown to cause problems, the chance always exists.

Proper Use of This Medicine

Miconazole usually comes with patient directions. Read them carefully before using this medicine.

Use this medicine at bedtime, unless otherwise directed by your doctor.

To help clear up your infection completely, *keep using this medicine for the full time of treatment* even though your condition may have improved. Also, keep using this medicine even if you begin to menstruate or if you have intercourse during the time of treatment.

If you miss a dose of this medicine, insert it as soon as possible. Then go back to your regular dosing schedule. But if you do not remember the missed dose until the next day, do not insert the missed dose at all. Instead, go back to your regular dosing schedule. If you have any questions about this, check with your doctor.

Precautions While Using This Medicine

To help cure the infection and to help prevent reinfection, good health habits are required. These include the following:

• Wear cotton panties (or panties or pantyhose with cotton crotches) instead of synthetic (for example, nylon, rayon) underclothes.

• Wear freshly laundered underclothes.

If you have any questions about this, check with your doctor, nurse, or pharmacist.

If you have any questions about douching during the time of treatment with this medicine, check with your doctor.

Since there may be some vaginal drainage while you are using this medicine, a sanitary napkin may be worn to protect your clothing.

Side Effects of This Medicine

Along with its needed effects, a medicine may cause some unwanted effects. Although not all of these side effects appear very often, when they do occur they may require medical attention. Check with your doctor if any of the following side effects occur:

More common

Vaginal burning, itching, or irritation not present before using this medicine

Rare

Skin rash or hives

Other side effects may occur which usually do not require medical attention. These side effects may go away during treatment as your body adjusts to the medicine. However, check with your doctor if any of the following side effects continue or are bothersome:

Less common or rare

Headache

Pelvic cramps

Other side effects not listed above may also occur in some patients. If you notice any other effects, check with your doctor.

MINOXIDIL (Systemic)
A commonly used brand name is Loniten.

Minoxidil (mi-NOX-i-dill) belongs to the general class of medicines called antihypertensives. It is used to treat high blood pressure. Minoxidil is available only with your doctor's prescription.

Before Using This Medicine

Minoxidil is a very strong medicine. In addition to its helpful effects in treating your medical problem, it has side effects that could be very bothersome. Before you take this medicine, be sure that you have discussed the use of it with your doctor.

In order to decide on the best treatment for your medical problem, your doctor should be told:

—if you have ever had any unusual reaction to minoxidil in the past. This medicine should not be taken if you are allergic to it.

—if you are pregnant, if you intend to become pregnant, or if you are breast-feeding an infant. Although minoxidil has not been shown to cause problems, the chance always exists.

—if you have any of the following medical problems:

Angina	Kidney disease
Heart or blood vessel disease	

—if you have recently had a heart attack or stroke.

—if you are now taking diuretics (water pills) or other antihypertensives (high blood pressure medicine).

Proper Use of This Medicine

Importance of Diet—When prescribing medicine for your condition, your doctor may also prescribe a personal diet for you. Such a diet may be low in sodium (salt). Medicine is usually more effective when this diet is properly followed.

Also, it may be very important for you to go on a reducing diet. However, check with your doctor before going on any diet.

Many patients who have high blood pressure will not notice any signs of the problem. In fact, many may feel normal. It is very important that you take your medicine exactly as directed and that you keep your doctor's appointments even if you feel well.

Remember that minoxidil will not cure your high blood pressure but it does control it. Therefore, you must continue to take it as directed if you expect to keep your blood pressure down. *You may have to take medicine for the rest of your life.* If high blood pressure is not treated, it can cause serious problems such as heart failure, blood vessel disease, stroke, or kidney disease.

In order to help remember to take your medicine, try to get into the habit of taking it at the same time each day.

This medicine is usually given together with certain other medicines. If you are using a combination of drugs, make sure that you take each medicine at the proper time and do not mix them. Ask your doctor, nurse, or pharmacist to help you plan a way to remember to take your medicines at the right time.

If you miss a dose of this medicine and remember it within a few hours, take it when you remember. However, if you do not remember until the next day, do not take the missed dose at all and do not double the next one. Instead, go back to your regular dosing schedule. If you have any questions about this, check with your doctor.

Precautions While Using This Medicine

It is important that your doctor check your progress at regular visits.

Do not take other medicines unless they have been discussed with your doctor. This especially includes over-the-counter (nonprescription) medicines for appetite control, asthma, colds, cough, hay fever, or sinus, since they may tend to increase your blood pressure.

Side Effects of This Medicine

Along with its needed effects, a medicine may cause some unwanted effects. Although not all of these side effects appear very often, when they do occur they may require medical attention. Check with your doctor if any of the following side effects occur:

More common

Bloating	Swelling of feet or
Flushing or redness	lower legs
of skin	Unusually rapid
Rapid or irregular	weight gain of
heartbeat	more than 5
	pounds (2 pounds
	in
	children)

Less common

Chest pains	Shortness of breath
Numbness or tingl-	
ing of hands,	
feet, or face	

Rare

Skin rash and
itching

Other side effects may occur which usually do not require medical attention. These side effects may go away during treatment as your body adjusts to the medicine. However, check with your doctor if any of the following side effects continue or are bothersome:

More common

Increase in hair growth, usually on face, arms, and back

Rare

Breast tenderness
Headache

This medicine causes a temporary increase in hair growth in most people. Hair may grow longer and darker in both men and women. This may first be noticed on the face several weeks after you start taking minoxidil. Later, new hair growth may be noticed on the back, arms, legs, and scalp. Talk to your doctor about shaving or using a hair remover during this time. After treatment with minoxidil has ended, the hair will stop growing, although it may take several months for the new hair growth to go away.

Other side effects not listed above may also occur in some patients. If you notice any other effects, check with your doctor.

MITHRAMYCIN (Systemic)
A commonly used brand name is Mithracin.

Mithramycin (mith-ra-MYE-sin) belongs to the group of medicines known as antineoplastics. It is given by injection to treat certain types of cancer. It is also used to treat hypercalcemia (too much calcium in the blood). This medicine is available only with a prescription and is to be administered by or under the immediate care of your doctor.

Before Using This Medicine

Mithramycin is a very strong medicine. In addition to its helpful effects in treating your medical problem, it has side effects that could be very serious. Before you receive this medicine, be sure that you have discussed the use of it with your doctor.

In order to decide on the best treatment for your medical problem, your doctor should be told:

—if you have ever had any unusual reaction to mithramycin in the past. This medicine should not be used if you are allergic to it.

—if you are pregnant, if you intend to become pregnant, or if you are breast-feeding an infant. Although mithramycin has not been shown to cause problems, the chance always exists.

—if you have any of the following medical problems:

Bleeding problems	Kidney disease
Blood disease	Liver disease

—if you are now taking any of the following medicines or types of medicine:

Acetaminophen	Cephaloridine
Aminoglycoside	Cephalothin
antibiotics (such	Cisplatin
as amikacin,	Dipyridamole
gentamicin,	Ethacrynic acid
kanamycin,	Furosemide
streptomycin,	Isoniazid
tobramycin)	Methotrexate
Amphotericin B	Polymyxin B
Aspirin or	Rifampin
medicines con-	Sulfinpyrazone
taining aspirin	Vancomycin
Capreomycin	

—if you are now taking bone marrow depressants such as:

Anticancer	Oxyphenbutazone
medicines	Penicillamine
Colchicine	Phenylbutazone
Gold compounds	

Proper Use of This Medicine

This medicine sometimes causes nausea, vomiting, and loss of appetite. However, it is very important that you continue to receive the medicine, even if you begin to feel ill. If you have any questions about this, check with your doctor.

Precautions While Using This Medicine

It is very important that your doctor check your progress at regular visits in order to make sure that this medicine does not cause unwanted effects.

Side Effects of This Medicine

Along with its needed effects, a medicine may cause some unwanted effects. Although not all of these side effects appear very often, when they do occur they may require medical attention. Check with your doctor if any of the following side effects occur:

Possible signs of overdose

Bloody or black	Unexplained
tarry stools	nosebleed
Flushing or redness	Unexplained sore
or swelling of	throat and fever
face	Unusual bleeding or
Skin rash or small	bruising
red spots on skin	Vomiting of blood

Other side effects may occur which usually do not require medical attention. These side effects may go away during treatment as your body adjusts to the medicine. However, check with your doctor if any of the following side effects continue or are bothersome:

More common

Diarrhea	Loss of appetite
Irritation or	
soreness of	
mouth	

May occur 1 to 2 hours after the injection is started and continue for 12 to 24 hours

Nausea or vomiting

Less common

Drowsiness	Pain, redness,
Fever	soreness, or swell-
Headache	ing at place of
Mental depression	injection
	Unusual tiredness or
	weakness

After you stop using this medicine, it may still produce some side effects that need attention. During this period of time check with your doctor if you notice any of the following side effects:

Bloody or black	Unexplained sore
tarry stools	throat and fever
Small red spots	Unusual bleeding or
on skin	bruising
Unexplained	Vomiting of blood
nosebleed	

Other side effects not listed above may also occur in some patients. If you notice any other effects, check with your doctor.

MITOMYCIN (Systemic)
A commonly used brand name is Mutamycin.

Mitomycin (mye-toe-MYE-sin) belongs to the group of medicines known as antineoplastics. It is used by injection to treat some kinds of cancer. Mitomycin is available only on prescription and is to be administered only by or under the immediate supervision of your doctor.

Before Using This Medicine

Mitomycin is a very strong medicine. In addition to its helpful effects in treating your medical problem, it has side effects that could be very serious. Before you receive this medicine, be sure that you have discussed the use of it with your doctor.

In order to decide on the best treatment for your medical problem, your doctor should be told:

—if you have ever had any unusual reaction to mitomycin in the past.

—if you are pregnant or if you intend to have children. This medicine may cause birth defects if either the male or female is taking it at the time of conception or if it is taken during pregnancy. It may also cause permanent sterility after it has been taken for a while. Be sure that you have discussed this with your doctor before taking this medicine.

—if you are breast-feeding an infant. Although mitomycin has not been shown to cause problems, the chance always exists.

—if you have any of the following medical problems:

Blood disease	Kidney disease
Infection	

—if you have been treated with x-rays or cancer drugs by another doctor.

Proper Use of This Medicine

This medicine is usually given together with certain other medicines. If you are using a combination of drugs, it is important that you receive each medicine at the proper time. If you are taking some of these medicines by mouth, ask your doctor, nurse, or pharmacist to help you plan a way to remember to take them at the right time.

This medicine often causes nausea, vomiting, and loss of appetite. However, it is very important that you continue to receive the medicine, even if you begin to feel ill. If you have any questions about this, check with your doctor.

Precautions While Using This Medicine

It is very important that your doctor check your progress at regular visits.

Side Effects of This Medicine

Along with its needed effects, a medicine may cause some unwanted effects. Although not all of these side effects appear very often, when they do occur they may require medical attention. Check with your doctor *immediately* if any of the following side effects occur:

More common

Unexplained fever, chills, or sore throat	Unusual bleeding or bruising

Less common

Blood in urine	Sores in the mouth and on the lips

Rare

Bloody vomit	Shortness of breath
Cough	

Other side effects may occur which usually do not require medical attention. These side effects may go away during treatment as your body adjusts to the medicine. However, check with your doctor if any of the following side effects continue or are bothersome:

More common

Loss of appetite
Nausea and
  vomiting

Less common

Loss of hair	Skin rash
Numbness or tingling in fingers and toes	

Rare

Blurred vision	Headache
Diarrhea	Mental confusion
Drowsiness	Swelling of feet or lower legs
Fainting spells	Tiredness

This medicine sometimes causes a temporary loss of hair. After treatment with mitomycin has ended, normal hair growth should return.

If mitomycin accidentally seeps out of the vein into which it is injected, it may damage the skin and cause scarring. Tell the doctor right away if you notice redness, pain, or swelling at the site of injection.

After you stop using this medicine, it may still produce some side effects that need attention. During this period of time check with your doctor if you notice any of the following:

Unexplained fever, chills, or sore throat	Unusual bleeding or bruising

Other side effects not listed above may also occur in some patients. If you notice any other effects, check with your doctor.

MITOTANE (Systemic)
A commonly used brand name is Lysodren.

Mitotane (MYE-toe-tane) is a medicine that acts on a part of the body called the adrenal cortex. It is used to treat some kinds of cancer which affect the adrenal cortex. Also, it is sometimes used when the adrenal cortex is overactive without being cancerous. Mitotane is available only with your doctor's prescription.

Before Using This Medicine

In order to decide on the best treatment for your medical problem, your doctor should be told:

—if you have ever had any unusual reaction to mitotane in the past.

—if you are pregnant, if you intend to become pregnant, or if you are breast-feeding an infant. Although mitotane has not been shown to cause problems, the chance always exists.

—if you have either of the following medical problems:

Infection
Liver disease

—if you have ever been treated with mitotane and had an allergic reaction to it.

—if you are taking cortisone or similar medicines by mouth or in any form such as ointments, creams, or eye drops.

Proper Use of This Medicine

Use this medicine only as directed by your doctor. Do not use more or less of it, and do not use it more often than your doctor ordered.

Do not stop using this medicine without first checking with your doctor.

If you miss a dose of this medicine, take the missed dose as soon as you remember it. If it is time for the next dose, do not take the missed dose at all and do not double the next one. Instead, go back to your regular dosing schedule and check with your doctor.

Precautions While Using This Medicine

It is very important that your doctor check your progress at regular visits.

This medicine may cause some people to become drowsy or less alert than they are normally. *Make sure you know how you react to this medicine before you drive, use machines, or do other jobs that require you to be alert.*

Check with your doctor right away if you get an injury, infection, or illness of any kind. This medicine may weaken your body's defenses against infection or inflammation.

Side Effects of This Medicine

Along with its needed effects, a medicine may cause some unwanted effects. Although not all of these side effects appear very often, when they do occur they may require medical attention. *Stop taking this medicine and check with your doctor immediately* if any of the following side effects occur:

More common

Darkening of skin	Mental depression
Diarrhea	Nausea and
Dizziness	vomiting
Drowsiness	Skin rash
Loss of appetite	Tiredness

Check with your doctor also if the following side effects occur:

Less common

Blood in urine	Seeing double
Blurred vision	

Other side effects may occur which usually do not require medical attention. These side effects may go away during treatment as your body adjusts to the medicine. However, check with your doctor if any of the following side effects continue or are bothersome:

Less common

Aching muscles	Fever
Dizziness or light-	Flushing
headedness when	Muscle twitching
getting up from	
a lying or sitting	
position	

Rare

Breast enlargement
in males

Other side effects not listed above may also occur in some patients. If you notice any other effects, check with your doctor.

MONOAMINE OXIDASE (MAO) INHIBITORS (Systemic)

This information applies to the following medicines:
Isocarboxazid (eye-soe-kar-BOX-a-zid)
Phenelzine (FEN-el-zeen)
Tranylcypromine (tran-ill-SIP-roe-meen)
This information does *not* apply to Pargyline.

Some commonly used brand names are:	Generic names:
Marplan	Isocarboxazid
Nardil	Phenelzine
Parnate	Tranylcypromine

This medicine belongs to the group of medicines called antidepressants. Specifically it is a monoamine oxidase (MAO) inhibitor antidepressant. It is used to relieve certain types of mental depression. This medicine is available only with your doctor's prescription.

Before Using This Medicine

In order to decide on the best treatment for your medical problem, your doctor should be told:

—if you have ever had any unusual reaction to monoamine oxidase inhibitors in the past. This medicine should not be taken if you are allergic to it.

—if you are pregnant, if you intend to become pregnant, or if you are breast-feeding an infant. Although this medicine has not been shown to cause problems, the chance always exists.

—if you have frequent headaches.

—if you have any of the following medical problems:

Alcoholism	High blood pressure
Angina (chest pain)	Kidney disease
Asthma or bron-	Liver disease
chitis	Mental disease
Diabetes	(history of)
Epilepsy	Overactive thyroid
Fever	Parkinson's disease
Headaches (severe	Pheochromocytoma
or frequent)	(PCC)
Heart disease	

—if you have recently had a stroke.

—if you are now taking or have taken within the past 2 weeks any of the following medicines or types of medicine:

Other monoamine	Tricyclic an-
oxidase (MAO)	tidepressants
inhibitors	(medicine for
	depression)

—if you are now taking any of the following medicines or types of medicine:

Asthma medicine	Medicine for
Barbiturates	reducing appetite
Blood pressure	Medicine for
medicine	seizures
Diuretics (water	Narcotics
pills)	Prescription pain
Levodopa	medicine
Medicine for	Sedatives, tran-
diabetes	quilizers,
Medicine for hay	or sleeping
fever, other aller-	medicine
gies, or colds	

Proper Use of This Medicine

Importance of Diet—When prescribing this medicine for your condition, your doctor will indicate certain foods and beverages that you should avoid. If a list of these foods and beverages is not given to you, ask your doctor, nurse, or pharmacist to provide one.

Take this medicine only as directed by your doctor. Do not take more of it, do not take it more often, and do not take it for a longer period of time than your doctor ordered.

Do not stop taking this medicine without first checking with your doctor. Your doctor may want you to reduce gradually the amount you are using before stopping completely.

Sometimes this medicine must be taken for several weeks before you begin to feel better. *Your doctor should check your progress at regular visits.*

If you miss a dose of this medicine and remember within 2 hours, take it right away and then go back to your regular dosing schedule. If you do not remember until later, do not take the missed dose at all and do not double the next one. Instead, go back to your regular dosing schedule. If you have any questions about this, check with your doctor or pharmacist.

Precautions While Using This Medicine

Check with your doctor or hospital emergency room immediately if severe headache, stiff neck, chest pains, rapid heartbeat, or nausea and vomiting occur while you are taking this medicine. These may be symptoms of a serious side reaction which should have a doctor's attention.

When taken with certain foods, drinks, or other medicines, MAO inhibitors can cause very dangerous reactions. To avoid such reactions, *obey the following rules of caution:*

• Do not eat foods that have a high tyramine content (most common in foods that are aged to increase their flavor), such as cheeses, sour cream, yogurt, pickled herring, chicken liver, canned figs, raisins, bananas, avocados, soy sauce, broad bean pods (fava bean pods), yeast extracts, or meats prepared with tenderizers.

• Do not drink alcoholic beverages, including beer and wines (especially chianti and other hearty red wines).

• Do not eat or drink any more than small amounts of caffeine-containing food or beverages such as chocolate, coffee, tea, or cola.

• Do not take any other medicine unless prescribed by your doctor. This especially includes over-the-counter (OTC) or nonprescription medicine such as that for colds (including nose drops), cough, asthma, hay fever, or appetite control.

After you stop using this medicine you must continue to obey the rules of caution concerning food, drink, and other medicine for at least 2 weeks since MAO inhibitors may continue to react with certain foods or other medicines for up to 14 days after you stop taking it.

This medicine may cause some people to become drowsy or less alert than they are normally. *Make sure you know how you react to this medicine before you drive, use machines, or do other jobs that require you to be alert.*

Dizziness, lightheadedness, or fainting may occur, especially when you get up from a lying or sitting position. *Getting up slowly may help.* When you get up from lying down, sit on the edge of the bed with your feet dangling for 1 or 2 minutes. Then stand up slowly. If the problem continues or gets worse, check with your doctor.

Caution: Diabetics—This medicine may affect blood sugar levels. While you are using this medicine, be especially careful in testing for sugar in your urine. If you have any questions about this, check with your doctor.

Before having any kind of surgery (including dental surgery) or emergency treatment, tell the doctor or dentist in charge that you are using this medicine or have used it within the past 2 weeks.

Your doctor may want you to carry an identification card stating that you are using this medicine.

Tell your doctor if you develop a fever since that may change the amount of medicine you have to take.

Caution: Patients with angina (chest pain)—This medicine may cause you to have an unusual feeling of health and energy. However, *do not suddenly increase the amount of exercise you get without discussing it with your doctor* since that could bring on an attack of angina.

Side Effects of This Medicine

Along with its needed effects, a medicine may cause some unwanted effects. Although not all of these side effects appear very often, when they do occur they may require medical attention. Check with your doctor *immediately* if any of the following side effects occur:

Less common

Rapid or pounding heartbeat

Rare

Chest pains	Nausea and
Headache (severe, pounding)	vomiting
	Stiff or sore neck

Check with your doctor also if any of the following side effects occur:

Less common

Diarrhea	Swelling of feet and lower legs
Fainting	Unusually active, excitable, and talkative

Rare

Dark urine	Yellowing of eyes and skin
Fever	
Skin rash	

Other side effects may occur which usually do not require medical attention. These side effects may go away during treatment as your body adjusts to the medicine. However, check with your doctor if any of the following side effects continue or are bothersome:

More common

Constipation	Drowsiness
Difficult urination	Dry mouth
Dizziness or lightheadedness, especially when getting up from a lying or sitting position	Tiredness and weakness

Less common or rare

Chills	Increased skin sensitivity to sunlight
Decreased sexual ability	Insomnia
Hallucinations (seeing, hearing, or feeling things that are not there)	Muscle twitching during sleep
	Nightmares
Increase in appetite and weight gain	Restlessness
	Shakiness

Other side effects not listed above may also occur in some patients. If you notice any other effects, check with your doctor.

MORPHINE (Systemic)

Morphine (mor-FEEN) is a medicine used to relieve pain. Morphine is used by injection and is available only with your doctor's prescription. Prescriptions cannot be refilled. A new prescription must be obtained from your doctor each time you need this medicine.

Before Using This Medicine

In order to decide on the best treatment for your medical problem, your doctor should be told:

—if you have ever had any unusual reaction to morphine in the past. This medicine should not be taken if you are allergic to it.

—if you are pregnant or if you intend to become pregnant while taking this medicine. Although morphine has not been shown to cause birth defects, the chance always exists.

—if you are breast-feeding an infant. Although morphine has not been shown to cause problems, it passes into the breast milk and may cause unwanted side effects.

—if you have any of the following medical problems:

Brain disease or injury	Kidney disease
Colitis	Liver disease
Emphysema, asthma, or chronic lung disease	Underactive adrenal gland (Addison's disease)
Enlarged prostate or problems with urination	Underactive thyroid Unusually slow or irregular heartbeat
Gallbladder disease or gallstones	

—if you are now taking other central nervous system (CNS) depressants such as:

Antihistamines or medicine for hay fever, other allergies, or colds	Sedatives, tranquilizers, or sleeping medicine
Barbiturates	Seizure medicine
Other narcotics	Tricyclic antidepressants (medicine for depression)
Other prescription pain medicine	

—if you are now taking prescription medicine for stomach cramps or spasms.

—if you are now taking or have taken within the past 2 weeks monoamine oxidase (MAO) inhibitors such as:

Isocarboxazid	Phenelzine
Pargyline	Tranylcypromine

Proper Use of This Medicine

Use this medicine only as directed by your doctor. Do not use more of it, do not use it more often, and do not use it for a longer period of time than your doctor ordered. If too much is used, it may become habit-forming.

Precautions While Using This Medicine

If you will be using this medicine for a long period of time (for example, for several months at a time), your doctor should check your progress at regular visits.

This medicine will add to the effects of alcohol and other medicines (CNS depressants) that slow down the nervous system. Some examples of CNS depressants are antihistamines or medicine for hay fever, other allergies, or colds; sedatives, tranquilizers, or sleeping medicine; prescription pain medicine or narcotics; barbiturates; medicine for seizures; tricyclic antidepressants (medicine for depression); or anesthetics, including some dental anesthetics. *Check with your doctor before taking any of the above while you are using this medicine.*

This medicine may cause some people to become drowsy or less alert than they are normally. *Make sure you know how you react to this medicine before you drive, use machines, or do other jobs that require you to be alert.*

Dizziness, lightheadedness, or fainting may occur, especially when you get up from a lying or sitting position. Getting up slowly may help lessen this problem.

Nausea may occur, especially after the first couple of doses. This effect will usually go away if you lie down for awhile.

Side Effects of This Medicine

Along with its needed effects, a medicine may cause some unwanted effects. Although not all of these side effects appear very often, when they do occur they may require medical attention. Check with your doctor if any of the following side effects occur:

Less common

Shortness of breath	Unusually slow
Troubled breathing	heartbeat

Other side effects may occur which usually do not require medical attention. These side effects may go away during treatment as your body adjusts to the medicine. However, check with your doctor if any of the following side effects continue or are bothersome:

More common

Constipation	Feeling faint
Dizziness	Lightheadedness
Drowsiness	Nausea or vomiting

Less common

Difficult urination or frequent urge to urinate	Unusual increase in sweating
Loss of appetite	Unusual tiredness or weakness
Redness or flushing of face	

Other side effects not listed above may also occur in some patients. If you notice any other effects, check with your doctor.

NALBUPHINE (Systemic)
A commonly used brand name is Nubain.

Nalbuphine (NAL-byoo-feen) is a medicine used to relieve pain. It is used by injection and is available only with your doctor's prescription.

Before Using This Medicine
In order to decide on the best treatment for your medical problem, your doctor should be told:

—if you have ever had any unusual reaction to nalbuphine in the past. This medicine should not be taken if you are allergic to it.

—if you are pregnant or if you intend to become pregnant while using this medicine. Nalbuphine crosses the placental barrier. Although it has not been shown to cause birth defects or other problems, the chance always exists. Therefore, use by pregnant women should be carefully considered.

—if you are breast-feeding an infant. Nalbuphine may pass into breast milk. Although it has not been shown to cause problems, the chance always exists. Therefore, use by nursing mothers should be carefully considered.

—if you have any of the following medical problems:

Brain disease or injury	Heart disease
Emphysema, asthma, or chronic lung disease	Kidney disease
	Liver disease
	Narcotic dependence or addiction
Gallbladder disease or gallstones	

—if you are now taking any of the following medicines or types of medicine:

Methadone or other narcotics when used for the treatment of narcotic dependence or addiction	Narcotics Propoxyphene

—if you are now taking other central nervous system (CNS) depressants such as:

Antihistamines or medicine for hay fever, other allergies, or colds	Sedatives, tranquilizers, or sleeping medicine
Barbiturates	Seizure medicine
Other prescription pain medicine	Tricyclic antidepressants (medicine for depression)

—if you are now taking or have taken within the past 2 weeks monoamine oxidase (MAO) inhibitors such as:

Isocarboxazid	Phenelzine
Pargyline	Tranylcypromine

Proper Use of This Medicine
Take this medicine only as directed by your doctor. Do not take more of it, do not take it more often, and do not take it for a longer period of time than your doctor ordered. If too much is taken, it may become habit-forming.

Precautions While Using This Medicine
If you will be taking this medicine for a long period of time (for example, for several months at a time), your doctor should check your progress at regular visits.

This medicine will add to the effects of alcohol and other medicines (CNS depressants) that slow down the nervous system. Some examples of CNS depressants are antihistamines or medicine for hay fever, other allergies, or colds; sedatives, tranquilizers, or sleeping medicine; prescription pain medicine or narcotics; barbiturates; medicine for seizures; tricyclic antidepressants (medicine for depression); or anesthetics, including some dental anesthetics. *Check with your doctor before taking any of the above while you are using this medicine.*

This medicine may cause some people to become drowsy, dizzy, or lightheaded, or to feel a false sense of well-being. *Make sure you know how you react to this medicine before you drive, use machines, or do other jobs that require you to be alert and clear-headed.*

Nausea may occur, especially after the first couple of doses. This effect usually goes away if you lie down for a while. However, if nausea or vomiting continues, check with your doctor.

Side Effects of This Medicine

Along with its needed effects, a medicine may cause some unwanted effects. Although not all of these side effects appear very often, when they do occur they may require medical attention. Check with your doctor if any of the following side effects occur:

Less common
    Shortness of breath
    Troubled breathing

Rare
    Hallucinations (see-   Itching, burning, or
      ing, hearing, or   skin rash
      feeling things that   Mental confusion or
      are not there)   depression
                            Unusually fast or
                              slow heart-
                              beat

Other side effects may occur which usually do not require medical attention. These side effects may go away during treatment as your body adjusts to the medicine. However, check with your doctor if any of the following side effects continue or are bothersome:

More common
    Drowsiness

Less common
    Constipation   Headache
    Dizziness or light-   Nausea or vomiting
      headedness   Unusual dryness of
    False sense of well-   mouth
      being   Unusual increase in
                              sweating

After you stop using this medicine, your body may need time to adjust. The length of time this takes depends on the amount of medicine you were using and how long you used it. During this period of time check with your doctor if you notice any of the following side effects:

    Loss of appetite   Stomach cramps
    Nervousness or
      restlessness

Other side effects not listed above may also occur in some patients. If you notice any other effects, check with your doctor.

NALIDIXIC ACID (Systemic)
A commonly used brand name is NegGram.

Nalidixic (nal-i-DIX-ik) acid belongs to the general family of medicines called anti-infectives. It is given by mouth to help the body overcome infections of the urinary tract. Nalidixic acid is available only with your doctor's prescription.

Before Using This Medicine

In order to decide on the best treatment for your medical problem, your doctor should be told:

—if you have had allergic reactions to oxolinic acid, a closely related medicine.

—if you are in the first 3 months of your pregnancy or if you intend to become pregnant, although nalidixic acid has not been shown to cause problems.

—if you are breast-feeding an infant. Nalidixic acid passes into the breast milk and may cause side effects in infants of mothers taking this medicine.

—if you have any of the following medical problems:

    Central nervous   Kidney disease
      system (brain or   Liver disease
      spinal cord)   Severe hardening of
      damage   the arteries in
    History of con-   the brain
      vulsive dis-
      orders (seizures,
      epilepsy)

—if you are taking either of the following medicines or types of medicines:

    Nitrofurantoin   Oral anticoagulants
                             (blood thinners
                             you take by
                             mouth)

Proper Use of This Medicine

Nalidixic acid is best taken with a full glass (8 ounces) of water on an empty stomach (either 1 hour before or 2 hours after meals). However, if this medicine causes nausea or upset stomach, it may be taken with food or milk.

If you are taking the oral liquid form of this medicine:

• Use a specially marked measuring spoon or other device to measure each dose accurately since the average household teaspoon may not' hold the right amount of liquid.

To help clear up your infection completely, *keep taking this medicine for the full time of treatment* even if you begin to feel better after a few days; *do not miss any doses.*

If you do miss a dose of this medicine, take it as soon as possible. However, if it is almost time for your next dose and your dosing schedule is:

• 3 or more doses a day—Space the missed dose and next dose 2 to 4 hours apart or double your next dose.

Then go back to your regular dosing schedule.

Do not give this medicine to infants under 3 months of age unless directed by your doctor.

Precautions While Using This Medicine

If your symptoms do not improve within 2 days or if they become worse, check with your doctor.

If you will be taking this medicine for more than 2 weeks, your doctor should check your progress at regular visits.

Some people who take nalidixic acid may become more sensitive to sunlight than they are normally. When you first begin taking this medicine, avoid too much sun or too much use of a sunlamp until you see how you react, especially if you tend to burn easily. You may still be more sensitive to sunlight or sunlamps for up to 1 year after stopping this medicine. If you have a severe reaction, check with your doctor.

Caution: Diabetics—This medicine may cause false test results with some urine sugar tests. Check with your doctor before changing your diet or the dosage of your diabetes medicine.

This medicine may cause some people to become drowsy or dizzy or may affect their vision. If any of these side effects occur, *use caution in driving, using machines, or doing other jobs that require you to be alert and to see clearly.*

Side Effects of This Medicine

Along with its needed effects, a medicine may cause some unwanted effects. Although not all of these side effects appear very often, when they do occur they may require medical attention. Check with your doctor if any of the following side effects occur:

More common

Blurred or decreased vision, double vision, change in color vision, overbrightness of lights, or halos around lights

Rare

Dark or amber urine	Unusual bleeding or bruising
Pale skin	Unusual tiredness or weakness
Pale stools	
Severe stomach pain	Yellowing of eyes or skin
Unexplained sore throat or fever	

Other side effects may occur which usually do not require medical attention. These side effects may go away during treatment as your body adjusts to the medicine. However, check with your doctor if any of the following side effects continue or are bothersome:

More common

Diarrhea	Rash
Itching	Vomiting
Nausea	

Less common

Dizziness	Increased sensitivity to sunlight
Drowsiness	

Other side effects not listed above may also occur in some patients. If you notice any other effects, check with your doctor.

NAPROXEN (Systemic)

Some commonly used brand names are Anaprox and Naprosyn.

Naproxen (na-PROX-en) is used to treat the symptoms of arthritis. It helps relieve inflammation, swelling, stiffness, and joint pain. Also, it is used as an analgesic to relieve pain. This medicine is available only with your doctor's prescription.

Before Using This Medicine

In order to decide on the best treatment for your medical problem, your doctor should be told:

—if you have ever had any unusual reaction to aspirin or other salicylates, fenoprofen, ibuprofen, meclofenamate, sulindac, or tolmetin.

—if you are pregnant, if you intend to become pregnant, or if you are breast-feeding an infant. Although naproxen has not been shown to cause problems in humans, the chance always exists.

—if you have any of the following medical problems:

Bleeding problems	Kidney disease
Heart disease	Stomach ulcer or
High blood pressure	other stomach problems

—if you are now taking any of the following medicines or types of medicine:

Anticoagulants blood thinners)	Inflammation medicine (for example, aspirin or other arthritis medicine)

Proper Use of This Medicine

When used for arthritis, this medicine must be taken regularly as ordered by your doctor in order for it to help you. Up to 2 weeks may pass before you begin to feel better and up to 4 weeks may pass before you feel the full effects of this medicine.

It is best to take this medicine 30 minutes before meals or 2 hours after meals so that it will get into the blood more quickly. However, to lessen stomach upset, your doctor may want you to take the medicine with food, milk, or antacids. If stomach upset (indigestion, nausea, vomiting, stomach pain, or diarrhea) continues or if you have any questions about how you should be taking this medicine, check with your doctor.

If you are taking this medicine regularly (for example, every day) and you miss a dose, take it as soon as possible. Then go back to your regular dosing schedule. However, if it is almost time for your next dose, do not take the missed dose at all and do not double the next one. Instead, go back to your regular dosing schedule. If you have any questions about this, check with your doctor.

Precautions While Using This Medicine

Your doctor should check your progress at regular visits in order to make sure that this medicine does not cause unwanted effects.

Stomach problems may be more likely to occur if you take aspirin regularly (for example, every day) or drink alcoholic beverages while being treated with this medicine. Therefore, *do not take aspirin regularly or drink alcoholic beverages while taking this medicine,* unless otherwise directed by your doctor.

Before having any kind of surgery (including dental surgery), tell the doctor or dentist in charge that you are taking this medicine.

This medicine may cause some people to become dizzy, lightheaded, drowsy, or less alert than they are normally. *Make sure you know how you react to this medicine before you drive, use machines, or do other jobs that require you to be alert.*

If you are taking naproxen sodium tablets:
• Caution: Patients on a sodium-restricted diet—This medicine contains 25 mg of sodium in each tablet. If you have any questions about this, check with your doctor or pharmacist.

Side Effects of This Medicine

Along with its needed effects, a medicine may cause some unwanted effects. Although not all of these side effects appear very often, when they do occur they may require medical attention. Check with your doctor if any of the following side effects occur:

Less common

Bloody or black tarry stools	Ringing or buzzing in ears or any loss of hearing
Blurred vision or any change in vision	Skin rash, hives, or itching
Decreased hearing	Swelling of feet or lower legs
Mental depression	Unusual weight gain

Rare

Bloody urine	Unexplained sore throat and fever
Difficult or painful urination	Unusual bleeding or bruising
Frequent urge to urinate	Yellowing of eyes or skin
Shortness of breath, troubled breathing, wheezing, or tightness in chest	

Other side effects may occur which usually do not require medical attention. These side effects may go away during treatment as your body adjusts to the medicine. However, check with your doctor if any of the following side effects continue or are bothersome:

More common

Constipation	Irritation or soreness of mouth
Diarrhea	
Heartburn	Nausea or vomiting
Indigestion	Stomach pain or discomfort

Less common

Dizziness or	Headache
lightheadedness	Unusual pounding
Drowsiness	heartbeat
	Unusual sweating

Other side effects not listed above may also occur in some patients. If you notice any other effects, check with your doctor.

NATAMYCIN (Ophthalmic)
A commonly used brand name is Natacyn.

Natamycin (na-ta-MYE-sin) belongs to the group of medicines called antifungals. It is used to treat some types of fungal infections of the eye. This medicine is available only with your doctor's prescription.

In order to decide on the best treatment for your medical problem, your doctor should be told:

—if you have ever had any unusual reaction to natamycin in the past. This medicine should not be used if you are allergic to it.

—if you are pregnant, if you intend to become pregnant, or if you are breast-feeding an infant, although natamycin has not been shown to cause problems.

Proper Use of This Medicine

To help clear up your eye infection completely, *keep using this medicine for the full time of treatment* even though your condition may have improved.

Shake well before using.

How to apply this medicine: First, wash hands. Tilt head back and pull lower eyelid away from eye to form a pouch. Drop the medicine into the pouch and gently close eyes. Do not blink. Keep eyes closed for 1 or 2 minutes to allow the medicine to be absorbed.

If you think you did not get the drop of medicine into your eye properly, use another drop.

To prevent contamination of the eye drops, do not touch the applicator tip to any surface (including the eye) and keep the container tightly closed.

If you miss a dose of this medicine, apply it as soon as possible. Then go back to your regular dosing schedule. But if it is almost time for your next dose, do not apply the missed dose at all. Instead, apply your next dose at the regularly scheduled time. Then continue with your regular dosing schedule. If you have any questions about this, check with your doctor.

Precautions While Using This Medicine

Your doctor should check your progress at regular visits.

If your eye condition has not improved after using this medicine for 7 to 10 days, or if it becomes worse, check with your doctor.

Side Effects of This Medicine

Along with its needed effects, a medicine may cause some unwanted effects. Although not all of these side effects appear very often, when they do occur they may require medical attention. Check with your doctor if the following side effect occurs:

Irritation of eye not present before using this medicine

Other side effects not listed above may also occur in some patients. If you notice any other effects, check with your doctor.

NEOMYCIN (Ophthalmic)
A commonly used brand name is Myciguent.

Neomycin (nee-oh-MYE-sin) belongs to the general family of medicines called antibiotics. Neomycin ophthalmic preparations are used to help the body overcome infections of the eye. They are available only with your doctor's prescription.

Before Using This Medicine

In order to decide on the best treatment for your medical problem, your doctor should be told:

—if you have had allergic reactions to any related antibiotics such as amikacin, gentamicin, kanamycin, neomycin (by mouth or by injection), streptomycin, or tobramycin.

—if you are pregnant, if you intend to become pregnant, or if you are breast-feeding an infant, although neomycin ophthalmic preparations have not been shown to cause problems.

Proper Use of This Medicine

To prevent contamination of the eye ointment, do not touch the applicator tip to any surface (including the eye). After using, wipe the tip of the ointment tube with a clean tissue and keep the tube tightly closed.

How to apply this medicine: First, wash hands. Then pull the lower eyelid away from eye to form a pouch. Squeeze a thin strip of ointment into the pouch. A 1-cm (approximately 1/3-inch) strip of ointment is usually enough unless otherwise directed by your doctor. Gently close eyes and keep them closed for 1 or 2 minutes to allow medicine to come into contact with the infection.

To help clear up your infection completely, *keep using this medicine for the full time of treatment,* even though your symptoms may have disappeared; *do not miss any doses.*

If you do miss a dose of this medicine, apply it as soon as possible. However, if it is almost time for your next application, skip the missed dose and go back to your regular dosing schedule.

Precautions While Using This Medicine

After application, eye ointments usually cause your vision to blur for a few minutes. In addition, occasional stinging or burning may be expected.

If your symptoms do not improve within a few days or if they become worse, check with your doctor.

Side Effects of This Medicine

Along with its needed effects, a medicine may cause some unwanted effects. Although not all of these side effects appear very often, when they do occur they may require medical attention. Stop using this medicine and check with your doctor if any of the following side effects occur:

Itching, rash, redness, swelling, or other sign of irritation not present before you started using this medicine

Other side effects not listed above may also occur in some patients. If you notice any other effects, check with your doctor.

NEOMYCIN (Oral)
Some commonly used brand names are Mycifradin and Neobiotic.

Oral neomycin (nee-oh-MYE-sin) belongs to the general family of medicines called antibiotics. It is given by mouth to help the body overcome infections of the bowels (diarrhea). Oral neomycin may also be used to help lessen the symptoms of hepatic coma, a complication of liver disease. In addition, it may be used before any surgery affecting the bowel to help prevent infection during surgery. Oral neomycin may also be used for other problems as determined by your doctor. This medicine is available only with your doctor's prescription.

Before Using This Medicine

In order to decide on the best treatment for your medical problem, your doctor should be told:

—if you have had allergic reactions to any related antibiotics such as amikacin, gentamicin, kanamycin, neomycin (by injection), streptomycin, or tobramycin.

—if you are pregnant, if you intend to become pregnant, or if you are breast-feeding an infant, although oral neomycin has not been shown to cause problems.

—if you have any of the following medical problems:

Blockage of the bowel	Myasthenia gravis
	Parkinsonism
Eighth-cranial-nerve disease (loss of hearing and/or balance)	Ulcers of the bowel
Kidney disease	

—if you are now taking any of the following medicines or types of medicine:

Amikacin	Gentamicin
Capreomycin	Kanamycin
Cephaloridine	Mercaptomerin
Cephalothin	Neomycin (by injection)
Cisplatin	
Colistimethate	Polymyxin B
Colistin	Streptomycin
Ethacrynic acid	Tobramycin
Furosemide	Vancomycin

Proper Use of This Medicine

This medicine may be taken without regard to meals.

If you are taking the oral liquid form of this medicine:

• Use a specially marked measuring spoon or other device to measure each dose accurately since the average household teaspoon may not hold the right amount of liquid.

Keep taking this medicine for the full time of treatment; do not miss any doses.

If you are taking this medicine for hepatic coma and you miss a dose, take it as soon as possible. However, if it is almost time for your next dose, do not take the missed dose or double your next dose. Instead, go back to your regular dosing schedule.

If you are taking this medicine for infections of the bowels or before any surgery affecting the bowels and you miss a dose, take it as soon as possible. However, if it is almost time for your next dose and your dosing schedule is:

• 1 dose every hour (for 4 hours)—Space the missed dose and the next dose 1/2 hour apart.

• 3 or more doses a day—Space the missed dose and the next dose 2 to 4 hours apart or double your next dose.

Then go back to your regular dosing schedule.

Precautions While Using This Medicine

If the symptoms of your infection do not improve within a few days or if they become worse, check with your doctor.

If this medicine causes any loss of hearing, a ringing or buzzing sound or a feeling of fullness in the ears, clumsiness, unsteadiness, dizziness, excessive thirst, or greatly decreased frequency of urination or amount of urine, stop taking it and check with your doctor as soon as possible.

Side Effects of This Medicine

Along with its needed effects, a medicine may cause some unwanted effects. Although not all of these side effects appear very often, when they do occur they may require medical attention. Stop taking this medicine and check with your doctor as soon as possible if any of the following side effects occur:

Rare

Any loss of hearing	Ringing or buzzing
Clumsiness	sound or a feeling
Dizziness	of fullness in the
Excessive thirst	ears
Greatly decreased	Unsteadiness
frequency of	
urination or	
amount of	
urine	

Other side effects may occur which usually do not require medical attention. These side effects may go away during treatment as your body adjusts to the medicine. However, check with your doctor if any of the following side effects continue or are bothersome:

More common

Irritation or	Nausea
soreness of the	Vomiting
mouth or rectal	
area	

Rare

Diarrhea	Light-colored,
Excessive gas	frothy, fatty-
	appearing stools
	Rash

Other side effects not listed above may also occur in some patients. If you notice any other effects, check with your doctor.

NEOMYCIN (Topical)
Some commonly used brand names are Herisan Antibiotic* and Myciguent.

---

*Not available in the United States.

Neomycin (nee-oh-MYE-sin) belongs to the general family of medicines called antibiotics. Neomycin topical preparations are used to help the body overcome infections of the skin. They are available without a prescription; however, your doctor may have special instructions on the proper use of topical neomycin for your medical problem.

Before Using This Medicine

In order to decide on the best treatment for your medical problem, your doctor should be told:

—if you have had allergic reactions to any related antibiotics such as amikacin, gentamicin, kanamycin, neomycin (by mouth or by injection), streptomycin, or tobramycin.

—if you are pregnant, if you intend to become pregnant, or if you are breast-feeding an infant, although neomycin topical preparations have not been shown to cause problems.

—if you are now taking any of the following medicines:

Amikacin	Neomycin (by
Gentamicin	mouth or by
Kanamycin	injection)
	Streptomycin
	Tobramycin

Proper Use of This Medicine

If you are using this medicine without a prescription, do not use it to treat deep wounds, puncture wounds, serious burns, or raw areas without first checking with your doctor or pharmacist.

Do not use this medicine in the eyes.

Before applying this medicine, wash the area to be treated with soap and water, and dry thoroughly.

If you are using the cream form of this medicine:

• Apply a generous amount of cream to the affected area, and rub in gently until cream disappears.

If you are using the ointment form of this medicine:

• Apply a generous amount of ointment to the affected area, and rub in gently.

After applying this medicine, the treated area may be covered with a gauze dressing if desired.

To help clear up your infection completely, *keep using this medicine for the full time of treatment,* even though your symptoms may have disappeared; *do not miss any doses.*

If you do miss a dose of this medicine, apply it as soon as possible. However, if it is almost time for your next application, skip the missed dose and go back to your regular dosing schedule.

Precautions While Using This Medicine

If there is no improvement in your skin problem after you have used this medicine for 1 week or if it becomes worse, check with your doctor.

Side Effects of This Medicine

Along with its needed effects, a medicine may cause some unwanted effects. Although not all of these side effects appear very often, when they do occur they may require medical attention. Stop using this medicine and check with your doctor if any of the following side effects occur:

More common
    Itching, rash, redness, swelling, or other sign of irritation not present before you started using this medicine
Rare
    Any loss of hearing

Other side effects not listed above may also occur in some patients. If you notice any other effects, check with your doctor.

NEOMYCIN, POLYMYXIN B, AND BACITRACIN (Ophthalmic)

Some commonly used brand names are:

Mycitracin	Neosporin
Neo-Polycin	Polyspectrin
	Pyocidin

Neomycin (nee-oh-MYE-sin), polymyxin (pol-i-MIX-in) B, and bacitracin (bass-i-TRAY-sin) is a combination antibiotic medicine used to help the body overcome infections of the eye. It is available only with your doctor's prescription.

Before Using This Medicine

In order to decide on the best treatment for your medical problem, your doctor should be told:

—if you have had allergic reactions to any related antibiotics such as amikacin, colistimethate, colistin, gentamicin, kanamycin, neomycin (by mouth or by injection), paromomycin, polymyxin B (by injection), streptomycin, or tobramycin.

—if you are pregnant, if you intend to become pregnant, or if you are breast-feeding an infant, although neomycin, polymyxin, and bacitracin ophthalmic preparations have not been shown to cause problems.

Proper Use of This Medicine

To prevent contamination of the eye ointment, do not touch the applicator tip to any surface (including the eye). After using, wipe the tip of the ointment tube with a clean tissue and keep the tube tightly closed.

How to apply this medicine: First, wash hands. Then pull the lower eyelid away from eye to form a pouch. Squeeze a thin strip of ointment into the pouch. A 1-cm (approximately 1/3-inch) strip of ointment is usually enough unless otherwise directed by your doctor. Gently close eyes and keep them closed for 1 or 2 minutes to allow medicine to come into contact with the infection.

To help clear up your infection completely, *keep using this medicine for the full time of treatment,* even though your symptoms may have disappeared; *do not miss any doses.*

If you do miss a dose of this medicine, apply it as soon as possible. However, if it is almost time for your next application, skip the missed dose and go back to your regular dosing schedule.

Precautions While Using This Medicine

After application, eye ointments usually cause your vision to blur for a few minutes.

If your symptoms do not improve within a few days or if they become worse, check with your doctor.

Side Effects of This Medicine

Along with its needed effects, a medicine may cause some unwanted effects. Although not all of these side effects appear very often, when they do occur they may require medical attention. Stop using this medicine and check with your doctor if any of the following side effects occur:

Itching, rash, redness, swelling, or other sign of irritation not present before you started using this medicine

Other side effects not listed above may also occur in some patients. If you notice any other effects, check with your doctor.

NEOMYCIN, POLYMYXIN B, AND BACITRACIN (Topical)
Some commonly used brand names are Mycitracin, Neo-Polycin, and Neosporin.

Neomycin (nee-oh-MYE-sin), polymyxin (pol-i-MIX-in) B, and bacitracin (bass-i-TRAY-sin) is a combination antibiotic medicine used to help the body overcome infections of the skin. It is available without a prescription; however, your doctor may have special instructions on the proper use of this medicine for your medical problem.

Before Using This Medicine

In order to decide on the best treatment for your medical problem, your doctor should be told:

—if you have had allergic reactions to any related antibiotics such as amikacin, colistimethate, colistin, gentamicin, kanamycin, neomycin (by mouth or by injection), paromomycin, polymyxin B (by injection), streptomycin, or tobramycin.

—if you are pregnant, if you intend to become pregnant, or if you are breast-feeding an infant, although neomycin, polymyxin, and bacitracin topical preparations have not been shown to cause problems.

—if you are now taking any of the following medicines:

Amikacin
Gentamicin
Kanamycin
Neomycin (by mouth or by injection)
Streptomycin
Tobramycin

Proper Use of This Medicine

If you are using this medicine without a prescription, do not use it to treat deep wounds, puncture wounds, serious burns, or raw areas without first checking with your doctor or pharmacist.

Do not use this medicine in the eyes.

Before applying this medicine, wash the area to be treated with soap and water, and dry thoroughly.

After applying this medicine, the treated area may be covered with a gauze dressing if desired.

To help clear up your infection completely, *keep using this medicine for the full time of treatment,* even though your symptoms may have disappeared; *do not miss any doses.*

If you do miss a dose of this medicine, apply it as soon as possible. However, if it is almost time for your next application, skip the missed dose and go back to your regular dosing schedule.

Precautions While Using This Medicine

If there is no improvement in your skin problem after you have used this medicine for 1 week or if it becomes worse, check with your doctor or pharmacist.

Side Effects of This Medicine

Along with its needed effects, a medicine may cause some unwanted effects. Although not all of these side effects appear very often, when they do occur they may require medical attention. Stop using this medicine and check with your doctor if any of the following side effects occur:

More common
Itching, rash, redness, swelling, or other sign of irritation not present before you started using this medicine
Rare
Any loss of hearing

Other side effects not listed above may also occur in some patients. If you notice any other effects, check with your doctor.

NEOMYCIN, POLYMYXIN B, AND GRAMICIDIN (Ophthalmic)

Some commonly used brand names are Neo-Polycin and Neosporin.

Neomycin (nee-oh-MYE-sin), polymyxin (pol-i-MIX-in) B, and gramicidin (gram-i-SYE-din) is a combination antibiotic medicine used to help the body overcome infections of the eye. It is available only with your doctor's prescription.

Before Using This Medicine

In order to decide on the best treatment for your medical problem, your doctor should be told:

—if you have had allergic reactions to any related antibiotics such as amikacin, colistimethate, colistin, gentamicin, kanamycin, neomycin (by mouth or by injection), paromomycin, polymyxin B (by injection), streptomycin, or tobramycin.

—if you are pregnant, if you intend to become pregnant, or if you are breast-feeding an infant, although neomycin, polymyxin, and gramicidin ophthalmic preparations have not been shown to cause problems.

Proper Use of This Medicine

Bottle is not full; this is to provide proper drop control.

To prevent contamination of the eye drops, do not touch applicator tip or dropper to any surface (including the eye), and keep the container tightly closed.

How to apply this medicine: First, wash hands. Then tilt head back and pull lower eyelid away from the eye to form a pouch. Drop medicine into pouch and gently close eyes. Do not blink. Keep eyes closed for 1 or 2 minutes to allow medicine to come into contact with the infection.

If you think you did not get the drop of medicine into your eye properly, use another drop.

To help clear up your infection completely, *keep using this medicine for the full time of treatment,* even though your symptoms may have disappeared; *do not miss any doses.*

If you do miss a dose of this medicine, apply it as soon as possible. However, if it is almost time for your next application, skip the missed dose and go back to your regular dosing schedule.

Precautions While Using This Medicine

After application of this medicine to the eye, occasional stinging or burning may be expected.

If your symptoms do not improve within a few days or if they become worse, check with your doctor.

Side Effects of This Medicine

Along with its needed effects, a medicine may cause some unwanted effects. Although not all of these side effects appear very often, when they do occur they may require medical attention. Stop using this medicine and check with your doctor if any of the following side effects occur:

Itching, rash, redness, swelling, or other sign of irritation not present before you started using this medicine

Other side effects not listed above may also occur in some patients. If you notice any other effects, check with your doctor.

NEOMYCIN, POLYMYXIN B, AND HYDROCORTISONE (Ophthalmic)

A commonly used brand name is Cortisporin.

Neomycin (nee-oh-MYE-sin), polymyxin (pol-i-MIX-in) B, and hydrocortisone (hye-droe-KOR-ti-sone) is a combination antibiotic and cortisone--like medicine. It is used to help the body overcome infections of the eye and to help provide relief from redness, irritation, and discomfort of certain eye problems. This medicine is available only with your doctor's prescription.

Before Using This Medicine

In order to decide on the best treatment for your medical problem, your doctor should be told:

—if you have had allergic reactions to any related antibiotics such as amikacin, colistimethate, colistin, gentamicin, kanamycin, neomycin (by mouth or by injection), paromomycin, polymyxin B (by injection), streptomycin, or tobramycin.

—if you are pregnant, if you intend to become pregnant, or if you are breast-feeding an infant, although neomycin, polymyxin, and hydrocortisone ophthalmic preparations have not been shown to cause problems.

—if you have any other eye infection or condition.

Proper Use of This Medicine

Bottle is not full; this is to provide proper drop control.

To prevent contamination of the eye drops, do not touch applicator tip or dropper to any surface (including the eye), and keep the container tightly closed.

How to apply this medicine: First, wash hands. Then tilt head back and pull lower eyelid away from the eye to form a pouch. Drop medicine into pouch and gently close eyes. Do not blink. Keep eyes closed for 1 or 2 minutes to allow medicine to come into contact with the infection.

If you think you did not get the drop of medicine into your eye properly, use another drop.

To help clear up your infection completely, *keep using this medicine for the full time of treatment,* even though your symptoms may have disappeared; *do not miss any doses.*

If you do miss a dose of this medicine, apply it as soon as possible. However, if it is almost time for your next application, skip the missed dose and go back to your regular dosing schedule.

Do not use any leftover medicine for future eye problems without checking with your doctor first, since this medicine should not be used on many different kinds of infection.

Precautions While Using This Medicine

After application of this medicine to the eye, occasional stinging or burning may be expected.

If you will be using this medicine for a long time (for example, longer than 6 weeks), your doctor should check your eyes at regular visits.

If your symptoms do not improve within a few days or if they become worse, check with your doctor.

Side Effects of This Medicine

Along with its needed effects, a medicine may cause some unwanted effects. Although not all of these side effects appear very often, when they do occur they may require medical attention. Stop using this medicine and check with your doctor if any of the following side effects occur:

Itching, rash, redness, swelling, or other sign of irritation not present before you started using this medicine

Other side effects not listed above may also occur in some patients. If you notice any other effects, check with your doctor.

NEOMYCIN, POLYMYXIN B, AND HYDROCORTISONE (Otic)

Some commonly used brand names are Cortisporin and Otobione.

Neomycin (nee-oh-MYE-sin), polymyxin (pol-i-MIX-in) B, and hydrocortisone (hye-droe-KOR-ti-sone) is a combination antibiotic and cortisone--like medicine. It is used to help the body overcome infections of the ear and to help provide relief from redness, irritation, and discomfort of certain ear problems. This medicine is available only with your doctor's prescription.

Before Using This Medicine

In order to decide on the best treatment for your medical problem, your doctor should be told:

—if you have had allergic reactions to any related antibiotics such as amikacin, colistimethate, colistin, gentamicin, kanamycin, neomycin (by mouth or by injection), paromomycin, polymyxin B (by injection), streptomycin, or tobramycin.

—if you are pregnant, if you intend to become pregnant, or if you are breast-feeding an infant, although neomycin, polymyxin, and hydrocortisone otic preparations have not been shown to cause problems.

—if you have any other ear infection or condition (including punctured eardrum).

Proper Use of This Medicine

Before applying this medicine, wash the area to be treated (including the ear canal) with soap and water, and dry thoroughly. The ear canal should be dried with a sterile cotton applicator.

You may warm the ear drops to body temperature (37 °C or 98.6 °F), but no higher, by holding the bottle in your hand for a few minutes before applying. If the medicine gets too warm, it may break down and not work at all.

To prevent contamination of the ear drops, do not touch the dropper to any surface (including the ear), and keep the container tightly closed.

How to apply this medicine: Lie down or tilt the head so that the infected ear faces up. Gently pull the earlobe up and back for adults (down and back for children) to straighten the ear canal. Drop medicine into the ear canal. Keep ear facing up for about 5 minutes to allow medicine to come into contact with the infection. A clean, soft cotton plug may be gently inserted into the ear opening to prevent the medicine from leaking out. However, your doctor may want you to keep a cotton plug moistened with this medicine in your ear for the full time of treatment. If you have any questions about this, check with your doctor.

To help clear up your infection completely, *keep using this medicine for the full time of treatment,* even though your symptoms may have disappeared; *do not miss any doses.*

If you do miss a dose of this medicine, apply it as soon as possible. However, if it is almost time for your next application, skip the missed dose and go back to your regular dosing schedule.

Do not use this medicine for more than 10 days unless otherwise directed by your doctor.

Precautions While Using This Medicine

If your symptoms do not improve within 1 week or if they become worse, check with your doctor.

Side Effects of This Medicine

Along with its needed effects, a medicine may cause some unwanted effects. Although not all of these side effects appear very often, when they do occur they may require medical attention. Stop using this medicine and check with your doctor if any of the following side effects occur:

Itching, rash, redness, swelling, or other sign of irritation not present before you started using this medicine

Other side effects not listed above may also occur in some patients. If you notice any other effects, check with your doctor.

NICOTINYL ALCOHOL (Systemic)
A commonly used brand name is Roniacol.

Nicotinyl (nik-oh-TIN-ill) alcohol belongs to the group of medicines called vasodilators. Vasodilators increase the size of blood vessels and are used to treat problems resulting from poor blood circulation. Nicotinyl alcohol is available only with your doctor's prescription.

Before Using This Medicine

In order to decide on the best treatment for your medical problem, your doctor should be told:

—if you have ever had any unusual reaction to nicotinyl alcohol in the past. This medicine should not be taken if you are allergic to it.

—if you are pregnant, if you intend to become pregnant, or if you are breast-feeding an infant. Although this medicine has not been shown to cause problems, the chance always exists.

—if you have any of the following medical problems:

Angina (chest pain)   High cholesterol
Glaucoma   levels
                                   Stomach ulcer

—if you have recently had a heart attack or stroke.

—if you smoke.

Proper Use of This Medicine

If you miss a dose of this medicine, take it as soon as you remember. If it is almost time for your next dose, do not take the missed dose at all and do not double the next one. Instead, go back to your regular dosing schedule. If you have any questions about this, check with your doctor.

Precautions While Using This Medicine

It may take some time for this medicine to work. If you feel that the medicine is not working, do not stop taking it on your own. Instead, check with your doctor.

The helpful effects of this medicine may be decreased if you smoke.

Side Effects of This Medicine

Along with its needed effects, a medicine may cause some unwanted effects. Although not all of these side effects appear very often, when they do occur they may require medical attention. Check with your doctor if any of the following side effects occur:

Rare

Swelling of feet or   Yellowing of eyes or
lower legs   skin

Other side effects may occur which usually do not require medical attention. These side effects may go away during treatment as your body adjusts to the medicine. However, check with your doctor if any of the following side effects continue or are bothersome:

More common

| Flushing | Warmth or tingling |

Less common or rare

Diarrhea	
Dizziness or faint-	Nausea and
ness	vomiting
Increased hair loss	Skin rash

Other side effects not listed above may also occur in some patients. If you notice any other effects, check with your doctor.

NITRATES (Systemic)

This information applies to the following medicines:

Erythrityl Tetranitrate (e-RI-thri-till)
Isosorbide Dinitrate (eye-soe-SOR-bide)
Pentaerythritol Tetranitrate (pen-ta-er-ITH-ri- tole)

This information does *not* apply to mannitol hexanitrate and nitroglycerin (glyceryl trinitrate).

Some commonly used brand names are:	Generic names:
Cardilate	Erythrityl Tetranitrate
Coronex* Dilatrate-SR Iso-Bid Isordil Isotrate Sorate Sorbide Sorbitrate	Isosorbide Dinitrate
Duotrate Kaytrate Pentraspan Pentritol Peritrate	Pentaerythritol Tetranitrate

*Not available in the United States.

This medicine belongs to the group of medicines called nitrates. It is used to improve the blood flow to the heart. Some dosage forms of nitrates are used to relieve the pain of angina attacks. Others are used to prevent such attacks. This medicine is available only with your doctor's prescription.

Before Using This Medicine

In order to decide on the best treatment for your medical problem, your doctor should be told:

—if you have ever had any unusual reaction to nitrates in the past. This medicine should not be taken if you are allergic to it.

—if you are pregnant, if you intend to become pregnant, or if you are breast-feeding an infant. Although this medicine has not been shown to cause problems, the chance always exists.

—if you have any of the following medical problems:

| Anemia (severe) | Overactive thyroid |

—if you have had a heart attack recently.

—if you are now taking any of the following medicines or types of medicine:

| Asthma medicine | Sinus medicine |
| High blood pressure medicine | |

Proper Use of This Medicine

Take this medicine exactly as directed by your doctor.

For patients taking the chewable tablets or sublingual (under-the-tongue) tablets to relieve an anginal attack:

• *When you begin to feel an attack of angina starting (chest pains or a tightness or squeezing in the chest), sit down. Then use a chewable tablet or dissolve a sublingual tablet under your tongue.* This medicine works best when you are standing or sitting; however, since you may become dizzy, lightheaded, or faint soon after taking a tablet, it is safer to sit rather than stand while the medicine is working. If you become dizzy or faint while sitting, take several deep breaths and bend forward with your head between your knees. Remain calm and you should feel better in a few minutes.

• *If you are taking the chewable tablet, it must be chewed well and held in the mouth for about 2 minutes.* This will allow the medicine to be absorbed through the lining of the mouth.

• *If you are taking the sublingual tablet, it should not be chewed or swallowed.* It works much faster when absorbed through the lining of the mouth. Do not eat, drink, or smoke while a tablet is dissolving.

• *This medicine usually gives relief in 2 to 5 minutes.* However, if the pain is not relieved within 10 minutes, use a second tablet. If the pain continues for another 10 minutes, a third tablet may be used. *If you still have the chest pains after using 3 tablets in a 15- to 30-minute period, call your doctor or go to a hospital without delay.*

- You may prevent anginal chest pains for up to 1 hour by using a chewable tablet or dissolving a sublingual tablet under the tongue 5 to 10 minutes before expected emotional stress or physical exertion that in the past seemed to bring on an attack.

For patients taking the tablet, extended-release capsule, or extended-release tablet form of this medicine:

- *This medicine is used to prevent angina attacks. It will not relieve an attack that is already started,* because it works too slowly (the extended-release form releases medicine gradually over a 6-hour period to provide its effect for 8 to 10 hours). Check with your doctor if you need a fast-acting medicine to relieve the pain of an angina attack.

- *Take this medicine with a full glass (8 ounces) of water on an empty stomach.* If taken either 1 hour before or 2 hours after meals, it will start working sooner.

- If you are taking the extended-release tablets, they are not to be broken, crushed, or chewed before they are swallowed. If broken up, they will not properly release the medicine.

- If you are taking this medicine regularly and you miss a dose, take it as soon as possible unless the next scheduled dose is within 2 hours (or within 6 hours for extended-release capsules or tablets). Then go back to your regular dosing schedule. Do not double doses. If you have any questions about this, check with your doctor.

Precautions While Using This Medicine

If you have been using this medicine regularly for several weeks, do not suddenly stop using it. Stopping suddenly may bring on attacks of angina. Check with your doctor for the best way to reduce gradually the amount you are taking before stopping completely.

Dizziness, lightheadedness, or a fainting feeling may occur, especially when you get up quickly from a lying or sitting position. Getting up slowly may help. *Drinking alcohol may make these effects much worse and may cause a serious drop in blood pressure.* Check with your doctor before drinking alcoholic beverages.

After taking a dose of this medicine you may get a headache that lasts for a short time. This is a common side effect which should become less

noticeable after you have taken the medicine for a while. If this effect continues or if the headaches are severe, check with your doctor.

Partially dissolved tablets have been found in the stools of a few patients taking the extended-release tablets of this medicine. Be alert to this possibility especially if you have frequent bowel movements, diarrhea, or digestive problems. Notify your doctor if any such tablets are discovered. The tablets must be properly digested in order to provide the correct dose of medicine.

Side Effects of This Medicine

Along with its needed effects, a medicine may cause some unwanted effects. Although not all of these side effects appear very often, when they do occur they may require medical attention. Check with your doctor if the following side effect occurs:

Rare

Skin rash

Other side effects may occur which usually do not require medical attention. These side effects may go away during treatment as your body adjusts to the medicine. However, check with your doctor if any of the following side effects continue or are bothersome:

More common

Dizziness, light-headedness, or fainting	Headache (severe or prolonged)
Flushing of face and neck	Nausea or vomiting Rapid heartbeat

Other side effects not listed above may also occur in some patients. If you notice any other effects, check with your doctor.

NITROFURANTOIN (Systemic)

Some commonly used brand names are:

Cyantin	Nephronex*
Furadantin	Nifuran*
Furatine*	Novofuran*
Macrodantin	

*Not available in the United States.

Nitrofurantoin (nye-troe-fyoor-AN-toyn) belongs to the general family of medicines called anti-infectives. It is given by mouth to help the body overcome infections of the urinary tract. Nitrofurantoin is available only with your doctor's prescription.

Before Using This Medicine

In order to decide on the best treatment for your medical problem, your doctor should be told:

—if you have had allergic reactions to any related medicines such as furazolidone or nitrofurazone.

—if you are pregnant and within a week or two of your delivery date. Nitrofurantoin should not be used during the last part of pregnancy since it may cause problems in the infant.

—if you are breast-feeding an infant. Nitrofurantoin passes into the breast milk in small amounts and may cause problems in an infant with glucose-6-phosphate dehydrogenase (G6PD) deficiency.

—if you have any of the following medical problems:

Glucose-6-phosphate dehydrogenase (G6PD) deficiency	Kidney disease (other than infection)
	Lung disease
	Nerve damage

—if you are now taking any of the following medicines:

Nalidixic acid	Sulfinpyrazone
Probenecid	

Proper Use of This Medicine

Nitrofurantoin is best taken with food or milk. This may lessen stomach upset and help your body absorb the medicine better.

If you are taking the oral liquid form of this medicine:

• Shake the oral liquid sharply (forcefully) befcre each dose to help make it pour more smoothly and to be sure the medicine is evenly mixed.

• Use a specially marked measuring spoon or other device to measure each dose accurately since the average household teaspoon may not hold the right amount of liquid.

• May be mixed with water, milk, fruit juices, or infants' formulas. If mixed with other liquids, take immediately after mixing. Be sure to drink all the liquid in order to get the full dose of medicine.

• To help keep this medicine from staining the teeth, rinse the mouth with water after swallowing the oral liquid form. The stain is not permanent, however.

To help clear up your infection completely, *keep taking this medicine for the full time of treatment* even if you begin to feel better after a few days; *do not miss any doses.*

If you do miss a dose of this medicine, take it as soon as possible. However, if it is almost time for your next dose and your dosing schedule is:

• 3 or more doses a day—Space the missed dose and the next dose 2 to 4 hours apart or double your next dose.

Then go back to your regular dosing schedule.

Do not give this medicine to infants under 1 month of age.

Precautions While Using This Medicine

If your symptoms do not improve within a few days or if they become worse, check with your doctor.

Caution: Diabetics—This medicine may cause false test results with urine sugar tests. Check with your doctor before changing your diet or the dosage of your diabetes medicine.

Side Effects of This Medicine

Along with its needed effects, a medicine may cause some unwanted effects. Although not all of these side effects appear very often, when they do occur they may require medical attention. Stop taking this medicine and check with your doctor if any of the following side effects occur:

More common

Chest pain, chills, cough, troubled breathing, or unexplained fever

Less common

Dizziness	Pale skin
Drowsiness	Unusual tiredness or weakness
Headache	
Numbness, tingling, or burning of face or mouth	

Rare

Yellowing of eyes or skin

Other side effects may occur which usually do not require medical attention. These side effects may go away during treatment as your body adjusts to the medicine. However, check with your doctor if any of the following side effects continue or are bothersome:

More common

Diarrhea	Rust-yellow to brown discoloration of urine
Loss of appetite	
Nausea	
	Vomiting

Less common

Discoloration of infants' or children's teeth (oral liquid only)	Itching Rash

This medicine may cause the urine to become rust-yellow to brown. This side effect does not require medical attention.

Other side effects not listed above may also occur in some patients. If you notice any other effects, check with your doctor.

NITROGLYCERIN (Systemic)

Some commonly used brand or other names are:

Glyceryl trinitrate	Nitrong
Nitro-Bid	Nitrospan
Nitroglyn	Nitrostat
Nitrol	

Nitroglycerin (nye-troe-GLI-ser-in) belongs to the group of medicines called nitrates. It is used to improve the supply of blood and oxygen to the heart. In some forms, this medicine is used to relieve the pain of angina attacks. In other forms, it is used to prevent such attacks. This medicine is available only with your doctor's prescription.

Before Using This Medicine

In order to decide on the best treatment for your medical problem, your doctor should be told:

—if you have ever had any unusual reaction to nitroglycerin in the past. This medicine should not be taken if you are allergic to it.

—if you have either of the following medical problems:

  Anemia (severe) Overactive thyroid

—if you are pregnant, if you intend to become pregnant, or if you are breast-feeding an infant. Although this medicine has not been shown to cause problems, the chance always exists.

—if you have recently had a heart attack.

—if you are now taking any of the following medicines or types of medicine:

  Asthma medicine Sinus medicine
  High blood pressure
   medicine

Proper Use of This Medicine

Use nitroglycerin exactly as directed by your doctor. It is effective only if taken correctly.

For patients taking the extended-release capsule or extended-release tablet form of this medicine:

• *This form of the medicine is used to prevent angina attacks. It will not relieve an attack that has already started, because it works too slowly.* Check with your doctor if you need a fast-acting form of this medicine to relieve the pain of an angina attack.

• *Take this medicine with a full glass (8 ounces) of water on an empty stomach.* If taken either 1 hour before or 2 hours after meals, it will start working sooner.

• The extended-release tablets are not to be broken, crushed, or chewed before they are swallowed, since if broken up, they will not properly release the medicine.

• If you are taking this medicine on a regular basis and you miss a dose, take it as soon as possible unless the next scheduled dose is within 6 hours. Then go back to your regular dosing schedule. Do not double doses. If you have any questions about this, check with your doctor.

For patients taking the sublingual (under-the-tongue) tablet form of this medicine:

• Testing the ability of a sublingual nitroglycerin tablet to relieve angina by the presence of a tingling or burning sensation, a feeling of warmth or flushing, or a headache, after a tablet has been dissolved under the tongue, is not completely reliable since some patients may be unable to detect these effects. Newer, stabilized sublingual nitroglycerin tablets are also making such potency testing less popular, since the stabilized tablets are less likely to produce these detectable effects.

• *When you begin to feel an attack of angina starting (chest pains or a tightness or squeezing in the chest), sit down. Then place a nitroglycerin tablet under your tongue and let it dissolve there.* This medicine works best when you are standing or sitting; however, since you may become dizzy, lightheaded, or faint soon after taking a tablet, it is safer to sit rather than stand while the medicine is working. If you become dizzy or faint while sitting, take several deep breaths and bend forward with your head between your knees.

• By remaining calm you will help relieve the attack sooner.

• You should feel better in a few minutes. This medicine should not be chewed or swallowed since it works much faster when absorbed through the lining of the mouth. Do not eat, drink, or smoke while a tablet is dissolving.

• *This medicine usually gives relief in 1 to 5 minutes.* However, if the pain is not relieved dissolve a second tablet under the tongue. If the pain continues for another 5 minutes, a third tablet may be used. *If you still have the chest pains after a total of 3 tablets in a 15-minute period, contact your doctor or go to a hospital emergency room without delay.*

• You may prevent anginal chest pains for up to 1 hour by putting a tablet under the tongue 5 to 10 minutes before expected emotional stress or physical exertion that in the past seemed to bring on an attack.

• When properly stored, sublingual nitroglycerin tablets retain their strength until the expiration date printed on the original label. However, because of patient usage, changing temperature and moisture, shaking, and repeated bottle opening, the tablets may be good for only 3 to 6 months. The "stabilized" sublingual tablets may stay good for a longer period of time.

• To help keep the nitroglycerin tablets at full strength:

—keep the medicine in the original glass, screw-cap bottle.

—remove the cotton plug that comes in the bottle and *do not* put it back.

—*put the cap on the bottle quickly and tightly after each use.*

—to select a tablet for use, pour several into the bottle cap, take one, and pour the others back into the bottle. Try not to hold them in the palm of your hand because they will pick up moisture and crumble.

—do not keep other medicines in the same bottle with the nitroglycerin since they will weaken the nitroglycerin effect.

—keep the medicine handy at all times but try not to carry the bottle close to the body. Medicine may lose strength because of body warmth. Instead, carry the tightly-closed bottle in your purse, jacket pocket, or other loose-fitting clothing whenever possible.

—store the bottle of nitroglycerin tablets in a cool, dry place. Average room temperature away from direct heat or direct sunlight is best. Do not store in the refrigerator or in a bathroom medicine cabinet because the moisture usually present in these areas may cause the tablets to crumble if the container is not tightly closed.

For patients using the ointment form of this medicine:

• *The ointment form of this medicine is used to prevent angina attacks. It will not relieve an attack that has already started* because it works too slowly. Check with your doctor if you need a fast-acting medicine to relieve the pain of an angina attack.

• *This medicine usually comes with patient instructions. Read them carefully before using.*

• Before applying a new dose of ointment, remove any ointment remaining on the skin from a previous dose; this will allow the fresh ointment to release the nitroglycerin properly.

• This medicine also comes with dose-measuring papers. Use them to measure the length of ointment squeezed from the tube and to apply the ointment to the skin. *Do not rub or massage the ointment on the skin; just spread in a thin, even layer, covering an area of the same size each time it is applied.*

• Each dose of ointment is best applied to a different area of skin to prevent irritation or other skin problems.

• If your doctor has ordered an occlusive dressing (for example, kitchen plastic wrap) to be applied over this medicine, make sure you know how to apply it. Since occlusive dressings increase the amount of medicine absorbed through the skin and the possibility of side effects, use them only as directed. If you have any questions about this, check with your doctor or pharmacist.

• Store the tube of nitroglycerin ointment in a cool place and keep it tightly closed.

Precautions While Using This Medicine

If you have been using nitroglycerin regularly for several weeks or more, do not suddenly stop using it. Stopping suddenly may bring on attacks of angina. Check with your doctor for the best way to reduce gradually the amount you are using before stopping completely.

Dizziness, lightheadedness, or a fainting feeling may occur, especially when you get up quickly from a lying or sitting position. Getting up slowly may help. *Drinking alcohol may make these effects much worse and may cause a serious drop in blood pressure.* Check with your doctor before drinking alcoholic beverages.

After using a dose of this medicine you may get a headache that lasts for a short time. This is a common side effect, which should become less noticeable after you have used the medicine for a while. If this effect continues, or if the headaches are severe, check with your doctor.

Side Effects of This Medicine

Along with its needed effects, a medicine may cause some unwanted effects. Although not all of these side effects appear very often, when they do occur they may require medical attention. Check with your doctor if the following side effect occurs:

Rare

Skin rash

Other side effects may occur which usually do not require medical attention. These side effects may go away during treatment as your body adjusts to the medicine. However, check with your doctor if any of the following side effects continue or are bothersome:

More common

Dizziness, light-headedness, or fainting
Flushing of face and neck

Headache (severe or prolonged)
Nausea or vomiting
Rapid heartbeat

Other side effects not listed above may also occur in some patients. If you notice any other effects, check with your doctor.

NYLIDRIN (Systemic)
A commonly used brand name is Arlidin.

Nylidrin (NYE-li-drin) belongs to the group of medicines called vasodilators. Vasodilators increase the size of blood vessels. Nylidrin is used to treat problems due to poor blood circulation. It is available only with your doctor's prescription.

Before Using This Medicine

In order to decide on the best treatment for your medical problem, your doctor should be told:

—if you have ever had any unusual reaction to nylidrin in the past. This medicine should not be taken if you are allergic to it.

—if you are pregnant, if you intend to become pregnant, or if you are breast-feeding an infant. Although nylidrin has not been shown to cause problems, the chance always exists.

—if you have any of the following medical problems:

Angina (chest pain)   Stomach ulcer
Heart disease

—if you have recently had a heart attack.

—if you smoke.

Proper Use of This Medicine

Nylidrin may cause you to have a rapid or pounding heartbeat. In order to keep this from affecting your nighttime sleep, do not take the last dose of the day at bedtime. However, it is best to plan your dose or doses according to a schedule that will least affect your sleep. Ask your doctor, nurse, or pharmacist to help you plan the best time to take this medicine.

If you miss a dose of this medicine, take the missed dose as soon as you remember. If it is almost time for the next dose, do not take the missed dose at all and do not double the next one. Instead, go back to your regular dosing schedule. If you have any questions about this, check with your doctor.

Precautions While Using This Medicine

It may take some time for this medicine to work. If you feel that the medicine is not working, do not stop taking it on your own. Instead, check with your doctor.

The helpful effects of this medicine may be decreased if you smoke. If you have any questions about this, check with your doctor.

Side Effects of This Medicine

Along with its needed effects, a medicine may cause some unwanted effects. Although not all of these side effects appear very often, when they do occur they may require medical attention. Check with your doctor *immediately* if any of the following side effects occur since they may indicate an overdose:

Blurred vision
Chest pain
Fever
Metallic taste

Unusual decrease in urination or inability to urinate

Check with your doctor also if the following side effects occur:

Less common

Dizziness
Rapid or irregular heartbeat

Weakness or tiredness

Other side effects may occur which usually do not require medical attention. These side effects may go away during treatment as your body adjusts to the medicine. However, check with your doctor if any of the following side effects continue or are bothersome:

Less common

Chilliness
Flushing or redness of face
Headache

Nausea and vomiting
Nervousness
Trembling

Other side effects not listed above may also occur in some patients. If you notice any other effects, check with your doctor.

NYSTATIN (Oral)
Some commonly used brand names are Mycostatin, Nadostine*, and Nilstat.

---

*Not available in the United States.

Nystatin (nye-STAT-in) belongs to the group of medicines called antifungals. The liquid form of this medicine is used to treat infections in the mouth and the tablet form is used to treat intestinal infections. This medicine is available only with your doctor's prescription.

Before Using This Medicine

In order to decide on the best treatment for your medical problem, your doctor should be told:

—if you have ever had any unusual reaction to nystatin in the past. This medicine should not be taken if you are allergic to it.

—if you are pregnant, if you intend to become pregnant, or if you are breast-feeding an infant. Although nystatin is not absorbed into the body and has not been shown to cause problems, the chance always exists.

Proper Use of This Medicine

To help clear up your infection completely, *keep taking this medicine for the full time of treatment* even though your condition may have improved; *do not miss any doses.*

If you do miss a dose of this medicine, take it as soon as possible. Then go back to your regular dosing schedule. If it is almost time for your next dose, do not take the missed dose at all and do not double the next one. Instead, go back to your regular dosing schedule. If you have any questions about this, check with your doctor.

If you are taking the liquid form of this medicine:

• Nystatin is to be taken by mouth even though it may come in a dropper bottle. If it does come in a dropper bottle, use the specially marked dropper to measure the correct amount of medicine.

• Shake well before using.

• Take this medicine by placing 1/2 of the dose in each side of your mouth. Hold the medicine in your mouth or swish it around in your mouth for as long as possible before swallowing.

Precautions While Using This Medicine

To help cure the infection and to help make sure it does not return, good health habits are required. If you have any questions about this, check with your doctor or pharmacist.

Side Effects of This Medicine

Along with its needed effects, a medicine may cause some unwanted effects. The following side effects may go away during treatment as your body adjusts to the medicine. However, check with your doctor if they continue or are bothersome:

More common with high doses

Diarrhea	Stomach pain
Nausea	Vomiting

Other side effects not listed above may also occur in some patients. If you notice any other effects, check with your doctor.

NYSTATIN (Topical)
Some commonly used brand names are:

Candex	Nilstat
Mycostatin	Nyaderm*
Nadostine*	

---

*Not available in the United States.

Nystatin (nye-STAT-in) belongs to the group of medicines called antifungals. Topical nystatin is applied to the skin to treat some types of fungal infections. This medicine is available only with your doctor's prescription.

Before Using This Medicine

In order to decide on the best treatment for your medical problem, your doctor should be told:

—if you have ever had any unusual reaction to nystatin in the past. This medicine should not be used if you are allergic to it.

—if you are pregnant, if you intend to become pregnant, or if you are breast-feeding an infant, although nystatin is not absorbed into the body and has not been shown to cause problems.

Proper Use of This Medicine

To help clear up your infection completely, *keep using this medicine for the full time of treatment* even though your condition may have improved.

Apply enough nystatin to cover the affected area.

If you are using the powder form of this medicine on the feet, sprinkle the powder between toes, on feet, and in socks and shoes.

Do not apply an occlusive dressing or airtight covering (for example, kitchen plastic wrap) over this medicine, since it may cause irritation of the skin. If you have any questions about this, check with your doctor.

If you miss a dose of this medicine, apply it as soon as possible. Then go back to your regular dosing schedule. But if it is almost time for your next dose, do not apply the missed dose at all. Instead, go back to your regular dosing schedule. If you have any questions about this, check with your doctor.

Precautions While Using This Medicine

To help cure the infection and to help prevent reinfection, good health habits are required. These include the following:

• Wash all towels and bedding after use.

• Use only freshly laundered clothes each time clothing is changed.

If you have any questions about this, check with your doctor, nurse, or pharmacist.

Side Effects of This Medicine

Along with its needed effects, a medicine may cause some unwanted effects. Although not all of these side effects appear very often, when they do occur they may require medical attention. Check with your doctor if the following side effect occurs:

Irritation of skin not present before using this medicine

Other side effects not listed above may also occur in some patients. If you notice any other effects, check with your doctor.

NYSTATIN (Vaginal)
Some commonly used brand names are:

Korostatin	Nadostine*
Mycostatin	Nilstat

*Not available in the United States.

Nystatin (nye-STAT-in) belongs to the group of medicines called antifungals. Vaginal nystatin tablets are used to treat fungal infections of the vagina. Also, they have been used as lozenges to treat fungal infections of the mouth. This medicine is available only with your doctor's prescription.

Before Using This Medicine

In order to decide on the best treatment for your medical problem, your doctor should be told:

—if you have ever had any unusual reaction to nystatin in the past. This medicine should not be used if you are allergic to it.

—if you are pregnant, if you intend to become pregnant, or if you are breast-feeding an infant, although nystatin is not absorbed into the body and has not been shown to cause problems.

Proper Use of This Medicine

Nystatin usually comes with patient directions. Read them carefully before using this medicine.

This medicine is usually inserted into the vagina with an applicator. However, if you are pregnant, check with your doctor before using the applicator to insert the vaginal tablet.

To help clear up your infection completely, *keep using this medicine for the full time of treatment* even though your condition may have improved. Also, keep using this medicine even if you begin to menstruate during the time of treatment.

If you miss a dose of this medicine, insert it as soon as possible. Then go back to your regular dosing schedule. But if it is almost time for your next dose, do not insert the missed dose at all. Instead, go back to your regular dosing schedule. If you have any questions about this, check with your doctor.

Precautions While Using This Medicine

To help cure the infection and to help prevent reinfection, good health habits are required. These include the following:

• Wear cotton panties (or panties or pantyhose with cotton crotches) instead of synthetic (for example, nylon, rayon) underclothes.

• Wear freshly laundered underclothes.

If you have any questions about this, check with your doctor, nurse, or pharmacist.

If you have any questions about douching or intercourse during the time of treatment with nystatin, check with your doctor.

Since there may be some vaginal drainage while you are using this medicine, a sanitary napkin may be worn to protect your clothing.

Side Effects of This Medicine

Along with its needed effects, a medicine may cause some unwanted effects. Although not all of these side effects appear very often, when they do occur they may require medical attention. Check with your doctor if the following side effect occurs:

Irritation of vagina not present before using this medicine

Other side effects not listed above may also occur in some patients. If you notice any other effects, check with your doctor.

NYSTATIN, NEOMYCIN, GRAMICIDIN, AND TRIAMCINOLONE (Topical)

Some commonly used brand names are:

Mycolog	Mytrex
Myco Triacet	Triamcinolone NNG

Nystatin (nye-STAT-in), neomycin (nee-oh-MYE-sin), gramicidin (gram-i-SYE-din), and triamcinolone (trye-am-SIN-oh-lone) is a combined antibiotic and cortisone-like medicine. It is used to help the body overcome infections of the skin and to help provide relief from the redness, itching, and discomfort of many skin problems. It is available only with your doctor's prescription.

Before Using This Medicine

In order to decide on the best treatment for your medical problem, your doctor should be told:

—if you have had allergic reactions to any related antibiotics such as amikacin, gentamicin, kanamycin, neomycin (by mouth or by injection), streptomycin, or tobramycin.

—if you are pregnant or if you intend to become pregnant while using this medicine. Use of cortisone-like medicines in large amounts or for a long time may cause problems in infants of mothers using this medicine.

—if you are breast-feeding an infant, although nystatin, neomycin, gramicidin, and triamcinolone topical preparations have not been shown to cause problems.

—if you have any other skin infection.

—if you are now taking any of the following medicines:

Amikacin	Neomycin (by
Gentamicin	mouth or by
Kanamycin	injection)
	Streptomycin
	Tobramycin

Proper Use of This Medicine

Do not use this medicine in or around the eyes.

Check with your doctor before using this medicine on any other skin problems since it should not be used on certain kinds of bacterial, viral, or fungal skin infections.

Before applying this medicine, wash the area to be treated with soap and water, and dry thoroughly.

Do not bandage or otherwise wrap the area of the skin being treated unless directed to do so by your doctor.

If you are using the cream form of this medicine:

• Apply a thin layer of cream to the affected area and rub in gently until cream disappears. Do not apply a thick layer; this only wastes medicine and does no more good than a thin layer.

If you are using the ointment form of this medicine:

• Apply a thin layer of ointment to the affected area and rub in gently. Do not apply a thick layer; this only wastes medicine and does no more good than a thin layer.

To help clear up your infection completely, *keep using this medicine for the full time of treatment* even though your symptoms may have disappeared; *do not miss any doses.* However, *do not use this medicine more often or for a longer period of time than your doctor ordered.* To do so may increase the chance of absorption through your skin and the chance of side effects. In addition, too much use, especially on thin skin areas (for example, face, armpits, groin), may result in thinning of the skin and stretch marks.

If you do miss a dose of this medicine, apply it as soon as possible. However, if it is almost time for your next application, skip the missed dose and go back to your regular dosing schedule.

Precautions While Using This Medicine

To help make sure your infection does not return, good health habits are required. If you have any questions about this, check with your doctor or pharmacist.

If there is no improvement in your skin problem after you have used this medicine for 1 to 2 weeks or if it becomes worse, check with your doctor.

This medicine may be absorbed through the skin and too much use can affect growth. *Children who must use this medicine should be followed closely by their doctor.*

Side Effects of This Medicine

Along with its needed effects, a medicine may cause some unwanted effects. Although not all of these side effects appear very often, when they do occur they may require medical attention. Stop using this medicine and check with your doctor if any of the following side effects occur:

More common

Blistering, burning, itching, peeling, rash, redness, swelling, or other sign of irritation not present before you started using this medicine

Very rare

Any loss of hearing

Other side effects not listed above may also occur in some patients. If you notice any other effects, check with your doctor.

OPIUM PREPARATIONS (Systemic)
Applies to:
Opium Tincture (OH-pee-um)
Paregoric (par-e-GOR-ik)

Opium preparations are used along with other measures to treat severe diarrhea. They are available only with your doctor's prescription.

Before Using This Medicine

In order to decide on the best treatment for your medical problem, your doctor should be told:
—if you have ever used a medicine like morphine, codeine, or papaverine and had an unusual reaction to it. This medicine should not be taken if you are allergic to it.

—if you are pregnant, if you intend to become pregnant, or if you are breast-feeding an infant. Although opium preparations have not been shown to cause problems, the chance always exists.

—if you have any of the following medical problems:

Addison's disease	Enlarged prostate
Alcoholism	Gallbladder disease
Colitis	or gallstones
Difficult urination	Heart disease
Emphysema, asth-	Hiatal hernia
ma, bronchitis,	Kidney disease
or other chron-	Liver disease
ic lung disease	Underactive thyroid

—if you are now taking ulcer medicine.

—if you are now taking other central nervous system (CNS) depressants such as:

Antihistamines or	Sedatives, tran-
medicine for	quilizers,
hay fever, other	or sleeping
allergies, or	medicine
colds	Seizure medicine
Barbiturates	Tricyclic an-
Other narcotics	tidepressants
Prescription pain	(medicine for
medicine	depression)

—if you are now taking or have taken within the past 2 weeks monoamine oxidase (MAO) inhibitors such as:

Isocarboxazid	Phenelzine
Pargyline	Tranylcypromine

Proper Use of This Medicine

Take this medicine only as directed by your doctor. Do not take more of it, do not take it more often, and do not take it for a longer period of time than your doctor ordered. If too much is taken, it may become habit-forming.

This medicine is to be taken by mouth even though it may come in a dropper bottle. The amount you should take is to be measured with the special dropper provided with your prescription and diluted with water just before you take each dose. This will cause it to turn milky in color, but the medicine will still work.

If your prescription is a liquid form but not in a dropper bottle and the directions on the bottle say to take by teaspoonful, it is not necessary to dilute it before using.

Keep this medicine out of the reach of children since overdose is especially dangerous in children.

Keep the container for this medicine tightly closed to prevent the alcohol from evaporating and the medicine from becoming stronger. Do not store this medicine in the refrigerator. If it does get cold and you notice any solid particles in it, throw it away.

If this medicine upsets your stomach, your doctor may want you to take it with food.

If you miss a dose of this medicine, take it as soon as possible. If it is almost time for your next dose, do not take the missed dose at all and do not double the next one. Instead, go back to your regular dosing schedule. If you have any questions about this, check with your doctor.

Precautions While Using This Medicine

Check with your doctor if your diarrhea does not stop after 1 or 2 days or if you develop a fever.

This medicine will add to the effects of alcohol and other medicines (CNS depressants) that slow down the nervous system. Some examples of CNS depressants are antihistamines or medicine for hay fever, other allergies, or colds; sedatives, tranquilizers, or sleeping medicine; prescription pain medicine or narcotics; barbiturates; medicine for seizures; tricyclic antidepressants (medicine for depression); or anesthetics, including some dental anesthetics. *Check with your doctor before taking any of the above while you are using this medicine.*

This medicine may cause some people to become dizzy, drowsy, or less alert than they are normally. Even if taken at bedtime, it may cause some people to feel drowsy or less alert on arising. *Make sure you know how you react to this medicine before you drive, use machines, or do other jobs that require you to be alert.*

If you have been taking this medicine regularly for a long time, *do not stop using it without first checking with your doctor.* Your doctor may want you to reduce gradually the amount you are using before stopping completely.

Side Effects of This Medicine

Along with its needed effects, a medicine may cause some unwanted effects. Although not all of these side effects appear very often, when they do occur they may require medical attention. Check with your doctor *immediately* if any of the following side effects are severe and occur suddenly since they may indicate a more severe and dangerous problem with your bowels:

Rare

Bloating	Nausea and
Constipation	vomiting
Loss of appetite	Stomach pain

Check with your doctor also if the following effects occur:

Rare

Shortness of breath	Troubled breathing
Skin rash or itching	Unusually slow
	heartbeat

Other side effects may occur which usually do not require medical attention. These side effects may go away during treatment as your body adjusts to the medicine. However, check with your doctor if any of the following side effects continue or are bothersome:

More common with large doses

Difficult urination	Redness or flushing
or frequent urge	of face
to urinate	Unusual increase in
Dizziness	sweating
Drowsiness	Unusual tiredness or
Faintness	weakness
Lightheadedness	

Other side effects not listed above may also occur in some patients. If you notice any other effects, check with your doctor.

ORPHENADRINE (Systemic)

Some commonly used brand names are:

Flexoject	Myolin	Ro-Orphena
Flexon	Neocyten	Tega-Flex
Marflex	Norflex	X-Otag

Orphenadrine (or-FEN-a-dreen) is a medicine that is used to help relax certain muscles in your body and relieve the pain and discomfort caused by strains, sprains, or other injury to your muscles. It is either taken by mouth in the form of tablets, or it is injected into a muscle or vein. This medicine is available only with your doctor's prescription.

Before Using This Medicine

In order to decide on the best treatment for your medical problem, your doctor should be told:

—if you have ever had any unusual reaction to orphenadrine in the past. This medicine should not be taken if you are allergic to it.

—if you are pregnant, if you intend to become pregnant while using this medicine, or if you are breast-feeding an infant. Although orphenadrine has not been shown to cause problems, the chance always exists.

—if you have any of the following medical problems:

Disease of the digestive tract, especially esophagus disease, stomach ulcer, intestinal blockage	Glaucoma Heart disease Myasthenia gravis Unusually fast or irregular heartbeat Urinary tract blockage
Enlarged prostate	

—if you are now taking other central nervous system (CNS) depressants such as:

Antihistamines or medicine for hay fever, other allergies, or colds	Prescription pain medicine Sedatives, tranquilizers, or sleeping medicine
Barbiturates Narcotics	Seizure medicine Tricyclic antidepressants (medicine for depression)

—if you are now taking or have taken within the past 2 weeks monoamine oxidase (MAO) inhibitors such as:

Isocarboxazid	Phenelzine
Pargyline	Tranylcypromine

Proper Use of This Medicine

If you miss a dose of this medicine and remember within an hour or so of the missed dose, take it right away. Then go back to your regular dosing schedule. But if you do not remember until later, do not take the missed dose at all and do not double the next one. Instead, go back to your regular dosing schedule. If you have any questions about this, check with your doctor.

Precautions While Using This Medicine

This medicine will add to the effects of alcohol and other medicines (CNS depressants) that slow down the nervous system. Some examples of CNS depressants are antihistamines or medicine for hay fever, other allergies, or colds; sedatives, tranquilizers, or sleeping medicine; prescription pain medicine or narcotics; barbiturates; medicine for seizures; tricyclic antidepressants (medicine for depression); or anesthetics, including some dental anesthetics. *Check with your doctor before taking any of the above while you are taking orphenadrine.*

This medicine may cause some people to have blurred vision or to become drowsy, dizzy, lightheaded, faint, or less alert than they are normally.*Make sure you know how you react to this medicine before you drive, use machines, or do other jobs that require you to be alert.*

Dryness of the mouth may occur while you are taking this medicine. Sucking on hard candy or ice chips or chewing gum may help relieve the dry mouth.

Side Effects of This Medicine

Along with its needed effects, a medicine may cause some unwanted effects. Although not all of these side effects appear very often, when they do occur they may require medical attention. Check with your doctor if any of the following side effects occur:

Less common

Mental confusion	Unusually fast or pounding heartbeat

Rare

Skin rash or itching

Other side effects may occur which usually do not require medical attention. These side effects may go away during treatment as your body adjusts to the medicine. However, check with your doctor if any of the following side effects continue or are bothersome:

More common

Dryness of mouth

Less common

Blurred vision	Lightheadedness
Constipation	Nausea or vomiting
Difficult urination	Nervousness or
Dizziness	restlessness
Drowsiness	Stomach cramps or
Fainting	discomfort
Headache	Trembling

Other side effects not listed above may also occur in some patients. If you notice any other effects, check with your doctor.

ORPHENADRINE AND APC (Systemic)
Some commonly used brand names are Norgesic and Norgesic Forte.

Orphenadrine (or-FEN-a-dreen) and APC is a combination medicine used to help relax certain muscles in your body and relieve the pain and discomfort caused by strains, sprains, or other injury to your muscles. APC is a combination of aspirin (AS-pir-in), phenacetin (fe-NASS-e-tin), and caffeine (KAF-een). Orphenadrine and APC combination is taken by mouth in the form of tablets and is available only with your doctor's prescription.

Before Using This Medicine

In order to decide on the best treatment for your medical problem, your doctor should be told:

—if you have ever had any unusual reaction to orphenadrine, acetaminophen, phenacetin, caffeine, aspirin or other salicylates including methyl salicylate (oil of wintergreen), or to other nonsteroidal anti-inflammatory agents such as fenoprofen, ibuprofen, indomethacin, naproxen, oxyphenbutazone, phenylbutazone, sulindac, or tolmetin.

—if you are pregnant or if you intend to become pregnant while using this combination medicine. Too much use of aspirin during the last 3 months of pregnancy may increase the length of pregnancy and may prolong labor. Aspirin taken during the last 2 weeks of pregnancy may cause the baby to have bleeding problems at birth. When phenacetin is used during pregnancy, it may cause side effects in the newborn infant. In addition, although orphenadrine, aspirin, phenacetin, and caffeine have not been shown to cause birth defects in humans, the chance always exists.

—if you are breast-feeding an infant. Although orphenadrine, aspirin, phenacetin, and caffeine have not been shown to cause problems, the chance always exists.

—if you have any of the following medical problems:

Anemia
Asthma, allergies, and nasal polyps (history of)
Disease of the digestive tract, especially esophagus disease, stomach ulcer, intestinal blockage
Enlarged prostate
Glaucoma
Glucose-6-phosphate dehydrogenase (G6PD) deficiency
Gout
Heart disease
Hemophilia or other bleeding problems
Hodgkin's disease
Hypoprothrombinemia
Kidney disease
Liver disease
Myasthenia gravis
Unusually fast or irregular heartbeat
Urinary tract blockage
Vitamin K deficiency

—if you are now taking any of the following medicines or types of medicine:

Antacids
Anticoagulants (blood thinners)
Gout medicine
Inflammation medicine (for example, arthritis medicine)
Insulin
Methotrexate
Oral hypoglycemics (diabetes medicine you take by mouth)
Spironolactone
Urine acidifiers (medicine to make your urine more acid)
Urine alkalizers (medicine to make your urine less acid)
Vitamin C

—if you are now taking other central nervous system (CNS) depressants such as:

Antihistamines or medicine for hay fever, other allergies, or colds
Barbiturates
Narcotics
Prescription pain medicine
Sedatives, tranquilizers, or sleeping medicine
Seizure medicine
Tricyclic antidepressants (medicine for depression)

—if you are now taking or have taken within the past 2 weeks monoamine oxidase (MAO) inhibitors such as:

Isocarboxazid
Pargyline
Phenelzine
Tranylcypromine

Proper Use of This Medicine

Take this medicine with food or a full glass (8 ounces) of water or milk to lessen stomach irritation.

Do not use this medicine if it has a strong vinegar-like odor, since this means the aspirin in the product is breaking down. If you have any questions about this, check with your doctor or pharmacist.

Use this medicine only as directed by your doctor. Do not use more of it, do not use it more often, and do not use it for a longer period of time than your doctor ordered. If too much is used, it may cause kidney damage.

Keep this medicine out of the reach of children since overdose is very dangerous in young children.

If you miss a dose of this medicine and remember within an hour or so of the missed dose, take it right away. Then go back to your regular dosing schedule. But if you do not remember until later, do not take the missed dose at all and do not double the next one. Instead, go back to your regular dosing schedule. If you have any questions about this, check with your doctor.

Precautions While Using This Medicine

Check the labels of all over-the-counter (OTC), nonprescription, and prescription medicines you now take. If any contain aspirin or other salicylates, phenacetin, or orphenadrine, be especially careful, since taking them while taking this medicine may lead to overdose. If you have any questions about this, check with your doctor or pharmacist.

Caution: Diabetics—This medicine contains aspirin and phenacetin which may cause false test results with urine sugar tests. If you have any questions about this, check with your doctor or pharmacist, especially if your diabetes is not well controlled.

This medicine will add to the effects of alcohol and other medicines (CNS depressants) that slow down the nervous system. Some examples of CNS depressants are antihistamines or medicine for hay fever, other allergies, or colds; sedatives, tranquilizers, or sleeping medicine; prescription pain medicine or narcotics; barbiturates; medicine for seizures; tricyclic antidepressants (medicine for depression); or anesthetics, including some dental anesthetics. In addition, stomach problems may be more likely to occur if you drink alcoholic beverages while being treated with this medicine. *Check with your doctor before taking any of the above while you are using this medicine.*

This medicine may cause some people to have blurred vision or to become drowsy, dizzy, lightheaded, faint, or less alert than they are normally. *Make sure you know how you react to this medicine before you drive, use machines, or do other jobs that require you to be alert.*

Dryness of the mouth may occur while you are taking this medicine. Sucking hard candy or ice chips or chewing gum may help relieve the dry mouth.

Do not take this medicine for 5 days before having any kind of surgery, including dental surgery, unless otherwise directed by your doctor. The aspirin in this product, if taken during this time, may cause bleeding problems.

Side Effects of This Medicine

Along with its needed effects, a medicine may cause some unwanted effects. Although not all of these side effects appear very often, when they do occur they may require medical attention. Check with your doctor if any of the following side effects occur:

Less common

Any loss of hearing	Stomach pain
Bloody or black tarry stools	Unusually fast or pounding heart-
Itching or skin rash	beat
Mental confusion	Wheezing, tightness
Nausea or vomiting	in chest, or shortness of breath

Possible signs of overdose

Dizziness or mental confusion	Ringing or buzzing in ear (continu-
Nausea or vomiting	ing)
Rapid breathing	Severe and continu- ing headache
	Stomach pain

Possible side effects with long-term use of APC

Bluish-colored fingernails or mucous membranes	Swelling of feet or lower legs
Cloudy urine	Unusual tiredness or weakness

Other side effects may occur which usually do not require medical attention. These side effects may go away during treatment as your body adjusts to the medicine. However, check with your doctor if any of the following side effects continue or are bothersome:

More common

Dryness of mouth
Indigestion

Less common

Blurred vision	Lightheadedness
Constipation	Nervousness or
Difficult urination	restlessness
Dizziness	Sleeplessness,
Drowsiness	nervousness,
Fainting	or jitters
Headache	Trembling

Other side effects not listed above may also occur in some patients. If you notice any other effects, check with your doctor.

OXOLINIC ACID (Systemic)
A commonly used brand name is Utibid.

Oxolinic (ox-oh-LIN-ik) acid belongs to the general family of medicines called anti-infectives. It is given by mouth to help the body overcome infections of the urinary tract. Oxolinic acid is available only with your doctor's prescription.

Before Using This Medicine

In order to decide on the best treatment for your medical problem, your doctor should be told:

—if you have had allergic reactions to nalidixic acid, a closely related medicine.

—if you are pregnant or if you intend to become pregnant, although oxolinic acid has not been shown to cause problems.

—if you are breast-feeding an infant. Oxolinic acid passes into the breast milk and may cause unwanted effects in infants of mothers taking this medicine.

—if you have either of the following medical problems:

History of con- vulsive disorders (seizures, epilepsy)	Kidney disease (other than infection)

—if you are now taking oral anticoagulants (blood thinners you take by mouth).

—if you are now taking central nervous system (CNS) stimulants such as:

Caffeine Medicine for ap- petite control	Medicine for hyperactive children Medicine for nar- colepsy

Proper Use of This Medicine

Oxolinic acid may be taken with food or antacids if it causes stomach upset.

To help clear up your infection completely, *keep taking this medicine for the full time of treatment* even if you begin to feel better after a few days; *do not miss any doses.*

If you do miss a dose of this medicine, take it as soon as possible. However, if it is almost time for your next dose, do not take the missed dose or double your next dose. Instead, go back to your regular dosing schedule.

Precautions While Using This Medicine

If your symptoms do not improve within 2 to 3 days or if they become worse, check with your doctor.

Some people who take oxolinic acid may become more sensitive to sunlight than they are normally. When you first begin taking this medicine, avoid too much sun or too much use of a sunlamp until you see how you react, especially if you tend to burn easily. You may still be more sensitive to sunlight or sunlamps after stopping this medicine. If you have a severe reaction, check with your doctor.

This medicine may also cause your eyes to become more sensitive to light than they are normally. Wearing sunglasses may help lessen the discomfort from bright light.

This medicine may cause some people to become drowsy or dizzy or may affect their vision. *Make sure you know how you react to this medicine before you drive, use machines, or do other jobs that require you to be alert and to see clearly.*

Side Effects of This Medicine

Along with its needed effects, a medicine may cause some unwanted effects. Although not all of these side effects appear very often, when they do occur they may require medical attention. Check with your doctor if any of the following side effects occur:

More common

Blurred vision, halos around lights, or other changes in vision Dizziness	Drowsiness Headache Insomnia Restlessness

Other side effects may occur which usually do not require medical attention. These side effects may go away during treatment as your body adjusts to the medicine. However, check with your doctor if any of the following side effects continue or are bothersome:

More common

Nausea
Vomiting

Less common

Constipation Diarrhea Itching	Loss of appetite Stomach pain or cramps

Rare

Increased sensitivity of the eyes and skin to sunlight	Metallic taste Swelling of arms or legs

Other side effects not listed above may also occur in some patients. If you notice any other effects, check with your doctor.

OXTRIPHYLLINE AND GUAIFENESIN
(Systemic)
Some commonly used brand names are Brondecon and Brondelate.

Oxtriphylline (ox-TRYE-fi-lin) and guaifenesin (gwye-FEN-e-sin) is a combination medicine that belongs to the group of medicines called bronchodilators. It is used in the treatment of bronchial asthma, chronic bronchitis, emphysema, and other lung diseases. It relieves wheezing, shortness of breath, and troubled breathing. This medicine is available only with your doctor's prescription.

Before Using This Medicine

In order to decide on the best treatment for your medical problem, your doctor should be told:

—if you have ever had any unusual reaction to aminophylline, caffeine, dyphylline, oxtriphylline, theobromine, or theophylline.

—if you are pregnant or if you intend to become pregnant while using this medicine. Use of oxtriphylline (contained in this combination medicine) during pregnancy may cause unwanted effects in the newborn infant. In addition, although oxtriphylline and guaifenesin combination has not been shown to cause birth defects or other problems, the chance always exists.

—if you are breast-feeding an infant. Theophylline passes into the breast milk and may cause irritability or other side effects in infants of mothers taking oxtriphylline.

—if you have any of the following medical problems:

Heart disease	Overactive thyroid
High blood pressure	Stomach ulcer (or
Kidney disease	history of)
Liver disease	

—if you are now taking any of the following medicines or types of medicine:

Clindamycin	Other medicine for
Erythromycin	asthma or
Lincomycin	breathing
Lithium	problems
	Propranolol
	Troleandomycin

Proper Use of This Medicine

Take this medicine only as directed by your doctor. Do not take more of it, do not take it more often, and do not take it for a longer period of time than your doctor ordered. To do so may increase the chance of side effects.

This medicine works best when taken with a glass of water on an empty stomach (either 30 minutes to 1 hour before meals or 2 hours after meals) since that way it will get into the blood sooner. However, in some cases your doctor may want you to take this medicine with meals or right after meals to lessen stomach upset. If you have any questions about how you should be taking this medicine, check with your doctor.

If you miss a dose of this medicine and remember within an hour or so of the missed dose, take it right away. Then go back to your regular dosing schedule. But if you do not remember until later, do not take the missed dose at all and do not double the next one. Instead, go back to your regular dosing schedule. If you have any questions about this, check with your doctor.

Precautions While Using This Medicine

Your doctor should check your progress at regular visits, especially for the first few weeks after you begin using this medicine.

The oxtriphylline in this medicine may add to the central nervous system stimulant effects of caffeine-containing beverages such as tea, coffee, cocoa, and cola drinks. *Avoid drinking large amounts of these beverages while using this medicine.* If you have any questions about this, check with your doctor.

Side Effects of This Medicine

Along with its needed effects, a medicine may cause some unwanted effects. Although not all of these side effects appear very often, when they do occur they may require medical attention. Check with your doctor if any of the following side effects occur:

Less common or rare

Skin rash or hives

Possible signs of overdose

Bloody or black tarry stools	Unusual tiredness or weakness
Cloudy urine	Unusually fast,
Increased urination	pounding, or
Mental confusion	irregular
Muscle twitching	heartbeat
Seizures	Vomiting up blood
Unusual thirst	or material that
	looks like coffee
	grounds

Other side effects may occur which usually do not require medical attention. These side effects may go away during treatment as your body

adjusts to the medicine. However, check with your doctor if any of the following side effects continue or are bothersome:

More common

Headache	Stomach pain
Irritability	Trouble in sleeping
Nausea	Vomiting
Nervousness or rest-	
lessness	

Less common

Diarrhea	Loss of appetite
Dizziness or light-	Unusually fast
headedness	breathing
Flushing or redness	
of face	

Other side effects not listed above may also occur in some patients. If you notice any other effects, check with your doctor.

OXYCODONE AND ACETAMINOPHEN
(Systemic)
Some commonly used brand names are Percocet-5 and Tylox.

Oxycodone and acetaminophen (ox-i-KOE-done and a-seat-a-MEE-noe-fen) is a combination of pain relievers. It is available only with your doctor's prescription. Since prescriptions cannot be refilled, a new prescription must be obtained from your doctor each time you need this medicine.

Before Using This Medicine

In order to decide on the best treatment for your medical problem, your doctor should be told:

—if you have ever had any unusual reaction to acetaminophen or oxycodone in the past. This medicine should not be taken if you are allergic to it.

—if you are pregnant, if you intend to become pregnant, or if you are breast-feeding an infant. Although oxycodone and acetaminophen have not been shown to cause problems, the chance always exists.

—if you have any of the following medical problems:

Brain disease	Enlarged prostate or
or injury	problems with
Colitis	urination
Emphysema,	Gallbladder disease
asthma, or	or gallstones
chronic lung	Kidney disease
disease	Liver disease

Underactive adrenal	Unusually slow or
gland (Addison's	irregular heart-
disease)	beat
Underactive thyroid	Virus infection
	of the liver

—if you are now taking other central nervous system (CNS) depressants such as:

Antihistamines or	Other prescription
medicine for hay	pain medicine
fever, otheraller-	Sedatives, tran-
gies, or colds	quilizers, or sleep-
Barbiturates	ing medicine
Other narcotics	Seizure medicine
	Tricyclic an-
	tidepressants
	(medicine for
	depression)

—if you are now taking prescription medicine for stomach cramps or spasms.

—if you are now taking or have taken within the past 2 weeks monoamine oxidase (MAO) inhibitors such as:

Isocarboxazid	Phenelzine
Pargyline	Tranylcypromine

Proper Use of This Medicine

Take this medicine only as directed by your doctor. Do not take more of it, do not take it more often, and do not take it for a longer period of time than your doctor ordered. If too much is taken, it may become habit-forming or cause liver damage.

Keep this medicine out of the reach of children since overdose is very dangerous in young children.

Precautions While Using This Medicine

Check the labels of all over-the-counter (OTC), nonprescription, and prescription medicines you now take. If any contain acetaminophen, oxycodone, or other narcotics, be especially careful, since taking them while taking this medicine may lead to overdose. If you have any questions about this, check with your doctor or pharmacist.

If you will be taking this medicine for a long period of time (for example, for several months at a time), your doctor should check your progress at regular visits.

This medicine will add to the effects of alcohol and other medicines (CNS depressants) that slow down the nervous system. Some examples of CNS depressants are antihistamines or medicine for hay fever, other allergies, or colds; sedatives, tranquilizers, or sleeping medicine; prescription pain medicine or narcotics; barbiturates; medicine for seizures; tricyclic antidepressants (medicine for depression); or anesthetics, including some dental anesthetics. In addition, there may be a greater risk of liver damage if large amounts of alcoholic beverages are used while you are taking this medicine. *Check with your doctor before taking any of the above while you are using this medicine.*

This medicine may cause some people to become drowsy or to feel a false sense of well-being. *Make sure you know how you react to this medicine before you drive, use machines, or do other jobs that require you to be alert and clear-headed.*

Dizziness, lightheadedness, or fainting may occur, especially when you get up from a lying or sitting position. Getting up slowly may help lessen this problem.

Nausea may occur, especially after the first couple of doses. This effect usually goes away if you lie down for a while. However, if nausea continues or is bothersome, check with your doctor.

Side Effects of This Medicine

Along with its needed effects, a medicine may cause some unwanted effects. Although not all of these side effects appear very often, when they do occur they may require medical attention. Check with your doctor if any of the following side effects occur:

Less common

Shortness of breath	Unusually slow
Troubled breathing	heartbeat

Rare

Itching or skin rash	Unusual tiredness or
Unexplained sore	weakness
throat and fever	Yellowing of eyes or
Unusual bleeding or	skin
bruising	

Other side effects may occur which usually do not require medical attention. These side effects may go away during treatment as your body adjusts to the medicine. However, check with your doctor if any of the following side effects continue or are bothersome:

More common

Dizziness	Lightheadedness
Drowsiness	Nausea or vomiting
Feeling faint	

Less common

Constipation	Loss of appetite
Difficult urination	Redness or flushing
False sense of well-	of face
being	Unusual increase in
Frequent urge to	sweating
urinate	

Other side effects not listed above may also occur in some patients. If you notice any other effects, check with your doctor.

OXYCODONE AND ASPIRIN (Systemic)
Some commonly used brand names are Percodan and Percodan-Demi.

Oxycodone (ox-i-KOE-done) and aspirin (AS-pir-in) is a combination of pain relievers. Oxycodone and aspirin combination is available only with your doctor's prescription. Since prescriptions cannot be refilled, a new prescription must be obtained from your doctor each time you need this medicine.

Before Using This Medicine

In order to decide on the best treatment for your medical problem, your doctor should be told:

—if you have ever had any unusual reaction to oxycodone, aspirin or other salicylates including methyl salicylate (oil of wintergreen), or other nonsteroidal anti-inflammatory agents such as fenoprofen, ibuprofen, indomethacin, naproxen, oxyphenbutazone, phenylbutazone, sulindac, or tolmetin.

—if you are pregnant or if you intend to become pregnant while using this medicine. Too much use of aspirin during the last 3 months of pregnancy may increase the length of pregnancy and may prolong labor. Also, aspirin taken during the last 2 weeks of pregnancy may cause the baby to have bleeding problems at birth. In addition, although aspirin and oxycodone have not been shown to cause birth defects, the chance always exists.

—if you are breast-feeding an infant. Although oxycodone and aspirin have not been shown to cause problems, the chance always exists. Therefore, use by nursing mothers should be carefully considered.

—if you have any of the following medical problems:

Anemia	Brain disease or in-
Asthma, allergies,	jury
and nasal polyps	Colitis
(history of)	

Emphysema, asthma, or chronic lung disease
Enlarged prostate or problems with urination
Gallbladder disease or gallstones
Gout
Hemophilia or other bleeding problems
Hodgkin's disease
Hypoprothrombinemia
Kidney disease
Liver disease
Ulcer or other stomach problems
Underactive adrenal gland (Addison's disease)
Underactive thyroid
Unusually slow or irregular heartbeat
Vitamin K deficiency

—if you are now taking any of the following medicines or types of medicine:

Antacids
Anticoagulants (blood thinners)
Gout medicine
Inflammation medicine (for example, arthritis medicine)
Insulin
Methotrexate
Oral hypoglycemics (diabetes medicine you take by mouth)
Prescription medicine for stomach cramps or spasms
Spironolactone
Urine acidifiers (medicine to make your urine more acid)
Urine alkalizers (medicine to make your urine less acid)
Vitamin C

—if you are now taking other central nervous system (CNS) depressants such as:

Antihistamines or medicine for hay fever, other allergies, or colds
Barbiturates
Other narcotics
Other prescription pain medicine
Sedatives, tranquilizers, or sleeping medicine
Seizure medicine
Tricyclic antidepressants (medicine for depression)

—if you are now taking or have taken within the past 2 weeks monoamine oxidase (MAO) inhibitors such as:

Isocarboxazid
Pargyline
Phenelzine
Tranylcypromine

Proper Use of This Medicine

Take this medicine with food or a full glass (8 ounces) of water or milk to lessen stomach irritation.

Do not use this medicine if it has a strong vinegar-like odor, since this means the aspirin in the product is breaking down. If you have any questions about this, check with your doctor or pharmacist.

Take this medicine only as directed by your doctor. Do not take more of it, do not take it more often, and do not take it for a longer period of time than your doctor ordered. If too much is taken, it may become habit-forming.

Keep this medicine out of the reach of children since overdose is very dangerous in young children.

Precautions While Using This Medicine

Check the labels of all over-the-counter (OTC), nonprescription, and prescription medicines you now take. If any contain oxycodone or other narcotics, or aspirin or other salicylates, be especially careful, since taking them while taking this medicine may lead to overdose. If you have any questions about this, check with your doctor or pharmacist.

Caution: Diabetics—This medicine contains aspirin which may cause false test results with urine sugar tests if you regularly take 8 or more tablets a day. Smaller doses or occasional use of aspirin usually does not affect urine sugar tests. If you have any questions about this, check with your doctor, nurse, or pharmacist, especially if your diabetes is not well controlled.

If you will be taking this medicine for a long period of time (for example, for several months at a time), your doctor should check your progress at regular visits.

Do not take this medicine for 5 days before any surgery, including dental surgery, unless otherwise directed by your doctor. Taking aspirin during this time may cause bleeding problems.

This medicine will add to the effects of alcohol and other medicines (CNS depressants) that slow down the nervous system. Some examples of CNS depressants are antihistamines or medicine for hay fever, other allergies, or colds; sedatives, tranquilizers, or sleeping medicine; prescription pain medicine or narcotics; barbiturates; medicine for seizures; tricyclic antidepressants (medicine for depression); or anesthetics, including some dental anesthetics. In addition, stomach problems may be more likely to occur if you drink alcoholic beverages while being treated with this medicine. *Check with your doctor before taking any of the above while you are using this medicine.*

This medicine may cause some people to become drowsy or to feel a false sense of well-being. *Make sure you know how you react to this medicine before you drive, use machines, or do other jobs that require you to be alert and clear-headed.*

Dizziness, lightheadedness, or fainting may occur, especially when getting up from a lying or sitting position. Getting up slowly may help lessen this problem.

Nausea may occur, especially after the first couple of doses. This effect usually goes away if you lie down for a while. However, if nausea or vomiting continues, check with your doctor.

Side Effects of This Medicine

Along with its needed effects, a medicine may cause some unwanted effects. Although not all of these side effects appear very often, when they do occur they may require medical attention. Check with your doctor if any of the following side effects occur:

More common

Nausea or vomiting
Stomach pain

Less common

Any loss of hearing	Troubled breathing
Bloody or black tarry stools	Unusually slow heartbeat
Itching or skin rash	Wheezing or tightness in chest
Shortness of breath	

Possible signs of overdose

Dizziness or mental confusion	Ringing or buzzing in ear (continuing)
Rapid breathing	Severe or continuing headache

Other side effects may occur which usually do not require medical attention. These side effects may go away during treatment as your body adjusts to the medicine. However, check with your doctor if any of the following side effects continue or are bothersome:

More common

Dizziness	Feeling faint
Drowsiness	Lightheadedness

Less common

Constipation	Loss of appetite
Difficult urination	Redness or flushing of face
False sense of well-being	Unusual increase in sweating
Frequent urge to urinate	Unusual tiredness or weakness
Indigestion	

Other side effects not listed above may also occur in some patients. If you notice any other effects, check with your doctor.

OXYMETAZOLINE (Nasal)

Some commonly used brand names are:

Afrin	St. Joseph
Duration	Decongestant for
Nafrine*	Children

---

*Not available in the United States.

Oxymetazoline (ox-i-met-AZ-oh-leen) is used for the temporary relief of nasal congestion or stuffiness caused by hay fever or other allergies, colds, or sinus trouble. This medicine is available without a prescription; however, your doctor may have special instructions on the proper use or dose for your medical condition.

Before Using This Medicine

In order to decide on the best treatment for your medical problem, your doctor should be told:

—if you have ever had any unusual reaction to nasal decongestants in the past. This medicine should not be used if you are allergic to it.

—if you are pregnant, if you intend to become pregnant, or if you are breast-feeding an infant. Although oxymetazoline has not been shown to cause problems, the chance always exists.

—if you have any of the following medical problems:

Blood vessel disease	High blood pressure
Diabetes	Overactive thyroid

—if you are now taking or have taken within the past 2 weeks monoamine oxidase (MAO) inhibitors such as:

Isocarboxazid	Phenelzine
Pargyline	Tranylcypromine

Proper Use of This Medicine

Use this medicine only as directed. Do not use more of it, do not use it more often, and do not use it for longer than 3 days without first checking with your doctor. To do so may make your runny or stuffy nose worse and may also increase the chance of side effects.

Wipe the tip of the applicator with a clean, damp tissue and replace the cap right after use. To avoid the spread of infection, do not use the bottle for more than one person.

If you are using the nose drops:

How to use: Blow nose gently. Tilt head back while standing or sitting up, or lie down on a bed and hang head over the side. Place the drops into each nostril and keep head tilted back for a few minutes to allow medicine to spread throughout the nose.

If you are using the nose spray:

How to use: Blow nose gently. With head upright, spray the medicine into each nostril. Sniff briskly while squeezing bottle quickly and firmly. For best results, spray once into each nostril, wait 2 to 5 minutes to allow medicine to work, then blow nose gently and thoroughly. Repeat until complete dose is used.

If you miss a dose of this medicine and remember within an hour or so of the missed dose, use it right away. Then go back to your regular dosing schedule. But if you do not remember until later, do not use the missed dose at all and do not double the next one. Instead, go back to your regular dosing schedule. If you have any questions about this, check with your doctor or pharmacist.

Side Effects of This Medicine

Along with its needed effects, a medicine may cause some unwanted effects. Although not all of these side effects appear very often, when they do occur they may require medical attention. When this medicine is used for short periods of time at low doses, side effects usually are rare. However, check with your doctor or pharmacist if any of the following occur:

Increase in runny
or stuffy nose

Possible signs of too much medicine being absorbed into the body

Headache or   Unusually fast, ir-
  lightheadedness   regular, or pound-
Trouble in sleeping   ing heartbeat
Unusual ner-
  vousness

Other side effects may occur which usually do not require medical attention. These side effects may go away during treatment as your body adjusts to the medicine. However, check with your doctor or pharmacist if any of the following side effects continue or are bothersome:

Burning, dryness,   Sneezing
  or stinging on in-
  side of nose

Other side effects not listed above may also occur in some patients. If you notice any other effects, check with your doctor or pharmacist.

PAPAVERINE (Systemic)
Some commonly used brand names are:

Cerebid	P-A-V	Pavatest
Cerespan	Pavabid	Pavatran
Dipav	Pavacap	Paverolan
Dylate	Pavacon	Ro-Papav
Hyobid	Pavadur	Sustaverine
Kavrin	Pavakey	Vasal
Myobid	Pavased	Vasospan
Orapav	Pavasule	

Papaverine (pa-PAV-er-een) belongs to the group of medicines called vasodilators. Vasodilators increase the size of blood vessels. Papaverine is used to treat problems resulting from poor blood circulation. It is available only with your doctor's prescription.

Before Using This Medicine

In order to decide on the best treatment for your medical problem, your doctor should be told:

—if you have ever had any unusual reaction to papaverine in the past. This medicine should not be taken if you are allergic to it.

—if you are pregnant, if you intend to become pregnant, or if you are breast-feeding an infant. Although papaverine has not been shown to cause problems, the chance always exists.

—if you have any of the following medical problems:

Angina (chest pain)   Heart disease
Glaucoma   Parkinson's disease

—if you have recently had a heart attack or stroke.

—if you are now taking levodopa.

—if you smoke.

Proper Use of This Medicine

If this medicine upsets your stomach, it may be taken with meals, milk, or antacids.

If you miss a dose of this medicine, take it as soon as you remember. If it is almost time for the next dose, do not take the missed dose at all and do not double the next one. Instead, go back to your regular dosing schedule. If you have any questions about this, check with your doctor.

For patients taking the extended-release capsule form of this medicine:

• The capsules are to be swallowed whole and must not be chewed or crushed. If the capsule is too large to swallow, mix the contents with a little jam and swallow it without chewing.

For patients taking the extended-release tablet form of this medicine:

• The tablets are to be swallowed whole and must not be chewed or crushed.

Precautions While Using This Medicine
It may take some time for this medicine to work. If you feel that the medicine is not working, do not stop taking it on your own. Instead, check with your doctor.

The helpful effects of this medicine may be decreased if you smoke. If you have any questions about this, check with your doctor.

Dizziness may occur, especially when you get up from a lying or sitting position or climb stairs. Getting up slowly may help. If this problem continues or gets worse, check with your doctor.

Side Effects of This Medicine
Along with its needed effects, a medicine may cause some unwanted effects. Although not all of these side effects appear very often, when they do occur they may require medical attention. Check with your doctor *immediately* if any of the following side effects occur:

Blurred or double vision	Weakness
Drowsiness	Yellowing of eyes and skin

For patients having papaverine injected:

• Check with your doctor if any of the following side effects occur:
    Redness, swelling, or pain at the place of injection

• Check with your doctor if any of the following side effects continue or are bothersome:

Deep breathing	Rapid heartbeat
Flushing of the face	

Other side effects not listed above may also occur in some patients. If you notice any other effects, check with your doctor.

PARALDEHYDE (Systemic)
A commonly used brand name is Paral.

Paraldehyde (par-AL-de-hyde) is taken by mouth, given by injection, or used rectally to treat nervous and mental conditions. It is used to calm or relax patients who are nervous or tense and to produce sleep. Also, it is used in the treatment of alcoholism and in some convulsive conditions. This medicine is available only with your doctor's prescription.

Before Using This Medicine
In order to decide on the best treatment for your medical problem, your doctor should be told:

—if you have ever had any unusual reaction to paraldehyde in the past. This medicine should not be used if you are allergic to it.

—if you are pregnant, if you intend to become pregnant, or if you are breast-feeding an infant. Although paraldehyde has not been shown to cause problems, the chance always exits.

—if you have any of the following medical problems:

Emphysema, asthma, bronchitis, or other chronic lung disease	Liver disease

—if you have gastroenteritis (stomach flu) or stomach ulcer. Your doctor may not want you to take this medicine by mouth since it may make your condition worse.

—if you have colitis. Your doctor may not want you to use the rectal form of this medicine since it may make your condition worse.

—if you are now taking other central nervous system (CNS) depressants such as:

Antihistamines or medicine for hay fever, other allergies, or colds	Prescription pain medicine
Barbiturates	Seizure medicine
Narcotics	Tricyclic antidepressants (medicine for depression)
Other sedatives, tranquilizers, or sleeping medicine	

—if you are now taking or have taken within the past 2 weeks monoamine oxidase (MAO) inhibitors such as:

Isocarboxazid   Phenelzine
Pargyline   Tranylcypromine

—if you are now taking disulfiram.

Proper Use of This Medicine

Use this medicine only as directed by your doctor. Do not use more of it, do not use it more often, and do not use it for a longer period of time than your doctor ordered. If too much is used, it may become habit-forming.

Do not use if liquid turns brownish in color or if it has a strong vinegar-like odor, since this means the paraldehyde is breaking down. If you have any questions about this, check with your doctor or pharmacist.

Keep this medicine away from the eyes and avoid getting it on the skin and clothing.

Keep away from heat, open flame, and sparks.

If you are taking this medicine regularly (for example, every day) and you miss a dose, take it right away if you remember within an hour or so of the missed dose. Then go back to your regular dosing schedule. But if you do not remember until later, do not take the missed dose at all and do not double the next one. Instead, go back to your regular dosing schedule. If you have any questions about this, check with your doctor.

If you are taking this medicine by mouth:

• *Do not use a plastic spoon, plastic glass, or any other plastic container to take this medicine,* since paraldehyde may react with the plastic. Use a metal spoon or glass container.

• *Take this medicine mixed in a glass of milk or iced fruit juice* to improve the taste and odor and to lessen stomach upset.

If you are using this medicine rectally:

• *Do not use paraldehyde in any plastic container* since it may react with the plastic.

• Before using paraldehyde rectally, make sure you understand exactly how to use it. Paraldehyde may need to be diluted. If you have any questions about this, check with your doctor or pharmacist.

Precautions While Using This Medicine

If you will be using this medicine regularly for a long period of time:

—your doctor should check your progress at regular visits.

—do not stop using it without first checking with your doctor. Your doctor may want you to reduce gradually the amount you are using before stopping completely.

This medicine will add to the effects of alcohol and other medicines (CNS depressants) that slow down the nervous system. Some examples of CNS depressants are antihistamines or medicine for hay fever, other allergies, or colds; sedatives, tranquilizers, or sleeping medicine; prescription pain medicine or narcotics; barbiturates; medicine for seizures; tricyclic antidepressants (medicine for depression); or anesthetics, including some dental anesthetics. *Check with your doctor before taking any of the above while you are using this medicine.*

If you think you may have taken an overdose, get emergency help at once. Taking an overdose of paraldehyde or taking alcohol or other CNS depressants with paraldehyde may lead to unconsciousness and possibly death. Some signs of an overdose are mental confusion, severe weakness, shortness of breath or troubled breathing, staggering, and unusually slow heartbeat.

This medicine may cause some people to become drowsy or less alert than they are normally. Even if taken at bedtime, it may cause some people to feel drowsy or less alert on arising. *Make sure you know how you react to this medicine before you drive, use machines, or do other jobs that require you to be alert.*

Side Effects of This Medicine

Along with its needed effects, a medicine may cause some unwanted effects. Although not all of these side effects appear very often, when they do occur they may require medical attention. Check with your doctor if any of the following side effects occur:

More common
   Skin rash

Rare
   Unusually slow
      heartbeat,
      shortness of
      breath, or trou-
      bled breathing

With long-term use
   Yellowing of eyes or
      skin

Other side effects may occur which usually do not require medical attention. These side effects may go away during treatment as your body adjusts to the medicine. However, check with your doctor if any of the following side effects continue or are bothersome:

More common

Drowsiness	Unpleasant breath
Nausea (when taken	odor
by mouth)	Vomiting (when
Stomach pain (when	taken by mouth)
taken by mouth)	

Less common

Clumsiness or	Dizziness
unsteadiness	"Hangover" effect

After you stop using this medicine, your body may need time to adjust. The length of time this takes depends on the amount of medicine you were using and how long you used it. During this period of time check with your doctor if you notice any of the following side effects:

Convulsions or	Muscle cramps
seizures	Nausea and
Hallucinations (see-	vomiting
ing, hearing, or	Stomach cramps
feeling things that	Trembling
are not there)	Unusual sweating

Paraldehyde will cause your breath to have a strong unpleasant odor. This effect will last until about one day after you have stopped using this medicine.

Other side effects not listed above may also occur in some patients. If you notice any other effects, check with your doctor.

PARGYLINE (Systemic)
A commonly used brand name is Eutonyl.

Pargyline (PAR-gi-leen) belongs to the group of medicines called antihypertensives. Specifically it is a monoamine oxidase (MAO) inhibitor. It is used to treat high blood pressure. This medicine is available only with your doctor's prescription.

Before Using This Medicine

In order to decide on the best treatment for your medical problem, your doctor should be told:

—if you have ever had any unusual reaction to pargyline in the past. This medicine should not be taken if you are allergic to it.

—if you are pregnant, if you intend to become pregnant, or if you are breast-feeding an infant. Although pargyline has not been shown to cause problems, the chance always exists.

—if you have frequent headaches.

—if you have any of the following medical problems:

Angina (chest pain)	Kidney disease
Asthma or bron-	Liver disease
chitis	Low blood pressure
Diabetes	Mental disease
Epilepsy	(history of)
Fever	Overactive thyroid
Glaucoma	Parkinson's disease
Headaches (severe	Pheochromocytoma
or frequent)	(PCC)
Heart disease	

—if you have recently had a stroke or heart attack.

—if you are now taking or have taken within the past 2 weeks any of the following medicines or types of medicine:

Other monoamine	Tricyclic an-
oxidase (MAO)	tidepressants
inhibitors	(medicine for
	depression)

—if you are now taking any of the following medicines or types of medicine:

Appetite sup-	Medicine for hay
pressants	fever, other aller-
Asthma medicine	gies, or colds
Barbiturates	Medicine for
Blood pressure	seizures
medicine	Narcotics
Carbamazepine	Prescription pain
Cyclobenzaprine	medicine
Levodopa	Sedatives, tran-
Medicine for	quilizers, or
diabetes	sleeping medicine

Proper Use of This Medicine

Importance of Diet—When prescribing medicine for your condition, your doctor may also prescribe a personal diet for you. Such a diet may be low in sodium (salt). Medicine is usually more effective when such a diet is properly followed.

Also, it may be very important for you to go on a reducing diet. However, check with your doctor before going on any diet.

Many patients who have high blood pressure will not notice any signs of the problem. In fact, many may feel normal. It is very important that you *take your medicine exactly as directed* and that you keep your doctor's appointments even if you feel well.

Remember that this medicine will not cure your high blood pressure but it does control it. Therefore, you must continue to take it as directed if you expect to keep your blood pressure down. *You may have to take medicine for the rest of your life.* If high blood pressure is not treated, it can cause serious problems such as heart failure, blood vessel disease, stroke, or kidney disease.

In order to help remember to take your medicine, try to get into the habit of taking it at the same time each day.

If you miss a dose of this medicine and remember within 2 hours, take it right away and then go back to your regular dosing schedule. If you do not remember until later, do not take the missed dose at all and do not double the next one. Instead, go back to your regular dosing schedule. If you have any questions about this, check with your doctor or pharmacist.

Precautions While Using This Medicine

Check with your doctor or hospital emergency room immediately if severe headache, stiff neck, chest pains, rapid heartbeat, or nausea and vomiting occur while you are taking this medicine. These may be symptoms of a serious side reaction which should have a doctor's attention.

When taken with certain foods, drinks, or other medicines, pargyline can cause very dangerous reactions. To avoid such reactions, *obey the following rules of caution:*

• Do not eat foods that have a high tyramine content (most common in foods that are aged to increase their flavor), such as cheeses, sour cream, yogurt, pickled herring, chicken liver, canned figs, raisins, bananas, avocados, soy sauce, broad bean pods (fava bean pods), yeast extracts, or meats prepared with tenderizers.

• Do not drink alcoholic beverages, including beer and wines (especially chianti and other hearty red wines).

• Do not eat or drink any more than small amounts of caffeine-containing food or beverages such as chocolate, coffee, tea, or cola.

• Do not take any other medicine unless prescribed by your doctor. This especially includes over-the-counter (OTC) or nonprescription medicine such as that for colds (including nose drops), cough, asthma, hay fever, sinus, or appetite control.

After you stop using this medicine you must continue to obey the rules of caution concerning food, drink, and other medicine for at least 2 weeks. This medicine may continue to react with certain foods or other medicines for up to 14 days after you stop taking it.

This medicine may cause some people to become drowsy or less alert than they are normally. *Make sure you know how you react to this medicine before you drive, use machines, or do other jobs that require you to be alert.*

Dizziness, lightheadedness, or fainting may occur, especially when you get up from a lying or sitting position. *Getting up slowly may help.* When you get up from lying down, sit on the edge of the bed with your feet dangling for 1 or 2 minutes. Then stand up slowly. If the problem continues or gets worse, check with your doctor.

Caution: Diabetics—This medicine may affect blood sugar levels. While you are using this medicine, be especially careful in testing for sugar in your urine. If you have any questions about this, check with your doctor.

Before having any kind of surgery (including dental surgery) or emergency treatment, tell the doctor or dentist in charge that you are using this medicine or have used it within the past 2 weeks.

Your doctor may want you to carry an identification card stating that you are using this medicine.

Tell your doctor if you develop a fever since that may change the amount of medicine you have to take.

Caution: Patients with angina (chest pain)—This medicine may cause you to have an unusual feeling of health and energy. However, *do not suddenly increase the amount of exercise you get without discussing it with your doctor* since that could bring on an attack of angina.

Side Effects of This Medicine

Along with its needed effects, a medicine may cause some unwanted effects. Although not all of these side effects appear very often, when they do occur they may require medical attention. Check with your doctor *immediately* if any of the following side effects occur:

Less common

Rapid or pounding heartbeat

Rare

Chest pains   Nausea and
Headache (severe)   vomiting
                     Stiff or sore neck

Check with your doctor also if any of the following side effects occur:

Less common

Diarrhea   Swelling of feet and
Fainting   lower legs

Rare

Dark urine   Yellowing of eyes
Fever   and skin

Other side effects may occur which usually do not require medical attention. These side effects may go away during treatment as your body adjusts to the medicine. However, check with your doctor if any of the following side effects continue or are bothersome:

More common

Constipation   Drowsiness
Difficult urination   Dry mouth
Dizziness or   Tiredness and
  lightheadedness,   weakness
  especially when
  getting up from a
  lying or sitting
  position

Less common or rare

Chills   Increased sensitivity
Hallucinations (see-   to sunlight
  ing, hearing, or   Insomnia
  feeling things that Muscle twitching
  are not there)   during sleep
Increase in appetite Nightmares
  and weight gain   Restlessness
                     Shakiness

Other side effects not listed above may also occur in some patients. If you notice any other effects, check with your doctor.

PEMOLINE (Systemic)
A commonly used brand name is Cylert.

Pemoline (PEM-oh-leen) belongs to the group of medicines called central stimulants. It is used for the treatment of behavior problems in children. This medicine is available only with your doctor's prescription.

Before Using This Medicine

In order to decide on the best treatment for your medical problem, your doctor should be told:

—if you have ever had any unusual reaction to pemoline in the past. This medicine should not be taken if you are allergic to it.

—if you have either of the following medical problems:

Kidney disease
Liver disease

Proper Use of This Medicine

Take this medicine only as directed by your doctor. Do not take more of it, do not take it more often, and do not take it for a longer period of time than your doctor ordered. If too much is taken, it may become habit-forming.

If you miss a dose of this medicine, take it as soon as possible. Then go back to your regular dosing schedule. But if you do not remember the missed dose until the next day, do not take it at all and do not double the next one. Instead, go back to your regular dosing schedule. If you have any questions about this, check with your doctor.

If you are taking the chewable tablet form of this medicine, these tablets may be chewed or swallowed whole.

Precautions While Using This Medicine

Your doctor should check your progress at regular visits in order to make sure that this medicine does not cause unwanted effects.

If you will be taking this medicine in large doses for a long period of time, do not stop taking it without first checking with your doctor. Your doctor may want you to reduce gradually the amount you are taking before stopping completely.

This medicine may cause some people to become dizzy or less alert than they are normally. *Make sure you know how you react to this medicine before doing things that require you to be alert.*

Side Effects of This Medicine

Along with its needed effects, a medicine may cause some unwanted effects. Although not all of these side effects appear very often, when they do occur they may require medical attention. Check with your doctor if any of the following side effects occur:

Rare

Yellowing of eyes or skin

Possible signs of overdose

Convulsions or seizures	Uncontrolled movements of the eyes or other parts of the body
Hallucinations (seeing hearing, or feeling things that are not there)	Unusual nervousness or restlessness
	Unusually fast heartbeat

Other side effects may occur which usually do not require medical attention. These side effects may go away during treatment as your body adjusts to the medicine. However, check with your doctor if any of the following side effects continue or are bothersome:

More common

Loss of appetite   Unusual weight loss
Trouble in sleeping

Less common

Dizziness	Mental depression
Drowsiness	Nausea
Headache	Skin rash
Increased irritability	Stomach ache

Other side effects not listed above may also occur in some patients. If you notice any other effects, check with your doctor.

PENICILLAMINE (Systemic)
Some commonly used brand names are Cuprimine and Depen.

Penicillamine (pen-i-SILL-a-meen) is used in the treatment of medical problems such as Wilson's disease (too much copper in the body) and rheumatoid arthritis. Also, it is used to prevent kidney stones. Penicillamine may also be used for other conditions as determined by your doctor. This medicine is available only with your doctor's prescription.

Before Using This Medicine

In addition to the helpful effects of this medicine, it has side effects that could be very serious. Before you take this medicine, be sure that you have discussed the use of it with your doctor.

In order to decide on the best treatment for your medical problem, your doctor should be told:

—if you are allergic to penicillin.

—if you are pregnant or if you intend to become pregnant while using this medicine. Penicillamine may cause birth defects if taken during pregnancy.

—if you are breast feeding an infant. Although penicillamine has not been shown to cause problems, the chance always exists.

—if you have kidney disease or a history of kidney disease (only for patients with rheumatoid arthritis).

—if you have had any problems with this medicine in the past.

—if you are now taking any of the following medicines or types of medicines:

Amodiaquine	Medicine containing iron
Chloroquine	
Gold injections	Medicine for cancer
Hydroxychloroquine	Oxyphenbutazone
	Phenylbutazone

Proper Use of This Medicine

Since penicillamine is taken in different ways for different medical problems, it is very important that you understand exactly why you are taking this medicine and how to take it. See below for information on specific medical problems. If you have any questions about this, check with your doctor.

Take this medicine regularly as directed. Do not stop taking it without first checking with your doctor, since stopping the medicine and then restarting it may increase the possibility of side effects.

If you miss a dose of this medicine and your dosing schedule is one dose to be taken:

Once a day—
Take the missed dose as soon as possible. Then go back to your regular dosing schedule. But if you do not remember the missed dose until the next day, do not take it at all and do not double the next one. Instead, go back to your regular dosing schedule.

Two times a day—
Take the missed dose as soon as possible. Then go back to your regular dosing schedule. However, if it is almost time for your next dose, do not take the missed dose at all and do not double the next one. Instead, go back to your regular dosing schedule.

More than two times a day—
If you remember within an hour or so of the missed dose, take it right away. Then go back to your regular dosing schedule. But if you do not remember until later, do not take the missed dose at all and do not double the next one. Instead, go back to your regular dosing schedule.

If you have any questions about this, check with your doctor.

If you are taking this medicine to prevent kidney stones:

• You should drink 2 full glasses (8 ounces each) of water at bedtime and another 2 full glasses (8 ounces each) during the night.

• It is very important that you follow any special instructions from your doctor such as following a low-methionine diet. If you have any questions about this, check with your doctor.

If you are taking this medicine for rheumatoid arthritis:

• Take this medicine on an empty stomach (at least 1 hour before meals and at least 1 hour before or after any other food, milk, or medicine).

• After you begin taking this medicine, 2 to 3 months may pass before you feel its effects.

If you are taking this medicine for Wilson's disease:

• Take this medicine on an empty stomach (at least 1/2 to 1 hour before meals or 2 hours after meals).

• It is very important that you follow any special instructions from your doctor such as following a low-copper diet. If you have any questions about this, check with your doctor.

• After you begin taking this medicine, 1 to 3 months may pass before you notice any improvement in your condition.

Precautions While Using This Medicine

Your doctor should check your progress at regular visits in order to make sure that this medicine does not cause unwanted effects.

Before having any kind of surgery (including dental surgery), tell the doctor or dentist in charge that you are taking this medicine.

If you are taking iron preparations (included also in some vitamin preparations), do not take them within 2 hours of the time you take this medicine.

Side Effects of This Medicine

Along with its needed effects, a medicine may cause some unwanted effects. Although not all of these side effects appear very often, when they do occur they may require medical attention. Check with your doctor if any of the following side effects occur:

More common

Fever	Swelling of lymph
Joint pain	glands
Skin rash, hives, or	
itching	

Less common

Bloody or cloudy	Unusual bleeding or
urine	bruising
Unexplained sore	Unusual tiredness or
throat and fever	weakness

Rare

Darkening of urine	Ringing or buzzing
Difficulty in	in ears
breathing, chew-	Spitting up blood
ing, talking, or	Ulcers, sores, or
swallowing	white spots in
Eye pain, blurred or	mouth
double vision, or	Unusual muscle
any change in	weakness
vision	Yellowing of eyes or
Pale stools	skin

Other side effects may occur which usually do not require medical attention. These side effects may go away during treatment as your body adjusts to the medicine. However, check with your doctor if any of the following side effects continue or are bothersome:

More common

Loss of appetite	Stomach pain
Nausea	Vomiting

Less common

Decreased or loss of	Diarrhea
taste	

Other side effects not listed above may also occur in some patients. If you notice any other effects, check with your doctor.

PENICILLINS (Systemic)

This information applies to the following medicines:

Amoxicillin (a-mox-i-SILL-in)
Ampicillin (am-pi-SILL-in)
Carbenicillin (kar-ben-i-SILL-in)
Cloxacillin (klox-a-SILL-in)
Cyclacillin (sye-kla-SILL-in)
Dicloxacillin (dye-klox-a-SILL-in)
Hetacillin (het-a-SILL-in)
Methicillin (meth-i-SILL-in)
Nafcillin (naf-SILL-in)
Oxacillin (ox-a-SILL-in)
Penicillin G (pen-i-SILL-in) G
Penicillin V
Ticarcillin (tye-kar-SILL-in)

Some commonly used brand names are:	Generic names:
Amoxil AmoxiCAN* Larotid Novamoxin* Penamox* Polymox Robamox Sumox Trimox Utimox Wymox	Amoxicillin
Amcill Ampicin* Ampilean* Omnipen Penbritin Pensyn Polycillin Principen Supen Totacillin	Ampicillin
Geocillin Geopen Pyopen	Carbenicillin
Bactopen* Cloxapen Cloxilean* Novocloxin* Orbenin* Tegopen	Cloxacillin
Cyclapen-W	Cyclacillin
Dycill Dynapen Pathocil Veracillin	Dicloxacillin
Versapen Versapen-K	Hetacillin
Azapen Celbenin Staphcillin	Methicillin
Nafcil Unipen	Nafcillin
Bactocill Prostaphlin	Oxacillin
Bicillin Crystapen* Crysticillin Duracillin Falapen* G-Recillin Kesso-Pen Megacillin* Novopen G* Penioral* Pentids Permapen Tu-Cillin Wycillin	Penicillin G
Betapen-VK Nadopen-V* Novopen-V* Penapar VK Penbec-V* Pen-Vee K Repen-VK Uticillin VK V-Cillin Veetids	Penicillin V
Ticar	Ticarcillin

*Not available in the United States.

Penicillins belong to the general family of medicines called antibiotics. They are given by mouth or by injection to help the body overcome infections. Carbenicillin by mouth is used only to help the body overcome infections of the urinary tract and prostate gland. Penicillin G and penicillin V are also used to prevent "strep" infections in patients with a history of rheumatic heart disease. Penicillins are available only with your doctor's prescription.

There are two kinds of penicillins: penicillinase-sensitive (amoxicillin; ampicillin; carbenicillin; cyclacillin; hetacillin, which breaks down into ampicillin in the body; penicillin G; penicillin V; and ticarcillin) and penicillinase-resistant (cloxacillin; dicloxacillin; methicillin; nafcillin; and oxacillin). Each is used to treat different kinds of infections. One kind of penicillin usually may not be used in place of the other.

Before Using This Medicine

In order to decide on the best treatment for your medical problem, your doctor should be told:

—if you have had allergic reactions to any of the penicillins, cephalosporins, or penicillamine.

—if you have had allergic reactions to procaine or other "caine-type" anesthetics (medicines which cause numbing) (applies only to penicillin G procaine given by injection into the muscle).

—if you are pregnant or if you intend to become pregnant, although penicillins have not been shown to cause problems.

—if you are breast-feeding an infant. Penicillins pass into the breast milk and may cause unwanted effects in infants of mothers taking any of these medicines.

—if you have any of the following medical problems:

History of general allergy (asthma, eczema, hay fever, hives)	Kidney disease (except nafcillin and oxacillin)

—if you are now taking any of the penicillins and are also taking any of the following medicines or types of medicine:

Chloramphenicol	Sulfonamides
Erythromycins	(sulfas)
Probenecid	Tetracyclines

—if you are now taking ampicillin or hetacillin and are also taking allopurinol.

Proper Use of This Medicine

Penicillins (except amoxicillin) are best taken with a full glass (8 ounces) of water on an empty stomach (either 1 hour before or 2 hours after meals) unless otherwise directed by your doctor.

If you are taking amoxicillin:

• Amoxicillin may be taken without regard to meals.

• The liquid form of this medicine may also be taken straight or mixed with formulas, milk, fruit juice, water, ginger ale, or other cold drinks. If mixed with other liquids, take immediately after mixing. Be sure to drink all the liquid in order to get the full dose of medicine.

If you are taking carbenicillin by mouth:

• This medicine usually comes with a drying agent in a small packet to help keep the tablets from breaking down. *Do not swallow the drying agent;* keep it in the bottle with the tablets until they are used up and then throw it away.

If you are taking penicillin G by mouth:

• Do not take acidic fruit juices (for example, orange or grapefruit juice) or other acidic beverages within 1 hour of the time you take penicillin G since this may keep the medicine from working as well.

If you are taking the oral liquid form of this medicine:

• This medicine is to be taken by mouth even though it may come in a dropper bottle. If this medicine does not come in a dropper bottle, use a specially marked measuring spoon or other device to measure each dose accurately since the average household teaspoon may not hold the right amount of liquid.

If you are taking the chewable tablet form of this medicine:

• Tablets should be chewed or crushed before they are swallowed.

To help clear up your infection completely, *keep taking this medicine for the full time of treatment* even if you begin to feel better after a few days; *do not miss any doses.* This is especially important if you have a "strep" infection since serious heart problems could develop later if your infection is not completely cleared up.

If you do miss a dose of this medicine, take it as soon as possible. However, if it is almost time for your next dose and your dosing schedule is:

• 2 doses a day—Space the missed dose and the next dose 5 to 6 hours apart.

• 3 or more doses a day—Space the missed dose and the next dose 2 to 4 hours apart or double your next dose.

Then go back to your regular dosing schedule.

Precautions While Using This Medicine

If your symptoms do not improve within a few days or if they become worse, check with your doctor.

Caution: Diabetics—Ampicillin, hetacillin, and penicillin G may cause false test results with some urine sugar tests. Check with your doctor before changing your diet or the dosage of your diabetes medicine.

Side Effects of This Medicine

Along with its needed effects, a medicine may cause some unwanted effects. Although not all of these side effects appear very often, when

they do occur they may require medical attention. Stop taking this medicine and check with your doctor if any of the following side effects occur:

More common (less common with carbenicillin and ticarcillin)

Hives	Rash
Itching	Wheezing

Other side effects may occur which usually do not require medical attention. These side effects may go away during treatment as your body adjusts to the medicine. However, check with your doctor if any of the following side effects continue or are bothersome:

More common with ampicillin, carbenicillin, cyclacillin, hetacillin, penicillin G, penicillin V, and ticarcillin

Diarrhea	Vomiting
Nausea	

Less common with amoxicillin, cloxacillin, dicloxacillin, methicillin, nafcillin, and oxacillin

Diarrhea	Vomiting
Nausea	

If you are taking carbenicillin by mouth:

• In addition to the side effects mentioned above, check with your doctor if the following side effect continues or is bothersome:

More common

Bitter or unpleasant
taste

If you are receiving methicillin by injection:

• In addition to the side effects mentioned above, check with your doctor immediately if any of the following side effects also occur:

More common

Blood in urine	Troubled breathing
Passage of large amounts of light-colored urine	Unusual tiredness or weakness
Swelling of the face and ankles	

In some patients penicillin G and penicillin V may cause the tongue to become darkened or discolored. These changes are only temporary and will go away when you stop taking these medicines.

Other side effects not listed above may also occur in some patients. If you notice any other effects, check with your doctor.

PENTAZOCINE (Systemic)
A commonly used brand name is Talwin.

Pentazocine (pen-TAZ-oh-seen) is a medicine used to relieve pain. It is available only with your doctor's prescription.

Before Using This Medicine

In order to decide on the best treatment for your medical problem, your doctor should be told:

—if you have ever had any unusual reaction to pentazocine in the past. This medicine should not be taken if you are allergic to it.

—if you are pregnant or if you intend to become pregnant while using this medicine. Pentazocine may cause unwanted side effects in the unborn infant or in the newborn infant.

—if you are breast-feeding an infant. Although pentazocine has not been shown to cause problems, the chance always exists.

—if you have any of the following medical problems:

Brain disease or injury	Gallbladder disease or gallstones
Emphysema, asthma, or chronic lung disease	History of convulsions or seizures
	Kidney disease
	Liver disease
Enlarged prostate or problems with urination	Narcotic dependence or addiction

—if you are now taking any of the following medicines or types of medicine:

Meperidine	Morphine
Methadone or other narcotics when used for the treatment of narcotic dependence or addiction	Prescription medicine for stomach cramps or spasms

—if you are now taking other central nervous system (CNS) depressants such as:

Antihistamines or medicine for hay fever, other allergies, or colds	Sedatives, tranquilizers, or sleeping medicine
Barbiturates	Seizure medicine
Narcotics	Tricyclic antidepressants (medicine for depression)
Other prescription pain medicine	

—if you are now taking or have taken within the past 2 weeks monoamine oxidase (MAO) inhibitors such as:

Isocarboxazid	Phenelzine
Pargyline	Tranylcypromine

Proper Use of This Medicine

Take this medicine only as directed by your doctor. Do not take more of it, do not take it more often, and do not take it for a longer period of time than your doctor ordered. If too much is taken, it may become habit-forming.

Precautions While Using This Medicine

If you will be taking this medicine for a long period of time (for example, for several months at a time), your doctor should check your progress at regular visits.

This medicine will add to the effects of alcohol and other medicines (CNS depressants) that slow down the nervous system. Some examples of CNS depressants are antihistamines or medicine for hay fever, other allergies, or colds; sedatives, tranquilizers, or sleeping medicine; prescription pain medicine or narcotics; barbiturates; medicine for seizures; tricyclic antidepressants (medicine for depression); or anesthetics, including some dental anesthetics. *Check with your doctor before taking any of the above while you are using this medicine.*

This medicine may cause some people to become drowsy, dizzy, or lightheaded, or to feel a false sense of well-being. *Make sure you know how you react to this medicine before you drive, use machines, or do other jobs that require you to be alert and clear-headed.*

Nausea may occur, especially after the first couple of doses. This effect usually goes away if you lie down for a while.

Side Effects of This Medicine

Along with its needed effects, a medicine may cause some unwanted effects. Although not all of these side effects appear very often, when they do occur they may require medical attention. Check with your doctor if any of the following side effects occur:

Less common

Hallucinations (seeing, hearing, or feeling things that are not there)	Mental confusion Shortness of breath Troubled breathing

Other side effects may occur which usually do not require medical attention. These side effects may go away during treatment as your body adjusts to the medicine. However, check with your doctor if any of the following side effects continue or are bothersome:

More common

Dizziness or lightheadedness	False sense of well-being
Drowsiness	Nausea or vomiting

Less common

Blurred vision or change in vision	Loss of appetite
	Nightmares
Constipation or diarrhea	Redness or flushing of face
Difficult urination	Sleeplessness
Frequent urge to urinate	Stomach cramps or pain
Headache	Unusual increase in sweating

Other side effects not listed above may also occur in some patients. If you notice any other effects, check with your doctor.

PENTAZOCINE AND ASPIRIN (Systemic)
A commonly used brand name is Talwin Compound.

Pentazocine (pen-TAZ-oh-seen) and aspirin (AS-pir-in) is a combination of pain relievers. It is available only with your doctor's prescription.

Before Using This Medicine

In order to decide on the best treatment for your medical problem, your doctor should be told:

—if you have ever had any unusual reaction to pentazocine or to aspirin or other salicylates including methyl salicylate (oil of wintergreen), or to other nonsteroidal anti-inflammatory agents such as fenoprofen, ibuprofen, indomethacin, naproxen, oxyphenbutazone, phenylbutazone, sulindac, or tolmetin.

—if you are pregnant or if you intend to become pregnant while using this medicine. Too much use of aspirin during the last 3 months of pregnancy may increase the length of pregnancy and may prolong labor. Also, aspirin taken during the last 2 weeks of pregnancy may cause the baby to have bleeding problems at birth. Pentazocine may cause unwanted side effects in the unborn infant or the newborn infant. In addition, although pentazocine and aspirin have not been shown to cause birth defects, the chance always exists.

—if you are breast-feeding an infant. Although pentazocine and aspirin have not been shown to cause problems, the chance always exists.

—if you have any of the following medical problems:

Anemia	Hemophilia or other
Asthma, allergies,	bleeding problems
and nasal polyps	History of convul-
(history of)	sions or seizures
Brain disease or	Hodgkin's disease
injury	Hypoprothrom-
Emphysema,	binemia
asthma, or	Kidney disease
chronic lung	Liver disease
disease	Narcotic
Enlarged prostate or	dependence or
problems with	addiction
urination	Ulcer or other
Gallbladder disease	stomach problems
or gallstones	Vitamin K deficiency
Gout	

—if you are now taking any of the following medicines or types of medicine:

Antacids	Morphine
Anticoagulants	Oral hypoglycemics
(blood thinners)	(diabetes medicine
Gout medicine	you take by
Inflammation	mouth)
medicine (for ex-	Prescription
ample, arthritis	medicine for
medicine)	stomach cramps
Insulin	or spasms
Meperidine	Spironolactone
Methadone or other	Urine acidifiers
narcotics when	(medicine to
used for the treat-	make your urine
ment of narcotic	more acid)
dependence or	Urine alkalizers
addiction	(medicine to
Methotrexate	make your urine
	less acid)
	Vitamic C

—if you are now taking other central nervous system (CNS) depressants such as:

Antihistamines or	Sedatives, tran-
medicine for hay	quilizers, or
fever, other	sleeping
allergies,	medicine
or colds	Seizure medicine
Barbiturates	Tricyclic an-
Narcotics	tidepressants
Other prescription	(medicine for
pain medicine	depression)

—if you are now taking or have taken within the past 2 weeks monoamine oxidase (MAO) inhibitors such as:

Isocarboxazid	Phenelzine
Pargyline	Tranylcypromine

Proper Use of This Medicine

Take this medicine with food or a full glass (8 ounces) of water or milk to lessen stomach irritation.

Do not use this medicine if it has a strong vinegar-like odor, since this means the aspirin is breaking down. If you have any questions about this, check with your doctor or pharmacist.

Take this medicine only as directed by your doctor. Do not take more of it, do not take it more often, and do not take it for a longer period of time than your doctor ordered. If too much is taken, it may become habit-forming.

Keep this medicine out of the reach of children since overdose is especially dangerous in young children.

Precautions While Using This Medicine

Check the labels of all over-the-counter (OTC) nonprescription and prescription medicines you now take. If any contain aspirin or other salicylates or pentazocine or other narcotics be especially careful, since taking them while taking this medicine may lead to overdose or other problems. If you have any questions about this, check with your doctor or pharmacist.

Caution: Diabetics—This medicine contains aspirin which may cause false test results with urine sugar tests if you regularly take 8 or more tablets a day. Smaller doses or occasional use of aspirin usually does not affect urine sugar tests. If you have any questions about this, check with your doctor, nurse, or pharmacist, especially if your diabetes is not well controlled.

If you will be taking this medicine for a long period of time (for example, for several months at a time), your doctor should check your progress at regular visits.

Do not take this medicine for 5 days before any surgery, including dental surgery, unless otherwise directed by your doctor. Taking aspirin at this time may cause bleeding problems.

This medicine will add to the effects of alcohol and other medicines (CNS depressants) that slow down the nervous system. Some examples of CNS depressants are antihistamines or medicine for hay fever, other allergies, or colds; sedatives, tranquilizers, or sleeping medicine; prescription pain medicine or narcotics; barbiturates; medicine for seizures; tricyclic antidepressants (medicine for depression); or anesthetics, including some dental anesthetics. In addition, stomach problems may be more likely to occur if you drink alcoholic beverages while being treated with this medicine. *Check with your doctor before taking any of the above while you are using this medicine.*

This medicine may cause some people to become drowsy, dizzy, or lightheaded, or to feel a false sense of well-being. *Make sure you know how you react to this medicine before you drive, use machines, or do other jobs that require you to be alert and clear-headed.*

Nausea may occur, especially after the first couple of doses. This effect usually goes away if you lie down for a while. However, if nausea or vomiting continues, check with your doctor.

Side Effects of This Medicine

Along with its needed effects, a medicine may cause some unwanted effects. Although not all of these side effects appear very often, when they do occur they may require medical attention. Check with your doctor if any of the following side effects occur:

More common

    Nausea or vomiting
    Stomach pain

Less common

Any loss of hearing	Itching or skin
Bloody or black	rash
tarry stools	Mental confusion
Hallucinations (see-	Shortness of breath
ing, hearing, or	Tightness in chest
feeling things that	Troubled breathing
are not there)	Wheezing

Possible signs of overdose

Dizziness or mental	Ringing or buzzing
confusion	in ear (continu-
Rapid breathing	ing)
	Severe or continuing
	headache

Other side effects may occur which usually do not require medical attention. These side effects may go away during treatment as your body adjusts to the medicine. However, check with your doctor if any of the following side effects continue or are bothersome:

More common

Dizziness	Indigestion
Drowsiness	Lightheadedness
False sense of	Nausea or vomiting
well-being	

Less common

Blurred vision or	Loss of appetite
change in vision	Nightmares
Constipation	Redness or flushing
Diarrhea	of face
Difficult urination	Sleeplessness
Frequent urge to	Stomach cramps or
urinate	pain
Headache	Unusual increase in
	sweating

Other side effects not listed above may also occur in some patients. If you notice any other effects, check with your doctor.

PENTOBARBITAL AND CARBROMAL
(Systemic)
A commonly used brand name is Carbrital.

Pentobarbital (pen-toe-BAR-bi-tal) and carbromal (kar-BROE-mal) combination is used in the treatment of insomnia or sleeplessness. It helps patients fall asleep and stay asleep through the night. Also, it is used as a sedative to calm or relax patients who are nervous or tense. This medicine is available only with your doctor's prescription.

Before Using This Medicine

In order to decide on the best treatment for your medical problem, your doctor should be told:

—if you have ever had any unusual reaction to barbiturates or bromides.

—if you are pregnant or if you intend to become pregnant while using this medicine. Too much use of pentobarbital (contained in this combination medicine) during pregnancy may cause the baby to become dependent on the medicine. This may lead to withdrawal side effects after birth. In addition, use of pentobarbital during pregnancy may cause bleeding problems in the newborn infant. Also, use of pentobarbital during late pregnancy may cause breathing problems in the newborn infant.

—if you are breast-feeding an infant. Pentobarbital and carbromal pass into the breast milk and may cause unwanted effects in infants of mothers taking this medicine.

—if you have any of the following medical problems:

Anemia	Diabetes
Asthma (or history	Heart or blood
of), emphysema,	vessel disease
or chronic lung	Hyperactivity
disease	(in children)

Kidney disease
Liver disease
Overactive thyroid

Porphyria (or
history of)
Underactive adrenal
glands

—if you are now taking any central nervous system (CNS) depressants such as:

Antihistamines or
medicine for
hay fever, other
allergies, or colds
Barbiturates
Narcotics
Prescription pain
medicine

Sedatives, tran-
quilizers,
or sleeping
medicine
Seizure medicine
Tricyclic an-
tidepressants
(medicine for
depression)

—if you are now taking or have taken within the past 2 weeks monoamine oxidase (MAO) inhibitors such as:

Isocarboxazid
Pargyline

Phenelzine
Tranylcypromine

—if you are now taking any of the following medicines or types of medicine:

Anticoagulants
(blood thinners)
Bromide-containing
medicine
Contraceptives, oral
(birth-control
pills)
Corticosteroids
(cortisone-like
medicines)

Cyclophosphamide
Digitalis
Digitoxin
Doxycycline
Estrogens
Griseofulvin
Phenytoin
Quinidine

Proper Use of This Medicine

Take this medicine only as directed by your doctor. Do not take more of it, do not take it more often, and do not take it for a longer period of time than your doctor ordered. If too much is taken, it may become habit-forming.

Keep this medicine out of the reach of children since overdose is especially dangerous in children.

Precautions While Using This Medicine

If you will be taking this medicine regularly for a long period of time:

—your doctor should check your progress at regular visits.

—do not stop taking it without first checking with your doctor. Your doctor may want you to reduce gradually the amount you are taking before stopping completely.

This medicine will add to the effects of alcohol and other medicines (CNS depressants) that slow down the nervous system. Some examples of CNS depressants are antihistamines or medicine for hay fever, other allergies, or colds; sedatives, tranquilizers, or sleeping medicine; prescription pain medicine or narcotics; barbiturates; medicine for seizures; tricyclic antidepressants (medicine for depression); or anesthetics, including some dental anesthetics. *Check with your doctor before taking any of the above while you are using this medicine.*

This medicine contains carbromal which is broken down into bromide in the body. Some other medicines, including over-the-counter (OTC) or nonprescription medicines, may contain bromide also. Taking them with this medicine may lead to an overdose. *Check with your doctor before taking any bromide-containing medicine while you are taking this medicine.*

If you think you may have taken an overdose, get emergency help at once. Taking an overdose of pentobarbital and carbromal combination or taking alcohol or other CNS depressants with this medicine may lead to unconsciousness and possibly death. Some signs of an overdose are mental confusion, severe weakness, shortness of breath or troubled breathing, staggering, and unusually slow heartbeat.

This medicine may cause some people to become dizzy, lightheaded, drowsy, or less alert than they are normally. Even if taken at bedtime, it may cause some people to feel drowsy or less alert on arising. *Make sure you know how you react to this medicine before you drive, use machines, or do other jobs that require you to be alert.*

Side Effects of This Medicine

Along with its needed effects, a medicine may cause some unwanted effects. Although not all of these side effects appear very often, when they do occur they may require medical attention. Check with your doctor if any of the following side effects occur:

Less common or rare

Swelling of eyelids,
face, or lips
Unexplained sore
throat and fever
Unusual bleeding or
bruising
Unusual excitement

Unusual tiredness or
weakness
Unusually slow
heartbeat
Wheezing or
tightness
in chest
Yellowing of eyes or
skin

Possible signs of overdose

Clumsiness or unsteadiness	Seeing or hearing things that are not there
Loss of memory	Shortness of breath or troubled breathing
Mental confusion	
Mood or mental changes	
	Skin rash or hives
	Speech problems

Other side effects may occur which usually do not require medical attention. These side effects may go away during treatment as your body adjusts to the medicine. However, check with your doctor if any of the following side effects continue or are bothersome:

More common

Dizziness or lightheadedness	Drowsiness "Hangover" effect

Less common

Diarrhea	Joint or muscle pain
Headache	Nausea or vomiting

After you stop using this medicine, your body may need time to adjust. The length of time this takes depends on the amount of medicine you were using and how long you used it. During this period of time check with your doctor if you notice any of the following side effects:

Convulsions or seizures	Increased dreaming
Feeling faint	Nightmares
Hallucinations (seeing, hearing, or feeling things that are not there)	Trembling
	Trouble in sleeping
	Unusual restlessness
	Unusual weakness

Other side effects not listed above may also occur in some patients. If you notice any other effects, check with your doctor.

PERPHENAZINE AND AMITRIPTYLINE
(Systemic)

Some commonly used brand names are Etrafon and Triavil.

Perphenazine (per-FEN-a-zeen) and amitriptyline (a-meeTRIP-ti-leen) is a combination of medicines used to treat certain mental and emotional conditions. This combination is available only with your doctor's prescription.

Before Using This Medicine

In order to decide on the best treatment for your medical problem, your doctor should be told:

—if you have ever had any unusual reaction to other phenothiazine medicines (such as chlorpromazine, fluphenazine, prochlorperazine, trifluoperazine, or thiothixene) or to other tricyclic antidepressants (such as desipramine, doxepin, imipramine, nortriptyline, or protriptyline) in the past. This medicine should not be taken if you are allergic to it.

—if you are pregnant or if you intend to become pregnant while using this medicine. Although perphenazine and amitriptyline have not been shown to cause birth defects, some side effects such as jaundice and muscle tremors have occured in a few newborn infants of mothers who received phenothiazines during pregnancy.

—if you are breast-feeding an infant. Perphenazine and amitriptyline have not been shown to cause problems during breast-feeding but the chance does exist since they pass into the breast milk.

—if you have any of the following medical problems:

Alcoholism	Heart or blood vessel disease
Asthma (history of) or other lung disease	Liver disease
	Parkinson's disease
Blood disease	Stomach or intestinal problems
Difficult urination	
Enlarged prostate	
Epilepsy	Thyroid disease
Glaucoma	

—if you are now taking any of the following medicines or types of medicine:

Amphetamines	Estrogens
Anticonvulsants (seizure medicine)	Guanethidine (high blood pressure medicine)
Asthma medicine	
Clonidine (high blood pressure medicine)	Levodopa
	Thyroid medicine
	Ulcer medicine
Epinephrine	

—if you are now taking central nervous system (CNS) depressants such as:

Antihistamines or medicine for hay fever, other allergies, or colds	Other tricyclic antidepressants (medicine for depression)
Barbiturates	Prescription pain medicine
Narcotics	Sedatives, tranquilizers, or sleeping medicine

—if you are now taking or have taken within the past two weeks monoamine oxidase (MAO) inhibitors such as:

Isocarboxazid   Phenelzine
Pargyline   Tranylcypromine

Proper Use of This Medicine

Do not take more of this medicine and do not take it more often than your doctor ordered. This is particularly important when it is given to children, since they may react very strongly to the effects of the medicine.

To lessen stomach upset, take this medicine immediately after meals or with food, unless your doctor has told you to take it on an empty stomach.

Sometimes this medicine must be taken for several weeks before its full effect is reached.

If you miss a dose of this medicine, take it as soon as possible. If it is 2 hours or less until your next dose, do not take the missed dose at all and do not double the next one. Instead, go back to your regular dosing schedule. If you have any questions about this, check with your doctor.

Precautions While Using This Medicine

Your doctor should check your progress at regular visits, especially for the first few months you take this medicine.

Do not stop taking this medicine without first checking with your doctor. Your doctor may want you to reduce gradually the amount you are taking before stopping completely.

Do not take this medicine within an hour of taking antacids or medicine for diarrhea. Taking them too close together may make this medicine less effective.

Before having any kind of surgery (including dental surgery) or emergency treatment, tell the doctor or dentist in charge that you are taking this medicine.

This medicine will add to the effects of alcohol and other medicines (CNS depressants) that slow down the nervous system. Some examples of CNS depressants are antihistamines or medicine for hay fever, other allergies, or colds; sedatives, tranquilizers, or sleeping medicine; prescription pain medicine or narcotics; barbiturates; medicine for seizures; tricyclic antidepressants (medicine for depres-

sion); or anesthetics, including some dental anesthetics. *Check with your doctor before taking any of the above while you are using this medicine.*

This medicine may cause some people to become drowsy or less alert than they are normally, especially during the first few weeks the medicine is being taken. Even if you take this medicine only at bedtime, you may feel drowsy or less alert on arising. *Make sure you know how you react to this medicine before you drive, use machines, or do other jobs that require you to be alert.*

Dizziness, lightheadedness, or fainting may occur, especially when you get up from a lying or sitting position. Getting up slowly may help. If the problem continues or gets worse, check with your doctor.

This medicine will often make you sweat less, causing your body temperature to increase. *Use extra care not to become overheated during exercise or hot weather while you are taking this medicine,* since overheating could possibly result in heat stroke. Also, hot baths or saunas may make you feel dizzy or faint while you are taking this medicine.

Your mouth may feel very dry while you are taking this medicine. To help relieve this feeling, chew sugarless gum or dissolve bits of ice in your mouth.

A few people who take this medicine may become more sensitive to sunlight than they are normally. When you first begin taking this medicine, avoid too much sun or too much use of a sunlamp until you see how you react. If you have a severe reaction, check with your doctor.

Side Effects of This Medicine

Along with its needed effects, a medicine may cause some unwanted effects. Although not all of these side effects appear very often, when they do occur they may require medical attention. Check with your doctor if any of the following side effects occur:

More common

Blurred vision	Tic-like (jerky)
Constipation	movements of
Irregular heartbeat	head, face,
Problems in	mouth, and neck
urinating	Trembling and
Shuffling walk	shaking of hands
	and fingers

Less common

Eye pain	Hallucinations (see-
Fainting	ing, hearing, or
Fine, worm-like	feeling things that
movements of	are not there)
tongue	Shakiness
	Unusually slow
	pulse

Rare

Seizures	Yellowing of eyes
Skin rash and	and skin
itching	
Unexplained sore	
throat and fever	

Other side effects may occur which usually do not require medical attention. These side effects may go away during treatment as your body adjusts to the medicine. However, check with your doctor if any of the following side effects continue or are bothersome:

More common

Dizziness	Increased skin sensi-
Drowsiness	tivity to sun
Dry mouth	Nasal congestion
Headache	Nausea and
Increased appetite	vomiting
for sweets	Tiredness or
	weakness

Less common

Changes in men-	Diarrhea
strual period	Insomnia
Decreased sexual	Swelling of breasts
ability	

This medicine may cause the urine to be discolored (pink to brownish red). This effect is not important and is to be expected during treatment with this medicine.

Other side effects not listed above may also occur in some patients. If you notice any other effects, check with your doctor.

PHENAZOPYRIDINE (Systemic)

Some commonly used brand names are:

Azo-100	Phenazodine
Azodine	Pyridiate
Azo-Standard	Pyridium
Di-Azo	Pyrodine
Phen-Azo	

Phenazopyridine (fen-az-oh-PEER-i-deen) is a medicine used to relieve the pain, burning, and discomfort caused by infection or irritation of the urinary tract. It is not an antibiotic and will not cure the infection itself. Phenazopyridine is available only with your doctor's prescription.

Before Using This Medicine

In order to decide on the best treatment for your medical problem, your doctor should be told:

—if you have ever had any unusual reaction to phenazopyridine in the past. This medicine should not be taken if you are allergic to it.

—if you are pregnant, if you intend to become pregnant, or if you are breast-feeding an infant. Although phenazopyridine has not been shown to cause problems, the chance always exists.

—if you have either of the following medical problems:

Hepatitis
Kidney disease

Proper Use of This Medicine

This medicine is best taken with meals or following meals to lessen stomach upset.

Do not use any left-over medicine for future urinary tract problems without first checking with your doctor. An infection may require additional medicine.

If you miss a dose of this medicine, take it as soon as possible. If it is almost time for your next dose, do not take the missed dose at all and do not double the next one. Instead, go back to your regular dosing schedule. If you have any questions about this, check with your doctor.

Precautions While Using This Medicine

This medicine causes the urine to turn reddish orange. This is to be expected while you are using this medicine. Also, the medicine may stain clothing.

Caution: Diabetics—This medicine may cause false test results with urine sugar tests and urine ketone tests. If you have any questions about this, check with your doctor, nurse, or pharmacist, especially if your diabetes is not well controlled.

Side Effects of This Medicine

Along with its needed effects, a medicine may cause some unwanted effects. Although not all of these side effects appear very often, when they do occur they may require medical attention. Check with your doctor if the following side effect occurs:

Yellowing of eyes
or skin

Other side effects may occur which usually do not require medical attention. These side effects may go away during treatment as your body adjusts to the medicine. However, check with your doctor if any of the following side effects continue or are bothersome:

| Dizziness | Indigestion |
| Headache | Stomach cramps or pain |

Other side effects not listed above may also occur in some patients. If you notice any other effects, check with your doctor.

PHENOTHIAZINES (Systemic)

This information applies to the following medicines:

Acetophenazine (a-set-oh-FEN-a-zeen)
Butaperazine (byoo-ta-PAIR-a-zeen)
Carphenazine (kar-FEN-a-zeen)
Chlorpromazine (klor-PROE-ma-zeen)
Fluphenazine (floo-FEN-a-zeen)
Mesoridazine (mez-oh-RID-a-zeen)
Perphenazine (per-FEN-a-zeen)
Piperacetazine (pi-per-a-SET-a-zeen)
Prochlorperazine (proe-klor-PAIR-a-zeen)
Promazine (PROE-ma-zeen)
Thioridazine (thye-oh-RID-a-zeen)
Trifluoperazine (trye-floo-oh-PAIR-a-zeen)
Triflupromazine (trye-floo-PROE-ma-zeen)

This information does *not* apply to the following medicines:

Ethopropazine
Methdilazine
Methotrimeprazine
Promethazine
Propiomazine
Thiethylperazine
Thiopropazate
Trimeprazine

Some commonly used brand names are:	Generic names:
Tindal	Acetophenazine
Repoise	Butaperazine
Proketazine	Carphenazine
Chloramead Chlor-Promanyl* Chlorprom* Promapar Promosol* Largactil* Thorazine	Chlorpromazine

Modecate* Moditen* Permitil Prolixin	Fluphenazine
Serentil	Mesoridazine
Phenazine* Trilafon	Perphenazine
Quide	Piperacetazine
Compazine Stemetil	Prochlorperazine
Norzine* Promanyl* Sparine	Promazine
Mellaril Novoridazine* Thioril*	Thioridazine
Clinazine* Novoflurazine* Pentazine* Solazine* Stelazine Terfluzine* Triflurin* Tripazine*	Trifluoperazine
Psyquil* Vesprin	Triflupromazine

*Not available in the United States.

Phenothiazines (fee-noe-THYE-a-zeens) are a family of medicines used to treat nervous, mental, and emotional conditions; some are used also to control anxiety, nausea and vomiting, and severe hiccups. Phenothiazines are available only with your doctor's prescription.

Before Using This Medicine

In order to decide on the best treatment for your medical problem, your doctor should be told:

—if you have ever had any unusual reaction to phenothiazine medicines in the past. This medicine should not be taken if you are allergic to it.

—if you are pregnant or if you intend to become pregnant while using this medicine. Although phenothiazines have not been shown to cause birth defects, some side effects such as jaundice and muscle tremors have occurred in a few newborns whose mothers received phenothiazines during pregnancy.

—if you are breast-feeding an infant. Phenothiazines have not been shown to cause problems during breast-feeding but the chance does exist since some phenothiazines are known to pass into the breast milk.

—if you have any of the following medical problems:

Alcoholism	Heart or blood
Blood disease	vessel disease
Difficult urination	Liver disease
Enlarged prostate	Lung disease
Glaucoma	Parkinson's disease
	Stomach ulcers

—if you are now taking any of the following medicines or types of medicine:

Amphetamines	Guanethidine (high
Anticonvulsants	blood pressure
(seizure medicine)	medicine)
Asthma medicine	Levodopa
Epinephrine	Ulcer medicine

—if you are now taking central nervous system (CNS) depressants such as:

Antihistamines or	Prescription pain
medicine for	medicine
hay fever, other	Sedatives, tran-
allergies, or colds	quilizers,
Barbiturates	or sleeping
Narcotics	medicine
	Tricyclic an-
	tidepressants
	(medicine for
	depression)

—if you are now taking or have taken within the past 2 weeks monoamine oxidase (MAO) inhibitors such as:

Isocarboxazid	Phenelzine
Pargyline	Tranylcypromine

Proper Use of This Medicine

Do not take more of this medicine or take it more often than your doctor ordered. This is particularly important when it is given to children, since they may react very strongly to the effects of the medicine.

Sometimes this medicine must be taken for several weeks before its full effect is reached in the treatment of certain mental and emotional conditions.

Do not stop taking this medicine without first checking with your doctor. Your doctor may want you to reduce gradually the amount you are taking before stopping completely, to prevent side effects or making your condition worse.

If you miss a dose of this medicine and your dosing schedule is one dose to be taken:

Once a day—
Take the missed dose as soon as possible. Then go back to your regular dosing schedule. But if you do not remember the missed dose until the next day, do not take it at all and do not double the next one. Instead, go back to your regular dosing schedule.

Two times a day—
Take the missed dose as soon as possible. Then go back to your regular dosing schedule. However, if it is almost time for your next dose, do not take the missed dose at all and do not double the next one. Instead, go back to your regular dosing schedule.

More than two times a day—
If you remember within an hour or so of the missed dose, take it right away. Then go back to your regular dosing schedule. But if you do not remember until later, do not take the missed dose at all and do not double the next one. Instead, go back to your regular dosing schedule.

If you have any questions about this, check with your doctor.

For patients taking this medicine by mouth:

• This medicine may be taken with food or a full glass (8 ounces) of water or milk to reduce stomach irritation.

• Do not take this medicine within an hour of taking antacids or medicine for diarrhea. Taking them too close together may make this medicine less effective.

• *If your medicine comes in a dropper bottle,* it must be diluted before you take it. Just before taking, measure each dose with the specially marked dropper and dilute it in 1/2 glass (4 ounces) of tomato or fruit juice, water, soup, coffee, tea, milk, or carbonated beverage.

• If you are taking the extended-release tablet form of this medicine each dose should be swallowed whole. Do not break, crush, or chew before swallowing.

For patients using the suppository form of this medicine:

• To insert suppository: First remove the foil wrapper and moisten the suppository with water. Lie down on left side with right knee bent, and push the suppository well up into the rectum with finger.

• If the suppository is too soft to insert because of storage in a warm place, before removing the foil wrapper chill the suppository in the refrigerator for 30 minutes or run cold water over it.

Precautions While Using This Medicine

Your doctor should check your progress at regular visits, especially for the first few months you take this medicine. This will allow your dosage to be changed if necessary to meet your needs.

This medicine will add to the effects of alcohol and other medicines (CNS depressants) that slow down the nervous system. Some examples of CNS depressants are antihistamines or medicine for hay fever, other allergies, or colds; sedatives, tranquilizers, or sleeping medicine; prescription pain medicine or narcotics; barbiturates; medicine for seizures; tricyclic antidepressants (medicine for depression); or anesthetics, including some dental anesthetics. *Check with your doctor before taking any of the above while you are using this medicine.*

This medicine may cause some people to become drowsy or less alert than they are normally, especially during the first few weeks the medicine is being taken. Even if you take this medicine only at bedtime, you may feel drowsy or less alert on arising. *Make sure you know how you react to this medicine before you drive, use machines, or do other jobs that require you to be alert.*

Dizziness, lightheadedness, or fainting may occur, especially when you get up from a lying or sitting position. Getting up slowly may help. If the problem continues or gets worse, check with your doctor.

Sometimes, patients may show signs of restlessness and excitement after taking this medicine. If this occurs, stop taking the medicine and check with your doctor.

This medicine will often make you sweat less, causing your body temperature to increase. *Use extra care not to become overheated during exercise or hot weather while you are taking this medicine,* since overheating could possibly result in heat stroke. Also, hot baths or saunas may make you feel dizzy or faint while you are taking this medicine.

A few people who take this medicine may become more sensitive to sunlight than they are normally. When you first begin taking this medicine, use sun screen lotions, or avoid too much sun or too much use of a sunlamp until you see how you react. If you have a severe reaction, check with your doctor.

If you are taking a liquid form of this medicine, try to avoid getting it on your skin or clothing because it may cause a skin rash or other irritation.

If you are receiving this medicine by injection:
• The effects of the long-acting injection form of this medicine may last for up to 6 weeks. The precautions and side effects information for this medicine applies during this period of time.

Side Effects of This Medicine

Along with its needed effects, a medicine may cause some unwanted effects. Although not all of these side effects appear very often, when they do occur they may require medical attention. Check with your doctor if any of the following side effects occur:

More common (occurring with increase of dosage)

Muscle spasms, especially of neck and back	Tic-like (jerky) movements of head, face, mouth, and neck
Restlessness	Trembling and
Shuffling walk	shaking of hands and fingers

Less common

Difficult urination	Fine, worm-like movements of tongue
Fainting	Skin rashes

Rare

Eye problems	Yellowing of eyes and skin
Unexplained sore throat and fever	

Other side effects may occur which usually do not require medical attention. These side effects may go away during treatment as your body adjusts to the medicine. However, check with your doctor if any of the following side effects continue or are bothersome:

More common

Blurred vision	Dry mouth
Constipation	Increased sensitivity of skin to sun
Decreased sweating	Nasal congestion
Dizziness	Unusually fast heartbeat (pulse)
Drowsiness	

Less common

Changes in menstrual period	Decreased sexual ability
	Swelling of breasts

This medicine may cause the urine to turn pinkish red to red or reddish brown; this is harmless and may be expected. If you have questions about this, ask your doctor or pharmacist.

Other side effects not listed above may also occur in some patients. If you notice any other effects, check with your doctor.

PHENOXYBENZAMINE (Systemic)
A commonly used brand name is Dibenzyline.

Phenoxybenzamine (fen-ox-ee-BEN-za-meen) belongs to the general class of medicines called antihypertensives. It is used to treat high blood pressure due to a disease called pheochromocytoma. It is also used to treat some problems due to poor blood circulation. Phenoxybenzamine is available only with your doctor's prescription.

Before Using This Medicine

In order to decide on the best treatment for your medical problem, your doctor should be told:

—if you have ever had any unusual reaction to phenoxybenzamine in the past. This medicine should not be taken if you are allergic to it.

—if you are pregnant, if you intend to become pregnant, or if you are breast-feeding an infant. Although phenoxybenzamine has not been shown to cause problems, the chance always exists.

—if you have any of the following medical problems:

Angina (chest pain)	Kidney disease
Heart or blood vessel disease	Lung infection

—if you have recently had a heart attack or stroke.

—if you are now taking the following medicines or types of medicine:

Epinephrine	Medicine for asthma or breathing problems

Proper Use of This Medicine

In order to help remember to take your medicine, try to get into the habit of taking it at the same time each day.

If you miss a dose of this medicine, take it as soon as you remember. However, if it is almost time for your next dose, do not take the missed dose at all and do not double the next one. Instead, go back to your regular dosing schedule. If you have any questions about this, check with your doctor.

Precautions While Using This Medicine

It is important that your doctor check your progress at regular visits.

Phenoxybenzamine may cause some people to become dizzy, drowsy, or less alert than they are normally. This is more likely to happen when you begin to take it or when you increase the amount of medicine you are taking. *Make sure you know how you react to this medicine before you drive, use machines, or do other jobs that require you to be alert.*

Dizziness, lightheadedness, or fainting may occur, especially when you get up from a lying or sitting position. Getting up slowly may help, but if the problem continues or gets worse, check with your doctor.

The dizziness, lightheadedness, or fainting is also more likely to occur if you drink alcohol, stand for long periods of time, exercise, or if the weather is hot. *While you are taking this medicine, be careful in the amount of alcohol you drink. Also, use extra care during exercise or hot weather or if you must stand for long periods of time.* Check with your doctor if you have any questions about this.

Before having any kind of surgery (including dental surgery) or emergency treatment, *tell the doctor or dentist in charge that you are using this medicine.*

Do not take other medicines unless they have been discussed with your doctor. This especially includes over-the-counter (nonprescription) medicines for appetite control, asthma, colds, cough, hay fever, or sinus.

Your mouth, nose, and throat may feel very dry while you are taking this medicine. To help relieve mouth dryness, chew sugarless gum or dissolve bits of ice in your mouth.

Side Effects of This Medicine

Along with its needed effects, a medicine may cause some unwanted effects. No serious side effects have been reported for this medicine. However, the following side effects may occur. Check with your doctor if they continue or are bothersome:

More common

Dizziness or lightheadedness, especially when getting up from a lying or sitting position	Pinpoint pupils Rapid heartbeat Stuffy nose

Less common

Confusion Drowsiness Dry mouth Headache Lack of energy	Sexual problems in males Tiredness Weakness

Rare

Diarrhea Nausea and vomiting	Skin rash and itching

Other side effects not listed above may also occur in some patients. If you notice any other effects, check with your doctor.

PHENYLBUTAZONE (Systemic)

This information applies to the following medicines:

Oxyphenbutazone (ox-i-fen-BYOO-ta-zone)
Phenylbutazone (fen-ill-BYOO-ta-zone)
Phenylbutazone, Buffered

Some commonly used brand names are:	Generic names:
Oxalid Tandearil	Oxyphenbutazone
Algoverine* Azolid Butagesic* Butazolidin Intrabutazone* Malgesic* Nadozone* Neo-Zoline* Novobutazone* Phenbutazone*	Phenylbutazone
Azolid-A Butazolidin Alka Phenylzone-A	Buffered Phenylbutazone

*Not available in the United States.

Oxyphenbutazone and phenylbutazone are used to treat the symptoms of certain types of arthritis or joint disease. They help relieve inflammation, swelling, stiffness, joint pain, and fever. These medicines are available only with your doctor's prescription.

Before Using This Medicine

Oxyphenbutazone and phenylbutazone are very strong medicines. In addition to their helpful effects in treating your medical problem, they have side effects that could be very serious. Before you take either one of these medicines, be sure that you have discussed the use of it with your doctor.

In order to decide on the best treatment for your medical problem, your doctor should be told:

—if you have ever had any unusual reaction to aspirin, dipyrone, oxyphenbutazone, phenylbutazone, or sulfinpyrazone.

—if you are pregnant or if you intend to become pregnant while using this medicine. Although oxyphenbutazone and phenylbutazone have not been shown to cause birth defects or other problems in humans, the chance always exists.

—if you are breast-feeding an infant. Phenylbutazone passes into the breast milk and may cause blood problems in infants of mothers taking this medicine. Although oxyphenbutazone has not been shown to cause problems, the chance always exists since it may also pass into the breast milk.

—if you have any of the following medical problems:

Asthma Blood disease Heart disease Inflammation of pancreas Inflammation of parotid gland Kidney disease Liver disease	Polymyalgia rheumatica or temporal arteritis Stomach ulcer or other stomach problems Ulcers, sores, or white spots in mouth

—if you are now taking any of the following medicines or types of medicine:

Amodiaquine Anticoagulants (blood thinners) Chloroquine Diabetes medicine you take by mouth Digitoxin Gold salts Heparin Hydroxychloroquine	Inflammation medicine (for example, other arthritis medicine) Iron preparations Isoniazid Methotrexate Penicillamine Phenytoin Sulfonamides (sulfa medicines) Tetracyclines

Proper Use of This Medicine

Take this medicine only as directed by your doctor. Do not take more of it, do not take it more often, and do not take it for a longer period of time than your doctor ordered. To do so may cause serious side effects.

Take this medicine with meals or a full glass (8 ounces) of milk to lessen stomach upset. If stomach upset (nausea, vomiting, stomach pain, or diarrhea) continues, check with your doctor.

If you miss a dose of this medicine and your dosing schedule is one dose to be taken:

Once or twice a day—
Take the missed dose as soon as possible. Then go back to your regular dosing schedule. But if you do not remember the missed dose until it is almost time for your next dose or until the next day, do not take the missed dose at all and do not double the next one. Instead, go back to your regular dosing schedule.

Three or more times a day—
If you remember within an hour or so of the missed dose, take it right away. Then go back to your regular dosing schedule. But if you do not remember until later, do not take the missed dose at all and do not double the next one. Instead, go back to your regular dosing schedule.

If you have any questions about this, check with your doctor.

Precautions While Using This Medicine

Your doctor should check your progress at regular visits in order to make sure that this medicine does not cause unwanted effects.

If you are taking buffered phenylbutazone and are also taking an iron preparation (included in some vitamin preparations), do not take these two medicines within 1 to 2 hours of each other. Taking them together may prevent the iron from being absorbed by your body.

This medicine may cause some people to become mentally confused, drowsy, or less alert than they are normally. *Make sure you know how you react to this medicine before you drive, use machines, or do other jobs that require you to be alert.*

Stomach problems may be more likely to occur if you take aspirin regularly (for example, every day) or drink alcoholic beverages while being treated with this medicine. Also, alcohol may add to the depressant side effects of this medicine. Therefore, *do not take aspirin regularly or drink alcoholic beverages while taking this medicine,* unless otherwise directed by your doctor.

Side Effects of This Medicine

Along with its needed effects, a medicine may cause some unwanted effects. Although not all of these side effects appear very often, when they do occur they may require medical attention. *Stop taking this medicine and check with your doctor immediately* if any of the following side effects occur:

More common

Swelling of feet or lower legs	Unusual weight gain

Rare

Bloody or black tarry stools	Unusual bleeding or bruising
Ulcers, sores, or white spots in mouth	Unusual tiredness or weakness
Unexplained sore throat and fever	

Check with your doctor also if any of the following side effects occur:

Less common
Skin rash

Rare

Bloody or cloudy urine	Indigestion or stomach pain
Difficult or painful urination	Mental depression, especially in elderly patients
Difficulty in breathing or wheezing	Ringing or buzzing in ears or any loss of hearing
Eye pain, blurred vision, or any change in vision	Swelling of neck or throat
Hives or itching of skin	Yellowing of eyes or skin

Other side effects may occur which usually do not require medical attention. These side effects may go away during treatment as your body adjusts to the medicine. However, check with your doctor if any of the following side effects continue or are bothersome:

More common

Diarrhea	Vomiting
Nausea	

Less common

Drowsiness	Mental confusion
Headache	Swelling of stomach
Irritability	

Some side effects may occur many days or weeks after you have stopped using this medicine. During this period of time check with your doctor *immediately* if you notice any of the following side effects:

Ulcers, sores, or white spots in mouth	Unusual bleeding or bruising
Unexplained sore throat and fever	Unusual tiredness or weakness

Other side effects not listed above may also occur in some patients. If you notice any other effects, check with your doctor.

PHENYLEPHRINE (Nasal)

Some commonly used brand names are:

Alcon-Efrin	Pyracort-D
Allerest	Rhinall
Contac	Sinarest
Coricidin	Super Anahist
Isophrin	Synasal
Neo-Mist	Vacon
Neo-Synephrine	

Phenylephrine (fen-ill-EF-rin) is used for the temporary relief of congestion or stuffiness in the nose caused by hay fever or other allergies, colds, or sinus trouble. This medicine is available without a prescription; however, your doctor may have special instructions on the proper use or dose for your medical condition.

Before Using This Medicine

In order to decide on the best treatment for your medical problem, your doctor should be told:

—if you have ever had any unusual reaction to nasal decongestants.

—if you are pregnant, if you intend to become pregnant, or if you are breast-feeding an infant. Although phenylephrine has not been shown to cause problems, the chance always exists.

—if you have any of the following medical problems:

Diabetes	High blood pressure
Heart or blood vessel disease	Overactive thyroid

—if you are now taking tricyclic antidepressants (medicine for depression).

—if you are now taking or have taken within the past 2 weeks monoamine oxidase (MAO) inhibitors such as:

Isocarboxazid	Phenelzine
Pargyline	Tranylcypromine

Proper Use of This Medicine

Use this medicine only as directed. Do not use more of it, do not use it more often, and do not use it for longer than 3 days without first checking with your doctor. To do so may make your runny or stuffy nose worse and may also increase the chance of side effects.

If you miss a dose of this medicine and you remember within an hour or so of the missed dose, use it right away. Then go back to your regular dosing schedule. But if you do not remember until later, do not use the missed dose at all and do not double the next one. Instead, go back to your regular dosing schedule. If you have any questions about this, check with your doctor or pharmacist.

If you are using the nose drops:

• How to use: Blow nose gently. Tilt head back while standing or sitting up, or lie down on a bed and hang head over the side. Place the drops into each nostril and keep head tilted back for a few minutes to allow medicine to spread throughout the nose.

• Rinse the dropper with hot water and dry with a clean tissue. Replace the cap right after use. To avoid the spread of infection, do not use the container for more than one person.

If you are using the nose spray:

• How to use: Blow nose gently. With head upright, spray the medicine into each nostril. Sniff briskly while squeezing bottle quickly and firmly. For best results, spray once or twice into each nostril and wait 3 to 5 minutes to allow medicine to work. Then, blow nose gently and thoroughly and repeat the sprays if needed.

• Rinse the tip of the spray bottle with hot water, taking care not to suck water into the bottle, and dry with a clean tissue. Replace the cap right after use. To avoid the spread of infection, do not use the container for more than one person.

If you are using the nose jelly:

• How to use: Blow nose gently. With your finger, place a small amount of jelly (about the size of a pea) up into each nostril. Sniff it well back into nose.

• Wipe the tip of the tube with a clean, damp tissue and replace the cap right after use.

Side Effects of This Medicine

Along with its needed effects, a medicine may cause some unwanted effects. Although not all of these side effects appear very often, when

they do occur they may require medical attention. When this medicine is used for short periods of time at low doses, side effects usually are rare. However, check with your doctor or pharmacist if any of the following occur:

Increase in runny or stuffy nose

Possible signs of too much medicine being absorbed into the body

Headache or dizziness	Unusual nervousness
Trembling	Unusual paleness
Trouble in sleeping	Unusually fast, irregular, or pounding heartbeat
Unusual increase in sweating	

Other side effects may occur which usually do not require medical attention. These side effects may go away during treatment as your body adjusts to the medicine. However, check with your doctor if any of the following side effects continue or are bothersome:

Burning, dryness, or stinging of inside of nose

Other side effects not listed above may also occur in some patients. If you notice any other effects, check with your doctor.

PHENYLEPHRINE (Ophthalmic)

Some commonly used brand names are:

Efricel	Phenoptic
Isopto Frin	Prefrin
Mydfrin	Soothe Eye
Neo-Synephrine	Tear-Efrin
Ocusol	

Ophthalmic phenylephrine (fen-ill-EF-rin) in strengths of 2.5 and 10% is used in the eye to dilate (enlarge) the pupil. It is used before eye examinations, before and after eye surgery, and to treat certain eye conditions. These preparations are available only with your doctor's prescription.

Ophthalmic phenylephrine in strengths of 0.15% and less is used to relieve minor irritation of the eye caused by allergy, dust, smoke, wind, and other irritants. These preparations are available without a prescription; however, your doctor may have special instructions on the proper use of phenylephrine for your eye problem.

Before Using This Medicine

In order to decide on the best treatment for your medical problem, your doctor should be told:

—if you have ever had any unusual reaction to phenylephrine in the past. This medicine should not be used if you are allergic to it.

—if you are pregnant, if you intend to become pregnant, or if you are breast-feeding an infant, although ophthalmic phenylephrine has not been shown to cause problems.

—if you have any of the following medical problems:

Diabetes	High blood pressure
Heart or blood vessel disease	

—if you are now taking any of the following medicines or types of medicine:

Guanethidine	Tricyclic antidepressants (medicine for depression)

—if you are now taking or have taken within the past 3 weeks monoamine oxidase (MAO) inhibitors such as:

Isocarboxazid	Phenelzine
Pargyline	Tranylcypromine

Proper Use of This Medicine

Do not use if the solution turns brown or becomes cloudy.

For patients using the 2.5 or 10% eye drops:

• *It is very important that you use this medicine only as directed.* Do not use more of it and do not use it more often than your doctor ordered. To do so may increase the chance of too much medicine being absorbed into the body and the chance of side effects. *This is especially important when this medicine is used in children or in patients with heart disease or high blood pressure,* since high doses of this medicine may cause an increase in blood pressure and irregular heartbeat.

• How to apply this medicine: First, wash hands. With middle finger, apply pressure to the inside corner of the eye (and continue to apply pressure for 1 or 2 minutes after the medicine has been placed in the eye). Tilt head back and with the index finger of the same hand, pull lower eyelid away from eye to form a pouch. Drop the medicine into the pouch and gently close eyes. Do not blink. Keep eyes closed for 1 or 2 minutes to allow the medicine to be absorbed.

• To prevent contamination of the eye drops, do not touch the applicator tip to any surface (including the eye) and keep the container tightly closed.

• If you miss a dose of this medicine, apply it as soon as possible. Then go back to your regular dosing schedule. But if it is almost time for your next dose, do not apply the missed dose at all. Instead, apply your next dose at the regularly scheduled time. Then continue with your regular dosing schedule. If you have any questions about this, check with your doctor.

Precautions While Using This Medicine

For patients using the 2.5 or 10% eye drops:

• After you apply this medicine to your eyes, your pupils will become unusually large. This may cause your eyes to become more sensitive to light than they are normally. Wearing sunglasses may help relieve the discomfort from bright light. If this effect continues for longer than 12 hours after you have stopped using this medicine, check with your doctor.

Side Effects of This Medicine

Along with its needed effects, a medicine may cause some unwanted effects. Although not all of these side effects appear very often, when they do occur they may require medical attention. Check with your doctor if any of the following side effects occur:

Less common with 10% solution; rare with 2.5% or weaker solution

Possible signs of too much medicine being absorbed into the body

Dizziness	Unusual paleness
Trembling	Unusually fast,
Unusual increase in	irregular, or
sweating	pounding heart-
	beat

Other side effects may occur which usually do not require medical attention. These side effects may go away during treatment as your body adjusts to the medicine. However, check with your doctor if any of the following side effects continue or are bothersome:

More common with 2.5 or 10% solution

Browache	Increased sensitivity
Headache	of eyes to light
	Watering of eyes

Less common

Irritation of eye not present before using this medicine

When you apply the 2.5 or 10% strength of this medicine, some burning or stinging of the eye may be expected.

Other side effects not listed above may also occur in some patients. If you notice any other effects, check with your doctor.

PHENYLPROPANOLAMINE (Systemic)
Some commonly used brand names are:

Coffee-Break	Obestat
Control	Pro-Dax 21
Delcopro	Propadrine
Diadax	Rhindecon
Dietac	

Phenylpropanolamine (fen-ill-proe-pa-NOLE-a-meen) is taken by mouth to relieve nasal congestion (stuffy nose).

Some phenylpropanolamine preparations are also used in the short-term treatment of obesity. For a few weeks (up to about 12), this medicine along with dieting can help patients lose weight. However, since its appetite-reducing effect does not last long, it is useful only for the first few weeks until new eating habits are established. It is not recommended for continuous use in diet control.

Some of these preparations are available only with your doctor's prescription. Others are available without a prescription; however, your doctor may have special instructions on the proper use of this medicine for your medical condition.

Before Using This Medicine

In order to decide on the best treatment for your medical problem, your doctor should be told:

—if you have ever had any unusual reaction to amphetamine, dextroamphetamine, ephedrine, epinephrine, isoproterenol, metaproterenol, methamphetamine, norepinephrine (levarterenol), phenylephrine, pseudoephedrine, or terbutaline.

—if you are pregnant, if you intend to become pregnant, or if you are breast-feeding an infant. Although phenylpropanolamine has not been shown to cause problems, the chance always exists.

—if you have any of the following medical problems:

Diabetes	High blood pressure
Heart or blood	Overactive thyroid
vessel disease	

—if you are now taking any of the following medicines or types of medicine:

Amphetamines	Tricyclic an-
Guanethidine	tidepressants
Medicine for	(medicine for
asthma or	depression)
breathing prob-	
blems	

—if you are now taking or have taken within the past 2 weeks monoamine oxidase (MAO) inhibitors such as:

Isocarboxazid	Phenelzine
Pargyline	Tranylcypromine

Proper Use of This Medicine

Take this medicine only as directed. Do not take more of it and do not take it more often than recommended on the label, unless otherwise directed by your doctor. To do so may increase the chance of side effects.

If this medicine causes trouble in sleeping, take the last dose for each day a few hours before bedtime. If you have any questions about this, check with your doctor.

If you are taking the extended-release capsule form of this medicine:

• Swallow the capsule whole.

• Do not break, crush, or chew before swallowing.

If you are taking this medicine for nasal congestion and you miss a dose, take it right away if you remember within an hour or so of the missed dose. Then go back to your regular dosing schedule. But if you do not remember until later, do not take the missed dose at all and do not double the next one. Instead, go back to your regular dosing schedule. If you have any questions about this, check with your doctor.

Precautions While Using This Medicine

If you are taking this medicine for nasal congestion and symptoms do not improve within 7 days or if you also have a high fever, check with your doctor. These signs may mean that you have other medical problems.

Side Effects of This Medicine

Along with its needed effects, a medicine may cause some unwanted effects. Although not all of these side effects appear very often, when they do occur they may require medical attention. Check with your doctor if any of the following side effects occur:

Rare

Tightness in chest	Unusually fast, pounding, or irregular heart-beat (with high doses)

Other side effects may occur which usually do not require medical attention. These side effects may go away during treatment as your body adjusts to the medicine. However, check with your doctor if any of the following side effects continue or are bothersome:

Less common—more common with high doses

Dizziness	Nervousness
Headache	Restlessness
Nausea	Trouble in sleeping

Other side effects not listed above may also occur in some patients. If you notice any other effects, check with your doctor.

PHENYLPROPANOLAMINE, PHENYLEPHRINE, PHENYLTOLOXAMINE, AND CHLORPHENIRAMINE (Systemic)

A commonly used brand names is Naldecon.

Phenylpropanolamine (fen-ill-proe-pa-NOLE-a-meen), phenylephrine (fen-ill-EF-rin), phenyltoloxamine (fen-ill-tole-OX-a-meen), and chlorpheniramine (klor-fen-IR-a-meen) is a combination antihistamine and decongestant. It is used to treat nasal congestion (stuffy nose) and other symptoms of hay fever and other types of allergy. This medicine is available only with your doctor's prescription.

Before Using This Medicine

In order to decide on the best treatment for your medical problem, your doctor should be told:

—if you have ever had any unusual reaction to chlorpheniramine, phenylephrine, phenylpropanolamine, phenyltoloxamine, or similar medicines in the past. This medicine should not be taken if you are allergic to it.

—if you are pregnant or if you intend to become pregnant while using this medicine. Although this medicine has not been shown to cause birth defects or other problems, the chance always exists.

—if you are breast-feeding an infant. This medicine may pass into the breast milk and cause unwanted effects in the infant.

—if you have any of the following medical problems:

Diabetes	High blood pressure
Enlarged prostate	Intestinal blockage
Glaucoma	Overactive thyroid
Heart disease	Stomach ulcer
	Urinary tract blockage

—if you are now taking any of the following medicines or types of medicine:

Amphetamines	Tricyclic an-
Guanethidine	tidepressants
Medicine for	(medicine for
asthma or	depression)
breathing prob-	
lems	

—if you are now taking any central nervous system (CNS) depressants such as:

Antihistamines or	Narcotics
medicine for hay	Prescription pain
fever, other	medicine
allergies,	Sedatives, tran-
or colds	quilizers,
Barbiturates	or sleeping
Medicines for	medicine
seizures	

—if you are now taking or have taken within the past 2 weeks monoamine oxidase (MAO) inhibitors such as:

Isocarboxazid	Phenelzine
Pargyline	Tranylcypromine

Proper Use of This Medicine

Take phenylpropanolamine, phenylephrine, phenyltoloxamine, and chlorpheniramine combination only as directed. Do not take more of it and do not take it more often than recommended on the label, unless otherwise directed by your doctor. To do so may increase the chance of side effects.

Do not give this medicine to premature or newborn infants, unless otherwise directed by your doctor.

Take this medicine with food or a glass of water or milk to lessen stomach irritation, if necessary.

If you are taking the long-acting tablet form of this medicine, the tablets are to be swallowed whole. Do not break, crush, or chew before swallowing.

If you must take this medicine regularly and you miss a dose, take the missed dose as soon as possible. However, if it is almost time for your next dose, do not take the missed dose at all

and do not double the next one. Instead, go back to your regular dosing schedule. If you have any questions about this, check with your doctor or pharmacist.

Precautions While Using This Medicine

The antihistamine in this medicine will add to the effects of alcohol and other medicines (CNS depressants) that slow down the nervous system. Some examples of CNS depressants are medicine for hay fever, other allergies, or colds; sedatives, tranquilizers, or sleeping medicine; prescription pain medicine or narcotics; barbiturates; medicine for seizures; tricyclic antidepressants (medicine for depression); or anesthetics, including some dental anesthetics. *Check with your doctor before taking any of the above while you are using this medicine.*

Chlorpheniramine and phenyltoloxamine may cause some people to become drowsy, dizzy, or less alert than they are normally. *Make sure you know how you react to this medicine before you drive, use machines, or do other jobs that require you to be alert.*

Other people may become nervous or restless or may have trouble in sleeping from the phenylpropanolamine and phenylephrine in this medicine. If you do have trouble in sleeping, take the last dose of this medicine for each day a few hours before bedtime. If you have any questions about this, check with your doctor.

Side Effects of This Medicine

Along with its needed effects, a medicine may cause some unwanted effects. Although not all of these side effects appear very often, when they do occur they may require medical attention. Check with your doctor if any of the following side effects occur:

Rare

Tightness in chest	Unusual weakness
Unexplained sore	Unusually fast,
throat and fever	irregular, or
Unusual bleeding or	pounding heart-
bruising	beat

Other side effects may occur which usually do not require medical attention. These side effects may go away during treatment as your body adjusts to the medicine. However, check with your doctor if any of the following side effects continue or are bothersome:

More common

Drowsiness	Thickening of the
	bronchial
	secretions

Less common—more common with high doses

Difficult or painful urination	Nausea, upset stomach, or stomach pain
Dizziness	Nervousness, restlessness, or trouble in sleeping (especially in children)
Dryness of mouth, nose, or throat	
Headache	
Loss of appetite	
	Skin rash
	Unusual increase in sweating

Other side effects not listed above may also occur in some patients. If you notice any other effects, check with your doctor.

PHYSOSTIGMINE (Ophthalmic)
Some commonly used brand names are Eserine and Isopto Eserine.

Physostigmine (fi-zoe-STIG-meen) is used in the eye to treat certain types of glaucoma and other eye conditions. This medicine is available only with your doctor's prescription.

Before Using This Medicine
In order to decide on the best treatment for your medical problem, your doctor should be told:

—if you have ever had any unusual reaction to physostigmine in the past. This medicine should not be used if you are allergic to it.

—if you are pregnant, if you intend to become pregnant, or if you are breast-feeding an infant, although physostigmine has not been shown to cause problems.

—if you are now using either of the following eye medicines:
  Echothiophate
  Isoflurophate

Proper Use of This Medicine
Use this medicine only as directed. Do not use more of it and do not use it more often than your doctor ordered. To do so may increase the chance of too much medicine being absorbed into the body and the chance of side effects.

If you miss a dose of this medicine and your dosing schedule is one dose to be applied:

Once a day—
Apply the missed dose as soon as possible. Then go back to your regular dosing schedule. But if you do not remember the missed dose until the next day, do not apply it at all. Instead, apply your regularly scheduled dose.

More than once a day—
Apply the missed dose as soon as possible. Then go back to your regular dosing schedule. But if it is almost time for your next dose, do not apply the missed dose at all. Instead, apply your next dose at the regularly scheduled time. Then continue with your regular dosing schedule.

If you have any questions about this, check with your doctor.

If you are using the eye-drop form of this medicine:

• Do not use if the solution becomes discolored.

• How to apply this medicine: First, wash hands. With middle finger, apply pressure to the inside corner of the eye (and continue to apply pressure for 1 or 2 minutes after the medicine has been placed in the eye). Tilt head back and with the index finger of the same hand, pull lower eyelid away from eye to form a pouch. Drop the medicine into the pouch and gently close eyes. Do not blink. Keep eyes closed for 1 or 2 minutes to allow the medicine to be absorbed.

• To prevent contamination of the eye drops, do not touch the applicator tip to any surface (including the eye) and keep the container tightly closed.

If you are using the ointment form of this medicine:

• How to apply this medicine: First, wash hands. Pull lower eyelid away from eye to form a pouch. Squeeze a thin strip of ointment into the pouch. A 1-cm (approximately 1/3-inch) strip of ointment is usually enough unless otherwise directed by your doctor. Gently close eyes and keep them closed for 1 or 2 minutes to allow the medicine to be absorbed.

• Immediately after applying the eye ointment, wash hands to remove any medicine that may be on them.

• To prevent contamination of the eye ointment, do not touch the applicator tip to any surface (including the eye), wipe the tip of the ointment tube with a clean tissue, and keep the tube tightly closed.

Precautions While Using This Medicine
Your doctor should check your eye pressure at regular visits.

For a short time after you apply this medicine, your vision may be blurred or there may be a change in your near or distant vision. *Make sure your vision is clear before you drive or do other jobs that require you to see well.*

Side Effects of This Medicine
Along with its needed effects, a medicine may cause some unwanted effects. Although not all of these side effects appear very often, when they do occur they may require medical attention. Check with your doctor if any of the following side effects occur:

Possible signs of too much medicine being absorbed into the body

Loss of bladder control	Unusual increase in sweating
Muscle weakness	Unusual tiredness or weakness
Nausea, vomiting, diarrhea, or stomach cramps or pain	Unusual watering of mouth
Shortness of breath, tightness in chest, or wheezing	Unusually slow or irregular heartbeat

Other side effects may occur which usually do not require medical attention. These side effects may go away during treatment as your body adjusts to the medicine. However, check with your doctor if any of the following side effects continue or are bothersome:

More common

Blurred vision or change in near or distant vision	Eye pain

Less common

Browache	Headache
Burning, redness, stinging, or other irritation of eyes	Twitching of eyelids Watering of eyes

Other side effects not listed above may also occur in some patients. If you notice any other effects, check with your doctor.

PILOCARPINE (Ophthalmic)
Some commonly used brand names are:

Adsorbocarpine	Ocusert
Almocarpine	Pilo
Isopto Carpine	Pilocar
Miocarpine*	Pilomiotin
	P. V. Carpine

*Not available in the United States.

Pilocarpine (pye-loe-KAR-peen) is used in the eye to treat glaucoma and other eye conditions. It is available only with your doctor's prescription.

Before Using This Medicine
In order to decide on the best treatment for your medical problem, your doctor should be told:

—if you have ever had any unusual reaction to pilocarpine in the past. This medicine should not be used if you are allergic to it.

—if you are pregnant, if you intend to become pregnant, or if you are breast-feeding an infant. Although pilocarpine has not been shown to cause problems, the chance always exists.

—if you have asthma.

Proper Use of This Medicine
Use this medicine only as directed. Do not use more of it and do not use it more often than your doctor ordered. To do so may increase the chance of too much medicine being absorbed into the body and the chance of side effects.

If you are using the eye drop form of this medicine:

• How to apply this medicine: First, wash hands. With middle finger, apply pressure to the inside corner of the eye (and continue to apply pressure for 1 or 2 minutes after the medicine has been placed in the eye). Tilt head back and with the index finger of the same hand, pull lower eyelid away from eye to form a pouch. Drop the medicine into the pouch and gently close eyes. Do not blink. Keep eyes closed for 1 or 2 minutes to allow the medicine to be absorbed.

• To prevent contamination of the eye drops, do not touch the applicator tip to any surface (including the eye) and keep the container tightly closed.

• If you miss a dose of this medicine, apply it as soon as possible. Then go back to your regular dosing schedule. But if it is almost time for your next dose, do not apply the missed dose at all. Instead, apply your next dose at the regularly scheduled time. Then continue with your regular dosing schedule. If you have any questions about this, check with your doctor.

If you are using the eye system form of this medicine:

• This medicine usually comes with patient directions. Read them carefully before using this medicine.

• If you think this medicine unit may be damaged, do not use it. If you have any questions about this, check with your doctor or pharmacist.

• If the unit seems to be releasing too much medicine into your eye, remove it and replace with a new unit. If you have any questions about this, check with your doctor.

Precautions While Using This Medicine

Your doctor should check your eye pressure at regular visits.

If you are using the eye drop form of this medicine:

• For a short time after you apply this medicine, your vision may be blurred or there may be a change in your near or distant vision. *Make sure your vision is clear before you drive or do other jobs that require you to see well.*

If you are using the eye system form of this medicine:

• For the first several hours after inserting this unit in the eye, your vision may be blurred or there may be a change in your near or distant vision. Therefore, insert this unit in the eye at bedtime, unless otherwise directed by your doctor. If this unit is inserted in the eye at any other time of the day, *make sure your vision is clear before you drive or do other jobs that require you to see well.*

Side Effects of This Medicine

Along with its needed effects, a medicine may cause some unwanted effects. Although not all of these side effects appear very often, when they do occur they may require medical attention. Check with your doctor if any of the following side effects occur:

Possible signs of too much medicine being absorbed into the body

Muscle tremors	Unusual increase in
Nausea, vomiting,	sweating
or diarrhea	Unusual watering
Troubled breathing	of mouth
or wheezing	

Other side effects may occur which usually do not require medical attention. These side effects may go away during treatment as your body adjusts to the medicine. However, check with your doctor if any of the following side effects continue or are bothersome:

More common

Blurred vision or	Eye pain
change in near or	
distant vision	

Less common

Headache	Twitching of eyelids
Irritation of eyes	

Other side effects not listed above may also occur in some patients. If you notice any other effects, check with your doctor.

POTASSIUM IODIDE (Systemic)
Some commonly used brand names are KI-N and Pima.

Potassium iodide (poe-TAS-ee-um EYE-oh-dide) is used for the treatment of chronic respiratory disease, certain types of thyroid disease, and some fungal infections. This medicine is available only with your doctor's prescription.

Before Using This Medicine

In order to decide on the best treatment for your medical problem, your doctor should be told:

—if you have ever had any unusual reaction to iodine or iodine-containing foods.

—if you are pregnant or if you intend to become pregnant while using this medicine. Taking potassium iodide during pregnancy may cause thyroid problems in the newborn infant.

—if you are breast-feeding an infant. Potassium iodide passes into the breast milk and may cause unwanted effects in infants of mothers taking this medicine.

—if you have any of the following medical problems:

Bronchitis	Overactive thyroid
Heart disease	(unless you are
Kidney disease	taking this medi-
Myotonia congenita	cine for this
	medical problem)
	Tuberculosis (TB)
	Underactive adrenal
	glands

—if you are now taking any of the following medicines or types of medicine:

Lithium	Spironolactone
Medicines contain-	Triamterene
ing potassium	

Proper Use of This Medicine

If potassium iodide upsets your stomach, *take it after meals or with food or milk* unless otherwise directed by your doctor. If stomach upset (nausea, vomiting, stomach pain, or diarrhea) continues, check with your doctor.

If you miss a dose of this medicine, take it as soon as possible. Then go back to your regular dosing schedule. However, if it is almost time for your next dose, do not take the missed dose at all and do not double the next one. Instead, go back to your regular dosing schedule. If you have any questions about this, check with your doctor.

If you are taking this medicine for a fungus infection, *keep taking it for the full course of treatment* even if you begin to feel better after a few days. This will help clear up your infection completely.

If you are taking the solution form of this medicine:

• Do not use if solution turns brownish yellow.

• Take potassium iodide in a full glass (8 ounces) of water or in fruit juice, milk, or broth to improve the taste and lessen stomach upset. Be sure to drink all of the liquid in order to get the full dose of medicine.

• If crystals form in potassium iodide solution, they may be dissolved by warming the closed container of solution in warm water and then gently shaking the container.

If you are taking the tablet form of this medicine:

• Before taking, dissolve each tablet in 1/2 glass (4 ounces) of water or milk. Be sure to drink all of the liquid in order to get the full dose of medicine.

If you are taking the enteric-coated tablet form of this medicine:

• Swallow the tablets whole. Do not crush, break, or chew before swallowing.

Precautions While Using This Medicine

Your doctor should check your progress at regular visits in order to make sure that this medicine does not cause unwanted effects.

Caution: Patients on a potassium-restricted diet—This medicine contains a large amount of potassium. If you have any questions about this, check with your doctor or pharmacist.

Side Effects of This Medicine

Along with its needed effects, a medicine may cause some unwanted effects. Although not all of these side effects appear very often, when they do occur they may require medical attention. When this medicine is used for short periods of time at low doses, side effects usually are rare. However, check with your doctor if any of the following side effects occur:

Bloody or black	Skin rash
tarry stools	Swelling of neck
Irregular heartbeat	or throat
Mental confusion	Unexplained fever
Numbness, tingling,	Unusual tiredness or
pain, or weakness	weakness
in hands or feet	Weakness and
	heaviness
	of legs

With long-term use

Burning of mouth	Soreness of teeth
or throat	and gums
Metallic taste in	Symptoms of head
mouth	cold
Severe headache	Unusual increase in
	salivation

Other side effects may occur which usually do not require medical attention. These side effects may go away during treatment as your body adjusts to the medicine. However, check with your doctor if any of the following side effects continue or are bothersome:

Diarrhea	Stomach pain
Nausea	Vomiting

Other side effects not listed above may also occur in some patients. If you notice any other effects, check with your doctor.

POTASSIUM PHOSPHATES (Systemic)

This information applies to the following medicines:

Dibasic Potassium Phosphate
Monobasic Potassium Phosphate
Potassium Phosphates

Some commonly used brand names are:	Generic names:
K-Phos Original	Monobasic Potassium Phosphates
Neutra-Phos-K	Potassium Phosphates

Potassium phosphates (poe-TAS-ee-um FOS-fates) are used as a dietary supplement for patients who are unable to get enough phosphorus in their regular diet, usually because of certain illnesses or diseases. In patients with hypercalcemia (too much calcium in the blood), potassium phosphates can be used to help the body lose calcium. Sometimes they are used to make the urine more acid to prevent the formation of stones in the urinary tract or to help treat urinary tract infections.

Some of these preparations are available only with your doctor's prescription. Others are available without a prescription; however, your doctor may have special instructions on the proper dose of potassium phosphates for your medical condition.

Before Using This Medicine

In order to decide on the best treatment for your medical problem, your doctor should be told:

—if you have ever had any unusual reaction to potassium phosphates in the past. This medicine should not be taken if you are allergic to it.

—if you are pregnant, if you intend to become pregnant, or if you are breast-feeding an infant. Although potassium phosphates have not been shown to cause problems, the chance always exists.

—if you have any of the following medical problems:

Heart disease	Underactive
Kidney disease	adrenal glands
Myotonia congenita	Underactive
Rickets	parathyroid
Softening of bones	glands

—if you are now taking any of the following medicines or types of medicine:

Antacids containing aluminum or magnesium	Medicine containing potassium
	Spironolactone
Aspirin or other salicylates	Triamterene
	Vitamin D
Medicine containing calcium	

Proper Use of This Medicine

Take this medicine only as directed. Do not take more of it and do not take it more often than recommended on the label, unless otherwise directed by your doctor.

Take this medicine immediately after meals or with food to lessen possible stomach upset or laxative action.

If you miss a dose of this medicine and you remember within an hour or so of the missed dose, take it right away. Then go back to your regular dosing schedule. But if you do not remember until later, do not take the missed dose at all and do not double the next one. Instead, go back to your regular dosing schedule. If you have any questions about this, check with your doctor.

If you are taking monobasic potassium phosphate tablets:

• Do not swallow tablets whole. Before taking, dissolve the tablets in 3/4 to 1 glass (6 to 8 ounces) of water. Let the tablets soak in water for 2 to 5 minutes and then stir until dissolved.

If you are taking potassium phosphates capsules for oral solution:

• Do not swallow capsules whole. Before taking, mix the contents of 1 capsule in 1/3 glass (about 2 1/2 ounces) of water or the contents of 2 capsules in 2/3 glass (about 5 ounces) of water and stir well.

If you are taking potassium phosphates for oral solution:

• If this medicine is not in solution, add the entire contents of 1 bottle (2 1/2 ounces) to enough water to make 1 gallon of solution. Shake for 2 or 3 minutes or until all the powder is dissolved.

• This solution may be chilled to improve flavor.

Precautions While Using This Medicine

Your doctor should check your progress at regular visits in order to make sure that this medicine does not cause unwanted effects.

If you are taking this medicine for hypercalcemia (too much calcium in the blood), your doctor may want you to follow a low-calcium diet. If you have any questions about this, check with your doctor.

Caution: Patients on a potassium-restricted diet—This medicine contains a large amount of potassium. If you have any questions about this, check with your doctor or pharmacist.

Side Effects of This Medicine

Along with its needed effects, a medicine may cause some unwanted effects. Although not all of these side effects appear very often, when they do occur they may require medical attention. Check with your doctor if any of the following side effects occur:

Less common or rare

Irregular heartbeat	Numbness or tin-
Mental confusion	gling around lips
Muscle cramps	Shortness of breath
Numbness, tingling,	or troubled
pain, or weakness	breathing
in hands or feet	Unusual tiredness
	Weakness or
	heaviness
	of legs

Other side effects may occur which usually do not require medical attention. These side effects may go away during treatment as your body adjusts to the medicine. However, check with your doctor if any of the following side effects continue or are bothersome:

Less common

Diarrhea	Stomach pain
Nausea	Vomiting

Other side effects not listed above may also occur in some patients. If you notice any other effects, check with your doctor.

POTASSIUM AND SODIUM PHOSPHATES
(Systemic)

This information applies to the following medicines:

Dibasic Potassium and Sodium Phosphates
Monobasic Potassium and Sodium Phosphates
Potassium and Sodium Phosphates

Some commonly used brand names are:	Generic names:
Uro-KP-Neutral	Dibasic Potassium and Sodium Phosphates
K-Phos M. F. K-Phos Neutral K-Phos No. 2	Monobasic Potassium and Sodium Phosphates
Neutra-Phos	Potassium and Sodium Phosphates

Potassium and sodium phosphates (poe-TAS-ee-um and SOE-dee-um FOS-fates) combination is used as a dietary supplement for patients who are unable to get enough phosphorus in their regular diet, usually because of certain illnesses or diseases. In patients with hypercalcemia (too much calcium in the blood), this medicine can be used to help the body lose calcium. Sometimes it is used to make the urine more acid to prevent the formation of stones in the urinary tract or to help treat urinary tract infections.

Some of these preparations are available only with your doctor's prescription. Others are available without a prescription; however, your doctor may have special instructions on the proper dose of this medicine for your medical condition.

Before Using This Medicine

In order to decide on the best treatment for your medical problem, your doctor should be told:

—if you have ever had any unusual reaction to potassium and sodium phosphates in the past. This medicine should not be taken if you are allergic to it.

—if you are pregnant, if you intend to become pregnant, or if you are breast-feeding an infant. Although potassium and sodium phosphates have not been shown to cause problems, the chance always exists.

—if you have any of the following medical problems:

Edema (swelling in feet or lower legs or fluid in lungs)	Myotonia congenita Rickets Softening of bones
Heart disease	Underactive
High blood pressure	adrenal glands
Kidney disease	Underactive
Liver disease	parathyroid glands

—if you are now taking any of the following medicines or types of medicine:

Antacids containing aluminum or magnesium	Medicine containing calcium
Aspirin or other salicylates	Medicine containing potassium
	Spironolactone
Cortisone-like medicine	Triamterene
	Vitamin D
High blood pressure medicine such as diazoxide, guanethidine, hydralazine, methyldopa, or reserpine	

Proper Use of This Medicine

Take this medicine only as directed. Do not take more of it and do not take it more often than recommended on the label, unless otherwise directed by your doctor.

Take this medicine immediately after meals or with food to lessen possible stomach upset or laxative action.

If you miss a dose of this medicine and you remember within an hour or so of the missed dose, take it right away. Then go back to your regular dosing schedule. But if you do not remember until later, do not take the missed dose at all and do not double the next one. Instead, go back to your regular dosing schedule. If you have any questions about this, check with your doctor.

If you are taking dibasic or monobasic potassium and sodium phosphates tablets:

• Take this medicine with a full glass (8 ounces) of water.

If you are taking potassium and sodium phosphates capsules for oral solution:

• Do not swallow capsules whole. Before taking, mix the contents of 1 capsule in 1/3 glass (about 2 1/2 ounces) of water or the contents of 2 capsules in 2/3 glass (about 5 ounces) of water and stir well.

If you are taking potassium and sodium phosphates for oral solution:

• If this medicine is not in solution, add the entire contents of 1 bottle (2 1/4 ounces) to enough water to make 1 gallon of solution. Shake for 2 or 3 minutes or until all the powder is dissolved.

• This solution may be chilled to improve flavor.

Precautions While Using This Medicine

Your doctor should check your progress at regular visits in order to make sure that this medicine does not cause unwanted effects.

If you are taking this medicine for hypercalcemia (too much calcium in the blood), your doctor may want you to follow a low-calcium diet. If you have any questions about this, check with your doctor.

Caution: Patients on a potassium- or sodium-restricted diet—This medicine contains a large amount of potassium and sodium. If you have any questions about this, check with your doctor or pharmacist.

Side Effects of This Medicine

Along with its needed effects, a medicine may cause some unwanted effects. Although not all of these side effects appear very often, when they do occur they may require medical attention. Check with your doctor if any of the following side effects occur:

Less common or rare

Decreased amount of urine	Shortness of breath or troubled breathing
Headache or dizziness	Swelling of feet or lower legs
Irregular heartbeat	Unusual thirst
Mental confusion	Unusual tiredness or weakness
Muscle cramps	
Numbness, tingling, pain, or weakness in hands or feet	Unusual weight gain
Numbness or tingling around lips	Unusually fast heartbeat
	Weakness or heaviness of legs

Other side effects may occur which usually do not require medical attention. These side effects may go away during treatment as your body adjusts to the medicine. However, check with your doctor if any of the following side effects continue or are bothersome:

Less common

Diarrhea	Stomach pain
Nausea	Vomiting

Other side effects not listed above may also occur in some patients. If you notice any other effects, check with your doctor.

POTASSIUM SUPPLEMENTS (Systemic)

This information applies to the following medicines:

Potassium Acetate (poe-TASS-ee-um)

Potassium Acetate, Potassium Bicarbonate, and Potassium Citrate

Potassium Bicarbonate and Citric Acid

Potassium Bicarbonate, Potassium Carbonate, and Potassium Chloride

Potassium Bicarbonate and Potassium Chloride

Potassium Bicarbonate, Potassium Chloride, and Citric Acid

Potassium Bicarbonate, Potassium Chloride, and Potassium Citrate

Potassium Chloride

Potassium Chloride and Potassium Gluconate

Potassium Citrate and Potassium Gluconate

Potassium Gluconate

This information does *not* apply to:

Potassium Citrate

Potassium Iodide

Potassium Permanganate

Potassium Phosphates

(see individual monographs)

Some commonly used brand names and other names are:	Generic names:
Potassium Triplex Tri-K Trikates	Potassium Acetate, Potassium Bicarbonate, and Potassium Citrate
K-Lyte	Potassium Bicarbonate and Citric acid
KEFF	Potassium Bicarbonate, Potassium Carbonate, and Potassium Chloride
Klorvess	Potassium Bicarbonate and Potassium Chloride
K-Lyte/Cl	Potassium Bicarbonate, Potassium Chloride, and Citric Acid
Kaochlor-Eff	Potassium Bicarbonate, Potassium Chloride, and Potassium Citrate
Kaochlor Kaon-Cl Kato Kay-Ciel K-Lor KLOR-10% KLOR-CON Klorvess Klotrix K-Lyte/Cl Slow-K	Potassium Chloride
Kolyum	Potassium Chloride and Potassium Gluconate
Twin-K	Potassium Citrate and Potassium Gluconate
Kaon	Potassium Gluconate

Potassium (poe-TASS-ee-um) is needed to maintain good health. Potassium supplements may be needed by patients who do not have enough potassium in their regular diet and by those who have lost too much potassium because of illness or treatment with certain medicines. Since too much potassium may also cause health problems, most potassium supplements are available only with your doctor's prescription.

Before Using This Medicine

In order to decide on the best treatment for your medical problem, your doctor should be told:

—if you have ever had any unusual reaction to potassium preparations in the past. This medicine should not be taken if you are allergic to it.

—if you are pregnant, if you intend to become pregnant, or if you are breast-feeding an infant. Although potassium supplements have not been shown to cause problems, the chance always exists. Therefore, use should be carefully considered.

—if you have any of the following medical problems:

Addison's disease (underactive adrenal glands) Diarrhea	Heart disease Intestinal blockage Kidney disease Stomach ulcer

—if you are now taking any of the following medicines or types of medicine:

Diuretics (water pills)   Laxatives

Heart medicine such as digitoxin or digoxin

—if you are now using salt substitutes or drinking low-salt milk.

Proper Use of This Medicine

Take this medicine only as directed by your doctor. Do not take more of it, do not take it more often, and do not take it for a longer period of time than your doctor ordered. *This is especially important if you are also taking both diuretics (water pills) and digitalis medicines for your heart.*

Take this medicine immediately after meals or with food to lessen possible stomach upset or laxative action.

If you miss a dose of this medicine and remember within 2 hours, take the missed dose right away with food or liquids. Then go back to your regular dosing schedule. However, if you do not remember until later, do not take the missed dose at all and do not double the next one. Instead, go back to your regular dosing schedule. If you have any questions about this, check with your doctor or pharmacist.

For patients taking the liquid form of this medicine:

• This medicine must be diluted in at least 1/2 glass (4 ounces) of cold water or juice to reduce possible stomach irritation or laxative effect.

For patients taking the soluble granule, soluble powder, or soluble tablet form of this medicine:

• This medicine must be completely dissolved in at least 1/2 glass (4 ounces) of cold water or juice to reduce possible stomach irritation or laxative effect.

• Allow any "fizzing" to stop before taking the dissolved medicine.

For patients taking the extended-release tablet form of this medicine:

• Swallow the tablets whole. Do not crush, chew, or suck on the tablet.

• If you have trouble swallowing tablets or if they seem to stick in your throat, check with your doctor. When this medicine is not properly released, it can cause irritation which may lead to ulcers.

For patients using juices to dilute or dissolve this medicine:

• If you are on a salt (sodium)-restricted diet, check with your doctor before using tomato juice to dilute your medicine. Tomato juice has a high salt (sodium) content.

Precautions While Using This Medicine

Your doctor should check your progress at regular visits.

Since salt substitutes and low-salt milk may contain potassium, do not use them unless told to do so by your doctor.

Check with your doctor at once if you notice blackish stools or other signs of stomach or intestinal bleeding. This medicine may cause such a condition to become worse, especially when taken in tablet form.

Side Effects of This Medicine

Along with its needed effects, a medicine may cause some unwanted effects. Although not all of these side effects appear very often, when they do occur they may require medical attention. *Stop taking this medicine and check with your doctor immediately if any of the following side effects occur:*

Rare

Irregular heartbeat
Mental confusion
Numbness or tingling in hands, feet, or lips
Shortness of breath or difficult breathing

Unexplained anxiety
Unusual tiredness or weakness
Weakness or heaviness of legs

Other side effects may occur which usually do not require medical attention. These side effects may go away during treatment as your body adjusts to the medicine. However, check with your doctor if any of the following side effects continue or are bothersome:

Less common

Diarrhea
Nausea

Stomach pain or discomfort
Vomiting

Other side effects not listed above may also occur in some patients. If you notice any other effects, check with your doctor.

PRAZOSIN (Systemic)
A commonly used brand name is Minipress.

Prazosin (PRA-zoe-sin) belongs to the general class of medicines called antihypertensives. It is used to treat high blood pressure. Prazosin is available only with your doctor's prescription.

Before Using This Medicine
In order to decide on the best treatment for your medical problem, your doctor should be told:

—if you have ever had any unusual reaction to prazosin in the past. This medicine should not be taken if you are allergic to it.

—if you are pregnant, if you intend to become pregnant, or if you are breast-feeding an infant. Although prazosin has not been shown to cause problems, the chance always exists.

—if you have any of the following medical problems:

Angina	Kidney disease
Heart disease	Mental depression

—if you are now taking any of the following medicines or types of medicine:

Diuretics (water pills)	Other antihypertensives (high blood pressure medicine)

Proper Use of This Medicine
Importance of Diet—Before prescribing medicine for your condition, your doctor will probably try to control your condition by prescribing a personal diet for you. Such a diet may be low in sodium (salt). Medicine is usually more effective when this diet is properly followed.

Also, it may be very important for you to go on a reducing diet. However, check with your doctor before going on any diet.

Many patients who have high blood pressure will not notice any signs of the problem. In fact, many may feel normal. It is very important that you take your medicine exactly as directed and that you keep your doctor's appointments even if you feel well.

Remember that prazosin will not cure your high blood pressure but it does control it. Therefore, you must continue to take it as directed if you expect to keep your blood pressure down. *You may have to take medicine for the rest of your life.* If high blood pressure is not treated, it can cause serious problems such as heart failure, blood vessel disease, stroke, or kidney disease.

In order to help remember to take your medicine, try to get into the habit of taking it at the same time each day.

If you miss a dose of this medicine, take it as soon as possible. If it is almost time for your next dose, do not take the missed dose at all and do not double the next one. Instead, go back to your regular dosing schedule. If you have any questions about this, check with your doctor.

Precautions While Using This Medicine
It is important that your doctor check your progress at regular visits.

Dizziness or drowsiness may occur after the first dose of this medicine. Taking the first dose at bedtime may prevent problems. *Avoid driving or performing hazardous tasks for the first 24 hours after you start taking this medicine or when the dose is increased. Make sure you know how you react to this medicine before you drive, use machines, or do other jobs that require you to be alert.*

Dizziness, lightheadedness, or fainting may occur, especially when you get up from a lying or sitting position. Getting up slowly may help lessen this problem. *If you begin to feel dizzy, lie down so that you do not faint.* Then sit for a few moments before standing to prevent the dizziness from returning.

The dizziness, lightheadedness, or fainting is also more likely to occur if you drink alcohol, stand for long periods of time, exercise, or if the weather is hot. *While you are taking this medicine, be careful in the amount of alcohol you drink. Also, use extra care during exercise or hot weather or if you must stand for long periods of time.* Check with your doctor if you have any questions about this.

Do not take other medicines unless they have been discussed with your doctor. This especially includes over-the-counter (nonprescription) medicines for appetite control, asthma, colds, cough, hay fever, or sinus, since they may tend to increase your blood pressure.

Side Effects of This Medicine
Along with its needed effects, a medicine may cause some unwanted effects. Although not all of these side effects appear very often, when they do occur they may require medical attention. Check with your doctor if any of the following side effects occur:

More common

Dizziness or light-
headedness, espe-
cially when get-
ting up from a
lying or sitting
position

Fainting
Irregular heartbeat

Less common

Chest pain
Shortness of breath

Swelling of feet or
lower legs
Weight gain

Rare

Inability to control
urination

Numbness or tin-
gling of hands or
feet

Other side effects may occur which usually do not require medical attention. These side effects may go away during treatment as your body adjusts to the medicine. However, check with your doctor if any of the following side effects continue or are bothersome:

More common

Drowsiness
Lack of energy

Less common

Blurred vision
Constipation
Diarrhea
Dry mouth
Hallucinations (see-
ing, hearing, or
feeling things that
are not there)
Headache
Loss of appetite

Mental depression
Nausea and
vomiting
Nervousness or
irritability
Skin rash or itching
Stomach pain
Stuffy nose
Unusually frequent
urination
Unusually vivid
dreams

Other side effects not listed above may also occur in some patients. If you notice any other effects, check with your doctor.

PRIMAQUINE (Systemic)

Primaquine (PRIM-a-kween) belongs to the group of medicines called antiprotozoals. It is used in the prevention and treatment of malaria. This medicine is available only with your doctor's prescription.

Before Using This Medicine

In order to decide on the best treatment for your medical problem, your doctor should be told:

—if you have ever had any unusual reaction to primaquine in the past. This medicine should not be taken if you are allergic to it.

—if you are pregnant, if you intend to become pregnant, or if you are breast-feeding an infant. Although primaquine has not been shown to cause problems, the chance always exists.

—if you have any of the following medical problems:

Family or personal
history of favism
or hemolytic
anemia
Glucose-6-
phosphate
dehydrogenase
(G6PD) deficiency

Lupus
erythematosus
Nicotinamide
adenine dinu-
cleotide (NADH)
methemoglobin
reductase
deficiency
Rheumatoid ar-
thritis

—if you are now taking any of the following medicines or types of medicine:

Dapsone
Dipyrone
Furazolidine
Gold salt injections
Medicine for cancer
Nitrofurantoin
Oxyphenbutazone

Penicillamine
Phenylbutazone
Quinacrine
Sulfonamides (sulfa
medicine)
Sulfoxone
Vitamin K

Proper Use of This Medicine

If you are taking primaquine for malaria, *keep taking it for the full time of treatment* in order to help prevent or clear up the infection completely.

If this medicine upsets your stomach, it may be taken with *meals or antacids.* If stomach upset (nausea, vomiting, or stomach pain) continues, check with your doctor.

If you miss a dose of this medicine, take it as soon as possible. Then go back to your regular dosing schedule. But if you do not remember the missed dose until the next day, do not take it at all and do not double the next one. Instead, go back to your regular dosing schedule. If you have any questions about this, check with your doctor.

Precautions While Using This Medicine

Your doctor should check your progress at regular visits in order to make sure that primaquine is not causing blood problems.

Side Effects of This Medicine

Along with its needed effects, a medicine may cause some unwanted effects. Although not all of these side effects appear very often, when they do occur they may require medical attention. Check with your doctor if any of the following side effects occur:

Less common—usually with high doses or in patients with nicotinamide adenine dinucleotide (NADH) methemoglobin reductase deficiency

Dizziness or light-headedness	Troubled breathing
	Unusual tiredness or weakness

Rare—more common in Sardinians and Negroes or individuals with a family or personal history of favism or hemolytic anemia

Darkening of urine	Unusual tiredness or weakness

Rare

Unexplained sore throat and fever

Other side effects may occur which usually do not require medical attention. These side effects may go away during treatment as your body adjusts to the medicine. However, check with your doctor if any of the following side effects continue or are bothersome:

More common

Nausea	Vomiting
Stomach pain or cramps	

Less common

Headache
Itching of skin

Other side effects not listed above may also occur in some patients. If you notice any other effects, check with your doctor.

PRIMIDONE (Systemic)
A commonly used brand name is Mysoline.

Primidone (PRI-mi-done) belongs to the group of medicines called anticonvulsants. It is used in the treatment of epilepsy to control certain types of seizures. Primidone is available only with your doctor's prescription.

Before Using This Medicine

In order to decide on the best treatment for your medical problem, your doctor should be told:

—if you have had any unusual reaction to any barbiturate medicine (for example amobarbital, butabarbital, pentobarbital, phenobarbital, secobarbital). This medicine should not be taken if you are allergic to it.

—if you are pregnant or if you intend to become pregnant while using this medicine. Although most mothers who take medicine for seizure control deliver normal babies, there are reports of increased birth defects when these medicines are used during pregnancy. It is not definitely known if any of these medicines are the cause of such problems. In addition, use of this medicine during pregnancy may cause bleeding problems in the newborn infant.

—if you are breast-feeding an infant. Primidone passes into the breast milk and may cause unwanted effects in infants of mothers taking this medicine.

—if you have been told by another doctor that you have any of the following medical problems:

Asthma, emphysema, or chronic lung disease	Kidney disease
	Liver disease
	Porphyria
Hyperactivity (in children)	

—if you are now taking any central nervous system (CNS) depressants such as:

Antihistamines or medicine for hay fever, other allergies, or colds	Prescription pain medicine
Narcotics	Sedatives, tranquilizers, or sleeping medicine
Other barbiturates	Tricyclic antidepressants (medicine for depression)
Other seizure medicine	

—if you are now taking or have taken within the past 2 weeks monoamine oxidase (MAO) inhibitors such as:

Isocarboxazid	Phenelzine
Pargyline	Tranylcypromine

—if you are now taking any of the following medicines or types of medicine:

Anticoagulants (blood thinners)	Digitalis
	Digitoxin
Corticosteroids (cortisone-like medicines)	Doxycycline
	Griseofulvin
	Phenytoin

Proper Use of This Medicine

Take this medicine every day in regularly spaced doses as ordered by your doctor.

If you miss a dose of this medicine, take it right away if you remember within an hour or so of the missed dose. Then go back to your regular dosing schedule. But if you do not remember until later, do not take the missed dose at all and do not double the next one. Instead, go back to your regular dosing schedule. If you have any questions about this, check with your doctor.

Precautions While Using This Medicine

It is very important that your doctor check your progress at regular visits, especially during the first few months you take primidone.

If you have been taking primidone regularly for several weeks, you should not suddenly stop taking it. Your doctor may want you to reduce gradually the amount you are taking before stopping completely.

Before having any kind of surgery (including dental surgery), tell the doctor or dentist in charge that you are using this medicine.

This medicine will add to the effects of alcohol and other medicines (CNS depressants) that slow down the nervous system. Some examples of CNS depressants are antihistamines or medicine for hay fever, other allergies, or colds; sedatives, tranquilizers, or sleeping medicine; prescription pain medicine or narcotics; barbiturates; medicine for seizures; tricyclic antidepressants (medicine for depression); or anesthetics, including some dental anesthetics. *Check with your doctor before taking any of the above while you are using this medicine.*

This medicine may cause some people to become dizzy, lightheaded, drowsy, or less alert than they are normally. Even if taken at bedtime, it may cause some people to feel drowsy or less alert on arising. *Make sure you know how you react to this medicine before you drive, use machines, or do other jobs that require you to be alert.*

Occasionally, children (and sometimes elderly patients) may show signs of restlessness and excitement after taking this medicine. If this occurs, check with your doctor.

Side Effects of This Medicine

Along with its needed effects, a medicine may cause some unwanted effects. Although not all of these side effects appear very often, when they do occur they may require medical attention. Check with your doctor if any of the following side effects occur:

Signs of intolerance or overdose

Change in vision	Shortness of breath
Mental confusion	or difficult
	breathing

Less common

Unusual excitement (especially in children)

Rare

Skin rash or hives	Wheezing or tight-
Swelling of eyelids	ness in chest
Unusual tiredness	
or weakness	

Other side effects may occur which usually do not require medical attention. These side effects may go away during treatment as your body adjusts to the medicine. However, check with your doctor if any of the following side effects continue or are bothersome:

More common

Clumsiness or	Dizziness
unsteadiness	Drowsiness

Less common

Decreased sexual	Nausea
ability	Vomiting
Headache	
Loss of appetite	

Other side effects not listed above may also occur in some patients. If you notice any other effects, check with your doctor.

PROBENECID (Systemic)

Some commonly used brand names are Benemid, Benuryl*, and Probalan.

---

*Not available in the United States.

Probenecid (proe-BEN-e-sid) is used in the treatment of chronic gout. Also, it is used to treat other medical problems that cause too much uric acid to be produced by the body. Sometimes it is used with certain kinds of antibiotics to make them more effective in the treatment of infections. This medicine is available only with your doctor's prescription.

Before Using This Medicine

In order to decide on the best treatment for your medical problem, your doctor should be told:

—if you have ever had any unusual reaction to probenecid in the past. This medicine should not be taken if you are allergic to it.

—if you are pregnant, if you intend to become pregnant, or if you are breast-feeding an infant. Although probenecid has not been shown to cause problems, the chance always exists.

—if you have any of the following medical problems:

Blood disease	Stomach ulcer
Kidney stones or disease	(history of)

—if you are now taking any of the following medicines or types of medicine:

Aminosalicylic acid	Indomethacin
Antibiotics (medicine for infection)	Methotrexate
	Nitrofurantoin
	Oral hypoglycemics
Aspirin or other salicylates	(diabetes medicine you take by mouth)
Dapsone	
Diuretics (water pills)	Pyrazinamide
	Sulfonamides
Ethacrynic acid	(sulfa medicine)
Furosemide	

Proper Use of This Medicine

If this medicine upsets your stomach, it may be taken with food or milk. If this does not work, an antacid may be taken. If stomach upset (nausea, vomiting, or loss of appetite) continues, check with your doctor.

If you are taking this medicine regularly and you miss a dose, take the missed dose as soon as possible. Then go back to your regular dosing schedule. If you do not remember the missed dose until it is almost time for the next dose, do not take the missed dose at all and do not double the next one. Instead, go back to your regular dosing schedule. If you have any questions about this, check with your doctor.

If you are taking this medicine for gout:

• This medicine will help prevent gout attacks but it will not relieve an attack that has already started. *Even if you take another medicine for gout attacks, continue to take this medicine also.* If you have any questions about this, check with your doctor.

• Drink at least 10 to 12 full glasses (8 ounces each) of fluids each day to help prevent kidney stones while taking this medicine, unless otherwise directed by your doctor.

Precautions While Using This Medicine

Your doctor should check your progress at regular visits.

Caution: Diabetics—Probenecid may cause false test results with copper sulfate urine sugar tests (Clinitest), but not with glucose enzymatic urine sugar tests (Clinistix). If you have any questions about this, check with your doctor or pharmacist.

Taking too much aspirin or other salicylates or drinking too much alcohol may lessen the effects of probenecid. Therefore, *do not take aspirin or other salicylates or drink alcoholic beverages while taking this medicine,* unless you have first checked with your doctor.

Side Effects of This Medicine

Along with its needed effects, a medicine may cause some unwanted effects. Although not all of these side effects appear very often, when they do occur they may require medical attention. Check with your doctor if any of the following side effects occur:

Less common

Bloody urine	Painful urination
Lower back pain	

Rare

Difficulty in breathing	Unusual bleeding or bruising
Skin rash or itching	Unusual tiredness or weakness
Unexplained fever	
Unexplained sore throat and fever	

Other side effects may occur which usually do not require medical attention. These side effects may go away during treatment as your body adjusts to the medicine. However, check with your doctor if any of the following side effects continue or are bothersome:

More common

Headache	Nausea
Loss of appetite	Vomiting

Less common

Dizziness	Frequent urge to urinate
Flushing or redness of face	Sore gums

Other side effects not listed above may also occur in some patients. If you notice any other effects, check with your doctor.

PROBUCOL (Systemic)
A commonly used brand name is Lorelco.

Probucol (proe-BYOO-kole) is used to lower cholesterol levels in the blood. This may help prevent medical problems caused by cholesterol clogging the blood vessels. Probucol is available only with your doctor's prescription.

Before Using This Medicine
Importance of Diet

Before prescribing medicine for your condition, your doctor will probably try to control your condition by prescribing a personal diet for you. Such a diet may be low in fats, sugars, and/or cholesterol. Many people are able to control their condition by carefully following their doctor's orders for proper diet and exercise. Medicine is prescribed only when additional help is needed and is effective only when a schedule of diet and exercise is properly followed.

Also, this medicine is less effective if you are greatly overweight. It may be very important for you to go on a reducing diet. However, check with your doctor before going on any diet.

In order to decide on the best treatment for your medical problem, your doctor should be told:

—if you have ever had any unusual reaction to probucol in the past. This medicine should not be taken if you are allergic to it.

—if you are pregnant, if you intend to become pregnant, or if you are breast-feeding an infant. Although probucol has not been shown to cause problems, the chance always exists.

—if you have any of the following medical problems:

Gallbladder disease or gallstones	Heart disease Liver disease

Proper Use of This Medicine
Many patients who have high cholesterol levels will not notice any signs of the problem. In fact, many may feel normal. *Take this medicine exactly as directed by your doctor, even though you may feel well.* Try not to miss any doses and do not take more medicine than your doctor ordered.

Remember that this medicine will not cure your condition but it does control it. Therefore, you must continue to take it as directed if you expect to keep your cholesterol levels down.

Follow carefully the special diet your doctor gave you. This is the most important part of controlling your condition, and is necessary if the medicine is to work properly.

This medicine works better when taken with meals.

If you miss a dose of this medicine, take it as soon as possible. If it is almost time for your next dose, do not take the missed dose at all and do not double the next one. Instead, go back to your regular dosing schedule. If you have any questions about this, check with your doctor.

Precautions While Using This Medicine
It is very important that your doctor check your progress at regular visits. This will allow your doctor to see if the medicine is working properly to lower your cholesterol levels and if you should continue to take it.

Do not stop taking this medicine without first checking with your doctor. When you stop taking this medicine, your blood fat levels may increase again. Your doctor may want you to follow a special diet to help prevent this.

Side Effects of This Medicine
Along with its needed effects, a medicine may cause some unwanted effects. Although not all of these side effects appear very often, when they do occur they may require medical attention. Check with your doctor if any of the following side effects occur:
Rare

Swellings on face, hands, or feet, or in mouth

Other side effects may occur which usually do not require medical attention. These side effects may go away during treatment as your body adjusts to the medicine. However, check with your doctor if any of the following side effects continue or are bothersome:
More common

Bloating Diarrhea	Nausea and vomiting Stomach pain

Less common or rare

Dizziness Headache Numbness or tingling of fingers, toes, or face	Unpleasant odor of perspiration Unusual increase in sweating

Other side effects not listed above may also occur in some patients. If you notice any other effects, check with your doctor.

PROCAINAMIDE (Systemic)

Some commonly used brand names are:

Procamide   Procopan
Procan   Pronestyl
Procan SR   Sub-Quin

Procainamide (proe-kane-A-mide) is most often used to restore irregular heartbeats to a normal rhythm and to slow an overactive heart. This allows the heart to work more efficiently. Procainamide is available only with your doctor's prescription.

Before Using This Medicine

In order to decide on the best treatment for your medical problem, your doctor should be told:

—if you have ever had any unusual reaction to procainamide, procaine, or a "caine-type" medicine in the past. This medicine should not be taken if you are allergic to them.

—if you are pregnant, if you intend to become pregnant, or if you are breast-feeding an infant. Although procainamide has not been shown to cause problems, the chance always exists.

—if you have any of the following medical problems:

Asthma   Kidney disease
History of lupus   Liver disease
  erythematosus   Myasthenia gravis

—if you are now taking any of the following medicines or types of medicine:

Antihypertensives   Medicine for
(high blood   myasthenia gravis
pressure   Other heart
medicine)   medicine

Proper Use of This Medicine

Take this medicine exactly as directed by your doctor, even though you may feel well. Do not miss any doses and do not take more medicine than ordered. *Do not stop taking this medicine without first checking with your doctor.*

This medicine should be taken with a glass of water on an empty stomach 1 hour before or 2 hours after meals so that it will be absorbed more quickly. However, your doctor may want you to take the medicine with food or milk to lessen stomach upset.

If you miss a dose of this medicine and remember within 1 hour or so of the missed dose, take it as soon as possible. Then go back to your regular dosing schedule. Do not double doses. If you have any questions about this, check with your doctor.

Precautions While Using This Medicine

It is important that your doctor check your progress at regular visits.

Before having any kind of surgery (including dental surgery) or emergency treatment, tell the doctor or dentist in charge that you are taking this medicine.

Your doctor may want you to carry a medical identification card or bracelet stating that you are using this medicine.

This medicine will break down and not work properly if it is exposed to too much moist air. Keep the container tightly closed and store in a dry place—not the bathroom medicine cabinet nor the refrigerator because of the moisture usually present in these areas.

If you begin to have symptoms of arthritis or pains with breathing, check with your doctor right away.

Side Effects of This Medicine

Along with its needed effects, a medicine may cause some unwanted effects. Although not all of these side effects appear very often, when they do occur they may require medical attention. Check with your doctor if any of the following side effects occur:

Less common

Fever   Pains with
Itching   breathing
Joint pain or swell- Skin rash
  ing
Rare
Fatigue   Mental confusion
Hallucinations (see- Mental depression
  ing, hearing, or   Unexplained fever
  feeling things that   and sore throat
  are not there)   Unusual bleeding or
                       bruising

Other side effects may occur which usually do not require medical attention. These side effects may go away during treatment as your body adjusts to the medicine. However, check with your doctor if any of the following side effects continue or are bothersome:

More common

Diarrhea   Nausea
Loss of appetite   Vomiting
Less common
Dizziness or light-
  headedness

Other side effects not listed above may also occur in some patients. If you notice any other effects, check with your doctor.

PROCARBAZINE (Systemic)

Some commonly used brand names are Matulane and Natulan*.

---

*Not available in the United States.

Procarbazine (pro-KAR-ba-zeen) belongs to the group of medicines known as alkylating agents. It is used to treat some kinds of cancer. Procarbazine is available only with your doctor's prescription.

Before Using This Medicine

Procarbazine is a very strong medicine. In addition to its helpful effects in treating your medical problem, it has side effects that could be very serious. Before you take this medicine, be sure that you have discussed the use of it with your doctor.

In order to decide on the best treatment for your medical problem, your doctor should be told:

—if you have ever had any unusual reaction to procarbazine in the past.

—if you are pregnant or if you intend to have children. This medicine may cause birth defects if either the male or female is taking it at the time of conception or if it is taken during pregnancy. It may also cause permanent sterility after it has been taken for a while. Be sure that you have discussed this with your doctor before taking this medicine.

—if you are breast-feeding an infant. Although procarbazine has not been shown to cause problems, the chance always exists.

—if you have any of the following medical problems:

Blood disease	Kidney disease
Diabetes	Liver disease

—if you have been treated with x-rays or cancer drugs by another doctor.

—if you are now taking or have taken within the past 2 weeks other monoamine oxidase (MAO) inhibitors such as:

Isocarboxazid	Phenelzine
Pargyline	Tranylcypromine

—if you are now taking or have taken within the past 2 weeks tricyclic antidepressants (medicine for depression).

—if you are now taking any of the following medicines or types of medicine:

Antihistamines or medicine for hay fever, other allergies, or colds	Blood pressure medicine
	Narcotics
Asthma medicine	Prescription pain medicine
Barbiturates	Sedatives, tranquilizers, or sleeping medicine

Proper Use of This Medicine

Use this medicine only as directed by your doctor. Do not use more or less of it and do not use it more often than your doctor ordered.

This medicine is sometimes given together with certain other medicines. If you are using a combination of drugs, make sure that you take each medicine at the right time and do not mix them. Ask your doctor, nurse, or pharmacist to help you plan a way to take your medicine at the right time.

This medicine commonly causes nausea and vomiting. Even if you begin to feel ill, *do not stop using this medicine without first checking with your doctor.* Taking this medicine with or after meals may lessen stomach upset.

If you miss a dose of this medicine and you remember it within a few hours, take it as soon as you remember it. Then go back to your regular dosing schedule. However, if several hours have passed or if it is almost time for the next dose, do not take the missed dose at all and do not double the next one. Instead, go back to your regular dosing schedule and check with your doctor.

Precautions While Using This Medicine

It is very important that your doctor check your progress at regular visits.

This medicine may cause some people to become drowsy or less alert than they are normally. *Make sure you know how you react to this medicine before you drive, use machines, or do other jobs that require you to be alert.*

Check with your doctor or hospital emergency room immediately if severe headache, stiff neck, chest pains, or rapid heartbeat, with nausea and vomiting occur while you are taking this medicine. These may be symptoms of a serious high blood pressure reaction which should have a doctor's attention.

When taken with certain foods, drinks, or other medicines, procarbazine can cause very dangerous reactions. To avoid such reactions, *obey the following rules of caution:*

—Do not eat foods that have a high tyramine content (most common in foods that are aged to increase their flavor), such as cheeses, sour cream, yogurt, pickled herring, chicken liver, canned figs, raisins, bananas, avocados, soy sauce, broad bean pods (fava beans), yeast extracts, or meats prepared with tenderizers.

—Do not drink alcoholic beverages, including beer and wines (especially chianti and other hearty red wines).

—Do not take any other medicine unless prescribed by your doctor. This especially includes over-the-counter (OTC) or nonprescription medicine such as that for colds (including nose drops), cough, asthma, hay fever, appetite control, or nausea.

After you stop using this medicine you must continue to obey the rules of caution concerning food, drink, and other medication for at least 2 weeks since procarbazine may continue to react with certain foods or other medicines for up to 14 days after you stop taking it.

Caution: Diabetics—Procarbazine may affect blood sugar levels. While you are using this medicine, be especially careful in testing for sugar in your urine. If you have any questions about this, check with your doctor.

If you are going to have surgery (including dental surgery) or emergency treatment tell the doctor in charge that you are using this medicine or have used it within the past 2 weeks.

Your doctor may want you to carry an identification card stating that you are using this medicine.

Side Effects of This Medicine

Along with its needed effects, a medicine may cause some unwanted effects. Although not all of these side effects appear very often, when they do occur they may require medical attention. *Stop taking this medicine and check with your doctor immediately* if the following side effects occur:

Rare

Chest pains	Severe headache
Rapid or irregular heartbeat	Stiff neck

Check with your doctor *immediately* if any of the following side effects occur:

More common

Black tarry stools	Unusual bleeding or bruising
Bloody vomit	
Unexplained fever, chills, or sore throat	

Less common

Diarrhea
Sores in the mouth and on the lips

Rare

Rash, hives, itching, or wheezing

Check with your doctor also if any of the following side effects occur:

More common

Continuing tiredness or weakness	Shortness of breath
Cough	Thickening of bronchial secretions

Less common

Convulsions	Nervousness
Hallucinations (seeing, hearing, or feeling things that are not there)	Nightmares
	Sleeplessness
	Tingling or numbness of the fingers or toes
Inability to sleep	Unsteadiness or awkwardness
Mental confusion	Yellowing of eyes and skin
Muscle twitching	

Rare

Dizziness or light-headedness when getting up from a lying or sitting position	Fainting

Other side effects may occur which usually do not require medical attention. These side effects may go away during treatment as your body adjusts to the medicine. However, check with your doctor if any of the following side effects continue or are bothersome:

More common

Drowsiness	Sweating
Muscle or joint pain	Tiredness
Nausea and vomiting	Weakness

Less common

Constipation	Feeling of warmth and redness in face
Darkening of skin	
Difficulty in swallowing	Headache
Dizziness	Loss of appetite
Dry mouth	Loss of hair
	Mental depression

Rare

Blurred vision	Hearing problems
Difficult urination	Hoarseness
Double vision	Increased sensitivity of skin to sunlight

Other side effects not listed above may also occur in some patients. If you notice any other effects, check with your doctor.

PROCHLORPERAZINE AND ISOPROPAMIDE (Systemic)

A commonly used brand name is Combid.

Prochlorperazine (proe-klor-PAIR-a-zeen) and isopropamide (eye-soe-PROE-pa-mide) is a combination of medicines used to relax the digestive system and to reduce stomach acid. It is used to treat stomach and intestinal problems such as ulcers and colitis. This combination is available only with your doctor's prescription.

Before Using This Medicine

In order to decide on the best treatment for your medical problem, your doctor should be told:

—if you have ever had any unusual reaction to iodine or phenothiazines in the past. This medicine should not be taken if you are allergic to it.

—if you are pregnant, if you intend to become pregnant, or if you are breast-feeding an infant. Although this medicine has not been shown to cause problems, the chance always exists.

—if you have any of the following medical problems:

Alcoholism	Hiatal hernia
Asthma	High blood pressure
Blood disease	Intestinal blockage
Bronchitis	Kidney disease
Difficult urination	Liver disease
Emphysema	Myasthenia gravis
Enlarged prostate	Overactive thyroid
Glaucoma	Parkinson's disease
Heart or circulation disease	Stomach ulcers
	Ulcerative colitis, severe

—if you are now taking any of the following medicines or types of medicine:

Amantadine	Haloperidol
Amphetamines	Heart medicine
Antacids	Levodopa
Anticonvulsants (seizure medicine)	Medicine for diarrhea
Asthma medicine	Medicine for Parkinson's disease
Epinephrine	
Guanethidine (high blood pressure medicine)	Ulcer medicine

—if you are now taking central nervous system (CNS) depressants such as:

Antihistamines or medicine for hay fever, other allergies, or colds	Sedatives, tranquilizers, or sleeping medicine
Barbiturates	Tricyclic antidepressants (medicine for depression)
Narcotics	
Prescription pain medicine	

—if you are now taking or have taken within the past 2 weeks monoamine oxidase (MAO) inhibitors such as:

Isocarboxazid	Phenelzine
Pargyline	Tranylcypromine

Proper Use of This Medicine

Take this medicine only as directed by your doctor. Do not take more of it, do not take it more often, and do not take it for a longer period of time than your doctor ordered.

If you miss a dose of this medicine, take it as soon as possible. If it is 2 hours or less until your next dose, do not take the missed dose at all and do not double the next one. Instead, go back to your regular dosing schedule. If you have any questions about this, check with your doctor.

Precautions While Using This Medicine

This medicine will add to the effects of alcohol and other medicines (CNS depressants) that slow down the nervous system. Some examples of CNS depressants are antihistamines or medicine for hay fever, other allergies, or colds; sedatives, tranquilizers, or sleeping medicine; prescription pain medicine or narcotics; barbiturates; medicine for seizures; tricyclic antidepressants (medicine for depression); or anesthetics, including some dental anesthetics. *Check with your doctor before taking any of the above while you are using this medicine.*

This medicine may cause some people to become drowsy or less alert than they are normally, especially during the first few weeks the medicine is being taken. Even if you take this medicine only at bedtime, you may feel drowsy or less alert on arising. *Make sure you know how you react to this medicine before you drive, use machines, or do other jobs that require you to be alert.*

Dizziness, lightheadedness, or fainting may occur, especially when you get up from a lying or sitting position. Getting up slowly may help. If the problem continues or gets worse, check with your doctor.

This medicine will often make you sweat less, causing your body temperature to increase. *Use extra care not to become overheated during exercise or hot weather while you are taking this medicine,* since overheating could possibly result in heat stroke. Also, hot baths or saunas may make you feel dizzy or faint while you are taking this medicine.

A few people who take this medicine may become more sensitive to sunlight than they are normally. When you first begin taking this medicine, avoid too much sun or too much use of a sunlamp until you see how you react. If you have a severe reaction, check with your doctor.

Your mouth, nose, and throat may feel very dry while you are taking this medicine. To help relieve mouth dryness, chew sugarless gum or dissolve bits of ice in your mouth.

Check with your doctor if you develop intestinal problems such as constipation. This is especially important if you are taking other medicine while you are taking this medicine, because if not corrected such problems may result in serious complications.

Do not take this medicine within 1 hour of taking antacids or medicine for diarrhea. Taking them too close together may make this medicine less effective.

Do not stop taking this medicine without first checking with your doctor. Your doctor may want you to reduce gradually the amount you are taking before stopping completely.

Side Effects of This Medicine

Along with its needed effects, a medicine may cause some unwanted effects. Although not all of these side effects appear very often, when they do occur they may require medical attention. Check with your doctor if any of the following side effects occur:

More common

Constipation
Mental confusion

Less common

Difficult urination	Shuffling walk
Fainting	Tic-like (jerky)
Fine, worm-like	movements of
movements of	head, face,
tongue	mouth, and neck
Restlessness	Trembling and
Skin rash	shaking of hands
	and fingers

Rare

Eye pain	Yellowing of eyes
Unexplained sore	and skin
throat and fever	

Other side effects may occur which usually do not require medical attention. These side effects may go away during treatment as your body adjusts to the medicine. However, check with your doctor if any of the following side effects continue or are bothersome:

More common

Bloated feeling	Dry mouth
Blurred vision	Increased skin sensi-
Decreased sweating	tivity to sun
Dizziness	Nasal congestion
Drowsiness	Unusually fast
	heartbeat

Less common

Changes in men-	Unusual tiredness
strual period	or weakness
Decreased sexual	
ability	

This medicine may cause the urine to be discolored (pink to brownish red). This effect is not important and is to be expected during treatment with this medicine.

Other side effects not listed above may also occur in some patients. If you notice any other effects, check with your doctor.

PROGESTINS (Systemic)

This information applies to the following medicines:

Dydrogesterone (dye-droe-JESS-ter-one)
Hydroxyprogesterone (hye-drox-ee-proe-JESS-terone)
Medroxyprogesterone (me-DROX-ee-proe-JESSte-rone)
Megestrol (me-JESS-trole)
Norethindrone (nor-eth-IN-drone)
Norethindrone Acetate
Norgestrel (nor-JESS-trel)
Progesterone (proe-JESS-ter-one)

Some commonly used brand names are:	Generic names:
Duphaston	Dydrogesterone
Delalutin	Hydrox-yprogesterone
Provera	Medrox-yprogesterone
Megace	Megestrol
Micronor Nor-Q.D. Norlutin	Norethindrone
Norlutate	Norethindrone Acetate
Ovrette	Norgestrel
Proluton Lipo-Lutin	Progesterone

Progestins (proe-JESS-tins) are sometimes called female hormones. They are produced by the body and are necessary during the childbearing years for the development of the milk-producing glands, and for the proper regulation of the menstrual cycle.

Progestins are prescribed for several reasons:

—for the proper regulation of the menstrual cycle

—to prevent pregnancy when used in birth-control pills

—in the treatment of selected cases of cancer of the breast, kidney, or uterus

—in testing the body's production of certain hormones

Progestins should not be used in pregnancy tests (except in special situations such as luteal phase defect) or in treatment of threatened miscarriage, since if used in the first 4 months of pregnancy they may cause birth defects.

Progestins are taken by mouth in tablet form when possible because of the greater convenience. However, to suit the individual needs of the patient better, they are sometimes given by intramuscular injection which provides a more constant and lasting effect.

Progestins are available only with your doctor's prescription.

Before Using This Medicine

To make the use of this medicine as safe and reliable as possible, you should understand how and when to take it and what effects may be expected. A paper with information for the patient will be given to you with your filled prescription, and will provide many details concerning the use of this medicine. Read this paper carefully and ask your doctor, nurse, or pharmacist if you need additional information or explanation.

In order to decide on the best treatment for your medical problem, your doctor should be told:

—if you have ever had any unusual reaction to this medicine in the past. This medicine should not be taken if you are allergic to it.

—if you are pregnant or if you suspect you are pregnant while using this medicine. Progestins may cause birth defects when used during the first 4 months of pregnancy and their use is not recommended during this time.

—if you are breast-feeding an infant. Although progestins have not been shown to cause problems, the chance always exists.

—if you have any of the following medical problems:

Asthma	Heart or circulation
Blood clots (or	disease
history of)	Kidney disease
Cancer (or history	Liver or gallbladder
of)	disease
Changes in vaginal	Mental depression
bleeding	Migraine headaches
Epilepsy	

Proper Use of This Medicine

Take this medicine only as directed by your doctor. Do not take more of it and do not take it for a longer period of time than your doctor ordered. Try to take the medicine at the same time each day to reduce the possibility of side effects and to allow it to work better. When used for birth control, this medicine should be taken every day of the year and 24 hours apart without interruption.

Nausea may occur during the first few weeks after you start taking this medicine. This effect usually disappears with continued use. If the nausea is bothersome, it can usually be prevented or reduced by taking each dose with food.

If you miss a dose of this medicine:
 • If you are *not* taking this medicine for birth control, take the missed dose as soon as possible. If it is almost time for your next dose, do not take the missed dose at all and do not double the next one. Instead, go back to your regular dosing schedule.
 • *If you are taking this medicine for birth control*, the safest thing to do when you miss 1 day's dose is to stop taking the medicine immediately and use another method of birth control until your period begins or until your doctor determines that you are not pregnant. This procedure is different from that used after missed doses of other birth control tablets which contain more than one hormone.

Precautions While Using This Medicine

It is very important that your doctor check your progress at regular visits. This will allow your dosage to be adjusted to your changing needs, and will allow any unwanted effects to be detected. These visits will usually be every 6 to 12 months, unless your doctor requires them more often.

Check with your doctor right away:
 —if vaginal bleeding continues for an unusually long time.
 —if you miss a menstrual period.
 —*if you suspect that you may have become pregnant. You should stop taking this medicine immediately* since continued use during pregnancy may cause birth defects in the child.

If you are taking this medicine for birth control:
 • *When you begin to use birth control tablets* your body will require several days to adjust before pregnancy will be prevented; therefore, you should *use a second method of birth control for the first cycle (or 3 weeks) to ensure full protection.*

 • Since one of the most important factors in the proper use of birth control tablets is taking every dose exactly on schedule, you should never let your tablet supply run out. Therefore, always keep 1 extra month's supply of tablets on hand. To keep the extra month's supply from becoming too old, use it next, after the pills now being used, and replace the extra supply each month on a regular schedule. The tablets will keep well when kept dry and at room temperature (light will fade some tablet colors but will not change their effect).

 • Keep the tablets in the container in which you received them. Most containers aid you in keeping track of dosage schedule.

 • The hormones in birth control tablets may cause birth defects. Since it takes a while for the effects of this medicine to wear off, birth defects may occur even though the tablets are no longer being used. Therefore, *when you stop using birth control tablets, it is very important that you wait at least 3 months before becoming pregnant. Be sure to use another method of birth control during that time.*

 • Caution: Your doctor has prescribed this medicine only for you after studying your health record and the results of your physical examination. Use of the tablets by other persons may be dangerous because of differences in health and body make-up. Therefore, do not give your birth control tablets to anyone else (and do not take tablets prescribed for someone else). Also, check with your doctor before taking any leftover birth control tablets from an old prescription, especially after a pregnancy. This medicine may be dangerous if your health has changed since your last physical examination.

Side Effects of This Medicine

Along with their needed effects, progestins sometimes cause some unwanted effects, such as blood clots and problems of the breasts, gallbladder, liver, and uterus.

The following side effects may be caused by blood clots but rarely occur; however, if they do occur they require immediate medical attention. If your doctor is not available, go to the nearest hospital emergency room.

Pains in chest, groin, or legs (especially in calves of legs)	Sudden loss of coordination
	Sudden loss of vision or change in vision
Severe, sudden headache	Sudden shortness of breath
Slurred speech (sudden)	

Other serious side effects which may occur and require medical attention, but usually not on an emergency basis, are:

Less common or rare

Changes in vaginal bleeding (spotting, breakthrough bleeding, prolonged or complete stoppage of bleeding)	Mental depression Pain in stomach or side Skin rash Yellowing of eyes or skin

Other side effects may occur which usually do not require medical attention. These side effects may go away during treatment as your body adjusts to the medicine. However, check with your doctor if any of the following side effects continue or are bothersome:

More common

Changes in appetite Changes in weight	Swelling of ankles and feet Unusual tiredness or weakness

Less common or rare

Acne Increased body and facial hair	Increased breast tenderness Nausea

Other side effects not listed above may also occur in some patients. If you notice any other effects, check with your doctor.

PROMETHAZINE (Systemic)

Some commonly used brand names are Historest, Phenergan, and Remsed.

Promethazine (proe-METH-a-zeen) belongs to the general class of medicines called antihistamines. It is used to relieve or prevent the symptoms of hay fever and other types of allergy. Since promethazine may cause drowsiness, it is used in some people to help them sleep.

Promethazine can be used to prevent motion sickness, nausea, vomiting, and dizziness. It may also be used for other conditions as determined by your doctor.

Promethazine is available only with your doctor's prescription.

Before Using This Medicine

In order to decide on the best treatment for your medical problem, your doctor should be told:

—if you have ever had any unusual reaction to promethazine or other phenothiazines in the past. This medicine should not be taken if you are allergic to it.

—if you are pregnant, if you intend to become pregnant, or if you are breast-feeding an infant. Although promethazine has not been shown to cause problems, the chance always exists.

—if you have any of the following medical problems:

Blood disease	Liver disease
Enlarged prostate	Lung disease
Glaucoma	Overactive thyroid
Heart disease	Reye's syndrome
High blood pressure	Stomach ulcer
Intestinal blockage	Urinary tract blockage

—if you are now taking any of the following medicines or types of medicine:

Guanethidine (high blood pressure medicine)	Medicine for epilepsy (anticonvulsants) Medicine for stomach ulcers or cramps

—if you are now taking any central nervous system (CNS) depressants such as:

Barbiturates Medicine for seizures Narcotics Other antihistamines or medicine for hay fever, other allergies, or colds	Prescription pain medicine Sedatives, tranquilizers, or sleeping medicine Tricyclic antidepressants (medicine for depression)

—if you are now taking or have taken within the past 2 weeks monoamine oxidase (MAO) inhibitors such as:

Isocarboxazid Pargyline	Phenelzine Tranylcypromine

Proper Use of This Medicine

If you are taking promethazine for motion sickness, take it at least 30 minutes before or, even better, 1 to 2 hours before you begin to travel.

Do not give this medicine to premature or newborn infants, unless otherwise directed by your doctor.

If you must take promethazine regularly and you miss a dose, take the missed dose as soon as possible. However, if it is almost time for your next dose, do not take the missed dose at all and do not double the next one. Instead, go back to your regular dosing schedule. If you have any questions about this, check with your doctor.

For patients taking promethazine by mouth:

• This medicine may be taken with food or a full glass (8 ounces) of water or milk to reduce stomach irritation.

For patients using the suppository form of promethazine:

• To insert suppository: First remove the foil wrapper and moisten the suppository with water. Lie down on side and push the suppository well up into the rectum with finger.

• If the suppository is too soft to insert because of storage in a warm place, before removing the foil wrapper chill the suppository in the refrigerator for 30 minutes or run cold water over it.

Precautions While Using This Medicine

If you will be taking this medicine for a long period of time (for example, for several months at a time), it is important that your doctor check your progress at regular visits.

Promethazine will add to the effects of alcohol and other medicines (CNS depressants) that slow down the nervous system. Some examples of CNS depressants are antihistamines or medicine for hay fever, other allergies, or colds; sedatives, tranquilizers, or sleeping medicine; prescription pain medicine or narcotics; barbiturates; medicine for seizures; tricyclic antidepressants (medicine for depression); or anesthetics, including some dental anesthetics. *Check with your doctor before taking any of the above while you are using this medicine.*

This medicine may cause some people to become drowsy or less alert than they are normally. Even if taken at bedtime, it may cause some people to feel drowsy or less alert on arising. *Make sure you know how you react to this medicine before you drive, use machines, or do other jobs that require you to be alert.*

A few people who take promethazine may become more sensitive to sunlight than they are normally. When you first begin taking this medicine, use sun screen lotions, or avoid too much sun or too much use of a sunlamp until you see how you react. If you have a severe reaction, check with your doctor.

When taking promethazine on a regular basis, make sure your doctor knows if you are taking large amounts of aspirin at the same time (as in arthritis). Effects of too much aspirin, such as dizziness or ringing in the ears, may be covered up by this medicine.

Side Effects of This Medicine

Along with its needed effects, a medicine may cause some unwanted effects. Although not all of these side effects appear very often, when they do occur they may require medical attention. Check with your doctor if the following side effects occur:

Rare

Unexplained fever and sore throat

Other side effects may occur which usually do not require medical attention. These side effects may go away during treatment as your body adjusts to the medicine. However, check with your doctor if any of the following side effects continue or are bothersome:

More common

Drowsiness

Less common or rare

Blurred vision	Nervousness,
Dizziness	restlessness, or
Dryness of mouth,	trouble in sleep-
nose, and throat	ing (especially
Increased sensitivity	in children)
of skin to sun	Skin rash
	Upset stomach or
	stomach pain

Other side effects not listed above may also occur in some patients. If you notice any other effects, check with your doctor.

PROPANTHELINE (Systemic)
A commonly used brand name is Pro-Banthine.

Propantheline (proe-PAN-the-leen) is a medicine that relieves cramping and spasms of the stomach, intestines, and bladder. Because it is thought to reduce the amount of acid formed in the stomach, it is often used to treat patients with stomach ulcers. This medicine is available only with your doctor's prescription.

Before Using This Medicine

In order to decide on the best treatment for your medical problem, your doctor should be told:

—if you have ever had any unusual reaction to propantheline in the past. This medicine should not be taken if you are allergic to it.

—if you are pregnant, if you intend to become pregnant, or if you are breast-feeding an infant. Although this medicine has not been shown to cause problems, the chance always exists.

—if you have any of the following medical problems:

Asthma	High blood pressure
Bronchitis	Intestinal blockage
Difficult urination	Kidney disease
Emphysema	Liver disease
Enlarged prostate	Myasthenia gravis
Glaucoma	Overactive thyroid
Heart disease	Severe ulcerative
Hiatal hernia	colitis

—if you are taking any of the following medicines or types of medicine:

Amantadine	Medicine for
Antacids	diarrhea
Antihistamines or	Medicine for
medicine for hay	Parkinson's
fever, other	disease
allergies,	Medicine for sleep
or colds	Nerve medicine
Haloperidol	Sedatives or
Heart medicine	tranquilizers
	Ulcer medicine

—if you are now taking or have taken within the past 2 weeks monoamine oxidase (MAO) inhibitors such as:

Isocarboxazid	Phenelzine
Pargyline	Tranylcypromine

Proper Use of This Medicine

Take this medicine about 1/2 to 1 hour before meals unless otherwise directed by your doctor.

If you miss a dose of this medicine, do not take the missed dose at all and do not double the next one. Instead, go back to your regular dosing schedule. If you have any questions about this, check with your doctor.

Precautions While Using This Medicine

This medicine will add to the effects of alcohol and other medicines (CNS depressants) that slow down the nervous system. Some examples of CNS depressants are antihistamines or medicine for hay fever, other allergies, or colds; sedatives, tranquilizers, or sleeping medicine; prescription pain medicine or narcotics; barbiturates; medicine for seizures; tricyclic antidepressants (medicine for depression); or anesthetics, including some dental anesthetics. *Check with your doctor before taking any of the above while you are using this medicine.*

Do not take this medicine within 1 hour of taking antacid or medicine for diarrhea. Taking them too close together may make propantheline less effective.

This medicine may cause your eyes to become more sensitive to light than they are normally. Wearing sunglasses may help lessen the discomfort from bright light.

This medicine may cause some people to become drowsy, dizzy, or less alert than they are normally. *Make sure you know how you react to this medicine before you drive, use machines, or do other jobs that require you to be alert.*

Propantheline will often reduce your tolerance of heat, since it makes you sweat less, causing your body temperature to increase. *Use extra care not to become overheated during exercise or hot weather while you are taking this medicine as this could possibly result in heat stroke.* Also, hot baths or saunas may make you feel dizzy or faint while you are taking this medicine.

Your mouth, nose, and throat may feel very dry while you are taking this medicine. *To help relieve mouth dryness, chew sugarless gum or dissolve bits of ice in your mouth.*

Check with your doctor if you develop intestinal problems such as constipation. This is especially important if you are taking other medicine while taking propantheline, because if the problems are not corrected serious complications may result.

Side Effects of This Medicine

Along with its needed effects, a medicine may cause some unwanted effects. Although not all of these side effects appear very often, when they do occur they may require medical attention. Check with your doctor if any of the following side effects occur:

More common

    Constipation

Less common

    Difficult urination

Rare

    Eye pain
    Skin rash

Other side effects may occur which usually do not require medical attention. These side effects may go away during treatment as your body adjusts to the medicine. However, check with your doctor if any of the following side effects continue or are bothersome:

More common

Bloated feeling	Headache
Dizziness	Rapid pulse
Dry mouth	Reduced sweating

Less common

Blurred vision	Nausea and
Decreased sexual	vomiting
ability	Nervousness
Drowsiness	Reduced sense of
Increased sensitivity	taste
of eyes to light	Tiredness
Mental confusion,	
especially in	
elderly	

Other side effects not listed above may also occur in some patients. If you notice any other effects, check with your doctor.

PROPOXYPHENE (Systemic)

Some commonly used brand names are:

Algodex*	Pro-65*
Darvon	Proxagesic
Depronal-SA*	Proxene
Dolene	SK-65
Novopropoxyn*	642*
Pargesic 65	

---

*Not available in the United States.

Propoxyphene (proe-POX-i-feen) is a medicine used to relieve pain. It is taken by mouth in the form of capsules, tablets, or liquid. Propoxyphene is available only with your doctor's prescription.

Before Using This Medicine

In order to decide on the best treatment for your medical problem, your doctor should be told:

—if you have ever had any unusual reaction to propoxyphene in the past. This medicine should not be taken if you are allergic to it.

—if you are pregnant or if you intend to become pregnant while using this medicine. Too much use of propoxyphene during pregnancy may cause the baby to become dependent on the medicine. This may lead to withdrawal side effects after birth. Be sure that you have discussed this with your doctor before taking this medicine. In addition, although propoxyphene has not been shown to cause birth defects, the chance always exists. Therefore, use during pregnancy should be carefully considered.

—if you are breast-feeding an infant. Propoxyphene passes into the breast milk. Although it has not been shown to cause problems, the chance always exists. Therefore, use by nursing mothers should be carefully considered.

—if you are now taking carbamazepine.

—if you are now taking other central nervous system (CNS) depressants such as:

Antihistamines or	Sedatives, tran-
medicine for hay	quilizers, or sleep-
fever, other aller-	ing medicine
gies, or colds	Seizure medicine
Barbiturates	Tricyclic an-
Narcotics	tidepressants
Other prescription	(medicine for
pain medicine	depression)

—if you are now taking or have taken within the past 2 weeks monoamine oxidase (MAO) inhibitors such as:

Isocarboxazid	Phenelzine
Pargyline	Tranylcypromine

Proper Use of This Medicine

Take this medicine only as directed by your doctor. Do not take more of it, do not take it more often, and do not take it for a longer period of time than your doctor ordered. If too much is taken, it may become habit-forming (causing mental or physical dependence) or lead to medical problems because of an overdose.

Keep this medicine out of reach of children since overdose is very dangerous in young children.

If you miss a dose of this medicine, do not double the next dose. Instead, go back to your regular dosing schedule. If you have any questions about this, check with your doctor.

Precautions While Using This Medicine

If you will be taking this medicine for a long period of time (for example, for several months at a time), your doctor should check your progress at regular visits.

This medicine will add to the effects of alcohol and other medicines (CNS depressants) that slow down the nervous system. Some examples of CNS depressants are antihistamines or medicine for hay fever, other allergies, or colds; sedatives, tranquilizers, or sleeping medicine; prescription pain medicine or narcotics; barbiturates; medicine for seizures; tricyclic antidepressants (medicine for depression); or anesthetics, including some dental anesthetics. *Check with your doctor before taking any of the above while you are using this medicine.*

If you think you may have taken an overdose, get emergency help right away. Taking an overdose of propoxyphene or taking alcohol or

Propoxyphene and Acetaminophen

CNS depressants along with propoxyphene may lead to signs of overdose, including unconsciousness or death. Signs of overdose include convulsions, mental confusion, severe nervousness or restlessness, seizures, severe dizziness, severe drowsiness, shortness of breath or troubled breathing, and severe weakness.

This medicine may cause some people to become drowsy, dizzy, or lightheaded, or to feel a false sense of well-being. *Make sure you know how you react to this medicine before you drive, use machines, or do other jobs that require you to be alert and clearheaded.*

Nausea may occur, especially after the first couple of doses. This effect usually goes away if you lie down for a while. However, if nausea or vomiting continues, check with your doctor.

Side Effects of This Medicine

Along with its needed effects, a medicine may cause some unwanted effects. Although not all of these side effects appear very often, when they do occur they may require medical attention. Check with your doctor *immediately* if any of the following side effects occur:

Less common
   Itching or skin rash

Possible signs of overdose
Convulsions	Seizures
Dizziness (severe)	Shortness of breath
Drowsiness (severe)	or troubled
Mental confusion	breathing
Nervousness or rest-	Unconsciousness
lessness (severe)	Weakness (severe)

Other side effects may occur which usually do not require medical attention. These side effects may go away during treatment as your body adjusts to the medicine. However, check with your doctor if any of the following side effects continue or are bothersome:

More common
Dizziness or light-	Drowsiness
headedness	Nausea or vomiting

Less common
Blurred vision or	Headache
other change in	Stomach pain
vision	Unusual tiredness or
Constipation	weakness
False sense of well-	
being	

After you stop taking this medicine, your body may need time to adjust. The length of time this takes depends on the amount of medicine you were using and how long you used it. During this period of time check with your doctor if you notice any of the following side effects:

Diarrhea	Runny nose
Fever	Shivering
Irritability	Stomach cramps
Nausea or vomiting	Sweating
Nervousness	Yawning
Restlessness	

Other side effects not listed above may also occur in some patients. If you notice any other effects, check with your doctor.

PROPOXYPHENE AND ACETAMINOPHEN
(Systemic)
Some commonly used brand names are:

Darvocet-N	SK-65-APAP
Dolacet	Wygesic
Dolene AP-65	

Propoxyphene (proe-POX-i-feen) and acetaminophen (a-seat-a-MEE-noe-fen) is a combination medicine used to relieve pain. It is available only with your doctor's prescription.

Before Using This Medicine

In order to decide on the best treatment for your medical problem, your doctor should be told:

—if you have ever had any unusual reaction to propoxyphene or acetaminophen in the past. This medicine should not be taken if you are allergic to it.

—if you are pregnant or if you intend to become pregnant while using this medicine. Too much use of propoxyphene during pregnancy may cause the baby to become dependent on the medicine. This may lead to withdrawal side effects after birth. Be sure that you have discussed this with your doctor before taking this medicine. In addition, although propoxyphene and acetaminophen have not been shown to cause birth defects, the chance always exists. Therefore, use during pregnancy should be carefully considered.

—if you are breast-feeding an infant. Propoxyphene and acetaminophen pass into the breast milk. Although they have not been shown to cause problems, the chance always exists. Therefore, use by nursing mothers should be carefully considered.

—if you have any of the following medical problems:

Kidney disease   Liver disease or cirrhosis of the liver

—if you are now taking carbamazepine.

—if you are now taking other central nervous system (CNS) depressants such as:

Antihistamines or medicine for hay fever, other allergies, or colds
Barbiturates
Narcotics
Other prescription pain medicine

Sedatives, tranquilizers, or sleeping medicine
Seizure medicine
Tricyclic antidepressants (medicine for depression)

—if you are now taking or have taken within the past 2 weeks monoamine oxidase (MAO) inhibitors such as:

Isocarboxazid   Phenelzine
Pargyline   Tranylcypromine

Proper Use of This Medicine

Keep this medicine out of the reach of children since overdose is very dangerous in young children.

Take this medicine only as directed by your doctor. Do not take more of it, do not take it more often, and do not take it for a longer period of time than your doctor ordered. If too much is taken, it may become habit-forming, cause liver damage, or lead to medical problems because of an overdose.

Precautions While Using This Medicine

Check the labels of all over-the-counter (OTC), nonprescription, and prescription medicines you now take. If any contain propoxyphene or acetaminophen be especially careful, since taking them while taking this medicine may lead to overdose. If you have any questions about this, check with your doctor or pharmacist.

If you will be taking this medicine for a long period of time (for example, for several months at a time), your doctor should check your progress at regular visits.

This medicine will add to the effects of alcohol and other medicines (CNS depressants) that slow down the nervous system. Some examples of CNS depressants are antihistamines or medicine for hay fever, other allergies, or colds; sedatives, tranquilizers, or sleeping

medicine; prescription pain medicine or narcotics; barbiturates; medicine for seizures; tricyclic antidepressants (medicine for depression); or anesthetics, including some dental anesthetics. In addition, there may be a greater risk of liver damage if large amounts of alcoholic beverages are used while you are taking acetaminophen. *Check with your doctor before taking any of the above while you are using this medicine.*

If you think you may have taken an overdose, get emergency help right away. Taking an overdose of propoxyphene or taking alcohol or CNS depressants along with propoxyphene may lead to signs of overdose, including unconsciousness or death. Signs of overdose include convulsions, mental confusion, severe nervousness or restlessness, seizures, severe dizziness, severe drowsiness, shortness of breath or troubled breathing, and severe weakness.

This medicine may cause some people to become drowsy, dizzy, or lightheaded, or to feel a false sense of well-being. *Make sure you know how you react to this medicine before you drive, use machines, or do other jobs that require you to be alert and clearheaded.*

Nausea may occur, especially after the first couple of doses. This effect usually goes away if you lie down for a while.

Side Effects of This Medicine

Along with its needed effects, a medicine may cause some unwanted effects. Although not all of these side effects appear very often, when they do occur they may require medical attention. Check with your doctor if any of the following side effects occur:

Rare

Itching or skin rash
Unexplained sore throat and fever
Unusual bleeding or bruising

Unusual tiredness or weakness
Yellowing of eyes or skin

Possible signs of overdose of acetaminophen

Diarrhea
Loss of appetite

Nausea or vomiting
Stomach cramps or pain

Possible signs of overdose of propoxyphene

Convulsions
Dizziness (severe)
Drowsiness (severe)
Mental confusion
Nervousness (severe)
Restlessness (severe)

Seizures
Shortness of breath or troubled breathing
Unconsciousness
Weakness (severe)

Other side effects may occur which usually do not require medical attention. These side effects may go away during treatment as your body adjusts to the medicine. However, check with your doctor if any of the following side effects continue or are bothersome:

More common

Dizziness or light-headedness	Drowsiness
	Nausea or vomiting

Less common

Blurred vision or other change in vision	Headache
	Stomach pain
Constipation	Unusual tiredness
False sense of well-being	Unusual weakness

After you stop using this medicine, your body may need time to adjust. The length of time this takes depends on the amount of medicine you were using and how long you used it. During this period of time check with your doctor if you notice any of the following side effects:

Diarrhea	Runny nose
Fever	Shivering
Irritability	Stomach cramps
Nausea or vomiting	Sweating
Nervousness	Yawning
Restlessness	

Other side effects not listed above may also occur in some patients. If you notice any other effects, check with your doctor.

PROPOXYPHENE AND APC (Systemic)
Some commonly used brand names are Darvon Compound, Dolene Compound-65, and SK-65 Compound.

Propoxyphene (proe-POX-i-feen) and APC is a combination medicine used to relieve pain. APC is the short name for aspirin (AS-pir-in), phenacetin (fe-NASS-e-tin), and caffeine (KAF-een). Propoxyphene and APC combination is available only with your doctor's prescription.

Before Using This Medicine

In order to decide on the best treatment for your medical problem, your doctor should be told:

—if you have ever had any unusual reaction to propoxyphene, acetaminophen, phenacetin, caffeine, or aspirin or other salicylates including methyl salicylate (oil of wintergreen) or to other nonsteroidal anti-inflammatory agents such as fenoprofen, ibuprofen, indomethacin, naproxen, oxyphenbutazone, phenylbutazone, sulindac, or tolmetin.

—if you are pregnant or if you intend to become pregnant while using this medicine. Too much use of propoxyphene during pregnancy may cause the baby to become dependent on the medicine. This may lead to withdrawal side effects after birth. Be sure that you have discussed this with your doctor before taking this medicine. Too much use of aspirin during the last 3 months of pregnancy may increase the length of pregnancy and prolong labor. Aspirin taken during the last 2 weeks of pregnancy may cause the baby to have bleeding problems at birth. When phenacetin is used during pregnancy, it may cause side effects in the newborn infant. In addition, although aspirin, phenacetin, caffeine, and propoxyphene have not been shown to cause birth defects in humans, the chance always exists.

—if you are breast-feeding an infant. Propoxyphene, aspirin, phenacetin, and caffeine pass into the breast milk. Although they have not been shown to cause problems, the chance always exists. Therefore, use by nursing mothers should be carefully considered.

—if you have any of the following medical problems:

Anemia	Hemophilia or other bleeding problems
Asthma, allergies, and nasal polyps (history of)	Hodgkin's disease
	Hypoprothrom-binemia
Glucose-6-phosphate dehydrogenase (G6PD) deficiency	Kidney disease
	Liver disease
	Ulcer or other stomach problems
Gout	Vitamin K deficiency

—if you are now taking any of the following medicines or types of medicine:

Antacids	Oral hypoglycemics (diabetes medicine you take by mouth)
Anticoagulants (blood thinners)	
Carbamazepine	
Corticosteroids (cortisone-like medicines)	Spironolactone
	Urine acidifiers (medicine to make your urine more acid)
Gout medicine	
Inflammation medicine (for example, arthritis medicine)	Urine alkalizers (medicine to make your urine less acid)
Insulin	
Methotrexate	Vitamin C

—if you are now taking other central nervous system (CNS) depressants such as:

Antihistamines or medicine for hay fever, other allergies, or colds	Sedatives, tranquilizers, or sleeping medicine
Barbiturates	Seizure medicine
Narcotics	Tricyclic antidepressants (medicine for depression)
Other prescription pain medicine	

—if you are now taking or have taken within the past 2 weeks monoamine oxidase (MAO) inhibitors such as:

Isocarboxazid	Phenelzine
Pargyline	Tranylcypromine

Proper Use of This Medicine

Take this medicine with food or a full glass (8 ounces) of water or milk to lessen stomach irritation.

Do not use this medicine if it has a strong vinegar-like odor, since this means the aspirin in the product is breaking down. If you have any questions about this, check with your doctor or pharmacist.

Take this medicine only as directed by your doctor. Do not take more of it, do not take it more often, and do not take it for a longer period of time than your doctor ordered. If too much is taken, it may become habit-forming, cause kidney damage, or lead to medical problems because of an overdose.

Keep this medicine out of the reach of children since overdose is very dangerous in young children.

Precautions While Using This Medicine

Check the labels of all over-the-counter (OTC), nonprescription, and prescription medicines you now take. If any contain propoxyphene, aspirin or other salicylates, or phenacetin be especially careful, since taking them while taking this medicine may lead to overdose. If you have any questions about this, check with your doctor, nurse, or pharmacist.

Caution: Diabetics—This medicine contains aspirin and phenacetin which may cause false test results with urine sugar tests. If you have any questions about this, check with your doctor, nurse, or pharmacist, especially if your diabetes is not well controlled.

If you will be taking this medicine for a long period of time (for example, for several months at a time), your doctor should check your progress at regular visits.

Do not take this medicine for 5 days before having surgery, including dental surgery, unless otherwise directed by your doctor. The aspirin in this product, if taken during this time, may cause bleeding problems.

This medicine will add to the effects of alcohol and other medicines (CNS depressants) that slow down the nervous system. Some examples of CNS depressants are antihistamines or medicine for hay fever, other allergies, or colds; sedatives, tranquilizers, or sleeping medicine; prescription pain medicine or narcotics; barbiturates; medicine for seizures; tricyclic antidepressants (medicine for depression); or anesthetics, including some dental anesthetics. In addition, stomach problems may be more likely to occur if you drink alcoholic beverages while being treated with this medicine. *Check with your doctor before taking any of the above while you are using this medicine.*

If you think you may have taken an overdose, get emergency help right away. Taking an overdose of propoxyphene or taking alcohol or CNS depressants along with propoxyphene may lead to signs of overdose, including unconsciousness or death. Signs of overdose include convulsions, mental confusion, severe nervousness or restlessness, seizures, severe dizziness, severe drowsiness, shortness of breath or troubled breathing, and severe weakness.

This medicine may cause some people to become drowsy, dizzy, or lightheaded, or to feel a false sense of well-being. *Make sure you know how you react to this medicine before you drive, use machines, or do other jobs that require you to be alert and clearheaded.*

Nausea may occur, especially after the first couple of doses. This effect usually goes away if you lie down for a while. However, if nausea or vomiting continues, check with your doctor.

Side Effects of This Medicine

Along with its needed effects, a medicine may cause some unwanted effects. Although not all of these side effects appear very often, when they do occur they may require medical attention. Check with your doctor if any of the following side effects occur:

Less common

Any loss of hearing	Shortness of breath
Bloody or black	Stomach pain
tarry stools	Tightness in chest
Itching or skin rash	Wheezing
Nausea or vomiting	

Possible signs of overdose of propoxyphene

Convulsions	Severe nervousness
Mental confusion	or restlessness
Seizures	Severe weakness
Severe dizziness	Shortness of breath
Severe drowsiness	or troubled
	breathing
	Unconsciousness

Possible signs of overdose of aspirin

Diarrhea	Severe or continuing
Dizziness or mental	headache
confusion	Stomach pain
Nausea or vomiting	Sweating
Rapid breathing	Thirst
Ringing or buzzing	Vision problems
in ear (continu-	
ing)	

Possible side effects with long-term use of APC

Bluish-colored	Swelling of feet or
fingernails or	lower legs
mucous	Unusual tiredness or
membranes	weakness
Cloudy urine	

Other side effects may occur which usually do not require medical attention. These side effects may go away during treatment as your body adjusts to the medicine. However, check with your doctor if any of the following side effects continue or are bothersome:

More common

Dizziness or light-	Drowsiness
headedness	Nausea or vomiting

Less common

Blurred vision or	Indigestion
other change in	Sleeplessness,
vision	nervousness, or
Constipation	jitters
False sense of well-	Stomach pain
being	Unusual tiredness or
Headache	weakness

After you stop using this medicine, your body may need time to adjust. The length of time this takes depends on the amount of medicine you were using and how long you used it. During this period of time check with your doctor if you notice any of the following side effects:

Diarrhea	Runny nose
Fever	Shivering
Irritability	Stomach cramps
Nausea or vomiting	Sweating
Nervousness	Yawning
Restlessness	

Other side effects not listed above may also occur in some patients. If you notice any other effects, check with your doctor.

PROPOXYPHENE AND ASPIRIN (Systemic)

Some commonly used brand names are Darvon with A.S.A. and Darvon-N with A.S.A.

Propoxyphene and aspirin (proe-POX-i-feen and AS-pir-in) is a combination medicine used to relieve pain. It is available only with your doctor's prescription.

Before Using This Medicine

In order to decide on the best treatment for your medical problem, your doctor should be told:

—if you have ever had any unusual reaction to propoxyphene or to aspirin or other salicylates including methyl salicylate (oil of wintergreen), or to other nonsteroidal anti-inflammatory agents such as fenoprofen, ibuprofen, indomethacin, naproxen, oxyphenbutazone, phenylbutazone, sulindac, or tolmetin.

—if you are pregnant or if you intend to become pregnant while using this medicine. Too much use of propoxyphene during pregnancy may cause the baby to become dependent on the medicine. This may lead to withdrawal side effects after birth. Be sure that you have discussed this with your doctor before taking this medicine. Too much use of aspirin during the last 3 months of pregnancy may increase the length of pregnancy and may prolong labor. Aspirin taken during the last 2 weeks of pregnancy may cause the baby to have bleeding problems at birth. In addition, although aspirin and propoxyphene have not been shown to cause birth defects in humans, the chance always exists.

—if you are breast-feeding an infant. Although aspirin and propoxyphene have not been shown to cause problems, the chance always exists. Therefore, use by nursing mothers should be carefully considered.

—if you have any of the following medical problems:

Anemia	Hodgkin's disease
Asthma, allergies, and nasal polyps (history of)	Hypoprothrom- binemia
	Kidney disease
Gout	Liver disease
Hemophilia or other bleeding problems	Ulcer or other stomach problems
	Vitamin K deficiency

—if you are now taking any of the following medicines or types of medicine:

Antacids	Methotrexate
Anticoagulants (blood thinners)	Oral hypoglycemics (diabetes medicine you take by mouth)
Carbamazepine	
Corticosteroids (cortisone-like medicine)	Spironolactone
	Urine acidifiers (medicine to make your urine more acid)
Gout medicine	
Inflammation medicine (for example, arthritis medicine)	Urine alkalizers (medicine to make your urine less acid)
Insulin	
	Vitamin C

—if you are now taking other central nervous system (CNS) depressants such as:

Antihistamines or medicine for hay fever, other allergies, or colds	Other prescription pain medicine
	Sedatives, tran- quilizers, or sleep- ing medicine
Barbiturates	
Narcotics	Seizure medicine
	Tricyclic an- tidepressants (medicine for depression)

—if you are now taking or have taken within the past 2 weeks monoamine oxidase (MAO) inhibitors such as:

Isocarboxazid	Phenelzine
Pargyline	Tranylcypromine

Proper Use of This Medicine

Take this medicine with food or a full glass (8 ounces) of water or milk to lessen stomach ir- ritation.

Do not use this medicine if it has a strong vinegar- like odor, since this means the aspirin is break- ing down. If you have any questions about this, check with your doctor or pharmacist.

Keep this medicine out of the reach of children since overdose is very dangerous in young children.

Take this medicine only as directed by your doc- tor. Do not take more of it, do not take it more often, and do not take it for a longer period of time than your doctor ordered. If too much is taken, it may become habit-forming or lead to medical problems because of an overdose.

Precautions While Using This Medicine

Check the labels of all over-the-counter (OTC), nonprescription, and prescription medicines you now take. If any contain propoxyphene or aspirin or other salicylates, be especially careful, since taking them while taking this medicine may lead to overdose. If you have any questions about this, check with your doctor or pharmacist.

Caution: Diabetics—This medicine contains aspirin which may cause false test results with urine sugar tests if you regularly take 8 or more tablets or capsules a day. Smaller doses or oc- casional use of aspirin usually do not affect urine sugar tests. If you have any questions about this, check with your doctor, nurse, or pharmacist, especially if your diabetes is not well controlled.

If you will be taking this medicine for a long period of time (for example, for several months at a time), your doctor should check your pro- gress at regular visits.

Do not take this medicine for 5 days before any surgery, including dental surgery, unless other- wise directed by your doctor. Taking aspirin during this time may cause bleeding problems.

This medicine will add to the effects of alcohol and other medicines (CNS depressants) that slow down the nervous system. Some examples of CNS depressants are antihistamines or medicine for hay fever, other allergies, or colds; sedatives, tranquilizers, or sleeping medicine; prescription pain medicine or nar- cotics; barbiturates; medicine for seizures; tricyclic antidepressants (medicine for depres- sion); or anesthetics, including some dental anesthetics. In addition, stomach problems may be more likely to occur if you drink alcoholic beverages while being treated with this medicine. *Check with your doctor before taking any of the above while you are using this medicine.*

If you think you may have taken an overdose, get emergency help right away. Taking an over- dose of propoxyphene or taking alcohol or CNS depressants along with propoxyphene may lead to signs of overdose, including unconsciousness or death. Signs of overdose include convulsions, mental confusion, severe nervousness or restlessness, seizures, severe dizziness, severe drowsiness, shortness of breath or troubled breathing, and severe weakness.

This medicine may cause some people to become drowsy, dizzy, or lightheaded, or to feel a false sense of well-being. *Make sure you know how you react to this medicine before you drive, use machines, or do other jobs that require you to be alert and clearheaded.*

Nausea may occur, especially after the first couple of doses. This effect usually goes away if you lie down for a while. However, if nausea or vomiting continues, check with your doctor.

Side Effects of This Medicine

Along with its needed effects, a medicine may cause some unwanted effects. Although not all of these side effects appear very often, when they do occur they may require medical attention. Check with your doctor if any of the following side effects occur:

More common
Nausea or vomiting
Stomach pain

Less common
Any loss of hearing   Shortness of breath
Bloody or black   Tightness in chest
  tarry stools   Wheezing
Itching or skin rash

Possible signs of overdose of propoxyphene
Convulsions   Severe nervousness
Mental confusion   or restlessness
Seizures   Severe weakness
Severe dizziness   Shortness of breath
Severe drowsiness   or troubled
                          breathing
                        Unconsciousness

Possible signs of overdose of aspirin
Diarrhea   Severe or continuing
Dizziness or mental   headache
  confusion   Stomach pain
Nausea or vomiting   Sweating
Rapid breathing   Thirst
Ringing or buzzing   Vision problems
  in ear (continu-
  ing)

Other side effects may occur which usually do not require medical attention. These side effects may go away during treatment as your body adjusts to the medicine. However, check with your doctor if the following side effects continue or are bothersome:

More common
Dizziness or light-   Indigestion
  headedness   Nausea or vomiting
Drowsiness

Less common
Blurred vision or   Headache
  other change in   Stomach pain
  vision   Unusual tiredness or
Constipation   weakness
False sense of well-
  being

After you stop using this medicine, your body may need time to adjust. The length of time this takes depends on the amount of medicine you were using and how long you used it. During this period of time check with your doctor if you notice any of the following side effects:

Diarrhea   Runny nose
Fever   Shivering
Irritability   Stomach cramps
Nausea or vomiting   Sweating
Nervousness   Yawning
Restlessness

Other side effects not listed above may also occur in some patients. If you notice any other effects, check with your doctor.

PSEUDOEPHEDRINE (Systemic)
Some commonly used brand names are:
Afrinol   Pseudofrin*
D-Feda   Robidrine*
Eltor*   Ro-Fedrin
Neobid   Sudafed
Novafed   Sudrin

*Not available in the United States.

Pseudoephedrine (soo-doe-e-FED-rin) is used for the relief of nasal congestion caused by the common cold, sinusitis, hay fever, and other respiratory allergies. Also, it is used for the relief of ear congestion caused by ear inflammation or infection. Some of these preparations are available only with your doctor's prescription. Others are available without a prescription; however, your doctor may have special instructions on the proper dose of pseudoephedrine for your medical condition.

Before Using This Medicine

In order to decide on the best treatment for your medical problem, your doctor should be told:

—if you have ever had any unusual reaction to medicines like pseudoephedrine such as amphetamines, ephedrine, epinephrine, isoproterenol, metaproterenol, norepinephrine (levarterenol), phenylephrine, phenylpropanolamine, or terbutaline.

—if you are pregnant or if you intend to become pregnant while using this medicine. Although pseudoephedrine has not been shown to cause problems, the chance always exists.

—if you are breast-feeding an infant. Pseudoephedrine passes into the breast milk and may cause unwanted effects in infants of mothers taking this medicine.

—if you have any of the following medical problems:

Diabetes	Heart or blood
Enlarged prostate	vessel disease
Glaucoma	High blood pressure
	Overactive thyroid

—if you are now taking any of the following medicines or types of medicine:

Alkavervir	Nadolol
Amphetamines	Propranolol
Digitalis glycosides	Protoveratrine A
(heart medicine)	Reserpine
Guanethidine	Tricyclic an-
Mecamylamine	tidepressants
Medicine for	(medicine for
asthma or	depression)
breathing prob-	Veratrum viride
lems	alkaloids
Methyldopa	
Metoprolol	

—if you are now taking or have taken within the past 2 weeks monoamine oxidase (MAO) inhibitors such as:

Isocarboxazid	Phenelzine
Pargyline	Tranylcypromine

Proper Use of This Medicine

Take this medicine only as directed. Do not take more of it and do not take it more often than recommended on the label, unless otherwise directed by your doctor. To do so may increase the chance of side effects.

To help prevent trouble in sleeping, *take the last dose of this medicine for each day a few hours before bedtime.* If you have any questions about this, check with your doctor.

If you miss a dose of this medicine and you remember within an hour or so of the missed dose, take it right away. Then go back to your regular dosing schedule. But if you do not remember until later, do not take the missed dose at all and do not double the next one. In-stead, go back to your regular dosing schedule. If you have any questions about this, check with your doctor.

If you are taking the extended-release capsule form of this medicine:

• Swallow the capsule whole.

• Do not crush, break, or chew before swallowing.

• If the capsule is too large to swallow, you may mix the contents of the capsule with jam or jelly and swallow without chewing.

If you are taking the extended-release tablet form of this medicine.

• Swallow the tablet whole.

• Do not break, crush, or chew before swallowing.

Precautions While Using This Medicine

If symptoms do not improve within 5 days or if you also have a high fever, check with your doctor since these signs may mean that you have other medical problems.

Side Effects of This Medicine

Along with its needed effects, a medicine may cause some unwanted effects. Although not all of these side effects appear very often, when they do occur they may require medical attention. Check with your doctor if any of the following side effects occur:

With high doses

Hallucinations (see-	Seizures
ing, hearing, or	Unusually slow
feeling things that	heartbeat, short-
are not there)	ness of breath, or
Irregular heartbeat	troubled
	breathing

Other side effects may occur which usually do not require medical attention. These side effects may go away during treatment as your body adjusts to the medicine. However, check with your doctor if any of the following side effects continue or are bothersome:

More common

Nervousness	Trouble in sleeping
Restlessness	

Less common

Difficult or painful	Troubled breathing
urination	Unusual increase in
Dizziness or light-	sweating
headedness	Unusual paleness
Headache	Unusually fast or
Nausea or vomiting	pounding heart-
Trembling	beat
	Weakness

Other side effects not listed above may also occur in some patients. If you notice any other effects, check with your doctor.

PYRAZINAMIDE (Systemic)

Pyrazinamide (peer-a-ZIN-a-mide) belongs to the general family of medicines called anti-infectives. It is used to help the body overcome tuberculosis (TB). It is given by mouth with one or more other medicines for TB. Pyrazinamide is available only with your doctor's prescription.

Before Using This Medicine

In order to decide on the best treatment for your medical problem, your doctor should be told:

—if you have had allergic reactions to ethionamide, isoniazid (INH), or niacin (nicotinic acid).

—if you are pregnant, if you intend to become pregnant, or if you are breast-feeding an infant, although pyrazinamide has not been shown to cause problems.

—if you have any of the following medical problems:

Diabetes   Liver disease
Gout (history of)

Proper Use of This Medicine

To help clear up your tuberculosis (TB) completely, *it is important that you keep taking this medicine for the full time of treatment* even if you begin to feel better after a few weeks. You may have to take it every day for as long as 1 to 2 years or more. *It is important that you do not miss any doses.*

If you do miss a dose of this medicine, take it as soon as possible. However, if it is almost time for your next dose, do not take the missed dose or double your next dose. Instead, go back to your regular dosing schedule.

Precautions While Using This Medicine

If your symptoms do not improve within 2 to 3 weeks or if they become worse, check with your doctor.

It is very important that your doctor check your progress at regular visits.

Caution: Diabetics—This medicine may cause false test results with urine ketone tests. Check with your doctor before changing your diet or the dosage of your diabetes medicine.

Side Effects of This Medicine

Along with its needed effects, a medicine may cause some unwanted effects. Although not all of these side effects appear very often, when they do occur they may require medical attention. Stop taking this medicine and check with your doctor if any of the following side effects occur:

More common

Loss of appetite   Yellowing of eyes
Unexplained fever   or skin
Unusual tiredness
  or weakness

Less common

Chills, pain and swelling of joints (especially great toe, ankle, knee), or tense, hot skin over affected joints

Other side effects may occur which usually do not require medical attention. These side effects may go away during treatment as your body adjusts to the medicine. However, check with your doctor if any of the following side effects continue or are bothersome:

Less common

Difficult urination   Vomiting
Nausea

Rare

Increased sensitivity   Itching
  to sunlight   Rash

Other side effects not listed above may also occur in some patients. If you notice any other effects, check with your doctor.

PYRILAMINE AND PENTOBARBITAL (Systemic)

Some commonly used brand names are Eme-Nil and Wans.

Pyrilamine (peer-ILL-a-meen) and pentobarbital (pen-toe-BAR-bi-tal) is a combination medicine used to treat nausea and vomiting. This medicine comes as a rectal suppository and is available only with your doctor's prescription.

Before Using This Medicine

In order to decide on the best treatment for your medical problem, your doctor should be told:

—if you have ever had any unusual reaction to barbiturates or antihistamines in the past. This medicine should not be used if you are allergic to it.

—if you are pregnant or if you intend to become pregnant while using this medicine. Too much use of barbiturates during pregnancy may cause the baby to become dependent on the medicine. This may lead to withdrawal side effects after birth. In addition, use of this medicine during pregnancy may cause bleeding problems in the newborn infant. Also, use of barbiturates during late pregnancy may cause breathing problems in the newborn infant. Barbiturates taken for epilepsy during pregnancy may increase the chance of birth defects.

—if you are breast-feeding an infant. Both pyrilamine and pentobarbital may pass into the breast milk and cause unwanted effects in the infant.

—if you have any of the following medical problems:

Asthma (or history of)	Kidney disease
	Liver disease
Emphysema or chronic lung disease	Overactive thyroid
	Porphyria (or history of)
Enlarged prostate	Stomach ulcer
Glaucoma	Underactive adrenal glands
Heart disease	
High blood pressure	Urinary tract blockage
Hyperactivity in children	
Intestinal blockage	

—if you are now taking any central nervous system (CNS) depressants such as:

Antihistamines or medicine for hay fever, other allergies, or colds	Sedatives, tranquilizers or sleeping medicine
Narcotics	Seizure medicine
Other barbiturates	Tricyclic antidepressants (medicine for depression)
Prescription pain medicine	

—if you are now taking or have taken within the past 2 weeks monoamine oxidase (MAO) inhibitors such as:

Isocarboxazid	Phenelzine
Pargyline	Tranylcypromine

—if you are now taking any of the following medicines or types of medicine:

Anticoagulants (blood thinners)	Cyclophosphamide
	Digitalis
Contraceptives, oral (birth-control pills)	Digitoxin
	Doxycycline
Corticosteroids (cortisone-like medicines)	Estrogens
	Phenytoin
	Quinidine

Proper Use of This Medicine

Pyrilamine and pentobarbital combination is used to treat nausea and vomiting. Use it only as directed by your doctor. Do not use more of it, do not use it more often, and do not use it for a longer period of time than your doctor ordered. If too much is used, it may become habit-forming.

Do not use this medicine to treat nausea and vomiting in children unless otherwise directed by your doctor. If you are giving this medicine to a child, be especially careful not to give more than is prescribed since side effects may be more serious in children.

How to insert suppository: First remove foil wrapper and moisten the suppository with water. Lie down on side and push the suppository well up into the rectum with finger. If the suppository is too soft to insert because of storage in a warm place, before removing the foil wrapper chill the suppository in the refrigerator for 30 minutes or run cold water over it.

Precautions While Using This Medicine

If you will be using this medicine regularly for a long period of time:

• Your doctor should check your progress at regular visits.

• Do not suddenly stop using it. Check with your doctor for the best way to reduce gradually the amount you are using before stopping completely.

This medicine will add to the effects of alcohol and other medicines (CNS depressants) that slow down the nervous system. Some examples of CNS depressants are antihistamines or medicine for hay fever, other allergies, or colds; sedatives, tranquilizers, or sleeping medicine; prescription pain medicine or narcotics; barbiturates; medicine for seizures; tricyclic antidepressants (medicine for depression); or anesthetics, including some dental anesthetics. *Check with your doctor before taking any of the above while you are using this medicine.*

This medicine may cause some people to become dizzy, lightheaded, drowsy, or less alert than they are normally. Even if used at bedtime, it may cause some people to feel drowsy or less alert on arising. *Make sure you know how you react to this medicine before you drive, use machines, or do other jobs that require you to be alert.*

When taking this medicine on a regular basis, make sure your doctor knows if you are taking large amounts of aspirin at the same time (as in arthritis). Effects of too much aspirin, such as ringing in the ears, may be covered up by this medicine.

Side Effects of This Medicine

Along with its needed effects, a medicine may cause some unwanted effects. Although not all of these side effects appear very often, when they do occur they may require medical attention. When this medicine is used for short periods of time at low doses, side effects usually are very rare. However, check with your doctor if any of the following side effects occur:

Rare

Mental confusion or depression	Unusual excitement
Shortness of breath or troubled breathing	Unusual tiredness or weakness
Skin rash or hives	Unusually slow heartbeat
Swelling of eyelids, face, or lips	Wheezing or tightness in chest
Unexplained sore throat and fever	Yellowing of eyes or skin
Unusual bleeding or bruising	

Other side effects may occur which usually do not require medical attention. These side effects may go away during treatment as your body adjusts to the medicine. However, check with your doctor if any of the following side effects continue or are bothersome:

More common

Clumsiness or unsteadiness	"Hangover" effect
Dizziness	Lightheadedness
Drowsiness	Thickening of the bronchial secretions

Less common

Blurred vision	Headache
Diarrhea	Joint or muscle pain
Difficult or painful urination	Slurred speech
Dryness of mouth, nose, and throat	Unusual increase in sweating
	Unusually fast heartbeat

After you stop using this medicine, your body may need time to adjust. The length of time this takes depends on the amount of medicine you were using and how long you used it. During this period of time check with your doctor if you notice any of the following side effects:

Feeling faint	Increased dreaming or nightmares
Hallucinations (seeing, hearing, or feeling things that are not there)	Trembling
	Trouble in sleeping
	Unusual restlessness
	Unusual weakness

Other side effects not listed above may also occur in some patients. If you notice any other effects, check with your doctor.

PYRITHIONE ZINC (Topical)
Some commonly used brand names are Danex, Head and Shoulders, and Zincon.

Pyrithione (peer-i-THYE-one) zinc is used as a shampoo to help control dandruff and seborrheic dermatitis of the scalp. This medicine is available without a prescription; however, your doctor may have special instructions on the proper use of this medicine for your medical condition.

Before Using This Medicine

In order to decide on the best treatment for your medical problem, your doctor should be told:

—if you have ever had any unusual reaction to pyrithione zinc in the past. This medicine should not be used if you are allergic to it.

—if you are pregnant, if you intend to become pregnant, or if you are breast-feeding an infant, although pyrithione zinc has not been shown to cause problems.

Proper Use of This Medicine

Before applying this shampoo, wet the hair and scalp with lukewarm water. Apply enough shampoo to the scalp to work up a lather and rub in well, then rinse. Apply the shampoo again and rinse thoroughly.

Keep this medicine away from the eyes. If you should accidentally get some in your eyes, flush them thoroughly with water.

Side Effects of This Medicine

Along with its needed effects, a medicine may cause some unwanted effects. Although not all of these side effects appear very often, when they do occur they may require medical attention. Check with your doctor if the following side effect occurs:

Irritation of skin

Other side effects not listed above may also occur in some patients. If you notice any other effects, check with your doctor.

PYRVINIUM (Systemic)
Some commonly used brand names are:

Pamovin*	Pyr-Pam*
Povan	Vanquin*

*Not available in the United States.

Pyrvinium (peer-VIN-ee-um) belongs to the group of medicines called anthelmintics. It is used to treat pinworm infections. Pyrvinium is available only with your doctor's prescription.

Before Using This Medicine

In order to decide on the best treatment for your medical problem, your doctor should be told:

—if you have ever had any unusual reaction to pyrvinium in the past. This medicine should not be taken if you are allergic to it.

—if you are pregnant, if you intend to become pregnant, or if you are breast-feeding an infant. Although pyrvinium has not been shown to cause problems, the chance always exists. Therefore, use should be carefully considered.

—if you have any of the following medical problems:

Inflammatory bowel disease	Kidney disease
	Liver disease

Proper Use of This Medicine

Take this medicine exactly as directed by your doctor. Read the instructions on the label and follow them carefully. The amount of medicine you need is based on your weight. You must take the exact amount if it is going to work.

Because pinworm infections may be easily transferred from person to person, all household members may have to be treated at the same time to prevent infection or reinfection. Make sure each family member takes the correct amount, since it may be different for each person.

To help cure the infection and to help prevent reinfection, good health habits to observe at all times are:

• Wash hands and under fingernails with soap and water before eating food or after using toilet facilities.

• Keep fingernails trimmed short.

• Keep hands and fingers away from the mouth.

• Wash or cook all raw fruits and vegetables before eating.

Special health habits that should be observed for 2 to 3 weeks after taking the medicine are:

• Change and wash underclothes, bed linens, towels, and night clothes daily.

• Disinfect toilet facilities daily.

• Vacuum (do not sweep) all floors and upholstered furniture daily.

• Take a shower or stand-up bath daily.

If you have any questions about this, check with your doctor.

Precautions While Using This Medicine

If your symptoms are not relieved in a few days, check with your doctor.

This medicine is a dye that will cause your stools to be red. This color is not harmful and will disappear in a few days. It may also stain teeth and clothing red. Nausea and vomiting may also occur occasionally and the vomit will be red in color.

• If you are taking the tablet form of this medicine, do not chew or crush them. Swallow the tablets whole. They are coated to prevent staining your teeth.

• If you are taking the oral liquid form of this medicine, be careful not to spill it. This medicine will stain any surface onto which it is spilled. Also, drinking it through a straw may help prevent staining of your teeth.

When you take this medicine, avoid too much sun or use of a sunlamp for a few days since you may become more sensitive to sunlight than usual. In case of a severe burn, check with your doctor.

Side Effects of This Medicine

Along with its needed effects, a medicine may cause some unwanted effects. Although not all of these side effects appear very often, when they do occur they may require medical attention. Check with your doctor if the following side effect occurs:

Rare

   Skin rash

Other side effects may occur which usually do not require medical attention. These side effects may go away during treatment as your body adjusts to the medicine. However, check with your doctor if any of the following side effects continue or are bothersome:

Rare

Diarrhea	Stomach cramps
Dizziness	Unusual sensitivity
Nausea and	of skin to
vomiting	sunlight

Other side effects not listed above may also occur in some patients. If you notice any other effects, check with your doctor.

QUINIDINE (Systemic)

Some commonly used brand names are:

Cardioquin	Quinate*
Cin-Quin	Quinidex Extentabs
Duraquin	Quinora
Quinaglute Dura-	
Tabs	

---

*Not available in the United States.

Quinidine (KWIN-i-deen) is most often used to restore irregular heartbeats to a normal rhythm and to slow an overactive heart. This allows the heart to work more efficiently. Do not confuse this medicine with quinine, which is a different medicine. Quinidine is available only with your doctor's prescription.

Before Using This Medicine

In order to decide on the best treatment for your medical problem, your doctor should be told:

—if you have experienced an unusual reaction to quinidine or quinine in the past. This medicine should not be taken if you are allergic to it.

—if you are pregnant, if you intend to become pregnant, or if you are breast-feeding an infant. Although quinidine has not been shown to cause problems, the chance always exists, since this medicine passes into the breast milk.

—if you have been told by another doctor that you have any of the following medical problems:

Asthma or em-	Low blood
physema	potassium
Blood disease	Myasthenia gravis
Kidney disease	Overactive thyroid
Liver disease	Psoriasis

—if you are now taking or have taken within the past 2 weeks any of the following medicines or types of medicine:

Acetazolamide	Other heart
Antacids (when	medicine (espe-
used frequently)	cially digoxin)
Anticoagulants	Phenytoin
(blood thinners)	(seizure medicine)
Barbiturates	Potassium sup-
Neostigmine	plements
	Sodium bicarbonate
	(baking soda)

Proper Use of This Medicine

Take this medicine exactly as directed by your doctor even though you may feel well. Do not miss taking any of the doses and do not take more medicine than ordered.

Take this medicine with a full glass (8 ounces) of water on an empty stomach 1 hour before or 2 hours after meals so that it will be absorbed more quickly. However, to lessen stomach upset, your doctor may want you to take the medicine with food or milk. If you have any questions about how you should be taking this medicine, check with your doctor.

If you miss a dose of this medicine and remember within 2 hours of the missed dose, take it as soon as possible. Then go back to your regular dosing schedule. Do not double doses. If you have any questions about this, check with your doctor.

For patients taking the extended-release tablet form of this medicine:

• Do not break or crush the tablets.

Precautions While Using This Medicine

It is most important that your doctor check your progress at regular visits.

Do not stop taking this medicine without first checking with your doctor, in order to avoid possible worsening of your condition.

Before having any kind of surgery (including dental surgery) or emergency treatment, *tell the doctor or dentist in charge that you are taking this medicine.*

Your doctor may want you to carry a medical identification card or bracelet stating that you are using this medicine.

Some people who are extra-sensitive to this medicine will have side effects after the first dose or first few doses. Check with your doctor right away if the following side effects occur: breathing difficulty, changes in vision, dizziness, fever, headache, ringing in ears, or skin rash.

Side Effects of This Medicine

Along with its needed effects, a medicine may cause some unwanted effects. Although not all of these side effects appear very often, when they do occur they may require medical attention. Check with your doctor if any of the following side effects occur:

Less common

Breathing difficulty	Fever
Dizziness,	Headache
lightheadedness,	Ringing in the ears
or fainting	Skin rash

Rare

Rapid heartbeat	Unusual bleeding
	or bruising

Other side effects may occur which usually do not require medical attention. These side effects may go away during treatment as your body adjusts to the medicine. However, check with your doctor if any of the following side effects continue or are bothersome:

More common

Bitter taste	Loss of appetite
Diarrhea	Nausea or vomiting
Flushing of skin	Stomach pain or
with itching	cramping

Less common

Change in vision	Mental confusion

Rare
Unusual tiredness
or weakness

Other side effects not listed above may also occur in some patients. If you notice any other effects, check with your doctor.

QUININE (Systemic)
Some commonly used brand names are Coco-Quinine, Kinine*, and Quine.

---

*Not available in the United States.

Quinine (KWYE-nine) belongs to the group of medicines called antiprotozoals. It is used in the treatment of malaria. Quinine may also be used for other conditions as determined by your doctor.

Do not confuse this medicine with quinidine, which is a different medicine used for heart problems. This medicine is available without a prescription; however, your doctor may have special instructions on the proper dose of quinine for your medical condition.

Before Using This Medicine

In order to decide on the best treatment for your medical problem, your doctor should be told:

—if you have ever had any unusual reaction to quinine or quinidine.

—if you are pregnant or if you intend to become pregnant while using this medicine. Quinine may cause birth defects if taken during pregnancy. Also, if too much of this medicine is taken during pregnancy, it may cause hearing problems in the baby.

—if you are breast-feeding an infant. Although quinine has not been shown to cause problems, the chance always exists since this medicine passes into the breast milk.

—if you have any of the following medical problems:

Asthma (or history	Hearing problems
of)	Heart disease
Eye disease	Myasthenia gravis
Glucose-6-	
phosphate	
dehydrogenase	
(G6PD) deficiency	

—if you are now taking any of the following medicines or types of medicine:

Acetazolamide	Medicine to make
Antacids containing	the urine less
aluminum	acid
Anticoagulants	Quinidine
(blood thinners)	Sodium bicarbonate
	(baking soda)

Proper Use of This Medicine

Take this medicine only as directed. Do not take more of it, do not take it more often, and do not take it for a longer period of time than recommended on the label, unless otherwise directed by your doctor. To do so may increase the chance of side effects.

Take this medicine with or after meals to lessen possible stomach upset, unless otherwise directed by your doctor. If you are to take this medicine at bedtime, take it with a snack or with a glass of water, milk, or other beverage.

If you are taking this medicine regularly (for example, every day) and you miss a dose, take it right away if you remember within an hour or so of the missed dose. Then go back to your regular dosing schedule. But if you do not remember until later, do not take the missed dose at all and do not double the next one. Instead, go back to your regular dosing schedule. If you have any questions about this, check with your doctor.

If you are taking this medicine for malaria, *keep taking it for the full time of treatment* to help clear up the infection completely, even if you begin to feel better after a few days.

Side Effects of This Medicine

Along with its needed effects, a medicine may cause some unwanted effects. Although not all of these side effects appear very often, when they do occur they may require medical attention. Check with your doctor if any of the following side effects occur:

More common

Blurred vision or any change in vision	Ringing or buzzing in ears or any loss of hearing
Dizziness	Severe headache

Less common

Skin rash, hives, or itching	Wheezing, shortness of breath, or troubled breathing

Rare

Unexplained sore throat and fever	Unusual tiredness or weakness
Unusual bleeding or bruising	

Other side effects may occur which usually do not require medical attention. These side effects may go away during treatment as your body adjusts to the medicine. However, check with your doctor if any of the following side effects continue or are bothersome:

Diarrhea	Stomach cramps or pain
Nausea	Vomiting

Other side effects not listed above may also occur in some patients. If you notice any other effects, check with your doctor.

QUININE AND AMINOPHYLLINE (Systemic)

Some commonly used brand names are Quinamm, Quinite, and Strema.

Quinine (KWYE-nine) and aminophylline (am-in-OFF-i-lin) combination is used to prevent and treat leg cramps, especially those occurring during sleeping hours. This medicine is available only with your doctor's prescription.

Before Using This Medicine

In order to decide on the best treatment for your medical problem, your doctor should be told:

—if you have ever had any unusual reaction to quinidine, quinine, aminophylline, caffeine, dyphylline, oxtriphylline, theobromine, or theophylline.

—if you are pregnant or if you intend to become pregnant while using this medicine. Quinine (in this combination medicine) may cause birth defects if taken during pregnancy. Also, if too much quinine is taken during pregnancy, it may cause hearing problems in the newborn infant. In addition, aminophylline (contained in this combination medicine) may cause unwanted effects in the newborn infant if taken during pregnancy. Although aminophylline has not been shown to cause birth defects, the chance always exists.

—if you are breast-feeding an infant. Theophylline passes into the breast milk and may cause irritability or other side effects in infants of mothers taking aminophylline (contained in this combination medicine). In addition, although quinine (in this combination medicine) has not been shown to cause problems, the chance always exists since this medicine passes into the breast milk.

—if you have any of the following medical problems:

Asthma (or history of)	Heart disease
Eye disease	High blood pressure
Glucose-6-phosphate dehydrogenase deficiency	Kidney disease
	Liver disease
	Myasthenia gravis
	Overactive thyroid
	Stomach ulcer
Hearing problems	(or history of)

—·if you are now taking any of the following medicines or types of medicine:

Acetazolamide	Medicine to make
Aminophylline	the urine less acid
Antacids containing	Propranolol
aluminum	Quinidine
Anticoagulants	Sodium bicarbonate
(blood thinners)	(baking soda)
Dyphylline	Theophylline
Lithium	

Proper Use of This Medicine

Take this medicine only as directed by your doctor. Do not take more of it, do not take it more often, and do not take it for a longer period of time than your doctor ordered.

Take this medicine with food or immediately after meals to lessen possible stomach upset.

Side Effects of This Medicine

Along with its needed effects, a medicine may cause some unwanted effects. Although not all of these side effects appear very often, when they do occur they may require medical attention. Check with your doctor if any of the following side effects occur:

More common

Blurred vision or	Ringing or buzzing
any change in	in ears or
vision	any loss of
Dizziness	hearing
	Severe headache

Less common
   Skin rash

Other side effects may occur which usually do not require medical attention. These side effects may go away during treatment as your body adjusts to the medicine. However, check with your doctor if any of the following side effects continue or are bothersome:

Diarrhea	Restlessness
Nausea	Stomach cramps or
Nervousness	pain
	Vomiting

Other side effects not listed above may also occur in some patients. If you notice any other effects, check with your doctor.

RAUWOLFIA ALKALOIDS (Systemic)

This information applies to the following medicines:
Deserpidine (de-SER-pi-deen)
Rauwolfia Serpentina (rah-WOOL-fee-a ser-pen-TEE-na)
Reserpine (re-SER-peen)

Some commonly used brand names are:	Generic names:
Harmonyl Raunormine*	Deserpidine
Raudixin Raulfia Raupoid Rauserpa	Rauwolfia Serpentina
Rau-Sed Reserpoid Sandril Serpasil	Reserpine

*Not available in the United States.

Rauwolfia alkaloids belong to the general class of medicines called antihypertensives. They are used to treat high blood pressure. They are also sometimes used to treat certain mental and emotional conditions as well as some other problems. These medicines are available only with your doctor's prescription.

Before Using This Medicine

In order to decide on the best treatment for your medical problem, your doctor should be told:

—if you have ever had any unusual reaction to rauwolfia alkaloids.

—if you are pregnant or if you intend to become pregnant while using this medicine. Too much use of rauwolfia alkaloids during pregnancy may cause unwanted effects in the baby. Be sure that you have discussed this with your doctor before taking this medicine. In addition, although rauwolfia alkaloids have not been shown to cause birth defects, the chance always exists.

—if you are breast-feeding an infant. Rauwolfia alkaloids pass into the breast milk and may cause unwanted effects in infants of mothers taking large doses of this medicine. Be sure you have discussed this with your doctor before taking this medicine.

—if you have any of the following medical problems:

Allergies or other breathing problems	Mental depression (or history of)
Asthma	Parkinson's disease
Epilepsy	Pheochromocytoma (PCC)
Gallstones	Stomach ulcer
Heart disease	Ulcerative colitis
Kidney disease	

—if you are now using any of the following medicines or types of medicine:

Digitalis glycosides (heart medicine)	Metoprolol
	Nadolol
Diuretics (water pills) or other antihypertensives (blood pressure medicine)	Nasal decongestants
	Phenylephrine
	Propranolol
	Quinidine
Levodopa	Tricyclic antidepressants (medicine for depression)
Methotrimeprazine	

—if you are now taking central nervous system (CNS) depressants such as:

Antihistamines or medicine for hay fever, other allergies, or colds	Prescription pain medicine
	Sedatives, tranquilizers, or sleeping medicine
Barbiturates	
Narcotics	Seizure medicine

—if you are now taking or have taken within the past 2 weeks monoamine oxidase (MAO) inhibitors such as:

Isocarboxazid	Phenelzine
Pargyline	Tranylcypromine

Proper Use of This Medicine

In order to help remember to take your medicine, try to get into the habit of taking it at the same time each day.

This medicine is sometimes given together with certain other medicines. If you are using a combination of drugs, make sure that you take each medicine at the proper time and do not mix them. Ask your doctor, nurse, or pharmacist to help you plan a way to remember to take your medicines at the right time.

If this medicine upsets your stomach, it may be taken with meals or milk. If stomach upset (nausea, vomiting, stomach cramps or pain) continues or gets worse, check with your doctor.

If you miss a dose of this medicine, do not take the missed dose at all and do not double the next one. Instead, go back to your regular dosing schedule. If you have any questions about this, check with your doctor.

For patients taking this medicine for high blood pressure:

• Importance of Diet—When prescribing medicine for your condition, your doctor may also prescribe a personal diet for you. Such a diet may be low in sodium (salt). Medicine is usually more effective when this diet is properly followed.

Also, it may be very important for you to go on a reducing diet. However, check with your doctor before going on any diet.

• Many patients who have high blood pressure will not notice any signs of the problem. In fact, many may feel normal. It is very important that you take your medicine exactly as directed and that you keep your doctor's appointments even if you feel well.

• Remember that this medicine will not cure your high blood pressure but it does control it. Therefore, you must continue to take it as directed if you expect to keep your blood pressure down. *You may have to take medicine for the rest of your life.* If high blood pressure is not treated, it can cause serious problems such as heart failure, blood vessel disease, stroke, or kidney disease.

Precautions While Using This Medicine

It is important that your doctor check your progress at regular visits.

In some patients, this medicine may cause mental depression. *Tell your doctor right away:*
—if you or anyone else notices unusual changes in your mood.
—if you start having early-morning sleeplessness or unusually vivid dreams or nightmares.

This medicine will add to the effects of alcohol and other medicines (CNS depressants) that slow down the nervous system. Some examples of CNS depressants are antihistamines or medicine for hay fever, other allergies, or colds; sedatives, tranquilizers, or sleeping medicine; prescription pain medicine or narcotics; barbiturates; medicine for seizures; tricyclic antidepressants (medicine for depression); or anesthetics, including some dental anesthetics. *Check with your doctor before taking any of the above while you are using this medicine.*

This medicine may cause some people to become drowsy or less alert than they are normally.

This is more likely to happen when you begin to take it or when you increase the amount of medicine you are taking. *Make sure you know how you react to this medicine before you drive, use machines, or do other jobs that require you to be alert.*

Dizziness, lightheadedness, or fainting may occur, especially when you get up from a lying or sitting position. Getting up slowly may lessen this problem.

Your mouth, nose, and throat may feel very dry while you are taking this medicine. To help relieve mouth dryness, chew sugarless gum or dissolve bits of ice in your mouth.

Before having any kind of surgery (including dental surgery) or emergency treatment, *tell the doctor or dentist in charge that you are taking this medicine.*

This medicine often causes stuffiness in the nose. However, do not use nasal decongestant medicines without first checking with your doctor or pharmacist.

Do not take other medicines unless they have been discussed with your doctor. This especially includes over-the-counter (nonprescription) medicines for appetite control, asthma, colds, cough, hay fever, or sinus, since they may tend to increase your blood pressure.

Side Effects of This Medicine

Along with its needed effects, a medicine may cause some unwanted effects. Although not all of these side effects appear very often, when they do occur they may require medical attention. Check with your doctor *immediately* if any of the following side effects occur:

More common

Drowsiness or faintness	Mental depression or inability
Headache	to concentrate
Impotence or decreased sexual interest	Nervousness or anxiety
Lack of energy or weakness	Vivid dreams or nightmares or early-morning sleeplessness

Less common

Black tarry stools	Stiffness
Bloody vomit	Stomach cramps or pain
Chest pain	
Irregular or slow heartbeat	Trembling and shaking of hands and fingers
Shortness of breath	

Rare

Painful or difficult urination	Unusual bleeding or bruising
Skin rash or itching	

Other side effects may occur which usually do not require medical attention. These side effects may go away during treatment as your body adjusts to the medicine. However, check with your doctor if any of the following side effects continue or are bothersome:

More common

Diarrhea	Dry mouth
Dizziness, especially when getting up from a lying or sitting position	Loss of appetite
	Nausea and vomiting
	Stuffy nose

Less common

Swelling of feet and lower legs

After you stop using this medicine, it may still produce some side effects that need attention. During this period of time check with your doctor *immediately* if you notice any of the following side effects:

Dizziness, drowsiness, or faintness	Mental depression or inability to concentrate
Impotence or decreased sexual interest	Nervousness or anxiety
Irregular or slow heartbeat	Vivid dreams or nightmares or early-morning sleeplessness
Lack of energy or weakness	

Other side effects not listed above may also occur in some patients. If you notice any other effects, check with your doctor.

RAUWOLFIA ALKALOIDS AND THIAZIDE DIURETICS (Systemic)

This information applies to the following medicines:

Deserpidine (de-SER-pi-deen) and Hydrochlorothiazide (hye-droe-klor-oh-THYE-a-zide)

Deserpidine and Methyclothiazide (meth-i-kloe-THYE-a-zide)

Rauwolfia Serpentina (rah-WOOL-fee-a ser-pen-TEE-na) and Bendroflumethiazide (ben-droe-floo-meth-EYE-a-zide)

Reserpine (re-SER-peen) and Benzthiazide (benz-THYE-a-zide)

Reserpine and Chlorothiazide (klor-oh-THYE-a-zide)

Reserpine and Chlorthalidone (klor-THAL-i-done)

Reserpine and Hydrochlorothiazide (hye-droe-klor-oh-THYE-a-zide)

Reserpine and Hydroflumethiazide (hye-droe-floo-meth-EYE-a-zide)

Reserpine and Methyclothiazide (meth-i-kloe-THYE-a-zide)

Reserpine and Polythiazide (pol-i-THYE-a-zide)

Reserpine and Quinethazone (kwin-ETH-a-zone)

Reserpine and Trichlormethiazide (trye-klor-meth-EYE-a-zide)

Some commonly used brand names are:	Generic names:
Oreticyl Oreticyl Forte	Deserpidine and Hydrochloro-thiazide
Enduronyl	Deserpidine and Methyclothiazide
Rauzide	Rauwolfia Serpen-tina and Bendro-flumethiazide
Exna-R	Reserpine and Benzthiazide
Diupres	Reserpine and Chlorothiazide
Demi-Regroton Regroton	Reserpine and Chlorthalidone
Hydropres Reserpazide Serpasil-Esidrix	Reserpine and Hydrochloro-thiazide
Salutensin Salutensin-Demi	Reserpine and Hydroflume-thiazide
Diutensen-R	Reserpine and Methyclothiazide
Renese-R	Reserpine and Polythiazide
Hydromox-R	Reserpine and Quinethazone
Metatensin Naquival	Reserpine and Trichlormethi-azide

Rauwolfia alkaloid and thiazide diuretic combinations are used in the treatment of high blood pressure. They are available only with your doctor's prescription.

Before Using This Medicine

In order to decide on the best treatment for your medical problem, your doctor should be told:

—if you are allergic to sulfonamides (sulfa drugs), thiazide diuretics (water pills), or rauwolfia alkaloids.

—if you are pregnant or if you intend to become pregnant while using this medicine. Too much use of it during pregnancy may cause unwanted effects in the baby. Be sure that you have discussed this with your doctor before taking this medicine. In addition, although this medicine has not been shown to cause birth defects, the chance always exists.

—if you are breast-feeding an infant. This medicine passes into the breast milk and may cause unwanted effects in infants of mothers taking large doses of it. Be sure you have discussed this with your doctor before taking this medicine.

—if you have any of the following medical problems:

Allergies or other breathing problems	Kidney disease Liver disease Mental depression (or history of)
Asthma	
Diabetes	
Epilepsy	Pancreas disease
Gallstones	Parkinson's disease
Gout	Pheochromocytoma (PCC)
Heart disease	Stomach ulcer
History of lupus erythematosus	Ulcerative colitis

—if you are now taking any of the following medicines or types of medicine:

Anticoagulants (blood thinners)	Gout medicine Levodopa
Colestipol	Lithium
Corticosteroids (cortisone-like medicines)	Methenamine Methotrimeprazine Nasal decongestants
Corticotropin (ACTH)	Phenylephrine Quinidine
Diabetes medicine	Tricyclic an-
Digitalis glycosides (heart medicine)	tidepressants (medicine for
Diuretics (water pills) or other antihypertensives (high blood pressure medicine)	depression)

—if you are now taking central nervous system (CNS) depressants such as:

Antihistamines or medicine for hay fever, other allergies, or colds	Prescription pain medicine Sedatives, tran-quilizers, or sleeping
Barbiturates	medicine
Narcotics	Seizure medicine

—if you are now taking or have taken within the past 2 weeks monoamine oxidase (MAO) inhibitors such as:

Isocarboxazid	Phenelzine
Pargyline	Tranylcypromine

Proper Use of This Medicine

Importance of Diet—When prescribing medicine for your condition, your doctor may also prescribe a personal diet for you. Such a diet may be low in sodium (salt). Medicine is usually more effective when this diet is properly followed.

Also, it may be very important for you to go on a reducing diet. However, check with your doctor before going on any diet.

Many patients who have high blood pressure will not notice any signs of the problem. In fact, many may feel normal. It is very important that you take your medicine exactly as directed and that you keep your doctor's appointments even if you feel well.

Remember that this medicine will not cure your high blood pressure but it does control it. Therefore, you must continue to take it as directed if you expect to keep your blood pressure down. *You may have to take medicine for the rest of your life.* If high blood pressure is not treated, it can cause serious problems such as heart failure, blood vessel disease, stroke, or kidney disease.

This medicine may cause you to have an unusual feeling of tiredness when you begin to take it. You may also notice an increase in the amount of urine or in your frequency of urination. After you have taken the medicine for a while, these effects should lessen. In general, in order to keep the increase in urine from affecting your sleep:

• If you are to take a single dose a day, take it in the morning after breakfast.

• If you are to take more than one dose a day, take the last dose no later than 6 p.m., unless otherwise directed by your doctor.

• However, it is best to plan your dose or doses according to a schedule that will least affect your personal activities and sleep. Ask your doctor, nurse, or pharmacist to help you plan the best time to take this medicine.

In order to help remember to take your medicine, try to get into the habit of taking it at the same time each day.

If this medicine upsets your stomach, it may be taken with meals or milk. If stomach upset (nausea, vomiting, stomach pain or cramps) continues, check with your doctor.

If you miss a dose of this medicine, take it as soon as possible. If it is almost time for your next dose, do not take the missed dose at all and do not double the next one. Instead, go back to your regular dosing schedule. If you have any questions about this, check with your doctor.

Precautions While Using This Medicine

It is important that your doctor check your progress at regular visits.

This medicine may cause a loss of potassium from your body.

• To help prevent this, your doctor may want you to:

—eat or drink foods that have a high potassium content (for example, orange or other citrus fruit juices), or

—take a potassium supplement, or

—take another medicine to help prevent the loss of the potassium in the first place.

• It is very important to follow these directions. Also, it is important not to change your diet on your own. This is more important if you are already on a special diet (as for diabetes), or if you are taking a potassium supplement or a medicine to reduce potassium loss. Extra potassium may not be necessary and, in some cases, too much potassium could be harmful.

Check with your doctor if you become sick and have severe or continuing vomiting or diarrhea. These problems may cause you to lose additional water and potassium.

Caution: Diabetics—This medicine may raise blood sugar levels. While you are using this medicine, be especially careful in testing for sugar in your urine. If you have any questions about this, check with your doctor.

A few people who take this medicine may become more sensitive to sunlight than they are normally. When you begin to take this medicine, avoid too much sun or use of a sunlamp until you see how you react, especially if you tend to burn easily. If you have a severe reaction, check with your doctor.

This medicine may cause some people to become drowsy or less alert than they are normally. This is more likely to happen when you begin to take it or when you increase the amount of medicine you are taking. *Make sure you know how you react to this medicine before you drive, use machines, or do other jobs that require you to be alert.*

Dizziness, lightheadedness, or fainting may occur, especially when you get up from a lying or sitting position. Getting up slowly may help but if the problem continues or gets worse, check with your doctor.

In some patients, this medicine may cause mental depression. *Tell your doctor right away:*

—if you or anyone else notices unusual changes in your moods.

—if you start having early-morning sleeplessness or unusually vivid dreams or nightmares.

This medicine will add to the effects of alcohol and other medicines (CNS depressants) that slow down the nervous system. Some examples of CNS depressants are antihistamines or medicine for hay fever, other allergies, or colds; sedatives, tranquilizers, or sleeping medicine; prescription pain medicine or narcotics; barbiturates; medicine for seizures; tricyclic antidepressants (medicine for depression); or anesthetics, including dental anesthetics. *Check with your doctor before taking any of the above while you are taking this medicine.*

Before having any kind of surgery (including dental surgery), or emergency treatment, *make sure the doctor or dentist in charge knows that you are taking this medicine.*

This medicine often causes stuffiness in the nose. However, do not use nasal decongestant medicines without first checking with your doctor or pharmacist.

Do not take other medicines unless they have been discussed with your doctor. This especially includes over-the-counter (nonprescription) medicines for appetite control, asthma, colds, cough, hay fever, or sinus, since they may tend to increase your blood pressure.

Your mouth, nose, and throat may feel very dry while you are taking this medicine. To help relieve mouth dryness, chew sugarless gum or dissolve bits of ice in your mouth.

Side Effects of This Medicine

Along with its needed effects, a medicine may cause some unwanted effects. Although not all of these side effects appear very often, when they do occur they may require medical attention. Check with your doctor *immediately* if any of the following side effects occur, *especially since some of them may mean that your body is losing too much potassium:*

Signs of too much potassium loss

Dryness of mouth   Muscle cramps or
Increased thirst   pain
                                      Nausea or vomiting

More common

Drowsiness or faint-   Mental depression
  ness   or inability to
Headache   concentrate
Impotence or   Nervousness or anx-
  decreased   iety
  sexual interest   Vivid dreams or
Lack of energy or   nightmares or
  weakness   early-morning
                                      sleeplessness

Less common

Black tarry stools   Shortness of breath
Bloody vomit   Stiffness
Chest pain   Trembling and
Irregular or slow   shaking of hands
  heartbeat   and fingers

Rare

Painful or difficult   Unexplained sore
  urination   throat and fever
Severe stomach pain   Unusual bleeding or
  with nausea and   bruising
  vomiting   Yellowing of eyes or
Skin rash or itching   skin

Other side effects may occur which usually do not require medical attention. These side effects may go away during treatment as your body adjusts to the medicine. However, check with your doctor if any of the following side effects continue or are bothersome:

More common

Diarrhea   Loss of appetite
Dizziness, especially   Stuffy nose
  when getting up
  from a lying or
  sitting posi-
  tion

After you stop using this medicine, it may still produce some side effects that need attention. During this period of time check with your doctor *immediately* if you notice any of the following side effects:

Dizziness, drowsiness, or faintness

Impotence or decreased sexual interest

Irregular or slow heartbeat

Lack of energy or weakness

Mental depression or inability to concentrate

Nervousness or anxiety

Vivid dreams or nightmares or early-morning sleeplessness

Other side effects not listed above may also occur in some patients. If you notice any other effects, check with your doctor.

RESERPINE AND HYDRALAZINE (Systemic)

A commonly used brand name is Serpasil-Apresoline.

The reserpine (re-SER-peen) and hydralazine (hye-DRAL-a-zeen) combination is used in the treatment of high blood pressure. It is available only with your doctor's prescription.

Before Using This Medicine

In order to decide on the best treatment for your medical problem, your doctor should be told:

—if you have ever had any unusual reaction to rauwolfia alkaloids or hydralazine in the past. This medicine should not be taken if you are allergic to it.

—if you are pregnant or if you intend to become pregnant while using this medicine. Too much use of it during pregnancy may cause unwanted effects in the baby. Be sure that you have discussed this with your doctor before taking this medicine. In addition, although this medicine has not been shown to cause birth defects in humans, the chance always exists.

—if you are breast-feeding an infant. This medicine passes into the breast milk and may cause unwanted effects in infants of mothers taking large doses of it. Be sure you have discussed this with your doctor before taking this medicine.

—if you have recently had a stroke.

—if you have any of the following medical problems:

Allergies or other breathing problems

Asthma

Epilepsy

Gallstones

Heart disease

Kidney disease

Mental depression (or history of)

Parkinson's disease

Pheochromocytoma (PCC)

Stomach ulcer

Ulcerative colitis

—if you are now taking any of the following medicines or types of medicine:

Digitalis glycosides (heart medicine)

Diuretics (water pills) or other antihypertensives (high blood pressure medicine)

Levodopa

Methotrimeprazine

Metoprolol

Nadolol

Nasal decongestants

Phenylephrine

Propranolol

Quinidine

Tricyclic antidepressants (medicine for depression)

—if you are now taking central nervous system (CNS) depressants such as:

Antihistamines or medicine for hay fever, other allergies, or colds

Barbiturates

Narcotics

Prescription pain medicine

Sedatives, tranquilizers, or sleeping medicine

Seizure medicine

—if you are now taking or have taken within the past 2 weeks monoamine oxidase (MAO) inhibitors such as:

Isocarboxazid

Pargyline

Phenelzine

Tranylcypromine

Proper Use of This Medicine

Importance of Diet—In addition to prescribing medicine for your condition, your doctor may also prescribe a personal diet for you. Such a diet may be low in sodium (salt). Medicine is usually more effective when this diet is properly followed.

Also, it may be very important for you to go on a reducing diet. However, check with your doctor before going on any diet.

Many people who have high blood pressure will not notice any signs of the problem. In fact, many may feel normal. It is very important that you take your medicine exactly as directed and that you keep your doctor's appointments even if you feel well.

Remember that this medicine will not cure your high blood pressure but it does control it. Therefore, you must continue to take it as directed if you expect to keep your blood pressure down. *You may have to take medicine for the rest of your life.* If high blood pressure is not treated, it can cause serious problems such as heart failure, blood vessel disease, stroke, or kidney disease.

In order to help remember to take your medicine, try to get into the habit of taking it at the same time each day.

If this medicine upsets your stomach, it may be taken with meals or milk. If stomach upset (nausea, vomiting, stomach pain, or cramps) continues, check with your doctor.

If you miss a dose of this medicine, take it as soon as possible. If it is almost time for your next dose, do not take the missed dose at all and do not double the next one. Instead, go back to your regular dosing schedule. If you have any questions about this, check with your doctor.

Precautions While Using This Medicine

It is important that your doctor check your progress at regular visits.

This medicine may cause some people to have headaches or to feel dizzy or drowsy. *Make sure you know how you react to this medicine before you drive, use machines, or do other jobs that require you to be alert.*

Dizziness, lightheadedness, or fainting may occur, especially when you get up from a lying or sitting position. Getting up slowly may help but if the problem continues or gets worse, check with your doctor.

The dizziness, lightheadedness, or fainting is also more likely to occur if you drink alcohol, stand for long periods of time, exercise, or if the weather is hot. *While you are taking this medicine, be careful in the amount of alcohol you drink. Also, use extra care during exercise or hot weather or if you must stand for long periods of time.* Check with your doctor if you have any questions about this.

In some patients, this medicine may cause mental depression. *Tell your doctor right away:*
—if you or anyone else notices unusual changes in your moods.
—if you start having early-morning sleeplessness or unusually vivid dreams or nightmares.

This medicine will add to the effects of alcohol and other medicines (CNS depressants) that slow down the nervous system. Some examples of CNS depressants are antihistamines or medicine for hay fever, other allergies, or cold; sedatives, tranquilizers, or sleeping medicine; prescription pain medicine or narcotics; barbiturates; medicine for seizures; tricyclic antidepressants (medicine for depression); or anesthetics, including dental anesthetics. *Check with your doctor before taking any of the above while you are taking this medicine.*

Before having any kind of surgery (including dental surgery), or emergency treatment, *make sure the doctor or dentist in charge knows that you are taking this medicine.*

This medicine often causes stuffiness in the nose. However, do not use nasal decongestant medicines without first checking with your doctor or pharmacist.

Do not take other medicines unless they have been discussed with your doctor. This especially includes over-the-counter (nonprescription) medicine for appetite control, asthma, colds, cough, hay fever, or sinus, since they may tend to increase your blood pressure.

Your mouth, nose, and throat may feel very dry while you are taking this medicine. To help relieve mouth dryness, chew sugarless gum or dissolve bits of ice in your mouth.

Side Effects of This Medicine

Along with its needed effects, a medicine may cause some unwanted effects. Although not all of these side effects appear very often, when they do occur they may require medical attention. Check with your doctor if any of the following side effects occur:

More common

Drowsiness or faintness	Mental depression or inability to concentrate
General feeling of body discomfort or weakness	Nervousness or anxiety
Headache	Vivid dreams or nightmares or early-morning sleeplessness
Impotence or decreased sexual interest	

Less common

Black tarry stools	Stiffness
Bloody vomit	Swelling of feet or lower legs
Chest pain	Swelling of the lymph glands
Irregular heartbeat	
Joint pain	
Numbness, tingling, pain, or weakness in hands or feet	Trembling and shaking of hands and fingers
Shortness of breath	Unexplained fever and sore throat
Skin rash or itching	

Rare

Painful or difficult urination	Unusual bleeding or bruising
Severe stomach pain with nausea and vomiting	Yellowing of eyes or skin

Other side effects may occur which usually do not require medical attention. These side effects may go away during treatment as your body adjusts to the medicine. However, check with your doctor if any of the following side effects continue or are bothersome:

More common

Diarrhea	Dry mouth
Dizziness, especially when getting up from a lying or sitting position	Loss of appetite Nausea or vomiting Stuffy nose

Less common

Constipation	Red, sore eyes
Flushing or redness of skin	

After you stop using this medicine, it may still produce some side effects that need attention. During this period of time check with your doctor if you notice any of the following side effects:

Dizziness, drowsiness, or faintness	Mental depression or inability to concentrate
General feeling of body discomfort or weakness	Nervousness or anxiety
Impotence or decreased sexual interest	Vivid dreams or nightmares or early-morning sleeplessness
Irregular or slow heartbeat	

Other side effects not listed above may also occur in some patients. If you notice any other effects, check with your doctor.

RESERPINE, HYDRALAZINE, AND HYDROCHLOROTHIAZIDE (Systemic)

Some commonly used brand names are Ser-Ap-Es and Tri-Hydroserpine.

Reserpine (re-SER-peen), hydralazine (hye-DRAL-a-zeen), and hydrochlorothiazide (hye-droe-klor-oh-THYE-a-zide) combinations are used in the treatment of high blood pressure. They are available only with your doctor's prescription.

Before Using This Medicine

In order to decide on the best treatment for your medical problem, your doctor should be told:

—if you are allergic to sulfonamides (sulfa drugs), thiazide diuretics (water pills), or rauwolfia alkaloids.

—if you are pregnant or if you intend to become pregnant while using this medicine. Too much use of it during pregnancy may cause unwanted effects in the baby. Be sure that you have discussed this with your doctor before taking this medicine. In addition, although this medicine has not been shown to cause birth defects in humans, the chance always exists.

—if you are breast-feeding an infant. This medicine passes into the breast milk and may cause unwanted effects in infants of mothers taking large doses of it. Be sure you have discussed this with your doctor before taking this medicine.

—if you have any of the following medical problems:

Allergies or other breathing problems	Kidney disease Liver disease Mental depression (or history of)
Asthma	Pancreas disease
Diabetes	Parkinson's disease
Epilepsy	Pheochromocytoma
Gallstones	(PCC)
Gout	Stomach ulcer
Heart disease	Ulcerative colitis
History of lupus erythematosus	

—if you are now taking any of the following medicines or types of medicine:

Anticoagulants (blood thinners)	Gout medicine Levodopa
Colestipol	Lithium
Corticosteroids (cortisone-like medicines)	Methenamine Methotrimeprazine Nasal decongestants
Corticotropin (ACTH)	Phenylephrine Quinidine
Diabetes medicine	Tricyclic antidepressants
Digitalis glycosides (heart medicine)	(medicine for depression)
Diuretics (water pills) or other antihypertensives (high blood pressure medicine)	

—if you are now taking central nervous system (CNS) depressants such as:

Antihistamines or medicine for hay fever, other allergies, or colds	Prescription pain medicine Sedatives, tranquilizers, or sleeping medicine
Barbiturates	
Narcotics	Seizure medicine

—if you are now taking or have taken within the past 2 weeks monoamine oxidase (MAO) inhibitors such as:

Isocarboxazid   Phenelzine
Pargyline   Tranylcypromine

Proper Use of This Medicine

Importance of Diet—When prescribing medicine for your condition, your doctor may also prescribe a personal diet for you. Such a diet may be low in sodium (salt). Medicine is usually more effective when a schedule of diet and exercise is properly followed.

Also, it may be very important for you to go on a reducing diet. However, check with your doctor before going on any diet.

Many patients who have high blood pressure will not notice any signs of the problem. In fact, many may feel normal. It is very important that you take your medicine exactly as directed and that you keep your doctor's appointments even if you feel well.

Remember that this medicine will not cure your high blood pressure but it does control it. Therefore, you must continue to take it as directed if you expect to keep your blood pressure down. *You may have to take medicine for the rest of your life.* If high blood pressure is not treated, it can cause serious problems such as heart failure, blood vessel disease, stroke, or kidney disease.

This medicine may cause you to have an unusual feeling of tiredness when you begin to take it. You may also notice an increase in the amount of urine or in your frequency of urination. After you have taken the medicine for a while, these effects should lessen. In general, in order to keep the increase in urine from affecting your sleep:

• If you are to take a single dose a day, take it in the morning after breakfast.

• If you are to take more than one dose a day, take the last dose no later than 6 p.m., unless otherwise directed by your doctor.

• However, it is best to plan your dose or doses according to a schedule that will least affect your personal activities and sleep. Ask your doctor, nurse, or pharmacist to help you plan the best time to take this medicine.

In order to help remember to take your medicine, try to get into the habit of taking it at the same time each day.

If this medicine upsets your stomach, it may be taken with meals or milk. If stomach upset (nausea, vomiting, stomach pain or cramps) continues, check with your doctor.

If you miss a dose of this medicine, take it as soon as possible. If it is almost time for your next dose, do not take the missed dose at all and do not double the next one. Instead, go back to your regular dosing schedule. If you have any questions about this, check with your doctor.

Precautions While Using This Medicine

It is important that your doctor check your progress at regular visits.

This medicine may cause some people to have headaches or to feel dizzy or drowsy. *Make sure you know how you react to this medicine before you drive, use machines, or do other jobs that require you to be alert.*

Dizziness, lightheadedness, or fainting may occur, especially when you get up from a lying or sitting position. Getting up slowly may help but if the problem continues or gets worse, check with your doctor.

In some patients, this medicine may cause mental depression. *Tell your doctor right away:*

—if you or anyone else notices unusual changes in your moods.

—if you start having early-morning sleeplessness or unusually vivid dreams or nightmares.

This medicine will add to the effects of alcohol and other medicines (CNS depressants) that slow down the nervous system. Some examples of CNS depressants are antihistamines or medicine for hay fever, other allergies, or colds; sedatives, tranquilizers, or sleeping medicine; prescription pain medicine or narcotics; barbiturates; medicine for seizures; tricyclic antidepressants (medicine for depression); or anesthetics, including dental anesthetics. *Check with your doctor before taking any of the above while you are taking this medicine.*

This medicine may cause a loss of potassium from your body.
• To help prevent this, your doctor may want you to:

—eat or drink foods that have a high potassium content (for example, orange or other citrus fruit juices), or

—take a potassium supplement, or

—take another medicine to help prevent the loss of the potassium in the first place.

• It is very important to follow these directions. Also, it is important not to change your diet on your own. This is more important if you are already on a special diet (as for diabetes), or if you are taking a potassium supplement or a medicine to reduce potassium loss. Extra potassium may not be necessary and, in some cases, too much potassium could be harmful.

Caution: Diabetics—This medicine may raise blood sugar levels. While you are using this medicine, be especially careful in testing for sugar in your urine. If you have any questions about this, check with your doctor.

A few people who take this medicine may become more sensitive to sunlight than they are normally. When you begin to take this medicine, avoid too much sun or use of a sunlamp until you see how you react, especially if you tend to burn easily. If you have a severe reaction, check with your doctor.

Before having any kind of surgery (including dental surgery), or emergency treatment, *make sure the doctor or dentist in charge knows that you are taking this medicine.*

This medicine often causes stuffiness in the nose. However, do not use nasal decongestant medicines without first checking with your doctor or pharmacist.

Do not take other medicines unless they have been discussed with your doctor. This especially includes over-the-counter (nonprescription) medicines for appetite control, asthma, colds, cough, hay fever, or sinus, since they may tend to increase your blood pressure.

Your mouth, nose, and throat may feel very dry while you are taking this medicine. To help relieve mouth dryness, chew sugarless gum or dissolve bits of ice in your mouth.

Side Effects of This Medicine

Along with its needed effects, a medicine may cause some unwanted effects. Although not all of these side effects appear very often, when they do occur they may require medical attention. Check with your doctor if any of the following side effects occur:

More common

Drowsiness or faintness	Headache
General feeling of body discomfort or weakness	Impotence or decreased sexual interest

Mental depression or inability to concentrate	Vivid dreams or nightmares or early-morning sleeplessness
Nervousness or anxiety	

Less common

Black tarry stools	Skin rash or itching
Bloody vomit	Stiffness
Chest pain	Swelling of the lymph glands
Irregular heartbeat	
Joint pain	Trembling and shaking of hands and fingers
Numbness, tingling, pain, or weakness in hands or feet	
	Unexplained fever and sore throat
Shortness of breath	

Rare

Painful or difficult urination	Unusual bleeding or bruising
Severe stomach pain with nausea and vomiting	Yellowing of eyes or skin

Other side effects may occur which usually do not require medical attention. These side effects may go away during treatment as your body adjusts to the medicine. However, check with your doctor if any of the following side effects continue or are bothersome:

More common

Diarrhea	Dry mouth
Dizziness, especially when getting up from a lying or sitting position	Loss of appetite
	Nausea or vomiting
	Stuffy nose

Less common

Constipation	Red, sore eyes
Flushing or redness of skin	

After you stop using this medicine, it may still produce some side effects that need attention. During this period of time check with your doctor if you notice any of the following side effects:

Dizziness, drowsiness, or faintness	Irregular heartbeat
	Mental depression or inability to concentrate
General feeling of body discomfort or weakness	Nervousness or anxiety
Impotence or decreased sexual interest	Vivid dreams or nightmares or early-morning sleeplessness

Other side effects not listed above may also occur in some patients. If you notice any other effects, check with your doctor.

RESORCINOL (Topical)

Resorcinol (re-SOR-si-nole) is applied to the skin to treat acne, seborrhea, and other skin disorders. This medicine is available only with your doctor's prescription.

Before Using This Medicine

In order to decide on the best treatment for your medical problem, your doctor should be told:

—if you have ever had any unusual reaction to resorcinol in the past. This medicine should not be used if you are allergic to it.

—if you are pregnant, if you intend to become pregnant, or if you are breast-feeding an infant, although resorcinol has not been shown to cause problems.

—if you are now using any topical acne preparation or preparation containing a peeling agent such as benzoyl peroxide, salicylic acid, sulfur, or tretinoin.

Proper Use of This Medicine

It is very important that you use this medicine only as directed. Do not use more of it, do not use it more often, and do not use it for a longer period of time than your doctor ordered. To do so may increase the chance of absorption through the skin and the chance of resorcinol poisoning.

Apply enough resorcinol to cover the affected areas, and rub in gently.

Immediately after using this medicine, wash your hands to remove any medicine that may be on them.

Keep this medicine away from the eyes. If you should accidentally get some in your eyes, flush them thoroughly with water.

If you miss a dose of this medicine, apply it as soon as possible. Then go back to your regular dosing schedule. But if it is almost time for your next dose, do not apply the missed dose at all. Instead, go back to your regular dosing schedule. If you have any questions about this, check with your doctor or pharmacist.

Precautions While Using This Medicine

This medicine may darken light-colored hair.

Side Effects of This Medicine

Along with its needed effects, a medicine may cause some unwanted effects. Although not all of these side effects appear very often, when they do occur they may require medical attention. Check with your doctor if any of the following side effects occur:

Irritation of skin not present before using this medicine

Possible signs of resorcinol poisoning

Diarrhea, nausea, stomach pain, or vomiting	Unusual drowsiness Unusual sweating Unusual tiredness
Dizziness	or weakness
Nervousness or restlessness	Unusually slow heartbeat, short-
Severe or con- tinuing headache	ness of breath, or troubled breathing

After you use this medicine for a few days, some redness and peeling of the skin may be expected.

Other side effects not listed above may also occur in some patients. If you notice any other effects, check with your doctor.

RESORCINOL AND SULFUR (Topical)

Some commonly used brand names are:

Acne-Dome	Exzit
Acnomel	pHisoAc
Cenac	Sulforcin

Resorcinol and sulfur (re-SOR-si-nole and SUL-fur) combination is applied to the skin to treat acne and similar skin conditions. This medicine is available without a prescription; however, your doctor may have special instructions on the proper use of this medicine for your medical condition.

Before Using This Medicine

In order to decide on the best treatment for your medical problem, your doctor should be told:

—if you have ever had any unusual reaction to resorcinol or sulfur in the past. This medicine should not be used if you are allergic to it.

—if you are pregnant, if you intend to become pregnant, or if you are breast-feeding an infant, although resorcinol and sulfur combination has not been shown to cause problems.

—if you are now using any topical acne preparation or preparation containing a peeling agent such as benzoyl peroxide, salicylic acid, or tretinoin.

—if you are now using any topical preparation containing mercury, such as ammoniated mercury ointment.

Proper Use of This Medicine

Use this medicine only as directed. Do not use more of it and do not use it more often than recommended on the label, unless otherwise directed by your doctor.

Before using this medicine, wash the affected areas thoroughly and gently pat dry. Then apply a small amount to the affected areas and spread on gently, but do not rub in.

Immediately after using this medicine, wash your hands to remove any medicine that may be on them.

Keep this medicine away from the eyes. If you should accidentally get some in your eyes, flush them thoroughly with water.

If you miss a dose of this medicine, apply it as soon as possible. Then go back to your regular dosing schedule. But if it is almost time for your next dose, do not apply the missed dose at all. Instead, go back to your regular dosing schedule. If you have any questions about this, check with your doctor or pharmacist.

Precautions While Using This Medicine

Do not use any topical acne preparation or preparation containing a peeling agent (for example, benzoyl peroxide, salicylic acid, or tretinoin) *on the same affected area as this medicine,* unless otherwise directed by your doctor. To do so may cause severe irritation of the skin.

Do not use any topical mercury-containing preparation such as ammoniated mercury ointment on the same affected area as this medicine. To do so may cause a foul odor, be irritating to the skin, and stain the skin black. If you have any questions about this, check with your doctor or pharmacist.

This medicine (depending on the product you are using) may darken light-colored hair. If you have any questions about this, check with your doctor or pharmacist.

Side Effects of This Medicine

Along with its needed effects, a medicine may cause some unwanted effects. Although not all of these side effects appear very often, when

they do occur they may require medical attention. Check with your doctor or pharmacist if the following side effect occurs:

Irritation of skin not present
before using this medicine

Other side effects may occur which usually do not require medical attention. However, check with your doctor or pharmacist if the following side effect continues or is bothersome:

Unusual dryness of skin

After you use this medicine for a few days, some redness and peeling of the skin may be expected.

Other side effects not listed above may also occur in some patients. If you notice any other effects, check with your doctor or pharmacist.

RIFAMPIN (Systemic)
Some commonly used brand names are:
Rifadin Rofact*
Rimactane

*Not available in the United States.

Rifampin (RIF-am-pin) belongs to the general family of medicines called antibiotics. It is given by mouth in combination with one or more other medicines to help the body overcome tuberculosis (TB). Rifampin is also given alone in patients who may carry meningitis bacteria (without feeling sick) and may spread them to others. Rifampin is available only with your doctor's prescription.

Before Using This Medicine

In order to decide on the best treatment for your medical problem, your doctor should be told:

—if you have ever had any unusual reaction to rifampin. This medicine should not be taken if you are allergic to it.

—if you are pregnant, if you intend to become pregnant, or if you are breast-feeding an infant, although rifampin has not been shown to cause problems in humans.

—if you have either of the following medical problems:
Alcoholism
Liver disease

—if you are taking any of the following medicines or types of medicine:

Aminosalicylates	Oral anticoagulants
Cortisone-like medicines	(blood thinners you take by mouth)
Dapsone	Oral contraceptives
Digitoxin (heart medicine)	(birth control pills)
Isoniazid	Probenecid
Methadone	Tolbutamide (diabetes medicine you take by mouth)

Proper Use of This Medicine

Rifampin is best taken with a full glass (8 ounces) of water on an empty stomach (either 1 hour before or 2 hours after a meal). However, if this medicine upsets your stomach, your doctor may want you to take it with food.

If you are giving this medicine to a child:
• Contents of the capsules may be mixed with applesauce or jelly. Be sure that the child takes all the food in order to get the full dose of medicine.

To help clear up your tuberculosis (TB) completely, *it is very important that you keep taking this medicine for the full time of treatment* even if you begin to feel better after a few weeks. You may have to take it every day for as long as 1 to 2 years or more. *It is important that you do not miss any doses.*

If you do miss a dose of this medicine, take it as soon as possible. However, if it is almost time for your next dose, do not take the missed dose or double your next dose. Instead, go back to your regular dosing schedule. *If this medicine is taken on an irregular schedule, side effects may occur more often and may be more serious than usual.* If you have any questions about this, check with your doctor or pharmacist.

Precautions While Using This Medicine

Do not take rifampin within 6 hours of the time you take aminosalicylates (another TB medicine) since they may keep rifampin from working as well.

This medicine will cause the urine, stool, saliva, sweat, and tears to turn reddish orange to reddish brown. This is to be expected while you are taking this medicine. Since this effect may cause soft contact lenses to become permanently discolored and standard cleaning solutions

may not take out all the discoloration, *it is best not to wear soft contact lenses while taking this medicine.* Hard contact lenses are not discolored by this medicine. If you have any questions about this, check with your doctor.

Oral contraceptives (birth control pills) may not work as well if you take them while you are taking rifampin. Unplanned pregnancies may occur. You should use a different means of birth control while you are taking rifampin. If you have any questions about this, check with your doctor or pharmacist.

If your symptoms do not improve within 2 to 3 weeks or if they become worse, check with your doctor.

It is very important that your doctor check your progress at regular visits.

If this medicine causes you to feel very tired or very weak or causes a loss of appetite, nausea, or vomiting, stop taking it and check with your doctor immediately. These may be early warning signs of more serious problems that could develop later.

Liver problems may be more likely to occur if you drink alcoholic beverages regularly while you are taking this medicine. Also, the regular use of alcohol may keep this medicine from working as well. Therefore, *you should not drink alcoholic beverages while you are taking this medicine.*

Side Effects of This Medicine

Along with its needed effects, a medicine may cause some unwanted effects. Although not all of these side effects appear very often, when they do occur they may require medical attention. Stop taking this medicine and check with your doctor *immediately* if any of the following side effects occur:

Less common

Chills	Muscle and bone
Difficult breathing	pain
Dizziness	Shivering
Headache	Unexplained fever

Rare

Greatly decreased frequency of urination or amount of urine	Unusual bruising or bleeding
	Unusual tiredness or weakness
Loss of appetite	Vomiting
Nausea	Yellowing of eyes or
Unexplained sore throat	skin

Other side effects may occur which usually do not require medical attention. These side effects may go away during treatment as your body adjusts to the medicine. However, check with your doctor if any of the following side effects continue or are bothersome:

More common

| Diarrhea | Stomach cramps |
| Reddish orange to reddish brown discoloration of urine, stools, saliva, sputum, sweat, and tears | |

Less common

| Itching | Redness |
| Rash | Sore mouth or tongue |

Other side effects not listed above may also occur in some patients. If you notice any other effects, check with your doctor.

RIFAMPIN AND ISONIAZID (Systemic)
A commonly used brand name is Rifamate.

Rifampin (RIF-am-pin) and isoniazid (eye-soe-NYE-a-zid) is a combination antibiotic and anti-infective medicine. It is given by mouth to help the body overcome tuberculosis (TB). It may be given alone or with one or more other medicines for TB. Rifampin and isoniazid is available only with your doctor's prescription.

Before Using This Medicine

In order to decide on the best treatment for your medical problem, your doctor should be told:

—if you have had allergic reactions to ethionamide, pyrazinamide, niacin (nicotinic acid), rifampin, or isoniazid.

—if you are pregnant, if you intend to become pregnant, or if you are breast-feeding an infant, although rifampin and isoniazid has not been shown to cause problems in humans.

—if you have any of the following medical problems:

| Alcoholism | Liver disease |
| Convulsive disorders such as seizures or epilepsy | Severe kidney disease |

—if you are now taking any of the following medicines or types of medicine:

Aluminum- and magnesium-containing antacids	Methadone
Aminosalicylates	Oral anticoagulants (blood thinners you take by mouth)
Cortisone-like medicines	Oral contraceptives (birth control pills)
Cycloserine	Phenytoin
Dapsone	Probenecid
Digitoxin (heart medicine)	Tolbutamide (diabetes medicine you take by mouth)
Disulfiram	

—if you have had any problems with rifampin or isoniazid in the past.

Proper Use of This Medicine

Rifampin and isoniazid is best taken with a full glass (8 ounces) of water on an empty stomach (either 1 hour before or 2 hours after a meal). However, if this medicine upsets your stomach, your doctor may want you to take it with food.

Antacids may also help; but do not take aluminum- or magnesium-containing antacids within 1 hour of the time you take rifampin and isoniazid since they may keep this medicine from working as well.

To help clear up your tuberculosis (TB) completely, *it is very important that you keep taking this medicine for the full time of treatment* even if you begin to feel better after a few weeks. You may have to take it every day for as long as 1 to 2 years or more. *It is important that you do not miss any doses.*

Your doctor may also want you to take pyridoxine (vitamin B_6) every day to help prevent or lessen some of the side effects of isoniazid. If so, *it is very important to take pyridoxine every day along with this medicine; do not miss any doses.*

If you do miss a dose of either of these medicines, take it as soon as possible. However, if it is almost time for your next dose, do not take the missed dose or double your next dose. Instead, go back to your regular dosing schedule. *If rifampin and isoniazid is taken on an irregular schedule, side effects may occur more often and may be more serious than usual.* If you have any questions about this, check with your doctor or pharmacist.

Precautions While Using This Medicine

Certain foods such as fish (tuna, skipjack, or Sardinella) or cheese (Swiss or Cheshire) may rarely cause reactions in some patients taking isoniazid-containing medicines. Check with your doctor if redness or itching of the skin, hot feeling, rapid or pounding heartbeat, sweating, chills or clammy feeling, headache, or lightheadedness occurs while you are taking this medicine.

Do not take rifampin and isoniazid within 6 hours of the time you take aminosalicylates (another TB medicine) since they may keep rifampin and isoniazid from working as well.

This medicine will cause the urine, stool, saliva, sweat, and tears to turn reddish orange to reddish brown. This is to be expected while you are taking this medicine. Since this effect may cause soft contact lenses to become permanently discolored and standard cleaning solutions may not take out all the discoloration, *it is best not to wear soft contact lenses while taking this medicine.* Hard contact lenses are not discolored by this medicine. If you have any questions about this, check with your doctor.

Oral contraceptives (birth control pills) may not work as well if you take them while you are taking rifampin and isoniazid. Unplanned pregnancies may occur. You should use a different means of birth control while you are taking this medicine. If you have any questions about this, check with your doctor or pharmacist.

If your symptoms do not improve within 2 to 3 weeks or if they become worse, check with your doctor.

It is very important that your doctor check your progress at regular visits. In addition, you should *check with your doctor immediately if blurred vision or any loss of vision, with or without eye pain, occurs during treatment.* He may want you to have your eyes checked by an ophthalmologist (eye doctor).

If this medicine causes you to feel very tired or very weak; or causes clumsiness; unsteadiness; a loss of appetite; nausea; numbness, tingling, burning, or pain in the hands and feet; or vomiting, stop taking it and check with your doctor immediately. These may be early warning signs of more serious liver or nerve problems that could develop later.

Caution: Diabetics—This medicine may cause false test results with some urine sugar tests.

Check with your doctor before changing your diet or the dosage of your diabetes medicine.

Liver problems may be more likely to occur if you drink alcoholic beverages regularly while you are taking this medicine. Also, the regular use of alcohol may keep this medicine from working as well. Therefore, *you should not drink alcoholic beverages while you are taking this medicine.*

Side Effects of This Medicine

Along with its needed effects, a medicine may cause some unwanted effects. Although not all of these side effects appear very often, when they do occur they may require medical attention. Stop taking this medicine and check with your doctor *immediately* if any of the following side effects occur:

More common

Clumsiness or unsteadiness	Unusual tiredness or weakness
Dark urine	Vomiting
Loss of appetite	Yellowing of eyes or skin
Nausea	
Numbness, tingling, burning, or pain in hands and feet	

Less common

Chills	Muscle and bone pain
Difficult breathing	Shivering
Dizziness	Unexplained fever
Headache	

Rare

Blurred vision or any loss of vision, with or without eye pain	Greatly decreased frequency of urination or amount of urine
	Unexplained sore throat
	Unusual bruising or bleeding

Other side effects may occur which usually do not require medical attention. These side effects may go away during treatment as your body adjusts to the medicine. However, check with your doctor if any of the following side effects continue or are bothersome:

More common

Diarrhea	Stomach cramps or upset
Reddish orange to reddish brown discoloration of urine, stools, saliva, sputum, sweat, and tears	

Less common

Enlargement of the breasts (males)	Rash
Itching	Redness
	Sore mouth or tongue

Other side effects not listed above may also occur in some patients. If you notice any other effects, check with your doctor.

SALICYLATES (Systemic)

This information applies to the following medicines:

Aspirin (AS-pir-in)
Buffered Aspirin
Carbaspirin (Karb-AS-pir-in)
Choline Salicylate (KOE-leen salicylate)
Sodium Salicylate

Some commonly used brand names are:	Generic names:
Bayer Aspirin Ecotrin Empirin Analgesic Measurin St. Joseph Aspirin	Aspirin
Ascriptin Bufferin CAMA Inlay-Tabs	Buffered Aspirin
Calurin	Carbaspirin
Arthropan	Choline Salicylate
Parbocyl Uracel	Sodium Salicylate

Salicylates are medicines used to relieve pain, reduce fever, and relieve redness and swelling caused by arthritis. Aspirin may also be used to lessen the chance of stroke in some men. Salicylates are available without a prescription; however, your doctor may have special instructions on the proper dose of these medicines for your medical condition.

Before Using This Medicine

In order to decide on the best treatment for your medical problem, your doctor should be told:

—if you have ever had any unusual reaction to aspirin or other salicylates including methyl salicylate (oil of wintergreen), or to other nonsteroidal anti-inflammatory agents such as fenoprofen, ibuprofen, indomethacin, naproxen, oxyphenbutazone, phenylbutazone, sulindac, or tolmetin.

—if you are pregnant or if you intend to become pregnant while using this medicine. Too much use of salicylates during the last 3 months of pregnancy may increase the length of pregnancy and may prolong labor.

Also, salicylates taken during the last 2 weeks of pregnancy may cause the baby to have bleeding problems at birth. In addition, although salicylates have not been shown to cause birth defects in humans, the chance always exists.

—if you are breast-feeding an infant. Although salicylates have not been shown to cause problems, the chance always exists. Therefore, use by nursing mothers should be carefully considered.

—if you have any of the following medical problems:

Anemia	Hodgkin's disease
Asthma, allergies, and nasal polyps (history of)	Hypoprothrombinemia
Gout	Kidney disease
Hemophilia or other bleeding problems	Liver disease
	Ulcer or other stomach problems
High blood pressure (for sodium salicylate only)	Vitamin K deficiency

—if you are now taking any of the following medicines or types of medicine:

Antacids	Insulin
Anticoagulants (blood thinners)	Methotrexate
Anti-emetics (medicine for nausea or vomiting)	Oral hypoglycemics (diabetes medicine you take by mouth)
Corticosteroids (cortisone-like medicine)	Spironolactone
	Urine acidifiers (medicine to make your urine more acid)
Gout medicine	
Inflammation medicine (for example, arthritis medicine)	Urine alkalizers (medicine to make your urine less acid)
	Vitamin C

Proper Use of This Medicine

Unless otherwise directed by your doctor:

• Do not take more of this medicine than recommended on the package label.

• Children up to 12 years of age should not take this medicine for more than 5 days in a row.

• Adults should not take this medicine for more than 10 days in a row.

If you have been directed to take this medicine for a longer period of time, it is important that your doctor check your progress at regular visits.

Keep this medicine out of the reach of children since overdose is very dangerous in young children.

For patients taking this medicine by mouth:

• *Take this medicine with food or a full glass (8 ounces) of water or milk* to lessen stomach irritation.

• *Do not use this medicine if it has a strong vinegar-like odor,* since this means the medicine is breaking down. If you have any questions about this, check with your doctor or pharmacist.

• If you have just had your tonsils removed, a tooth pulled, or other oral surgery and you are to take aspirin during the next 7 days, be sure to swallow the aspirin whole. Do not chew aspirin during this period.

• Do not place the tablets directly on a tooth or gum surface because they may cause a burn.

• There are several different forms of salicylate tablets. If you are taking:

—*chewable aspirin tablets,* they may be chewed, dissolved in liquid, crushed, or swallowed whole.

—*enteric-coated tablets of aspirin or sodium salicylate,* they are to be swallowed whole.

—*extended-release aspirin tablets* (not the enteric-coated tablets), and they are too large to swallow whole, you may gently break or crumble them but do not grind them up.

If you have any questions about how to take your medicine, check with your pharmacist.

For patients using the suppository form of aspirin:

• How to insert suppository: First remove the foil wrapper and moisten the suppository with water. Lie down on side and push the suppository well up into rectum with finger.

• Too much use of aspirin suppositories may cause irritation of the rectum. Check with your doctor if this occurs.

Precautions While Using This Medicine

Check with your doctor:

—if your symptoms do not improve or if they become worse.

—if you are taking this medicine to bring down a fever, and the fever lasts for more than 3 days or returns.

Check the labels of all over-the-counter (OTC), nonprescription, and prescription medicines you now take. If any contain aspirin or other salicylates be especially careful, since taking them while taking this medicine may lead to overdose. If you have any questions about this, check with your doctor or pharmacist.

Caution: Diabetics—False urine sugar test results may occur if you are regularly taking:

—8 or more 325-mg (5 grain) doses of aspirin, buffered aspirin, or sodium salicylate a day.

—8 or more 382-mg doses of carbaspirin a day.

—4 or more teaspoonsful (each teaspoonful containing 870 mg) of choline salicylate a day.

Smaller doses or occasional use of salicylates usually do not affect urine sugar tests. If you have any questions about this, check with your doctor, nurse, or pharmacist, especially if your diabetes is not well controlled.

Do not take a salicylate for 5 days before any surgery, including dental surgery, unless otherwise directed by your doctor. Taking a salicylate during this time may cause bleeding problems.

If you are taking buffered aspirin or carbaspirin, and you are also taking a tetracycline antibiotic, do not take the two medicines within 1 hour of each other. Taking them together may prevent the tetracycline from being absorbed by your body. If you have any questions about this, check with your doctor or pharmacist.

If you have high blood pressure and are on a low salt diet, do not take sodium salicylate without first checking with your doctor or pharmacist.

For patients taking this medicine by mouth:

• Stomach problems may be more likely to occur if you drink alcoholic beverages while being treated with this medicine, especially if you are taking it in high doses or for a long time. Check with your doctor if you have any questions about this.

Side Effects of This Medicine

Along with its needed effects, a medicine may cause some unwanted effects. Although not all of these side effects appear very often, when they do occur they may require medical attention. When this medicine is used for short periods of time at low doses, side effects usually are rare. However, check with your doctor or pharmacist if any of the following occur:

More common

Nausea or vomiting
Stomach pain

Less common

Any loss of hearing	Shortness of breath
Bloody or black tarry stools	Tightness in chest
	Wheezing
Itching or skin rash	

Possible signs of overdose

Diarrhea	Severe or continuing headache
Dizziness or mental confusion	Stomach pain
Nausea or vomiting	Sweating
Rapid breathing	Thirst
Ringing or buzzing in ear (continuing)	Vision problems

Other side effects may occur which usually do not require medical attention. These side effects may go away during treatment as your body adjusts to the medicine. However, check with your doctor or pharmacist if the following side effect continues or is bothersome:

Indigestion

Other side effects not listed above may also occur in some patients. If you notice any other effects, check with your doctor or pharmacist.

SALICYLIC ACID (Topical)

Some commonly used brand names are:

Calicylic	Keralyt
Domerine	Mediplast
Fomac	Saligel
Hydrisalic	Sebisol
Ionil	Xseb

Salicylic acid (sal-i-SILL-ik AS-id) is used topically to treat many skin disorders such as acne, psoriasis, seborrheic dermatitis, calluses, corns, and warts, depending on the strength of the preparation. Some of these preparations are available only with your doctor's prescription. Others are available without a prescription; however, your doctor may have special instructions on the proper use of salicylic acid for your medical condition.

Before Using This Medicine

In order to decide on the best treatment for your medical problem, your doctor should be told:

—if you have ever had any unusual reaction to salicylic acid in the past. This medicine should not be used if you are allergic to it.

—if you are pregnant, if you intend to become pregnant, or if you are breast-feeding an infant, although salicylic acid has not been shown to cause problems.

—if you have blood vessel disease or diabetes (only for patients using the plaster form of salicylic acid)

—if you are now using any topical acne preparation or preparation containing a peeling agent such as benzoyl peroxide, resorcinol, sulfur, or tretinoin.

Proper Use of This Medicine

It is very important that you use this medicine only as directed. Do not use more of it, do not use it more often, and do not use it for a longer period of time than recommended on the label, unless otherwise directed by your doctor. To do so may increase the chance of absorption through the skin and the chance of salicylic acid poisoning.

If your doctor has ordered an occlusive dressing (for example, kitchen plastic wrap) to be applied over this medicine, make sure you know how to apply it. Since an occlusive dressing will increase the amount of medicine absorbed through your skin and the possibility of salicylic acid poisoning, use it only as directed. If you have any questions about this, check with your doctor.

Unless your hands are being treated, wash them immediately after applying this medicine to remove any medicine that may be on them.

Keep this medicine away from the eyes and other mucous membranes such as the mouth and inside of the nose.

If you miss a dose of this medicine, apply it as soon as possible. Then go back to your regular dosing schedule. But if it is almost time for your next dose, do not apply the missed dose at all. Instead, go back to your regular dosing schedule. If you have any questions about this, check with your doctor or pharmacist.

If you are using the cream, lotion, or ointment form of this medicine:

• Apply enough medicine to cover the affected area, and rub in gently.

If you are using the topical foam form of this medicine:

- For best results, do not wet the skin before applying this medicine.

- Apply enough foam to cover the affected area, and rub in gently. Allow the medicine to remain on the skin for 3 to 5 minutes, then rinse well with lukewarm water and pat dry.

- Do not use any soap or other skin cleansers on the affected area while using this medicine.

If you are using the gel form of this medicine:

- Before using salicylic acid gel, apply wet packs to the affected areas for at least 5 minutes. If you have any questions about this, check with your doctor or pharmacist.

- Apply enough gel to cover the affected areas, and rub in gently.

If you are using the plaster form of this medicine:

- How to apply the salicylic acid plaster: First, cut off the length of plaster needed to cover only the affected area. Remove the gauze from the plaster before applying. If the gauze sticks to the plaster, dampen with a wet cloth. Then apply the plaster to the affected area. Make sure the plaster does not touch any healthy tissue.

- Do not use this plaster on irritated or infected skin.

If you are using the shampoo form of this medicine:

- Before applying this medicine, wet the hair and scalp with lukewarm water. Apply enough medicine to work up a lather and rub well into the scalp for 2 or 3 minutes, then rinse. Apply the medicine again and rinse thoroughly.

If you are using the soap form of this medicine:

- Work up a lather with the soap, using hot water, and scrub the entire affected area with a washcloth or facial brush.

- If you are to use this soap in a foot bath, work up rich suds in hot water and soak the feet for 10 to 15 minutes. Then pat dry without rinsing.

Precautions While Using This Medicine

Do not use any topical acne preparation or preparation containing a peeling agent (for example, benzoyl peroxide, resorcinol, sulfur, or tretinoin) *on the same affected area as this medicine,* unless otherwise directed by your doctor. To do so may cause severe irritation of the skin.

Side Effects of This Medicine

Along with its needed effects, a medicine may cause some unwanted effects. Although not all of these side effects appear very often, when they do occur they may require medical attention. Check with your doctor or pharmacist if any of the following side effects occur:

Irritation of skin not present
before using this medicine

Possible signs of salicylic acid poisoning

Dizziness
Mental confusión
Rapid breathing

Ringing or buzzing
in ears, contin-
uing
Severe or continuing
headache

When you apply the gel form of this medicine, a mild temporary stinging may be expected.

Other side effects not listed above may also occur in some patients. If you notice any other effects, check with your doctor or pharmacist.

SALICYLIC ACID AND SULFUR (Topical)
Some commonly used brand names are:

Acne-Dome
Acno
Antiseb
BUF
Exzit
Fostex
Klaron
Meted

Pernox
Rezamid
SAStid
Sebex
Sebulex
Therac
Vanseb

Salicylic acid (sal-i-SILL-ik AS-id) and sulfur (SUL-fur) combination may be applied to the skin to treat acne and other skin disorders or used on the scalp as a shampoo to treat dandruff and other scalp disorders. This medicine is available without a prescription; however, your doctor may have special instructions on the proper use of this medicine for your medical condition.

Before Using This Medicine

In order to decide on the best treatment for your medical problem, your doctor should be told:

—if you have ever had any unusual reaction to salicylic acid or sulfur in the past. This medicine should not be used if you are allergic to it.

—if you are pregnant, if you intend to become pregnant, or if you are breast-feeding an infant, although salicylic acid and sulfur combination has not been shown to cause problems.

—if you are now using any topical acne preparation or preparation containing a peeling agent such as benzoyl peroxide, resorcinol, or tretinoin.

—if you are now using any topical preparation containing mercury, such as ammoniated mercury ointment.

Proper Use of This Medicine

Use this medicine only as directed. Do not use more of it and do not use it more often than recommended on the label, unless otherwise directed by your doctor.

Immediately after using this medicine, wash your hands to remove any medicine that may be on them.

Keep this medicine away from the eyes. If you should accidentally get some in your eyes, flush them thoroughly with water.

If you miss a dose of this medicine, apply or use it as soon as possible. Then go back to your regular dosing schedule. But if it is almost time for your next dose, do not apply or use the missed dose at all. Instead, go back to your regular dosing schedule. If you have any questions about this, check with your doctor or pharmacist.

If you are using the skin cleanser form of this medicine:

• After wetting the skin, apply this medicine with your fingertips or a wet sponge and rub in gently to work up a lather. Then rinse thoroughly and pat dry.

If you are using the lotion form of this medicine:

• Apply a small amount of this medicine to the affected areas, and rub in gently.

If you are using the shampoo form of this medicine:

• Wet the hair and scalp with lukewarm water. Then apply enough medicine to work up a lather and rub into the scalp. Continue rubbing the lather into the scalp for several minutes or allow it to remain on the scalp for about 5 minutes, depending on the product being used, then rinse. Apply the medicine again and rinse thoroughly.

If you are using the bar soap form of this medicine:

• After wetting the skin, use this medicine to wash the face and other affected areas. Then rinse thoroughly and pat dry.

Precautions While Using This Medicine

Do not use any topical acne preparation or preparation containing a peeling agent (for example, benzoyl peroxide, resorcinol, or tretinoin) *on the same affected area as this medicine,* unless otherwise directed by your doctor. To do so may cause severe irritation of the skin.

Do not use any topical mercury-containing preparation such as ammoniated mercury ointment on the same affected area as this medicine. To do so may cause a foul odor, be irritating to the skin, and stain the skin black. If you have any questions about this, check with your doctor or pharmacist.

Side Effects of This Medicine

Along with its needed effects, a medicine may cause some unwanted effects. Although not all of these side effects appear very often, when they do occur they may require medical attention. Check with your doctor or pharmacist if the following side effect occurs:

Irritation of skin not present before using this medicine

Other side effects may occur which usually do not require medical attention. However, check with your doctor or pharmacist if the following side effect continues or is bothersome:

Unusual dryness of skin

After you use this medicine for a few days, some redness and peeling of the skin may be expected.

Other side effects not listed above may also occur in some patients. If you notice any other effects, check with your doctor or pharmacist.

SALICYLIC ACID, SULFUR, AND COAL TAR (Topical)

Some commonly used brand names are:

Antiseb-T	Sebutone
Sebex-T	Vanseb-T

Salicylic acid (sal-i-SILL-ik AS-id), sulfur (SUL-fur), and coal tar (kole tar) combination is used as a shampoo to treat dandruff, seborrheic dermatitis, and psoriasis of the scalp. This medicine is available without a prescription; however, your doctor may have special instructions on the proper use of this medicine for your medical condition.

Before Using This Medicine

In order to decide on the best treatment for your medical problem, your doctor should be told:

—if you have ever had any unusual reaction to salicylic acid, sulfur, or coal tar in the past. This medicine should not be used if you are allergic to it.

—if you are pregnant, if you intend to become pregnant, or if you are breast-feeding an infant, although salicylic acid, sulfur, and coal tar combination has not been shown to cause problems.

—if you are now using any topical preparation containing mercury, such as ammoniated mercury ointment.

Proper Use of This Medicine

Use this medicine only as directed. Do not use it more often than recommended on the label, unless otherwise directed by your doctor.

Before using this medicine, wet the hair and scalp with lukewarm water. Then apply a generous amount to the scalp and work up a rich lather. Rub the lather into the scalp for 5 minutes, then rinse. Apply the medicine again and rinse thoroughly.

Immediately after using this medicine, wash your hands to remove any medicine that may be on them.

Keep this medicine away from the eyes. If you should accidentally get some in your eyes, flush them thoroughly with water.

Precautions While Using This Medicine

Do not use any topical mercury-containing preparation such as ammoniated mercury ointment on the same affected area as this medicine. To do so may cause a foul odor, be irritating to the skin, and stain the skin black. If you have any questions about this, check with your doctor or pharmacist.

This medicine may temporarily discolor blond, bleached, or tinted hair.

Side Effects of This Medicine

Along with its needed effects, a medicine may cause some unwanted effects. Although not all of these side effects appear very often, when they do occur they may require medical attention. Check with your doctor or pharmacist if the following side effect occurs:

   Irritation of skin not present
      before using this medicine

Other side effects not listed above may also occur in some patients. If you notice any other effects, check with your doctor or pharmacist.

SELENIUM SULFIDE (Topical)

Some commonly used brand names are:

Exsel	Selsun Blue
Iosel	Sul-Blue
Selsun	

Selenium sulfide (se-LEE-nee-um SUL-fide) is used as a shampoo to treat dandruff and seborrheic dermatitis of the scalp. Some of these preparations are available only with your doctor's prescription. Others are available without a prescription; however, your doctor may have special instructions on the proper use of this medicine for your medical problem.

Before Using This Medicine

In order to decide on the best treatment for your medical problem, your doctor should be told:

—if you have ever had any unusual reaction to selenium sulfide in the past. This medicine should not be used if you are allergic to it.

—if you are pregnant, if you intend to become pregnant, or if you are breast-feeding an infant, although selenium sulfide has not been shown to cause problems.

Proper Use of This Medicine

Use this medicine only as directed. Do not use it more often than recommended on the label, unless otherwise directed by your doctor.

Before using this medicine, wet the hair and scalp with lukewarm water. Then apply enough medicine to the scalp to work up a lather. Allow the lather to remain on the scalp for 2 to 3 minutes, then rinse. Apply the medicine again. Then *rinse thoroughly to lessen the possibility of hair discoloration.*

Also, if you use this medicine before or after bleaching, tinting, or permanent-waving your hair, rinse your hair for at least 5 minutes in cool running water after using the medicine.

Do not use this medicine if blistered, raw, or oozing areas are present on your scalp, unless otherwise directed by your doctor.

Keep this medicine away from the eyes. If you should accidentally get some in your eyes, flush them thoroughly with water.

Side Effects of This Medicine

Along with its needed effects, a medicine may cause some unwanted effects. Although not all of these side effects appear very often, when they do occur they may require medical attention. Check with your doctor or pharmacist if the following side effect occurs:

Irritation of skin

Other side effects may occur which usually do not require medical attention. Check with your doctor or pharmacist if any of the following side effects continue or are bothersome:

More common

Unusual dryness or oiliness of hair or scalp

Less common

Increase in normal hair loss

Other side effects not listed above may also occur in some patients. If you notice any other effects, check with your doctor or pharmacist.

SODIUM FLUORIDE (Systemic)

Some commonly used brand names are:

Denta-Fl	Flura	Pedi-Dent
Flo-Tab	Karidium	Pediaflor
Fluorident	Luride	Stay-Flo
Fluoritab	Luride-SF	Studaflor
Fluorodex	Nafeen	

Fluoride has been found to be helpful in reducing the number of cavities in the teeth. It is usually present naturally in drinking water. However, some areas of the country do not have a high enough level in the water to prevent cavities. To make up for this, extra fluorides may be added to the diet. Some children may require both dietary fluorides and fluoride treatments by the dentist. Use of a fluoride toothpaste or rinse may be helpful, as well.

Taking fluorides does not replace good dental habits. These include eating a good diet, brushing teeth often, and having regular dental checkups.

This medicine is available only with your physician's or dentist's prescription.

Before Using This Medicine

In order to decide on the best treatment for your medical problem, your physician or dentist should be told:

—if you have ever had any unusual reaction to medicines containing fluorides.

—if you have an underactive thyroid gland.

Proper Use of This Medicine

Take this medicine only as directed by your physician or dentist. Do not take more of it and do not take it more often than ordered. Taking even slightly too much fluoride over a period of time may cause unwanted effects.

If you miss a dose of this medicine, take it as soon as you remember. However, if it is almost time for the next dose, do not take the missed dose at all and do not double the next one. Instead, go back to your regular dosing schedule. If you have any questions about this, check with your physician or dentist.

For patients taking the chewable tablet form of this medicine:

• Tablets should be chewed or crushed before they are swallowed.

• This medicine works best if it is taken at bedtime, after the teeth have been thoroughly brushed.

For patients taking the oral liquid form of this medicine:

• This medicine is to be taken by mouth even though it comes in a dropper bottle. The amount to be taken is to be measured with the specially marked dropper.

• *Always store this medicine in the original plastic container.* Fluoride will affect glass and should not be stored in glass containers.

• This medicine may be dropped directly into the mouth or mixed with cereal, fruit juice, or other food.

Precautions While Using This Medicine

The level of fluoride present in the water is different in different parts of the country. If you move to another area, check with a physician or dentist in the new area as soon as possible to see if this medicine is still needed or if the dose needs to be changed.

Inform your physician or dentist as soon as possible if you notice white, brown, or black spots on the teeth. These are signs of too much fluoride.

Keep this medicine out of reach of children, since overdose is especially dangerous in children.

Side Effects of This Medicine

Along with its needed effects, a medicine may cause some unwanted effects. Although not all of these side effects appear very often, when they do occur they may require medical attention. When the correct amount of this medicine is used, side effects usually are rare. However, *stop taking this medicine and check with your physician immediately* if any of the following side effects occur as they may be symptoms of overdose:

Black tarry stools	Stomach cramps or
Bloody vomit	pain
Diarrhea	Tremors
Drowsiness	Unusual excitement
Faintness	Unusual increase in
Nausea and	saliva
vomiting	Watery eyes
Shallow breathing	Weakness

Check with your physician or dentist also if the following side effects occur:

Constipation	Sores in the mouth
Loss of appetite	and on the lips
Pain and aching of	Stiffness
bones	Weight loss
Skin rash	White, brown, or
	black discolor-
	ation of teeth

Other side effects not listed above may also occur in some patients. If you notice any other effects, check with your physician or dentist.

SODIUM PHOSPHATES (Systemic)

This information applies to the following medicines:

Sodium Phosphate
Sodium Phosphates

Sodium phosphates (SOE-dee-um FOS-fates) are used as a dietary supplement for patients who are unable to get enough phosphorus in their regular diet, usually because of certain illnesses or diseases. In patients with hypercalcemia (too much calcium in the blood), sodium phosphates can be used to help the body lose calcium.

This medicine is available only with your doctor's prescription.

Before Using This Medicine

In order to decide on the best treatment for your medical problem, your doctor should be told:

—if you have ever had any unusual reaction to sodium phosphates in the past. This medicine should not be taken if you are allergic to it.

—if you are pregnant, if you intend to become pregnant, or if you are breast-feeding an infant. Although sodium phosphates have not been shown to cause problems, the chance always exists.

—if you have any of the following medical problems:

Edema (swelling of	Liver disease
feet or lower legs	Rickets
or fluid in lungs)	Seizures
Heart disease	Softening of bones
High blood pressure	Underactive
Kidney disease	parathyroid
	glands

—if you are now taking any of the following medicines or types of medicine:

Antacids containing	High blood pressure
aluminum or	medicine such as
magnesium	diazoxide,
Cortisone-like	guanethidine,
medicine	hydralazine,
Digitalis glycosides	methyldopa, or
(heart medicine)	reserpine
	Medicine containing
	calcium
	Vitamin D

Proper Use of This Medicine

Take this medicine only as directed. Do not take more of it and do not take it more often than your doctor ordered.

Take this medicine immediately after meals or with food to lessen possible stomach upset or laxative action.

If you miss a dose of this medicine and you remember within an hour or so of the missed dose, take it right away. Then go back to your regular dosing schedule. But if you do not remember until later, do not take the missed dose at all and do not double the next one. Instead, go back to your regular dosing schedule. If you have any questions about this, check with your doctor.

Precautions While Using This Medicine

Your doctor should check your progress at regular visits in order to make sure that this medicine does not cause unwanted effects.

If you are taking this medicine for hypercalcemia (too much calcium in the blood), your doctor may want you to follow a low-calcium diet. If you have any questions about this, check with your doctor.

Caution: Patients on a sodium-restricted diet—This medicine contains a large amount of sodium. If you have any questions about this, check with your doctor or pharmacist.

Side Effects of This Medicine

Along with its needed effects, a medicine may cause some unwanted effects. Although not all of these side effects appear very often, when they do occur they may require medical attention. Check with your doctor if any of the following side effects occur:

Less common or rare

Headache or dizziness	Shortness of breath or troubled breathing
Decreased urination	
Mental confusion	Swelling of feet or lower legs
Muscle cramps	
Numbness, tingling, pain, or weakness in hands or feet	Unusual thirst
	Unusual tiredness or weakness
	Unusual weight gain
	Unusually fast heartbeat

Other side effects may occur which usually do not require medical attention. These side effects may go away during treatment as your body adjusts to the medicine. However, check with your doctor if any of the following side effects continue or are bothersome:

Less common

Diarrhea	Stomach pain
Nausea	Vomiting

Other side effects not listed above may also occur in some patients. If you notice any other effects, check with your doctor.

SPIRONOLACTONE (Systemic)
A commonly used brand name is Aldactone.

Spironolactone (speer-on-oh-LAK-tone) is a diuretic and antihypertensive agent. It is commonly used to treat high blood pressure. It is used also to help reduce the amount of water in the body by increasing the flow of urine. This medicine is available only with your doctor's prescription.

Before Using This Medicine

In order to decide on the best treatment for your medical problem, your doctor should be told:

—if you have ever had any unusual reaction to spironolactone in the past. This medicine should not be taken if you are allergic to it.

—if you are pregnant, if you intend to become pregnant, or if you are breast-feeding an infant. Although spironolactone has not been shown to cause problems, the chance always exists.

—if you have any of the following medical problems:

Diabetes	Kidney disease
Heart disease	Liver disease

—if you are now taking any of the following medicines or types of medicine:

Ammonium chloride	Other diuretics (water pills) or antihypertensives (high blood pressure medicine)
Carbenoxolone	
Laxatives	
Lithium	
	Potassium supplements

Proper Use of This Medicine

This medicine may cause you to have an unusual feeling of tiredness when you begin to take it. You may also notice an increase in the amount of urine or in your frequency of urination. After taking the medicine for a while, these effects should lessen. In order to keep the increase in urine from affecting your nighttime sleep:

• If you are to take a single dose a day, take it in the morning after breakfast.

• If you are to take more than one dose a day, take the last dose no later than 6 p.m., unless otherwise directed by your doctor.

• However, it is best to plan your dose or doses according to a schedule that will least affect your personal activities and sleep. Ask your doctor, nurse, or pharmacist to help you plan the best time to take this medicine.

In order to help remember to take your medicine, try to get into the habit of taking it at the same time each day.

If this medicine upsets your stomach, it may be taken with meals or milk. If stomach upset (nausea, vomiting, stomach pain or cramps) continues, check with your doctor.

If you miss a dose of this medicine, take it as soon as possible. If it is almost time for your next dose, do not take the missed dose at all and do not double the next one. Instead, go back to your regular dosing schedule. If you have any questions about this, check with your doctor.

For patients taking taking this medicine for high blood pressure:

•Importance of Diet—When prescribing medicine for your condition, your doctor may also prescribe a personal diet for you. Such a diet may be low in sodium (salt). Medicine is usually more effective when this diet is properly followed.

Also, it may be very important for you to go on a reducing diet. However, check with your doctor before going on any diet.

•Many patients who have high blood pressure will not notice any signs of the problem. In fact, many may feel normal. It is very important that you take your medicine exactly as directed and that you keep your doctor's appointments even if you feel well.

•Remember that this medicine will not cure your high blood pressure but it does control it. Therefore, you must continue to take it as directed if you expect to keep your blood pressure down. *You may have to take medicine for the rest of your life.* If high blood pressure is not treated, it can cause serious problems such as heart failure, blood vessel disease, stroke, or kidney disease.

Precautions While Using This Medicine

It is important that your doctor check your progress at regular visits.

This medicine does not cause a loss of potassium from your body as other diuretics (water pills) do. Therefore, it is not necessary for you to get extra potassium in your diet and too much potassium could even be harmful. Since salt substitutes and low-salt milk may contain potassium, do not use them unless told to do so by your doctor.

Check with your doctor if you become sick and have severe or continuing vomiting or diarrhea. These problems may cause you to lose additional water, which could be harmful, or to lose potassium, which could lessen the medicine's helpful effects.

Before having any kind of surgery (including dental surgery) or emergency treatment, tell the doctor or dentist in charge that you are taking this medicine.

Do not take other medicines unless they have been discussed with your doctor. This especially includes over-the-counter (nonprescription) medicines for appetite control, asthma, colds, cough, hay fever, or sinus, since they may tend to increase your blood pressure.

Side Effects of This Medicine

Along with its needed effects, a medicine may cause some unwanted effects. Although not all of these side effects appear very often, when they do occur they may require medical attention. *Check with your doctor if any of the following side effects occur, especially since some of them may mean that your body has too much potassium:*

Signs of too much potassium

Irregular heartbeat	Unexplained anxiety
Mental confusion	Unusual tiredness or
Numbness or tin-	weakness
gling in hands,	Weakness or
feet, or lips	heaviness of
Shortness of breath	legs
or difficult	
breathing	

Uncommon or rare

Fever
Skin rash or itching

Other side effects may occur which usually do not require medical attention. These side effects may go away during treatment as your body adjusts to the medicine. However, *check with your doctor if any of the following side effects continue or are bothersome, especially since some of them may mean that your body has too little sodium:*

Signs of too little sodium

Drowsiness	Increased thirst
Dryness of mouth	Lack of energy

More common

Nausea and
vomiting
Stomach cramps
and diarrhea

Less common

Breast tenderness in	Inability to have or
women	keep an erection
Clumsiness	Increased hair
Deepening of voice	growth in women
in women	Irregular menstrual
Enlargement of	periods
breasts in men	Unusual sweating
Headache	

This medicine sometimes causes enlarged breasts in men, especially when they take large doses of it for a long time. Breasts usually decrease in size gradually over several months after this medicine is stopped. If you have any questions about this, check with your doctor.

Other side effects not listed above may also occur in some patients. If you notice any other effects, check with your doctor.

SPIRONOLACTONE AND HYDROCHLOROTHIAZIDE (Systemic)
A commonly used brand name is Aldactazide.

Spironolactone (speer-on-oh-LAK-tone) and hydrochlorothiazide (hye-droe-klor-oh-THYE-a-zide) is a combination of diuretics. It is commonly used to treat high blood pressure. It is used also to help reduce the amount of water in the body by increasing the flow of urine. This medicine is available only with your doctor's prescription.

Before Using This Medicine
In order to decide on the best treatment for your medical problem, your doctor should be told:

—if you are allergic to sulfonamides (sulfa drugs), thiazide diuretics (water pills), or spironolactone.

—if you are pregnant or if you intend to become pregnant while using this medicine. When this medicine is used during pregnancy, it may cause side effects in the newborn infant. In addition, although this medicine has not been shown to cause birth defects, the chance always exists.

—if you have any of the following medical problems:

Diabetes	Kidney disease
Gout	Liver disease
Heart disease	Pancreas disease
History of lupus erythematosus	

—if you are now taking any of the following medicines or types of medicine:

Ammonium chloride	Lithium
Carbenoxolone	Methenamine
Colestipol	Oral anticoagulants
Corticosteroids (cortisone-like medicines)	(blood thinners you take by mouth)
Corticotropin (ACTH)	Other diuretics (water pills) or antihypertensives
Diabetes medicine	(high blood
Digitalis glycosides (heart medicine)	pressure medicine)
Gout medicine	Potassium supplements
Laxatives	

Proper Use of This Medicine
This medicine may cause you to have an unusual feeling of tiredness when you begin to take it. You may also notice an increase in the amount of urine or in your frequency of urination.

After you have taken the medicine for a while, these effects should lessen. In general, in order to keep the increase in urine from affecting your sleep:

• If you are to take a single dose a day, take it in the morning after breakfast.

• If you are to take more than one dose a day, take the last dose no later than 6 p.m., unless otherwise directed by your doctor.

• However, it is best to plan your dose or doses according to a schedule that will least affect your personal activities and sleep. Ask your doctor, nurse, or pharmacist to help you plan the best time to take this medicine.

In order to help remember to take your medicine, try to get into the habit of taking it at the same time each day.

If this medicine upsets your stomach, it may be taken with meals or milk. If stomach upset (nausea, vomiting, stomach pain or cramps) continues, check with your doctor.

If you miss a dose of this medicine, take it as soon as possible. If it is almost time for your next dose, do not take the missed dose at all and do not double the next one. Instead, go back to your regular dosing schedule. If you have any questions about this, check with your doctor.

For patients taking this medicine for high blood pressure:

• Importance of Diet—When prescribing medicine for your condition, your doctor may also prescribe a personal diet for you. Such a diet may be low in sodium (salt). Medicine is usually more effective when this diet is properly followed.

Also, it may be very important for you to go on a reducing diet. However, check with your doctor before going on any diet.

• Many patients who have high blood pressure will not notice any signs of the problem. In fact, many may feel normal. It is very important that you take your medicine exactly as directed and that you keep your doctor's appointments even if you feel well.

• Remember that this medicine will not cure your high blood pressure but it does control it. Therefore, you must continue to take it as directed if you expect to keep your blood pressure down. *You may have to take medicine for the rest of your life.* If high blood pressure is not treated, it can cause serious problems such as heart failure, blood vessel disease, stroke, or kidney disease.

Precautions While Using This Medicine

It is important that your doctor check your progress at regular visits.

This medicine may cause a loss or increase of potassium in your body. Your doctor may have special instructions about eating or drinking foods or beverages that have a high potassium content (for example, orange or other citrus fruit juices), taking a potassium supplement, or using salt substitutes. It is important not to change your diet on your own. Tell your doctor if you are already on a special diet (as for diabetes), or if you are taking a potassium supplement or using salt substitutes. Check with your doctor, nurse, or pharmacist if you need a list of foods which are high in potassium or if you have any questions.

Check with your doctor if you become sick and have severe or continuing vomiting or diarrhea. These problems may cause you to lose additional water and potassium.

Caution: Diabetics—This medicine may raise blood sugar levels. While you are using this medicine, be especially careful in testing for sugar in your urine. If you have any questions about this, check with your doctor.

A few people who take this medicine may become more sensitive to sunlight than they are normally. When you begin to take this medicine, avoid too much sun or use of a sunlamp until you see how you react, especially if you tend to burn easily. If you have a severe reaction, check with your doctor.

Before having any kind of surgery (including dental surgery) or emergency treatment, *tell the doctor or dentist in charge that you are taking this medicine.*

For patients taking this medicine for high blood pressure:

• *Do not take other medicines unless they have been discussed with your doctor.* This especially includes over-the-counter (nonprescription) medicines for appetite control, asthma, colds, cough, hay fever, or sinus, since they may tend to increase your blood pressure.

Side Effects of This Medicine

Along with its needed effects, a medicine may cause some unwanted effects. Although not all of these side effects appear very often, when they do occur they may require medical atten-

tion. *Check with your doctor if any of the following side effects occur, especially since some of them may mean that your body has too much or is losing too much potassium:*

Signs of changes in potassium

Dryness of mouth	Nausea or vomiting
Increased thirst	Numbness or tingling in hands, feet, or lips
Irregular heartbeats	
Mood or mental changes	Unusual tiredness or weakness
Muscle cramps or pain	Weak pulse

Rare

Severe stomach pain with nausea and vomiting	Unusual bleeding or bruising
Skin rash or hives	Yellowing of eyes or skin
Unexplained sore throat and fever	

Other side effects may occur which usually do not require medical attention. These side effects may go away during treatment as your body adjusts to the medicine. However, check with your doctor if any of the following side effects continue or are bothersome:

More common

Loss of appetite	Upset stomach
Stomach cramps and diarrhea	

Less common

Breast tenderness in women	Inability to have or keep an erection
Clumsiness	Increased body hair growth in women
Deepening of voice in women	Increased sensitivity of skin to sunlight
Dizziness or lightheadedness when getting up from a lying or sitting position	Irregular menstrual periods
	Lack of energy
Enlargement of breasts in men	Mental confusion
	Unusual sweating
Headache	

This medicine sometimes causes enlarged breasts in men, especially when they take large doses of it for a long time. Breasts usually decrease in size gradually over several months after this medicine is stopped. If you have any questions about this, check with your doctor.

Other side effects not listed above may also occur in some patients. If you notice any other effects, check with your doctor.

SUCCINIMIDE-TYPE ANTICONVULSANTS
(Systemic)

This information applies to the following medicines:

Ethosuximide (eth-oh-SUX-i-mide)
Methsuximide (meth-SUX-i-mide)
Phensuximide (fen-SUX-i-mide)

Some commonly used brand names are:	Generic names:
Zarontin	Ethosuximide
Celontin	Methsuximide
Milontin	Phensuximide

This medicine belongs to the group of medicines called anticonvulsants. It is used to control certain seizures in the treatment of epilepsy. This medicine is available only with your doctor's prescription.

Before Using This Medicine

In order to decide on the best treatment for your medical problem, your doctor should be told:

—if you have had any unusual reactions to anticonvulsant medicines in the past. This medicine should not be taken if you are allergic to it.

—if you are pregnant, if you intend to become pregnant, or if you are breast-feeding an infant. Although succinimide-type anticonvulsants have not been shown to cause problems, the chance always exists, since there have been problems with other anticonvulsants.

—if you have any of the following medical problems:

Blood disease   Liver disease
Kidney disease

—if you are now taking medicine for mental illness or depression.

—if you are now taking other anticonvulsant medicine.

Proper Use of This Medicine

This medicine must be taken every day in regularly spaced doses as ordered by your doctor.

If this medicine upsets your stomach, take it with food or milk unless otherwise directed by your doctor.

If you miss a dose of this medicine and remember within 4 hours, take it as soon as possible. Then go back to your regular dosing schedule. Do not double doses. If you have any questions about this, check with your doctor.

Precautions While Using This Medicine

Your doctor should check your progress at regular visits, especially during the first few months you take this medicine. During this time the amount of medicine you are taking may have to be changed often to meet your individual needs.

If you have been taking this medicine regularly, do not stop taking it without first checking with your doctor. Your doctor may want you to reduce gradually the amount you are taking before stopping completely. Stopping this medicine suddenly may cause seizures.

This medicine may cause some people to become drowsy or less alert than they are normally. *Make sure you know how you react to this medicine before you drive, use machines, or do other jobs that require you to be alert.* After you have taken this medicine for a while this effect may lessen.

Your doctor may want you to carry a medical identification card or bracelet stating that you are taking this medicine.

Side Effects of This Medicine

Along with its needed effects, a medicine may cause some unwanted effects. Although not all of these side effects appear very often, when they do occur they may require medical attention. Check with your doctor if any of the following side effects occur:

Less common

Mood or mental changes

Rare

Skin rash or itching	Unusual bleeding or
Swollen lymph glands	bruising
Unexplained sore throat and fever	

Other side effects may occur which usually do not require medical attention. These side effects may go away during treatment as your body adjusts to the medicine. However, check with your doctor if any of the following side effects continue or are bothersome:

More common

Loss of appetite	Stomach cramps
Nausea and vomiting	

Less common

Dizziness	Irritability
Drowsiness	Tiredness
Headache	

Other side effects not listed above may also occur in some patients. If you notice any other effects, check with your doctor.

SULFASALAZINE (Systemic)

Some commonly used brand names are:

Azulfidine   Salazopyrin*
S.A.S.-500

---

*Not available in the United States.

Sulfasalazine (sul-fa-SAL-a-zeen), a sulfonamide or sulfa medicine, belongs to the general family of medicines called anti-infectives. It is given by mouth to help control inflammatory bowel disease such as enteritis or colitis. Sulfasalazine is available only with your doctor's prescription.

Before Using This Medicine

In order to decide on the best treatment for your medical problem, your doctor should be told:

—if you have had allergic reactions to any of the sulfonamides, furosemide or thiazide diuretics (water pills), dapsone, sulfoxone, oral hypoglycemics (diabetes medicine you take by mouth), glaucoma medicine you take by mouth (for example, acetazolamide, dichlorphenamide, ethoxzolamide, methazolamide), or salicylates (for example, aspirin).

—if you are pregnant or if you intend to become pregnant, although sulfasalazine has not been shown to cause birth defects and other problems do not usually occur.

—if you are breast-feeding an infant. Sulfonamides pass into the breast milk in small amounts and may cause unwanted effects in infants with glucose-6-phosphate dehydrogenase (G6PD) deficiency.

—if you have any of the following medical problems:

Blockage of   Kidney disease
  stomach, intes-   Liver disease
  tines, or urinary Porphyria
  tract
Blood problems
Glucose-6-
  phosphate
  dehydrogenase
  (G6PD) deficiency

—if you are now taking any of the following medicines or types of medicine:

Digoxin (heart   Oral hypoglycemics
  medicine)   (diabetes medicine
Folic acid   you take by
Methenamine   mouth)
Methotrexate   Oxyphenbutazone
Oral anticoagulants   Phenylbutazone
  (blood thinners   Phenytoin
  you take by   Probenecid
  mouth)   Sulfinpyrazone

—if you are now taking medicine to make your urine more alkaline such as:

Sodium bicarbonate   Sodium citrate,
  (baking soda)   potassium citrate,
Sodium citrate   and citric acid
Sodium citrate and
  citric acid

Proper Use of This Medicine

Sulfasalazine is best taken after meals or with food to lessen stomach upset. If stomach upset continues or is bothersome, check with your doctor.

Each dose of sulfasalazine should also be taken with a full glass (8 ounces) of water. Several additional glasses of water should be taken every day, unless otherwise directed by your doctor. Drinking extra water will help to prevent unwanted side effects of the sulfonamide.

If you are taking the enteric-coated tablet form of this medicine:

• Swallow tablets whole. Do not break or crush.

Keep taking this medicine for the full time of treatment even if you begin to feel better after a few days; *do not miss any doses.*

If you do miss a dose of this medicine, take it as soon as possible. However, if it is almost time for your next dose, do not take the missed dose or double your next dose. Instead, go back to your regular dosing schedule.

Do not give sulfasalazine to infants under 2 years of age unless directed by your doctor.

Precautions While Using This Medicine

If your symptoms (including diarrhea) do not improve within a month or two or if they become worse, check with your doctor.

It is important that your doctor check your progress at regular visits.

Before having any kind of surgery (including dental surgery) with a general anesthetic, tell the doctor or dentist in charge that you are taking a sulfonamide.

Some people who take sulfonamides may become more sensitive to sunlight than they are normally. When you begin to take this medicine, avoid too much sun or too much use of a sunlamp until you see how you react, especially if you tend to burn easily. You may still be more sensitive to sunlight or sunlamps for many months after you stop taking this medicine. If you have a severe reaction, check with your doctor.

Side Effects of This Medicine

Along with its needed effects, a medicine may cause some unwanted effects. Although not all of these side effects appear very often, when they do occur they may require medical attention. Stop taking this medicine and check with your doctor if any of the following side effects occur:

More common

Continuing headache	Itching
	Rash
Increased sensitivity to sunlight	

Less common

Aching of joints and muscles	Unexplained sore throat or fever
Difficulty in swallowing	Unusual bleeding or bruising
Pale skin	Unusual tiredness or weakness
Redness, blistering, peeling, or loosening of skin	Yellowing of eyes or skin

Rare

Blood in urine	Swelling of front part of neck
Lower-back pain	
Pain or burning while urinating	

Other side effects may occur which usually do not require medical attention. These side effects may go away during treatment as your body adjusts to the medicine. However, check with your doctor if any of the following side effects continue or are bothersome:

More common

Diarrhea	Loss of appetite
Dizziness	Nausea
Headache	Vomiting

In some patients this medicine may cause the urine to become orange-yellow. This side effect does not require medical attention.

Other side effects not listed above may also occur in some patients. If you notice any other effects, check with your doctor.

SULFINPYRAZONE (Systemic)
Some commonly used brand names are Anturan*, Anturane, and Zynol*.

*Not available in the United States.

Sulfinpyrazone (sul-fin-PEER-a-zone) is taken by mouth to treat chronic gout. It is available only with your doctor's prescription.

Before Using This Medicine

In order to decide on the best treatment for your medical problem, your doctor should be told:

—if you have ever had any unusual reaction to dipyrone, oxyphenbutazone, or phenylbutazone.

—if you are pregnant, if you intend to become pregnant, or if you are breast-feeding an infant. Although sulfinpyrazone has not been shown to cause problems, the chance always exists.

—if you have any of the following medical problems:

Blood disease (or history of)	Stomach ulcer or other stomach
Kidney disease	problems (or history of)

—if you are now taking any of the following medicines or types of medicine:

Aspirin or other salicylates	Nitrofurantoin
	Oral hypoglycemics
Coumarin-type anticoagulants (blood thinners)	(diabetes medicine you take by mouth)
Diuretics (water pills)	Pyrazinamide
	Sulfonamides (sulfa
Insulin	medicine)

Proper Use of This Medicine

In order for sulfinpyrazone to help you, it must be taken regularly as ordered by your doctor.

Sulfinpyrazone is used to help prevent gout attacks. It will not relieve an attack that has already started. *Even if you take another medicine for gout attacks, continue to take this medicine also.* If you have any questions about this, check with your doctor.

If this medicine upsets your stomach, it may be taken with food or milk. If this does not work, an antacid may be taken. If stomach upset (nausea, vomiting, or stomach pain) continues, check with your doctor.

To help prevent kidney stones from forming while taking sulfinpyrazone, *drink at least 10 to 12 full glasses (8 ounces each) of fluids each day* unless otherwise directed by your doctor.

If you miss a dose of this medicine, take it as soon as possible. Then go back to your regular dosing schedule. However, if you do not remember the missed dose until it is almost time for your next dose, do not take the missed dose at all and do not double the next one. Instead, go back to your regular dosing schedule. If you have any questions about this, check with your doctor.

Precautions While Using This Medicine

Your doctor should check your progress at regular visits in order to make sure that this medicine does not cause unwanted effects.

Taking aspirin or other salicylates or drinking too much alcohol may lessen the effects of sulfinpyrazone. Therefore, *do not take aspirin or other salicylates or drink alcoholic beverages while taking this medicine,* unless you have first checked with your doctor.

Side Effects of This Medicine

Along with its needed effects, a medicine may cause some unwanted effects. Although not all of these side effects appear very often, when they do occur they may require medical attention. Check with your doctor if any of the following side effects occur:

Less common

Skin rash

Rare

Bloody or black tarry stools	Unexplained sore throat and fever
Bloody urine	Unusual bleeding or bruising
Difficult or painful urination	Unusual tiredness or weakness
Lower back pain	

Other side effects may occur which usually do not require medical attention. These side effects may go away during treatment as your body adjusts to the medicine. However, check with your doctor if any of the following side effects continue or are bothersome:

More common

Nausea	Vomiting
Stomach pain	

Other side effects not listed above may also occur in some patients. If you notice any other effects, check with your doctor.

SULFONAMIDES (Ophthalmic)

This information applies to the following medicines:

Sulfacetamide (sul-fa-SEE-ta-mide)
Sulfisoxazole (sul-fi-SOX-a-zole)

Some commonly used brand names are:	Generic names:
Bleph	
Cetamide	
Isopto Cetamide	
Optosulfex*	Sulfacetamide
Sulamyd	
Sulf-10	
Gantrisin	Sulfisoxazole

*Not available in the United States.

Sulfonamides (sul-FON-a-mides) or sulfa drugs belong to the general family of medicines called anti-infectives. Sulfonamide ophthalmic preparations are used to help the body overcome infections of the eye. They are available only with your doctor's prescription.

Before Using This Medicine

In order to decide on the best treatment for your medical problem, your doctor should be told:

—if you have had allergic reactions to any of the sulfonamides, furosemide or thiazide diuretics (water pills), dapsone, sulfoxone, oral hypoglycemics (diabetes medicine you take by mouth), or glaucoma medicine you take by mouth (for example, acetazolamide, dichlorphenamide, ethoxzolamide, methazolamide).

—if you are pregnant, if you intend to become pregnant, or if you are breast-feeding an infant, although sulfonamide ophthalmic preparations have not been shown to cause problems.

—if you are now using silver preparations such as silver nitrate or mild silver protein in the eye.

Proper Use of This Medicine

If you are using the eye drop form of this medicine:

• Bottle is not full; this is to provide proper drop control.

• To prevent contamination of the eye drops, do not touch the applicator tip to any surface (including the eye), and keep the container tightly closed.

• How to apply this medicine: First, wash hands. Then tilt head back and pull lower eyelid away from eye to form a pouch. Drop medicine into the pouch and gently close eyes. Do not blink. Keep eyes closed for 1 or 2 minutes to allow medicine to come into contact with the infection.

• If you think you did not get the drop of medicine into your eye properly, use another drop.

If you are using the eye ointment form of this medicine:

• To prevent contamination of the eye ointment, do not touch the applicator tip to any surface (including the eye). After using, wipe the tip of the ointment tube with a clean tissue and keep the tube tightly closed.

• How to apply this medicine: First, wash hands. Then pull the lower eyelid away from eye to form a pouch. Squeeze a thin strip of ointment into the pouch. A 1.25- to 2.5-cm (approximately 1/2- to 1-inch) strip of ointment is usually enough unless otherwise directed by your doctor. Gently close eyes and keep them closed for 1 or 2 minutes to allow medicine to come into contact with the infection.

To help clear up your infection completely, *keep using this medicine for the full time of treatment,* even though your symptoms may have disappeared; *do not miss any doses.*

If you do miss a dose of this medicine, apply it as soon as possible. However, if it is almost time for your next application, skip the missed dose and go back to your regular dosing schedule.

Precautions While Using This Medicine

After application, eye ointments usually cause your vision to blur for a few minutes.

After application of this medicine to the eye, occasional stinging or burning may be expected.

If your symptoms do not improve within a few days or if they become worse, check with your doctor.

Side Effects of This Medicine

Along with its needed effects, a medicine may cause some unwanted effects. Although not all of these side effects appear very often, when

they do occur they may require medical attention. Check with your doctor if any of the following side effects occur:

Itching, redness, swelling, or other sign of irritation not present before you started using this medicine

Other side effects not listed above may also occur in some patients. If you notice any other effects, check with your doctor.

SULFONAMIDES (Systemic)

This information applies to the following medicines:

Sulfacytine (sul-fa-SYE-teen)
Sulfamethoxazole (sul-fa-meth-OX-a-zole)
Sulfamethoxazole and Trimethoprim (sul-fa-meth-OX-a-zole and trye-METH-oh-prim)
Sulfisoxazole (sul-fi-SOX-a-zole)

Some commonly used brand names are:	Generic names:
Renoquid	Sulfacytine
Gantanol Methoxal Methoxanol	Sulfamethoxazole
Bactrim Septra	Sulfamethoxazole and Trimethoprim
Gantrisin Lipo Gantrisin Novosoxazole* Sosol Sulfalar Sulfizin Sulfizole*	Sulfisoxazole

*Not available in the United States.

Sulfonamides (sul-FON-a-mides) or sulfa medicines belong to the general family of medicines called anti-infectives. They are given by mouth to help the body overcome infections. Sulfonamides are available only with your doctor's prescription.

Before Using This Medicine

In order to decide on the best treatment for your medical problem, your doctor should be told:

—if you have had allergic reactions to any of the sulfonamides, furosemide or thiazide diuretics (water pills), dapsone, sulfoxone, oral hypoglycemics (diabetes medicine you take by mouth), or glaucoma medicine you take by mouth (for example, acetazolamide, dichlorphenamide, ethoxzolamide, methazolamide).

—if you are pregnant or if you intend to become pregnant, although sulfonamides have not been shown to cause birth defects, and other problems do not usually occur.

—if you are breast-feeding an infant. Sulfonamides pass into the breast milk in small amounts and may cause unwanted effects in infants with glucose-6-phosphate dehydrogenase (G6PD) deficiency.

—if you have any of the following medical problems:

Glucose-6-phosphate dehydrogenase (G6PD) deficiency	Kidney disease Liver disease Porphyria

—if you are now taking any of the following medicines or types of medicine:

Aminobenzoic acid (PABA)	Oxyphenbutazone
Methenamine	Penicillins
Methotrexate	Phenylbutazone
Oral anticoagulants (blood thinners you take by mouth)	Phenytoin
	Probenecid
	Sulfinpyrazone
Oral hypoglycemics (diabetes medicine you take by mouth)	

—if you are now taking medicine to make your urine more alkaline such as:

Sodium bicarbonate (baking soda)	Sodium citrate, potassium citrate, and citric acid
Sodium citrate	
Sodium citrate and citric acid	

Proper Use of This Medicine

Sulfonamides are best taken with a full glass (8 ounces) of water on an empty stomach (either 1 hour before or 2 hours after meals). *Several additional glasses of water should be taken every day,* unless otherwise directed by your doctor. Drinking extra water will help to prevent unwanted side effects of sulfonamides.

If you are taking the oral liquid form of this medicine:

• Use a specially marked measuring spoon or other device to measure each dose accurately since the average household teaspoon may not hold the right amount of liquid.

To help clear up your infection completely, *keep taking this medicine for the full time of treatment* even if you begin to feel better after a few days; *do not miss any doses.*

If you do miss a dose of this medicine, take it as soon as possible. However, if it is almost time for your next dose and your dosing schedule is:

• 2 doses a day—Space the missed dose and the next dose 5 to 6 hours apart.

• 3 or more doses a day—Space the missed dose and the next dose 2 to 4 hours apart or double your next dose.

Then go back to your regular dosing schedule.

Do not give sulfonamides to infants under 1 month of age unless otherwise directed by your doctor. However, sulfacytine should not be given to children under 14 years of age.

Precautions While Using This Medicine

If your symptoms do not improve within a few days or if they become worse, check with your doctor.

It is important that your doctor check your progress at regular visits if you will be taking this medicine for a long time.

Before having any kind of surgery (including dental surgery) with a general anesthetic, tell the doctor or dentist in charge that you are taking a sulfonamide.

Some people who take sulfonamides may become more sensitive to sunlight than they are normally. When you begin to take this medicine, avoid too much sun or too much use of a sunlamp until you see how you react, especially if you tend to burn easily. You may still be more sensitive to sunlight or sunlamps for many months after you stop taking this medicine. If you have a severe reaction, check with your doctor.

Side Effects of This Medicine

Along with its needed effects, a medicine may cause some unwanted effects. Although not all of these side effects appear very often, when they do occur they may require medical attention. Stop taking this medicine and check with your doctor if any of the following side effects occur:

More common

Increased sensitivity to sunlight	Itching Rash

Less common

Aching of joints and muscles	Unexplained sore throat or fever
Difficulty in swallowing	Unusual bleeding or bruising
Pale skin	Unusual tiredness or weakness
Redness, blistering, peeling, or loosening of skin	Yellowing of eyes or skin

Rare

Blood in urine	Swelling of front part of neck
Lower-back pain	
Pain or burning while urinating	

Other side effects may occur which usually do not require medical attention. These side effects may go away during treatment as your body adjusts to the medicine. However, check with your doctor if any of the following side effects continue or are bothersome:

More common

Diarrhea	Loss of appetite
Dizziness	Nausea
Headache	Vomiting

Other side effects not listed above may also occur in some patients. If you notice any other effects, check with your doctor.

SULFONAMIDES (Vaginal)

This information applies to the following medicines:

Sulfanilamide (sul-fa-NILL-a-mide), Aminacrine (am-in-AK-rin), and Allantoin (al-AN-toyn)
Sulfathiazole (sul-fa-THYE-a-zole),
 Sulfacetamide (sul-fa-SEE-ta-mide),
 and Sulfabenzamide (sul-fa-BENZ-a-mide)
Sulfisoxazole (sul-fi-SOX-a-zole)
Sulfisoxazole, Aminacrine, and Allantoin

Some commonly used brand names are:	Generic names:
AVC	
Femguard	
Nil	Sulfanilamide,
Tricholan	Aminacrine,
Vagidine	and Allantoin
Vagimine	
Vagitrol	

Sultrin	Sulfathiazole,
Trysul	Sulfacetamide, and Sulfabenzamide
Koro-Sulf	Sulfisoxazole
Vagilia	Sulfisoxazole, Aminacrine, and Allantoin

Vaginal sulfonamides (sulfas), including sulfonamide-containing combination medicines, are used to help the body overcome infections of the vagina and to help provide relief from the itching, irritation, burning, odor, pain, or discharge of certain vaginal problems. Vaginal sulfonamides are available only with your doctor's prescription.

Before Using This Medicine

In order to decide on the best treatment for your medical problem, your doctor should be told:

—if you have had allergic reactions to any of the sulfonamides, furosemide or thiazide diuretics (water pills), dapsone, sulfoxone, oral hypoglycemics (diabetes medicine you take by mouth), or glaucoma medicine you take by mouth (for example, acetazolamide, dichlorphenamide, ethoxzolamide, methazolamide).

—if you are pregnant, if you intend to become pregnant, or if you are breast-feeding an infant, although vaginal sulfonamides have not been shown to cause problems.

Proper Use of This Medicine

This medicine usually comes with patient directions. Read them carefully before using this medicine.

This medicine is usually inserted into the vagina with an applicator. However, if you are pregnant, check with your doctor before using the applicator.

Use of tampons is not recommended since they may absorb too much of this medicine. Also, tampons may be more likely to come out of the vagina if you use them during treatment with this medicine.

To help clear up your infection completely, *keep using this medicine for the full time of treatment* even though your symptoms may have disappeared. You should keep using this medicine even if you begin to menstruate during treatment; *do not miss any doses.*

If you do miss a dose of this medicine, insert it as soon as possible. However, if it is almost time for your next dose, skip the missed dose and go back to your regular dosing schedule.

Precautions While Using This Medicine

If you are using an aminacrine-containing medicine:

• Since this medicine may stain underclothing, a sanitary napkin or minipad may be worn for protection.

• After the first few applications of this medicine to the vagina, a mild, temporary stinging or burning may be expected.

If your symptoms do not improve within a few days or if they become worse, check with your doctor.

Good health habits are also required to help clear up your infection completely and to help prevent reinfection. These include wearing cotton panties or panties or pantyhose with cotton crotches instead of synthetic underclothes (for example, nylon or rayon). If you have any questions about this, check with your doctor, pharmacist, or nurse.

If you have intercourse while using this medicine, it may be desirable that your partner wear a condom (prophylactic) to prevent reinfection. Also, it may be necessary for your partner to be treated at the same time you are being treated. If you have any questions about this, check with your doctor or pharmacist.

Side Effects of This Medicine

Along with its needed effects, a medicine may cause some unwanted effects. Although not all of these side effects appear very often, when they do occur they may require medical attention. Stop using this medicine and check with your doctor if any of the following side effects occur:

Itching, rash, redness, swelling, or other sign of irritation not present before you started using this medicine

Other side effects not listed above may also occur in some patients. If you notice any other effects, check with your doctor.

SULFONAMIDES AND PHENAZOPYRIDINE
(Systemic)

This information applies to the following medicines:

Sulfamethoxazole (sul-fa-meth-OX-a-zole) and
  Phenazopyridine (fen-az-oh-PEER-i-deen)
Sulfisoxazole (sul-fi-SOX-a-zole) and
  Phenazopyridine

Some commonly used brand names are:	Generic names:
Azo Gantanol	Sulfamethoxazole and Phenazopyridine
Azo Gantrisin Azo-Soxazole Azosul Azo-Sulfizin Suldiazo	Sulfisoxazole and Phenazopyridine

---

Sulfonamides and phenazopyridine, combination products containing a sulfa medicine and a urinary pain reliever, belong to the general family of medicines called anti-infectives. They are given by mouth to help the body overcome infections of the urinary tract and to help relieve the pain, burning, and irritation of these infections. Sulfonamides and phenazopyridine are available only with your doctor's prescription.

Before Using This Medicine

In order to decide on the best treatment for your medical problem, your doctor should be told:

—if you have had allergic reactions to any of the sulfonamides, furosemide or thiazide diuretics (water pills), dapsone, sulfoxone, oral hypoglycemics (diabetes medicine you take by mouth), or glaucoma medicine you take by mouth (for example, acetazolamide, dichlorphenamide, ethoxzolamide, methazolamide).

—if you are pregnant or if you intend to become pregnant, although sulfonamides and phenazopyridine have not been shown to cause birth defects, and other problems do not usually occur.

—if you are breast-feeding an infant. Sulfonamides pass into the breast milk in small amounts and may cause unwanted effects in infants with glucose-6-phosphate dehydrogenase (G6PD) deficiency.

—if you have any of the following medical problems:

Glucose-6-phosphate dehydrogenase (G6PD) deficiency	Hepatitis or other liver disease Kidney disease Porphyria

—if you are now taking any of the following medicines or types of medicine:

Aminobenzoic acid (PABA)	Oxyphenbutazone
Methenamine	Penicillins
Methotrexate	Phenylbutazone
Oral anticoagulants (blood thinners you take by mouth)	Phenytoin
	Probenecid
Oral hypoglycemics (diabetes medicine you take by mouth)	Sulfinpyrazone

—if you are now taking medicine to make your urine more alkaline such as:

Sodium bicarbonate (baking soda)	Sodium citrate, potassium citrate, and citric acid
Sodium citrate	
Sodium citrate and citric acid	

Proper Use of This Medicine

Sulfonamides and phenazopyridine are best taken with a full glass (8 ounces) of water on an empty stomach (either 1 hour before or 2 hours after meals). However, this medicine may be taken with meals or following meals if it upsets your stomach.

Several additional glasses of water should be taken every day, unless otherwise directed by your doctor. Drinking extra water will help to prevent unwanted side effects of the sulfonamide. Also, this will help the medicine clear up your infection sooner by flushing out the bacteria.

To help clear up your infection completely, *keep taking this medicine for the full time of treatment* even if you begin to feel better after a few days; *do not miss any doses.*

If you do miss a dose of this medicine, take it as soon as possible. However, if it is almost time for your next dose, do not take the missed dose or double your next dose. Instead, go back to your regular dosing schedule.

Do not give sulfonamides and phenazopyridine to infants and children under 12 years of age unless otherwise directed by your doctor.

Do not use any left-over medicine for future urinary tract problems without first checking with your doctor. Another infection may require a different medicine.

Precautions While Using This Medicine

This medicine causes the urine to turn reddish orange. This is to be expected while you are using this medicine. Also, the medicine may stain clothing. If you have any questions about removing the stain, check with your doctor or pharmacist.

Caution: Diabetics—This medicine may cause false test results with some urine sugar tests and urine ketone tests. Check with your doctor before changing your diet or the dosage of your diabetes medicine.

If your symptoms do not improve within a few days or if they become worse, check with your doctor.

Before having any kind of surgery (including dental surgery) with a general anesthetic, tell the doctor or dentist in charge that you are taking a sulfonamide.

Some people who take sulfonamides may become more sensitive to sunlight than they are normally. When you first begin taking this medicine, avoid too much sun or too much use of a sunlamp until you see how you react, especially if you tend to burn easily. You may still be more sensitive to sunlight or sunlamps for many months after stopping this medicine. If you have a severe reaction, check with your doctor.

Side Effects of This Medicine

Along with its needed effects, a medicine may cause some unwanted effects. Although not all of these side effects appear very often, when they do occur they may require medical attention. Stop taking this medicine and check with your doctor if any of the following side effects occur:

More common

Increased sensitivity to sunlight	Itching
	Rash

Less common

Aching of joints and muscles	Unexplained sore throat or fever
Difficulty in swallowing	Unusual bleeding or bruising
Pale skin	Unusual tiredness or weakness
Redness, blistering, peeling, or loosening of skin	Yellowing of eyes or skin

Rare

Lower-back pain	Swelling of front part of neck

Other side effects may occur which usually do not require medical attention. These side effects may go away during treatment as your body adjusts to the medicine. However, check with your doctor if any of the following side effects continue or are bothersome:

More common

Diarrhea	Loss of appetite
Dizziness	Nausea
Headache	Vomiting

Less common

Indigestion	Stomach cramps or pain

This medicine causes the urine to become reddish orange. This side effect does not require medical attention.

Other side effects not listed above may also occur in some patients. If you notice any other effects, check with your doctor.

SULFUR (Topical)

Sulfur (SUL-fur) is applied to the skin to treat acne, scabies, seborrheic dermatitis, and other skin disorders. Some of these preparations are available only with your doctor's prescription. Others are available without a prescription; however, your doctor may have special instructions on the proper use of sulfur for your medical condition.

Before Using This Medicine

In order to decide on the best treatment for your medical problem, your doctor should be told:

—if you have ever had any unusual reaction to sulfur in the past. This medicine should not be used if you are allergic to it.

—if you are pregnant, if you intend to become pregnant, or if you are breast-feeding an infant, although sulfur has not been shown to cause problems.

—if you are now using any topical acne preparation or preparation containing a peeling agent such as benzoyl peroxide, resorcinol, salicylic acid, or tretinoin.

—if you are now using any topical preparation containing mercury, such as ammoniated mercury ointment.

Proper Use of This Medicine

Use this medicine only as directed. Do not use it more often and do not use it for a longer period of time than recommended on the label, unless otherwise directed by your doctor.

Keep this medicine away from the eyes. If you should accidentally get some in your eyes, flush them thoroughly with water.

If you miss a dose of this medicine, apply or use it as soon as possible. Then go back to your regular dosing schedule. But if it is almost time for your next dose, do not apply or use the missed dose at all. Instead, go back to your regular dosing schedule. If you have any questions about this, check with your doctor or pharmacist.

If you are using the ointment form of this medicine:

• Before applying sulfur ointment, wash the affected areas with soap and water and dry thoroughly. Then apply enough ointment to cover the affected areas and rub in gently.

If you are using the soap form of this medicine:

• Work up a rich lather with the soap, using hot water. Wash the affected areas and rinse thoroughly. Apply the lather again, and rub in gently for a few minutes. Remove excess lather with a towel or tissue without rinsing.

Precautions While Using This Medicine

Do not use any topical acne preparation or preparation containing a peeling agent (for example, benzoyl peroxide, resorcinol, salicylic acid, or tretinoin), *on the same affected area as this medicine,* unless otherwise directed by your doctor. To do so may cause severe irritation of the skin.

Do not use any topical mercury-containing preparation such as ammoniated mercury ointment on the same affected area as this medicine. To do so may cause a foul odor, be irritating to the skin, and stain the skin black. If you have any questions about this, check with your doctor or pharmacist.

Side Effects of This Medicine

Along with its needed effects, a medicine may cause some unwanted effects. Although not all of these side effects appear very often, when they do occur they may require medical attention. Check with your doctor or pharmacist if the following side effect occurs:

Irritation of skin not present before using this medicine

After you use this medicine for a few days, some redness and peeling of the skin may be expected.

Other side effects not listed above may also occur in some patients. If you notice any other effects, check with your doctor or pharmacist.

SULINDAC (Systemic)
A commonly used brand name is Clinoril.

Sulindac (sul-IN-dak) is used to treat the symptoms of arthritis. It helps relieve inflammation, swelling, stiffness, and joint pain. This medicine is available only with your doctor's prescription.

Before Using This Medicine
In order to decide on the best treatment for your medical problem, your doctor should be told:

—if you have ever had any unusual reaction to aspirin or other salicylates, fenoprofen, ibuprofen, meclofenamate, naproxen, or tolmetin.

—if you are pregnant, if you intend to become pregnant, or if you are breast-feeding an infant. Although sulindac has not been shown to cause problems in humans, the chance always exists.

—if you have any of the following medical problems:

Bleeding problems	Kidney disease
Heart disease	Stomach ulcer or
High blood pressure	other stomach problems

—if you are now taking any of the following medicines or types of medicine:

Anticoagulants (blood thinners)	Inflammation medicine (for example, aspirin or other arthritis medicine)
	Probenecid

Proper Use of This Medicine
In order for this medicine to help you, it must be taken regularly as ordered by your doctor. Up to 2 to 3 weeks may pass before you feel the full effects of this medicine.

It is best to take this medicine 30 minutes before meals or 2 hours after meals so that it will get into the blood more quickly. However, to lessen stomach upset, your doctor may want you to take the medicine with food, milk, or antacids. If stomach upset (indigestion, nausea, vomiting, stomach pain, or diarrhea) continues or if you have any questions about how you should be taking this medicine, check with your doctor.

If you miss a dose of this medicine, take it as soon as possible. Then go back to your regular dosing schedule. However, if it is almost time for your next dose, do not take the missed dose at all and do not double the next one. Instead, go back to your regular dosing schedule. If you have any questions about this, check with your doctor.

Precautions While Using This Medicine
Your doctor should check your progress at regular visits in order to make sure that this medicine does not cause unwanted effects.

Stomach problems may be more likely to occur if you take aspirin regularly (for example, every day) or drink alcoholic beverages while being treated with this medicine. Therefore, *do not take aspirin regularly or drink alcoholic beverages while taking this medicine,* unless otherwise directed by your doctor.

Before having any kind of surgery (including dental surgery), tell the doctor or dentist in charge that you are taking this medicine.

This medicine may cause some people to become dizzy. *Make sure you know how you react to this medicine before you drive, use machines, or do other jobs that require you to be alert.*

Side Effects of This Medicine
Along with its needed effects, a medicine may cause some unwanted effects. Although not all of these side effects appear very often, when they do occur they may require medical attention. Check with your doctor if any of the following side effects occur:

More common
Skin rash

Less common

Itching of skin	Swelling of feet or
Ringing or buzzing in ears	lower legs
	Unusual weight gain

Rare

Bloody or black tarry stools	Unexplained sore throat and fever
Blurred vision or any change in vision	Unusual bleeding or bruising
Decreased hearing	Yellowing of eyes or skin
Shortness of breath, troubled breathing, wheezing, or tightness in chest	

Other side effects may occur which usually do not require medical attention. These side effects may go away during treatment as your body adjusts to the medicine. However, check with your doctor if any of the following side effects continue or are bothersome:

More common

Constipation	Indigestion
Diarrhea	Nausea
Dizziness	Stomach pain or
Headache	discomfort

Less common

Bloated feeling or	Loss of appetite
gas	Nervousness
Irritation or sore-	Vomiting
ness of mouth	

Other side effects not listed above may also occur in some patients. If you notice any other effects, check with your doctor.

TAMOXIFEN (Systemic)
A commonly used brand name is Nolvadex.

Tamoxifen (ta-MOX-i-fen) is a medicine that blocks the effects of the hormone estrogen in the body. It is used to treat some cases of breast cancer. Also, it is sometimes used to treat women who have problems with their menstrual cycles (periods) or who cannot become pregnant. Tamoxifen is available only with your doctor's prescription.

Before Using This Medicine

In order to decide on the best treatment for your medical problem, your doctor should be told:

—if you have ever had any unusual reaction to tamoxifen in the past.

—if you are pregnant, if you intend to become pregnant, or if you are breast-feeding an infant. Although tamoxifen has not been shown to cause problems, the chance always exists.

—if you have a blood disease, or cataracts or eye problems.

Proper Use of This Medicine

Use this medicine only as directed by your doctor. Do not use more or less of it, and do not use it more often than your doctor ordered.

This medicine commonly causes nausea and vomiting. However, it may have to be taken for several weeks or months to be effective. Even if

you begin to feel ill, *do not stop using this medicine without first checking with your doctor.*

If you miss a dose of this medicine, do not take the missed dose at all and do not double the next one. Instead, go back to your regular dosing schedule and check with your doctor.

Precautions While Using This Medicine

It is very important that your doctor check your progress at regular visits.

Side Effects of This Medicine

Along with its needed effects, a medicine may cause some unwanted effects. Although not all of these side effects appear very often, when they do occur they may require medical attention. Check with your doctor if any of the following side effects occur:

Rare

Blurred vision	Mental confusion
Marked weakness or	Pain or swelling in
sleepiness	legs
	Shortness of breath

Other side effects may occur which usually do not require medical attention. These side effects may go away during treatment as your body adjusts to the medicine. However, check with your doctor if any of the following side effects continue or are bothersome:

More common

Bone pain	Nausea and
Hot flushes	vomiting
	Weight gain

Less common

Changes in	Skin rash or dryness
menstrual	Vaginal bleeding or
period	discharge
Headache	
Itching in genital	
area	

Rare

Dizziness	Loss of hair
Excessive growth of	Mental depression
hair	Milk production
Increased sensitivity	and leaking from
to sunlight	breasts
Lightheadedness	Swelling of hands
Loss of appetite	or feet

Other side effects not listed above may also occur in some patients. If you notice any other effects, check with your doctor.

TERBUTALINE (Systemic)
Some commonly used brand names are Brethine and Bricanyl.

Terbutaline (ter-BYOO-ta-leen) is taken by mouth or given by injection to treat bronchial asthma, bronchitis, and emphysema. It relieves wheezing, shortness of breath, and troubled breathing. This medicine is available only with your doctor's prescription.

Before Using This Medicine
In order to decide on the best treatment for your medical problem, your doctor should be told:

—if you have ever had any unusual reaction to medicines like terbutaline such as amphetamines, ephedrine, epinephrine, isoproterenol, metaproterenol, norepinephrine (levarterenol), phenylephrine, phenylpropanolamine, or pseudoephedrine.

—if you are pregnant, if you intend to become pregnant, or if you are breast-feeding an infant. Although terbutaline has not been shown to cause problems, the chance always exists.

—if you have any of the following medical problems:

Diabetes	High blood pressure
Heart disease	Overactive thyroid
	Seizures (history of)

—if you are now taking any of the following medicines or types of medicine:

Amphetamines	Propranolol
Other medicine for	
asthma or	
breathing	
problems	

Proper Use of This Medicine
Take this medicine only as directed. Do not take more of it and do not take it more often than your doctor ordered. To do so may increase the chance of side effects.

If you miss a dose of this medicine and remember within an hour or so of the missed dose, take it right away. Then go back to your regular dosing schedule. But if you do not remember until later, do not take the missed dose at all and do not double the next one. Instead, go back to your regular dosing schedule. If you have any questions about this, check with your doctor.

Precautions While Using This Medicine
If you still have trouble breathing after taking this medicine, or if your condition gets worse, *check with your doctor at once.*

Side Effects of This Medicine
Along with its needed effects, a medicine may cause some unwanted effects. The following side effects may go away during treatment as your body adjusts to the medicine; however, check with your doctor if they continue or are bothersome:

More common

Nervousness	Trembling
Restlessness	

Less common

Dizziness or light-	Nausea or vomiting
headedness	Unusual increase
Drowsiness	in sweating
Headache	Unusually fast or
Muscle cramps	pounding heart-
or twitching	beat
	Weakness

Other side effects not listed above may also occur in some patients. If you notice any other effects, check with your doctor.

TERPIN HYDRATE (Systemic)

Terpin hydrate (TER-pin HYE-drate) is used to relieve cough due to colds and mild bronchial irritations. It loosens mucus or phlegm (pronounced flem) in the lungs.

This medicine is usually not used for the chronic cough that occurs with smoking, asthma, or emphysema or when there is an unusually large amount of mucus or phlegm with the cough.

Terpin hydrate is available without a prescription; however, your doctor may have special instructions on the proper dose of this medicine for your medical condition.

Before Using This Medicine
In order to decide on the best treatment for your medical problem, your doctor should be told:

—if you have ever had any unusual reaction to terpin hydrate in the past. This medicine should not be taken if you are allergic to it.

—if you are pregnant or if you intend to become pregnant while using this medicine. This medicine contains 42.5% of alcohol. Too much use of alcohol during pregnancy may cause birth defects. In addition, although terpin hydrate has not been shown to cause birth defects or other problems, the chance always exists.

—if you are breast-feeding an infant. The alcohol in this medicine passes into the breast milk. Although the amount of alcohol in recommended doses of this medicine does not usually cause problems, the chance always exists.

Proper Use of This Medicine

Take this medicine only as directed. Do not take more of it and do not take it more often than recommended on the label, unless otherwise directed by your doctor. If too much is taken, it may become habit-forming since this medicine contains a large amount of alcohol.

To help loosen mucus or phlegm (flem) in the lungs, *drink a glass of water after each dose of this medicine,* unless otherwise directed by your doctor.

If you miss a dose of this medicine, take it as soon as possible. Then go back to your regular dosing schedule. But if it is almost time for your next dose, do not take the missed dose at all. Instead, take your next dose at the regularly scheduled time. Then continue with your regular dosing schedule. If you have any questions about this, check with your doctor or pharmacist.

Precautions While Using This Medicine

If your cough has not improved after 7 days or if you have a high fever with the cough, check with your doctor. These signs may mean that you have other medical problems.

If crystals form in this solution, dissolve them by warming the closed container of solution in warm water and then gently shaking it.

The alcohol in this medicine will add to the effects of other alcohol and medicines (CNS depressants) that slow down the nervous system. Some examples of CNS depressants are antihistamines or medicine for hay fever, other allergies, or colds; sedatives, tranquilizers, or sleeping medicine; prescription pain medicine or narcotics; barbiturates; medicine for seizures; tricyclic antidepressants (medicine for depression); or anesthetics, including some dental anesthetics. *Check with your doctor before taking any of the above while you are using this medicine.*

Side Effects of This Medicine

Along with its needed effects, a medicine may cause some unwanted effects. Although no serious side effects have been reported for terpin hydrate, the following side effects may be noticed by some patients. Check with your doctor if any of these effects continue or are bothersome:

Less common or rare

Nausea	Vomiting
Stomach pain	

Other side effects not listed above may also occur in some patients. If you notice any other effects, check with your doctor.

TERPIN HYDRATE AND CODEINE
(Systemic)
A commonly used brand name is Cortussis.

Terpin hydrate (TER-pin HYE-drate) and codeine (KOE-deen) combination medicine is used to relieve coughs due to colds. It is usually not used for chronic cough that occurs with smoking, asthma, or emphysema or when there is an unusually large amount of mucus or phlegm (pronounced flem) with the cough.

In some states this medicine is available only with your doctor's prescription. In other states, it is available without a prescription; however, your doctor may have special instructions on the proper dose of this medicine for your medical condition.

In the states where this medicine is available without a prescription, you must ask your pharmacist for it, show personal identification, and sign a record book showing that you bought the medicine, since codeine is a narcotic.

Before Using This Medicine

In order to decide on the best treatment for your medical problem, your doctor should be told:

—if you have ever had any unusual reaction to terpin hydrate or codeine in the past. This medicine should not be taken if you are allergic to it.

—if you are pregnant or if you intend to become pregnant while using this medicine. This medicine contains a large amount of alcohol. Too much use of alcohol during pregnancy may cause birth defects. In addition, although terpin hydrate and codeine have not been shown to cause birth defects or other problems, the chance always exists. Be sure you have discussed this with your doctor before taking this medicine.

—if you are breast-feeding an infant. The alcohol and codeine in this medicine pass into the breast milk. Although the amount of alcohol and codeine in recommended doses of this medicine does not usually cause problems, the chance always exists. Therefore, use by nursing mothers should be carefully considered.

—if you have any of the following medical problems:

Brain injury or disease
Colitis
Emphysema, asthma, or chronic lung disease
Enlarged prostate or problems with urination
Gallbladder disease or gallstones

Kidney disease
Liver disease
Underactive adrenal gland (Addison's disease)
Underactive thyroid
Unusually slow or irregular heartbeat

—if you are now taking central nervous system (CNS) depressants such as:

Antihistamines or medicine for hay fever, other allergies, or colds
Barbiturates
Narcotics
Prescription pain medicine

Sedatives, tranquilizers, or sleeping medicine
Seizure medicine
Tricyclic antidepressants (medicine for depression)

—if you are now taking prescription medicine for stomach cramps or spasms.

—if you are now taking or have taken within the past 2 weeks monoamine oxidase (MAO) inhibitors such as:

Isocarboxazid
Pargyline

Phenelzine
Tranylcypromine

Proper Use of This Medicine

Take this medicine only as directed. Do not take more of it, do not take it more often, and do not take it for a longer period of time than recommended on the label, unless otherwise directed by your doctor. If too much is taken, it may become habit-forming.

Precautions While Using This Medicine

If your cough has not improved after 7 days or if you have a high fever with the cough, check with your doctor. These signs may mean that you have other medical problems.

If crystals form in the solution, dissolve them by warming the closed container of solution in warm water and then gently shaking it.

The alcohol and codeine in this medicine will add to the effects of other alcohol and medicines (CNS depressants) that slow down the nervous system. Some examples of CNS depressants are antihistamines or medicine for hay fever, other allergies, or colds; sedatives, tranquilizers, or sleeping medicine; prescription pain medicine or narcotics; barbiturates; medicine for seizures; tricyclic antidepressants (medicine for depression); or anesthetics, including some dental anesthetics. *Check with your doctor before taking any of the above while you are using this medicine.*

This medicine may cause some people to become drowsy or less alert than they are normally. *Make sure you know how you react to this medicine before you drive, use machines, or do other jobs that require you to be alert.*

Dizziness, lightheadedness, or fainting may occur, especially when you get up from a lying or sitting position. Getting up slowly may help. If the problem continues or gets worse, check with your doctor.

Nausea may occur, especially after the first couple of doses. This effect usually goes away if you lie down for a while. However, if nausea continues, check with your doctor.

Side Effects of This Medicine

Along with its needed effects, a medicine may cause some unwanted effects. Although not all of these side effects appear very often, when they do occur they may require medical attention. Check with your doctor if any of the following side effects occur:

Rare

Shortness of breath
Troubled breathing
Unusual excitement (especially in children)

Unusually slow heartbeat

Other side effects may occur which usually do not require medical attention. These side effects may go away during treatment as your body adjusts to the medicine. However, check with your doctor if any of the following side effects continue or are bothersome:

More common
Constipation
Drowsiness

Less common

Difficult urination	Nausea or vomiting
Dizziness	Redness or flushing
Feeling faint	of face
Frequent urge to	Stomach pain
urinate	Unusual increase in
Lightheadedness	sweating
Loss of appetite	Unusual tiredness or
	weakness

Other side effects not listed above may also occur in some patients. If you notice any other effects, check with your doctor.

TESTOLACTONE (Systemic)
A commonly used brand name is Teslac.

Testolactone (tess-toe-LAK-tone) belongs to the general group of medicines called antineoplastics. It is used to treat some cases of breast cancer. Testolactone is available only with your doctor's prescription.

Before Using This Medicine

In order to decide on the best treatment for your medical problem, your doctor should be told:

—if you have ever had any unusual reaction to testolactone in the past.

—if you are pregnant, if you intend to become pregnant, or if you are breast-feeding an infant. Although testolactone has not been shown to cause problems, the chance always exists.

—if you have heart or kidney disease.

Proper Use of This Medicine

Use this medicine only as directed by your doctor. Do not use more or less of it, and do not use it more often than your doctor ordered.

This medicine sometimes causes nausea and vomiting. However, it may have to be taken for several weeks or months to be effective. Even if you begin to feel ill, *do not stop using this medicine without first checking with your doctor.*

If you miss a dose of this medicine, take it as soon as you remember. However, if it is almost time for the next dose, do not take the missed dose at all and do not double the next one. Instead, go back to your regular dosing schedule and check with your doctor. If you miss more than one dose, check with your doctor.

Precautions While Using This Medicine

It is very important that your doctor check your progress at regular visits.

Side Effects of This Medicine

Along with its needed effects, a medicine may cause some unwanted effects. Although not all of these side effects appear very often, when they do occur they may require medical attention. Check with your doctor if the following side effect occurs:

Numbness or tingling of fingers, toes, or face

Other side effects may occur which usually do not require medical attention. These side effects may go away during treatment as your body adjusts to the medicine. However, check with your doctor if any of the following side effects continue or are bothersome:

Less common

Diarrhea	Pain or swelling in
Loss of appetite	feet or lower legs
Nausea and	legs
vomiting	Swelling or redness
Pain or redness at	of the tongue
the place of injec-	
tion	

Rare

Changes in finger-	Loss of hair
nails or toe-	Skin rash
nails	

Other side effects not listed above may also occur in some patients. If you notice any other effects, check with your doctor.

TETRACYCLINES (Ophthalmic)

This information applies to the following medicines:

Chlortetracycline (klor-te-tra-SYE-kleen)
Tetracycline (te-tra-SYE-kleen)

Some commonly used brand names are:	Generic names:
Aureomycin	Chlortetracycline
Achromycin	Tetracycline

Tetracyclines belong to the general family of medicines called antibiotics. Tetracycline ophthalmic preparations are used to help the body overcome infections of the eye. They are available only with your doctor's prescription.

Before Using This Medicine

In order to decide on the best treatment for your medical problem, your doctor should be told:

—if you have had allergic reactions to any related antibiotics such as demeclocycline, doxycycline, methacycline, minocycline, oxytetracycline, or tetracycline (by mouth or by injection).

—if you are pregnant, if you intend to become pregnant, or if you are breast-feeding an infant, although tetracycline ophthalmic preparations have not been shown to cause problems.

Proper Use of This Medicine

If you are using the eye drop form of this medicine:

• Bottle is not full; this is to provide proper drop control.

• To prevent contamination of the eye drops, do not touch the applicator tip to any surface (including the eye), and keep the container tightly closed.

• How to apply this medicine: First, wash hands. Then tilt head back and pull lower eyelid away from eye to form a pouch. Drop medicine into the pouch and gently close eyes. Do not blink. Keep eyes closed for 1 or 2 minutes to allow medicine to come into contact with the infection.

• If you think you did not get the drop of medicine into your eye properly, use another drop.

If you are using the eye ointment form of this medicine:

• To prevent contamination of the eye ointment, do not touch the applicator tip to any surface (including the eye). After using, wipe the tip of the ointment tube with a clean tissue and keep the tube tightly closed.

• How to apply this medicine: First wash hands. Then pull the lower eyelid away from eye to form a pouch. Squeeze a thin strip of ointment into the pouch. A 1-cm (approximately 1/3-inch) strip of ointment is usually enough unless otherwise directed by your doctor. Gently close eyes and keep them closed for 1 or 2 minutes to allow medicine to come into contact with the infection.

To help clear up your infection completely, *keep using this medicine for the full time of treatment,* even though your symptoms may have disappeared; *do not miss any doses.*

If you do miss a dose of this medicine, apply it as soon as possible. However, if it is almost time for your next application, skip the missed dose and go back to your regular dosing schedule.

Precautions While Using This Medicine

After application, this medicine usually causes your vision to blur for a few minutes.

If your symptoms do not improve within a few days or if they become worse, check with your doctor.

Side Effects of This Medicine

There have not been any common or important side effects reported with this medicine. However, if you notice any unusual effects, check with your doctor.

TETRACYCLINES (Systemic)

This information applies to the following medicines:
Demeclocycline (dem-e-kloe-SYE-kleen)
Doxycycline (dox-i-SYE-kleen)
Methacycline (meth-a-SYE-kleen)
Minocycline (mi-noe-SYE-kleen)
Oxytetracycline (ox-i-te-tra-SYE-kleen)
Tetracycline (te-tra-SYE-kleen)

Some commonly used brand names are:	Generic names:
Declomycin	Demeclocycline
Doxychel Doxy-Tabs Vibramycin Vibra-Tabs	Doxycycline
Rondomycin	Methacycline
Minocin Ultramycin*	Minocycline
Oxlopar Oxy-Kesso-Tetra Terramycin Tetramine	Oxytetracycline

Achromycin
Bio-Tetra*
Bristacycline
Cyclopar
Medicycline*
Neo-Tetrine*
Novotetra*   Tetracycline
Panmycin
Retet
Robitet
Sumycin
Tetracrine*
Tetracyn

*Not available in the United States.

Aminosalicylate	Iron supplements
calcium	Laxatives
Antacids	(magnesium-
Calcium sup-	containing)
plements such	Magnesium
as calcium glu-	salicylate
conate, calcium	Penicillins
lactate, or dical-	Sodium bicarbonate
cium phosphate	(baking soda)

—if you are now taking doxycycline and are also taking any of the following medicines or types of medicine:

Barbiturates   Phenytoin
Carbamazepine

Tetracyclines belong to the general family of medicines called antibiotics. They are given by mouth or by injection to help the body overcome infections and are also given by mouth to help control acne. Demeclocycline and doxycycline may also be used for other problems as determined by your doctor. Tetracyclines are available only with your doctor's prescription.

Before Using This Medicine

In order to decide on the best treatment for your medical problem, your doctor should be told:

—if you have had allergic reactions to any of the tetracyclines or combination medicines containing a tetracycline.

—if you have had allergic reactions to lidocaine, procaine, or other "caine-type" anesthetics (medicines which cause numbing) (applies only to oxytetracycline and tetracycline given by injection into the muscle).

—if you are pregnant, if you intend to become pregnant, or if you are breast-feeding an infant. Tetracyclines may cause the unborn infant's teeth to become discolored and may slow down the growth of the infant's teeth and bones if they are taken during the last half of pregnancy. In addition, tetracyclines pass into the breast milk and may cause these same effects in infants of mothers taking these medicines.

—if you have either of the following medical problems:

Kidney disease   Liver disease
(does not apply to
doxycycline or
minocycline)

—if you have diabetes insipidus (water diabetes) and you are taking demeclocycline.

—if you are now taking any of the tetracyclines and are also taking any of the following medicines or types of medicine:

Proper Use of This Medicine

Tetracyclines should be taken with a full glass (8 ounces) of water to prevent irritation of the esophagus (tube between the throat and stomach) or stomach. In addition, most tetracyclines (except doxycycline and minocycline) are best taken on an empty stomach (either 1 hour before or 2 hours after meals). However, if this medicine still upsets your stomach, your doctor may want you to take it with food.

If you are taking the oral liquid form of this medicine:

• Use a specially marked measuring spoon or other device to measure each dose accurately, since the average household teaspoon may not hold the right amount of liquid.

Do not take milk, milk formulas, or other dairy products within 1 to 2 hours of the time you take tetracyclines (except doxycycline and minocycline) by mouth since they may keep this medicine from working as well.

If you are taking doxycycline or minocycline:

• These medicines may be taken with food or milk if they upset your stomach.

To help clear up your infection completely, *keep taking this medicine for the full time of treatment* even if you begin to feel better after a few days; *do not miss any doses.* This is especially important if you have a "strep" infection, since serious heart problems could develop later if your infection is not completely cleared up.

If you do miss a dose of this medicine, take it as soon as possible. However, if it is almost time for your next dose and your dosing schedule is:

• 1 dose a day (for example, for acne)—Space the missed dose and the next dose 10 to 12 hours apart.

• 2 doses a day—Space the missed dose and the next dose 5 to 6 hours apart.

• 3 or more doses a day—Space the missed dose and the next dose 2 to 4 hours apart or double your next dose.

Then go back to your regular dosing schedule.

If this medicine has changed color, taste, or looks different, has become outdated (old), has been stored incorrectly (too warm or too damp), or otherwise appears to have broken down, do not use it. To do so may cause serious side effects. Discard by flushing it down the toilet. If you have any questions about this, check with your doctor or pharmacist.

Do not give tetracyclines to infants or children under 8 years of age unless directed by your doctor since they may cause permanently discolored teeth and other problems.

Precautions While Using This Medicine

If your symptoms do not improve within a few days (or a few weeks or months for acne patients) or if they become worse, check with your doctor.

Do not take aminosalicylate calcium; antacids; calcium supplements such as calcium gluconate, calcium lactate, or dicalcium phosphate; magnesium salicylate; magnesium-containing laxatives such as Epsom salt; or sodium bicarbonate (baking soda) within 1 to 2 hours of the time you take any of the tetracyclines by mouth. In addition, do not take iron preparations (included also in some vitamin preparations) within 2 to 3 hours of the time you take tetracyclines by mouth. To do so may keep this medicine from working as well.

Before having surgery (including dental surgery) with a general anesthetic, tell the doctor or dentist in charge that you are taking a tetracycline. This does not apply to doxycycline.

Some people who take tetracyclines may become more sensitive to sunlight than they are normally. When you first begin taking this medicine, avoid too much sun or too much use of a sunlamp until you see how you react, especially if you tend to burn easily. You may still be more sensitive to sunlight or sunlamps for 2 weeks to several months or more after stopping this medicine. If you have a severe reaction, check with your doctor.

If you are taking minocycline:

• In addition to the precautions mentioned above, minocycline may cause some people to become dizzy, lightheaded, or unsteady. *Make sure you know how you react to this medicine before you drive, use machines, or do other jobs that require coordination.* If these reactions are especially bothersome, check with your doctor.

Side Effects of This Medicine

Along with its needed effects, a medicine may cause some unwanted effects. In some infants and children, tetracyclines may cause the teeth to become discolored. Even though this may not happen right away, check with your doctor if you notice this effect or if you have any questions about it.

Other side effects may occur which usually do not require medical attention. These side effects may go away during treatment as your body adjusts to the medicine. However, check with your doctor if any of the following side effects continue or are bothersome:

More common

Cramps or burning of the stomach	Itching of the rectal or genital areas
Diarrhea	Nausea
Increased sensitivity to sunlight (rare with minocycline)	Sore mouth or tongue
	Vomiting

In some patients tetracyclines may cause the tongue to become darkened or discolored. These changes are only temporary and will go away when you stop taking this medicine.

If you are taking demeclocycline:

• In addition to the side effects mentioned above, check with your doctor also if any of the following side effects occur:

Less common

Excessive thirst	Unusual tiredness or weakness
Greatly increased frequency of urination or amount of urine	

If you are taking minocycline:

• In addition to the side effects mentioned above, check with your doctor also if any of the following side effects continue or are bothersome:

More common
> Dizziness, light-
> headedness, or
> unsteadiness

Other side effects not listed above may also occur in some patients. If you notice any other effects, check with your doctor.

TETRACYCLINES (Topical)

This information applies to the following medicines:

Chlortetracycline (klor-te-tra-SYE-kleen)
Tetracycline (te-tra-SYE-kleen)

Some commonly used brand names are:	Generic names:
Aureomycin	Chlortetracycline
Achromycin Topicycline	Tetracycline

Tetracyclines belong to the general family of medicines called antibiotics. Tetracycline topical preparations are used to help the body overcome infections of the skin and to help control acne. Topical ointment dosage forms of the tetracyclines are available without a prescription; however, your doctor may have special instructions on the proper use of this medicine for your medical problem. The topical liquid dosage form of tetracycline is available only with your doctor's prescription.

Before Using This Medicine

In order to decide on the best treatment for your medical problem, your doctor should be told:

—if you have had allergic reactions to any related antibiotics such as demeclocycline, doxycycline, methacycline, minocycline, oxytetracycline, or tetracycline (by mouth or by injection).

—if you are pregnant, if you intend to become pregnant, or if you are breast-feeding an infant, although tetracycline topical preparations have not been shown to cause problems.

Proper Use of This Medicine

Before applying this medicine, wash the area to be treated with soap and water, and dry thoroughly.

If you are using the ointment form of this medicine:

• Avoid getting this medicine on your clothing since it may stain.

• If you are using this medicine without a prescription, do not use it to treat deep wounds, puncture wounds, or serious burns without first checking with your doctor or pharmacist.

• Do not use this medicine in the eyes.

• After applying this medicine, the treated area may be covered with a gauze dressing if desired.

If you are using the topical liquid form of this medicine:

• This medicine usually comes with patient instructions. Read these instructions carefully before using this medicine.

• Do not use this medicine in the eyes, nose, or mouth.

• The presence of the floating plastic plug in the liquid means that the medicine has been mixed properly. *Do not remove the plastic plug.*

• Bottle contains approximately an 8-week supply of medicine if used only on the face and neck or approximately a 4-week supply if used on the face and neck plus other involved areas.

• This medicine may cause slight yellowing of the skin, especially in people with light complexions. The color may be removed by washing.

• Treated areas of the skin will glow (fluoresce) under ultraviolet (UV) light.

• After application, stinging or burning of the skin may occur and may last up to a few minutes or more.

• You may continue your normal use of cosmetics while you are using this medicine.

To help clear up your infection completely, *keep using this medicine for the full time of treatment,* even though your symptoms may have disappeared; *do not miss any doses.*

If you do miss a dose of this medicine, apply it as soon as possible. However, if it is almost time for your next application, skip the missed dose and go back to your regular dosing schedule.

Precautions While Using This Medicine

If there is no improvement in your skin problem after you have used this medicine for 1 week (or longer for acne patients) or if it becomes worse, check with your doctor or pharmacist.

Side Effects of This Medicine

Along with its needed effects, a medicine may cause some unwanted effects. Although not all of these side effects appear very often, when they do occur they may require medical attention. Check with your doctor if any of the following side effects occur:

> Pain, redness, swelling, or other sign of irritation not present before you started using this medicine

Other side effects not listed above may also occur in some patients. If you notice any other effects, check with your doctor.

THEOPHYLLINE, EPHEDRINE, AND BARBITURATES (Systemic)

This information applies to the following medicines:

Theophylline (thee-OFF-i-lin), Ephedrine (e-FED-rin), and Amobarbital (am-oh-BAR-bi-tal)
Theophylline, Ephedrine, and Butabarbital (byoo-ta-BAR-bi-tal)
Theophylline, Ephedrine, and Phenobarbital (fee-noe-BAR-bi-tal)

Some commonly used brand names are:

Asminyl	Thedrizem
Asma-lief	Theodrine
Phedral	Theofed
Tedfern	Theofenal
Tedral	Theoral
Thalfed	Theotabs

Theophylline, ephedrine, and barbiturates (bar-BI-tyoo-rates) is a combination medicine that belongs to the group of medicines called bronchodilators. It is used in the treatment of bronchial asthma, asthmatic bronchitis, and other respiratory (lung) conditions. It relieves wheezing, shortness of breath, and troubled breathing.

Some preparations of this medicine are available only with your doctor's prescription. Others are available without a prescription; however, your doctor may have special instructions on the proper dose of this medicine for your medical condition.

Before Using This Medicine

In order to decide on the best treatment for your medical problem, your doctor should be told:

—if you have ever had any unusual reaction to aminophylline, caffeine, dyphylline, oxtriphylline, theobromine, or theophylline.

—if you have ever had any unusual reaction to ephedrine or medicines like ephedrine such as amphetamines, epinephrine, isoproterenol, metaproterenol, norepinephrine (levarterenol), phenylephrine, phenylpropanolamine, pseudoephedrine, or terbutaline.

—if you have ever had any unusual reaction to barbiturates.

—if you are pregnant or if you intend to become pregnant while using this medicine. When barbiturates (contained in this combination medicine) are used during pregnancy, they may cause side effects in the newborn infant. Also, too much use of barbiturates during pregnancy may cause the baby to become dependent on the medicine. This may lead to withdrawal side effects after birth. Use of theophylline (contained in this combination medicine) during pregnancy may cause unwanted effects in the newborn infant. In addition, although the theophylline, ephedrine, and barbiturates in this combination medicine have not been shown to cause birth defects, the chance always exists.

—if you are breast-feeding an infant. The theophylline, ephedrine, and barbiturates in this combination medicine pass into the breast milk and may cause unwanted effects in infants of mothers taking this medicine.

—if you have any of the following medical problems:

Diabetes	Kidney disease
Enlarged prostate	Liver disease
Heart or blood	Overactive thyroid
vessel disease	Porphyria (or
High blood pressure	history of)
Hyperactivity	Stomach ulcer
(in children)	(or history of)

—if you are now taking any of the following medicines or types of medicine:

Amphetamines	Estrogens
Anticoagulants	Griseofulvin
(blood thinners)	Guanethidine
Clindamycin	Lincomycin
Contraceptives, oral	Lithium
(birth-control	Methylergonovine
pills)	Other medicine for
Corticosteroids	asthma or
(cortisone-like	breathing
medicines)	problems
Cyclophosphamide	Phenytoin
Digitalis glycosides	Propranolol
(heart medicine)	Quinidine
Doxycycline	Troleandomycin
Ergonovine	
Erythromycin	

—if you are now taking central nervous system (CNS) depressants such as:

Antihistamines or medicine for hay fever, other allergies, or colds	Prescription pain medicine
Barbiturates	Sedatives, tranquilizers, or sleeping medicine
Narcotics	Seizure medicine
	Tricyclic antidepressants (medicine for depression)

—if you are now taking or have taken within the past 2 weeks monoamine oxidase (MAO) inhibitors such as:

Isocarboxazid	Phenelzine
Pargyline	Tranylcypromine

Proper Use of This Medicine

Take this medicine only as directed. Do not take more of it and do not take it more often than recommended on the label, unless otherwise directed by your doctor. If too much is taken, the barbiturate in this medicine may become habit-forming.

This medicine works best when taken with a glass of water on an empty stomach (either 30 minutes to 1 hour before meals or 2 hours after meals) since that way it will get into the blood sooner. However, in some cases your doctor may want you to take this medicine with meals or right after meals to lessen stomach upset. If you have any questions about how you should be taking this medicine, check with your doctor.

If you miss a dose of this medicine and you remember within an hour or so of the missed dose, take it right away. Then go back to your regular dosing schedule. But if you do not remember until later, do not take the missed dose at all and do not double the next one. Instead, go back to your regular dosing schedule. If you have any questions about this, check with your doctor or pharmacist.

If you are taking the extended-release tablet form of this medicine, swallow the tablet whole. Do not crush, break, or chew before swallowing.

Precautions While Using This Medicine

The theophylline in this medicine may add to the central nervous system stimulant effects of caffeine-containing beverages such as tea, coffee, cocoa, and cola drinks. *Avoid drinking large amounts of these beverages while taking this medicine.* If you have any questions about this, check with your doctor.

The barbiturate in this medicine will add to the effects of alcohol and other medicines (CNS depressants) that slow down the nervous system. Some examples of CNS depressants are antihistamines or medicine for hay fever, other allergies, or colds; sedatives, tranquilizers, or sleeping medicine; prescription pain medicine or narcotics; barbiturates; medicine for seizures; tricyclic antidepressants (medicine for depression); or anesthetics, including some dental anesthetics. *Check with your doctor before taking any of the above while you are using this medicine.*

This medicine may cause some people to become dizzy, lightheaded, drowsy, or less alert than they are normally. *Make sure you know how you react to this medicine before you drive, use machines, or do other jobs that require you to be alert.*

Side Effects of This Medicine

Along with its needed effects, a medicine may cause some unwanted effects. Although not all of these side effects appear very often, when they do occur they may require medical attention. Check with your doctor or pharmacist if the following side effect occurs:

Rare

Skin rash or hives

Other side effects may occur which usually do not require medical attention. These side effects may go away during treatment as your body adjusts to the medicine. However, check with your doctor or pharmacist if any of the following side effects continue or are bothersome:

More common

Drowsiness	Nervousness or restlessness
Headache	
Irritability	Stomach pain
Nausea or vomiting	Trouble in sleeping

Less common

Diarrhea	Flushing or redness of face
Difficult urination	
Dizziness or lightheadedness	Loss of appetite
Feeling of warmth	Unusually fast or pounding heartbeat

Other side effects not listed above may also occur in some patients. If you notice any other effects, check with your doctor.

THEOPHYLLINE, EPHEDRINE, GUAIFENESIN, AND BARBITURATES
(Systemic)

[Former name of Guaifenesin—Glyceryl Guaiacolate]

This information applies to the following medicines:

Theophylline (theo-OFF-i-lin), Ephedrine (e-FED-rin), Guaifenesin (gwye-FEN-e-sin), and Butabarbital (byoo-ta-BAR-bi-tal)
Theophylline, Ephedrine, Guaifenesin, and Phenobarbital (fee-noe-BAR-bi-tal)

Some commonly used brand names are:

Broncholate	Luftodil
Bronkolixir	Mudrane GG
Bronkotabs	Quibron Plus
Duovent	Verequad

Theophylline, ephedrine, guaifenesin, and barbiturates (bar-BI-tyoo-rates) is a combination medicine that belongs to the group of medicines called bronchodilators. It is used in the treatment of bronchial asthma, chronic bronchitis, emphysema, and other lung diseases. It relieves wheezing, shortness of breath, and troubled breathing. Some of these preparations are available only with your doctor's prescription. Others are available without a prescription; however, your doctor may have special instructions on the proper use of this medicine for your medical condition.

Before Using This Medicine

In order to decide on the best treatment for your medical problem, your doctor should be told:

—if you have ever had any unusual reaction to aminophylline, caffeine, dyphylline, oxtriphylline, theobromine, or theophylline.

—if you have ever had any unusual reaction to ephedrine or medicines like ephedrine such as amphetamines, epinephrine, isoproterenol, metaproterenol, norepinephrine (levarterenol), phenylephrine, phenylpropanolamine, pseudoephedrine, or terbutaline.

—if you have ever had any unusual reaction to barbiturates.

—if you are pregnant or if you intend to become pregnant while using this medicine. When barbiturates (contained in this combination medicine) are used during pregnancy, they may cause side effects in the newborn infant. Also, too much use of barbiturates during pregnancy may cause the baby to become dependent on the medicine. This may lead to withdrawal side effects after birth. Use of theophylline (contained in this combination medicine) during pregnancy may cause unwanted effects in the newborn infant. In addition, although the theophylline, ephedrine, guaifenesin, and barbiturates in this combination medicine have not been shown to cause birth defects, the chance always exists.

—if you are breast-feeding an infant. The theophylline, ephedrine, and barbiturates in this combination medicine pass into the breast milk and may cause unwanted effects in infants of mothers taking this medicine.

—if you have any of the following medical problems:

Diabetes	Kidney disease
Enlarged prostate	Liver disease
Heart or blood	Overactive thyroid
vessel disease	Porphyria (or
High blood pressure	history of)
Hyperactivity	Stomach ulcer
(in children)	(or history of)

—if you are now taking any of the following medicines or types of medicine:

Amphetamines	Estrogens
Anticoagulants	Griseofulvin
(blood thinners)	Guanethidine
Clindamycin	Lincomycin
Contraceptives, oral	Lithium
(birth-control	Methylergonovine
pills)	Other medicine for
Corticosteroids	asthma or
(cortisone-like	breathing
medicines)	problems
Cyclophosphamide	Phenytoin
Digitalis glycosides	Propranolol
(heart medicine)	Quinidine
Doxycycline	Troleandomycin
Ergonovine	
Erythromycin	

—if you are now taking central nervous system (CNS) depressants such as:

Antihistamines or	Sedatives, tran-
medicine for hay	quilizers, or sleep-
fever, other aller-	ing medicine
gies, or colds	Seizure medicine
Barbiturates	Tricyclic an-
Narcotics	tidepressants
Prescription pain	(medicine for
medicine	depression)

—if you are now taking or have taken within the past 2 weeks monoamine oxidase (MAO) inhibitors such as:

Isocarboxazid	Phenelzine
Pargyline	Tranylcypromine

Proper Use of This Medicine

Take this medicine only as directed. Do not take more of it and do not take it more often than recommended on the label, unless otherwise directed by your doctor. If too much is taken, the barbiturate in this medicine may become habit-forming.

This medicine works best when taken with a glass of water on an empty stomach (either 30 minutes to 1 hour before meals or 2 hours after meals) since that way it will get into the blood sooner. However, in some cases your doctor may want you to take this medicine with meals or right after meals to lessen stomach upset. If you have any questions about how you should be taking this medicine, check with your doctor.

If you miss a dose of this medicine and you remember within an hour or so of the missed dose, take it right away. Then go back to your regular dosing schedule. But if you do not remember until later, do not take the missed dose at all and do not double the next one. Instead, go back to your regular dosing schedule. If you have any questions about this, check with your doctor or pharmacist.

Precautions While Using This Medicine

The theophylline in this medicine may add to the central nervous system stimulant effects of caffeine-containing beverages such as tea, coffee, cocoa, and cola drinks. *Avoid drinking large amounts of these beverages while taking this medicine.* If you have any questions about this, check with your doctor.

The barbiturate in this medicine will add to the effects of alcohol and other medicines (CNS depressants) that slow down the nervous system. Some examples of CNS depressants are antihistamines or medicine for hay fever, other allergies, or colds; sedatives, tranquilizers, or sleeping medicine; prescription pain medicine or narcotics; barbiturates; medicine for seizures; tricyclic antidepressants (medicine for depression); or anesthetics, including some dental anesthetics. *Check with your doctor before taking any of the above while you are using this medicine.*

This medicine may cause some people to become dizzy, lightheaded, drowsy, or less alert than they are normally. *Make sure you know how you react to this medicine before you drive, use machines, or do other jobs that require you to be alert.*

Side Effects of This Medicine

Along with its needed effects, a medicine may cause some unwanted effects. Although not all of these side effects appear very often, when they do occur they may require medical attention. Check with your doctor or pharmacist if the following side effect occurs:

Rare
   Skin rash or hives

Other side effects may occur which usually do not require medical attention. These side effects may go away during treatment as your body adjusts to the medicine. However, check with your doctor or pharmacist if any of the following side effects continue or are bothersome:

More common

Drowsiness	Nervousness or
Headache	restlessness
Irritability	Stomach pain
Nausea or vomiting	Trouble in sleeping

Less common

Diarrhea	Flushing or redness
Difficult urination	of face
Dizziness or	Loss of appetite
lightheadedness	Unusually fast or
Feeling of warmth	pounding heart-beat

Other side effects not listed above may also occur in some patients. If you notice any other effects, check with your doctor or pharmacist.

THEOPHYLLINE, EPHEDRINE, AND HYDROXYZINE (Systemic)

Some commonly used brand names are:

Asminorel	Marax
E.T.H. Compound	Theophozine
Hydrophed	Theozine

Theophylline (thee-OFF-i-lin), ephedrine (e-FED-rin), and hydroxyzine (hye-DROX-i-zeen) is a combination medicine that belongs to the group of medicines called bronchodilators. It is used in the treatment of bronchial asthma, chronic bronchitis, emphysema, and other lung diseases. It relieves wheezing, shortness of breath, and troubled breathing. This medicine is available only with your doctor's prescription.

Before Using This Medicine

In order to decide on the best treatment for your medical problem, your doctor should be told:

—if you have ever had any unusual reaction to aminophylline, caffeine, dyphylline, oxtriphylline, theobromine, or theophylline.

—if you have ever had any unusual reaction to ephedrine or medicines like ephedrine such as amphetamines, epinephrine, isoproterenol, metaproterenol, norepinephrine (levarterenol), phenylephrine, phenylpropanolamine, pseudoephedrine, or terbutaline.

—if you are pregnant or if you intend to become pregnant while using this medicine. Use of theophylline (contained in this combination medicine) during pregnancy may cause unwanted effects in the newborn infant. In addition, although the theophylline, ephedrine, and hydroxyzine in this combination medicine have not been shown to cause birth defects in humans, the chance always exists.

—if you are breast-feeding an infant. The theophylline, ephedrine, and possibly hydroxyzine in this combination medicine pass into the breast milk and may cause unwanted effects in infants of mothers taking this medicine.

—if you have any of the following medical problems:

Diabetes	Kidney disease
Enlarged prostate	Liver disease
Heart or blood vessel disease	Overactive thyroid Stomach ulcer
High blood pressure	(or history of)

—if you are now taking any of the following medicines or types of medicine:

Amphetamines	Lithium
Clindamycin	Methylergonovine
Digitalis glycosides (heart medicine)	Other medicine for asthma or
Ergonovine	breathing
Erythromycin	problems
Guanethidine	Propranolol
Lincomycin	Troleandomycin

—if you are now taking central nervous system (CNS) depressants such as:

Antihistamines or medicine for hay fever, other allergies, or colds	Prescription pain medicine
	Sedatives, tranquilizers, or sleeping medicine
Barbiturates	
Medicine for seizures	Tricyclic antidepressants (medicine for depression)
Narcotics	

—if you are now taking or have taken within the past 2 weeks monoamine oxidase (MAO) inhibitors such as:

Isocarboxazid	Phenelzine
Pargyline	Tranylcypromine

Proper Use of This Medicine

Take this medicine only as directed. Do not take more of it and do not take it more often than your doctor ordered. To do so may increase the chance of side effects.

This medicine works best when taken with a glass of water on an empty stomach (either 30 minutes to 1 hour before meals or 2 hours after meals) since that way it will get into the blood sooner. However, in some cases your doctor may want you to take this medicine with meals or right after meals to lessen stomach upset. If you have any questions about how you should be taking this medicine, check with your doctor.

If you miss a dose of this medicine and you remember within an hour or so of the missed dose, take it right away. Then go back to your regular dosing schedule. But if you do not remember until later, do not take the missed dose at all and do not double the next one. Instead, go back to your regular dosing schedule. If you have any questions about this, check with your doctor.

Precautions While Using This Medicine

The theophylline in this medicine may add to the central nervous system stimulant effects of caffeine-containing beverages such as tea, coffee, cocoa, and cola drinks. *Avoid drinking large amounts of these beverages while taking this medicine.* If you have any questions about this, check with your doctor.

The hydroxyzine in this medicine will add to the effects of alcohol and other medicines (CNS depressants) that slow down the nervous system. Some examples of CNS depressants are antihistamines or medicine for hay fever, other allergies, or colds; sedatives, tranquilizers, or sleeping medicine; prescription pain medicine or narcotics; barbiturates; medicine for seizures; tricyclic antidepressants (medicine for depression); or anesthetics, including dental anesthetics. *Check with your doctor before taking any of the above while you are taking this medicine.*

This medicine may cause some people to become dizzy, lightheaded, drowsy, or less alert than they are normally. *Make sure you know how you react to this medicine before you drive, use machines, or do other jobs that require you to be alert.*

Side Effects of This Medicine

Along with its needed effects, a medicine may cause some unwanted effects. Although not all of these side effects appear very often, when they do occur they may require medical attention. Check with your doctor if the following side effect occurs:

Rare

Skin rash or hives

Other side effects may occur which usually do not require medical attention. These side effects may go away during treatment as your body adjusts to the medicine. However, check with your doctor if any of the following side effects continue or are bothersome:

More common

Drowsiness	Nervousness or
Headache	restlessness
Irritability	Stomach pain
Nausea or vomiting	Trouble in sleeping

Less common

Diarrhea	Flushing or redness
Difficult urination	of face
Dizziness or	Loss of appetite
lightheadedness	Unusually fast or
Feeling of warmth	pounding heart-
	beat

Other side effects not listed above may also occur in some patients. If you notice any other effects, check with your doctor.

THEOPHYLLINE AND GUAIFENESIN
(Systemic)
[Formerly called Theophylline and Glyceryl Guaiacolate]

Some commonly used brand names are:

Asbron G	Glyceryl T	Slo-Phyllin GG
Asma	Hylate	Synophylate-
Cerylin	Lanophyllin-	GG
Dialixir	GG	Theo-Col
Glybron	Quibron	Theo-Guaia

Theophylline (thee-OFF-i-lin) and guaifenesin (gwye-FEN-e-sin) is a combination medicine that belongs to the group of medicines called bronchodilators. It is used in the treatment of bronchial asthma, chronic bronchitis, emphysema, and other lung diseases. It relieves wheezing, shortness of breath, and troubled breathing. This medicine is available only with your doctor's prescription.

Before Using This Medicine

In order to decide on the best treatment for your medical problem, your doctor should be told:

—if you have ever had any unusual reaction to aminophylline, caffeine, dyphylline, oxtriphylline, theobromine, or theophylline.

—if you are pregnant or if you intend to become pregnant while using this medicine. Use of theophylline (contained in this combination medicine) during pregnancy may cause unwanted effects in the newborn infant. In addition, although theophylline and guaifenesin combination has not been shown to cause birth defects or other problems, the chance always exists.

—if you are breast-feeding an infant. Theophylline (contained in this combination medicine) passes into the breast milk and may cause irritability or other side effects in infants.

—if you have any of the following medical problems:

Heart disease	Liver disease
High blood pressure	Overactive thyroid
Kidney disease	Stomach ulcer (or
	history of)

—if you are now taking any of the following medicines or types of medicine:

Clindamycin	Other medicine for
Erythromycin	asthma or
Lincomycin	breathing
Lithium	problems
	Propranolol
	Troleandomycin

Proper Use of This Medicine

Take this medicine only as directed. Do not take more of it, do not take it more often, and do not take it for a longer period of time than your doctor ordered. To do so may increase the chance of side effects.

This medicine works best when taken with a glass of water on an empty stomach (either 30 minutes to 1 hour before meals or 2 hours after meals) since that way it will get into the blood sooner. However, in some cases your doctor may want you to take this medicine with meals or right after meals to lessen stomach upset. If you have any questions about how you should be taking this medicine, check with your doctor.

If you miss a dose of this medicine and remember within an hour or so of the missed dose, take it right away. Then go back to your regular dosing schedule. But if you do not remember until later, do not take the missed dose at all and do

not double the next one. Instead, go back to your regular dosing schedule. If you have any questions about this, check with your doctor.

Precautions While Using This Medicine

Your doctor should check your progress at regular visits, especially for the first few weeks after you begin taking this medicine.

The theophylline in this medicine may add to the central nervous system stimulant effects of caffeine-containing beverages such as tea, coffee, cocoa, and cola drinks. *Avoid drinking large amounts of these beverages while taking this medicine.* If you have any questions about this, check with your doctor.

Side Effects of This Medicine

Along with its needed effects, a medicine may cause some unwanted effects. Although not all of these side effects appear very often, when they do occur they may require medical attention. Check with your doctor if any of the following side effects occur:

Rare

Skin rash or hives

Possible signs of overdose of theophylline

Bloody or black tarry stools	Unusual tiredness or weakness
Cloudy urine	Unusually fast,
Increased urination	pounding, or irregular heartbeat
Mental confusion	ular heartbeat
Muscle twitching	Vomiting blood or
Seizures	material that
Unusual thirst	looks like coffee grounds

Other side effects may occur which usually do not require medical attention. These side effects may go away during treatment as your body adjusts to the medicine. However, check with your doctor if any of the following side effects continue or are bothersome:

More common

Headache	Stomach pain
Irritability	Trouble in sleeping
Nausea	Vomiting
Nervousness or restlessness	

Less common

Diarrhea	Loss of appetite
Dizziness or lightheadedness	Unusually fast breathing
Flushing or redness of face	

Other side effects not listed above may also occur in some patients. If you notice any other effects, check with your doctor.

THIAZIDE DIURETICS (Systemic)

This information applies to the following medicines:

Bendroflumethiazide (ben-droe-floo-meth-EYE-a-zide)
Benzthiazide (benz-THYE-a-zide)
Chlorothiazide (klor-oh-THYE-a-zide)
Chlorthalidone (klor-THAL-i-doan)
Cyclothiazide (sye-kloe-THYE-a-zide)
Hydrochlorothiazide (hye-droe-klor-oh-THYE-a-zide)
Hydroflumethiazide (hye-droe-floo-meth-EYE-a-zide)
Methyclothiazide (meth-ee-kloe-THYE-a-zide)
Metolazone (me-TOLE-a-zone)
Polythiazide (pol-i-THYE-a-zide)
Quinethazone (kwin-ETH-a-zone)
Trichlormethiazide (trye-klor-meth-EYE-a-zide)

Some commonly used brand names are:	Generic names:
Naturetin	Bendroflumethiazide
Aquastat Aquatag Exna Hydrex	Benzthiazide
Diuril SK-Chlorothiazide	Chlorothiazide
Hygroton Novothalidone* Uridon	Chlorthalidone
Anhydron	Cyclothiazide
Esidrix Hydro-Aquil HydroDIURIL Novohydrazide* Oretic	Hydrochlorothiazide
Diucardin Saluron	Hydroflumethiazide
Aquatensen Duretic Enduron	Methyclothiazide
Diulo Zaroxolyn	Metolazone
Renese	Polythiazide
Hydromox	Quinethazone
Metahydrin Naqua	Trichlormethiazide

*Not available in the United States.

This medicine is a thiazide or thiazide-like diuretic. It is commonly used to treat high blood pressure. It is used also to help reduce the amount of water in the body by increasing the flow of urine. Thiazide diuretics may also be used for other conditions as determined by your doctor. They are available only with your doctor's prescription.

Before Using This Medicine

In order to decide on the best treatment for your medical problem, your doctor should be told:

—if you are allergic to sulfonamides (sulfa drugs) or any of the thiazide diuretics.

—if you are pregnant or if you intend to become pregnant while using this medicine. When this medicine is used during pregnancy, it may cause side effects in the newborn infant. In addition, although this medicine has not been shown to cause birth defects, the chance always exists.

—if you are breast-feeding an infant. Although thiazide diuretics have not been shown to cause problems, the chance always exists.

—if you have any of the following medical problems:

Diabetes	Kidney disease
Gout	Liver disease
History of lupus erythematosus	Pancreas disease

—if you are now taking any of the following medicines or types of medicine:

Colestipol	Lithium
Corticosteroids (cortisone-like medicines)	Methenamine
	Oral anticoagulants (blood thinners you take by mouth)
Corticotropin (ACTH)	
Diabetes medicine	
Digitalis glycosides (heart medicine)	Other diuretics (water pills) or antihypertensives (high blood pressure medicine)
Gout medicine	

Proper Use of This Medicine

This medicine may cause you to have an unusual feeling of tiredness when you begin to take it. You may also notice an increase in the amount of urine or in your frequency of urination. After taking the medicine for a while, these effects should lessen. In order to keep the increase in urine from affecting your nighttime sleep:

—if you are to take a single dose a day, take it in the morning after breakfast.

—if you are to take more than one dose a day, take the last dose no later than 6 p.m., unless otherwise directed by your doctor.

However, it is best to plan your dose or doses according to a schedule that will least affect your personal activities and sleep. Ask your doctor, nurse, or pharmacist to help you plan the best time to take this medicine.

In order to help remember to take your medicine, try to get into the habit of taking it at the same time each day.

If you miss a dose of this medicine, take it as soon as possible. If it is almost time for your next dose, do not take the missed dose at all and do not double the next one. Instead, go back to your regular dosing schedule. If you have any questions about this, check with your doctor.

For patients taking this medicine for high blood pressure:

• Importance of Diet—When prescribing medicine for your condition, your doctor may also prescribe a personal diet for you. Such a diet may be low in sodium (salt). Medicine is usually more effective when this diet is properly followed.

Also, it may be very important for you to go on a reducing diet. However, check with your doctor before going on any diet.

• Many patients who have high blood pressure will not notice any signs of the problem. In fact, many may feel normal. It is very important that you take your medicine exactly as directed and that you keep your doctor's appointments even if you feel well.

• Remember that this medicine will not cure your high blood pressure but it does control it. Therefore, you must continue to take it as directed if you expect to keep your blood pressure down. *You may have to take medicine for the rest of your life.* If high blood pressure is not treated, it can cause serious problems such as heart failure, blood vessel disease, stroke, or kidney disease.

Precautions While Using This Medicine

It is important that your doctor check your progress at regular visits.

This medicine may cause a loss of potassium from your body. To help prevent this, your doctor may want you to:

—eat or drink foods that have a high potassium content (for example, orange or other citrus fruit juices), or

—take a potassium supplement, or

—take another medicine to help prevent the loss of the potassium in the first place.

It is very important to follow these directions. Also, it is important not to change your diet on your own. This is more important if you are already on a special diet (as for diabetes), or if you are taking a potassium supplement or a medicine to reduce potassium loss. Extra potassium may not be necessary and, in some cases, too much potassium could be harmful.

Check with your doctor if you become sick and have severe or continuing vomiting or diarrhea. These problems may cause you to lose additional water and potassium.

Caution: Diabetics—Thiazide diuretics may raise blood sugar levels. While you are using this medicine, be especially careful in testing for sugar in your urine. If you have any questions about this, check with your doctor.

A few people who take this medicine may become more sensitive to sunlight than they are normally. When you begin to take this medicine, avoid too much sun or use of a sunlamp until you see how you react, especially if you tend to burn easily. If you have a severe reaction, check with your doctor.

For patients taking this medicine for high blood pressure:

• *Do not take other medicines unless they have been discussed with your doctor.* This especially includes over-the-counter (nonprescription) medicines for appetite control, asthma, colds cough, hay fever, or sinus.

Side Effects of This Medicine

Along with its needed effects, a medicine may cause some unwanted effects. Although not all of these side effects appear very often, when they do occur they may require medical attention. Check with your doctor if any of the following side effects occur:

Rare

Severe stomach pain with nausea and vomiting	Unusual bleeding or bruising
Skin rash or hives	Yellowing of eyes or skin
Unexplained sore throat and fever	

Signs of too much potassium loss

Dryness of mouth	Irregular heartbeats
Increased thirst	Mood or mental changes

Muscle cramps or pain	Unusual tiredness or weakness
Nausea or vomiting	Weak pulse

Other side effects may occur which usually do not require medical attention. These side effects may go away during treatment as your body adjusts to the medicine. However, check with your doctor if any of the following side effects continue or are bothersome:

Less common

Diarrhea	Increased sensitivity of skin to sunlight
Dizziness or light-headedness when getting up from a lying or sitting position	Loss of appetite
	Upset stomach

Other side effects not listed above may also occur in some patients. If you notice any other effects, check with your doctor.

THIOGUANINE (Systemic)

Thioguanine (thye-oh-GWON-een) belongs to the group of medicines known as antimetabolites. It is used to treat some kinds of cancer as well as some noncancerous conditions. It is used also in some situations to reduce the body's natural immunity. Thioguanine is available only with your doctor's prescription.

Before Using This Medicine

Thioguanine is a very strong medicine. In addition to its helpful effects in treating your medical problem, it has side effects that could be very serious. Before you take this medicine, be sure that you have discussed the use of it with your doctor.

In order to decide on the best treatment for your medical problem, your doctor should be told:

—if you have ever had any unusual reaction to thioguanine in the past.

—if you are pregnant or if you intend to have children. This medicine may cause birth defects if either the male or female is taking it at the time of conception or if it is taken during pregnancy. It may also cause permanent sterility after it has been taken for a while. Be sure that you have discussed this with your doctor before taking this medicine.

—if you are breast-feeding an infant. Although thioguanine has not been shown to cause problems, the chance always exists.

—if you have any of the following medical problems:

Blood disease   Kidney disease
Gout   Kidney stones
Infection   Liver disease

—if you are taking gout medicine.

—if you have been treated with x-rays or cancer drugs by another doctor.

Proper Use of This Medicine

Use this medicine only as directed by your doctor. Do not use more or less of it, and do not use it more often than your doctor ordered.

This medicine is sometimes given together with certain other medicines. If you are using a combination of drugs, make sure that you take each medicine at the right time and do not mix them. Ask your doctor, nurse, or pharmacist to help you plan a way to take your medicine at the right time.

Do not stop using this medicine without first checking with your doctor.

If you miss a dose of this medicine, do not take the missed dose at all and do not double the next one. Instead, go back to your regular dosing schedule and check with your doctor.

Precautions While Using This Medicine

It is very important that your doctor check your progress at regular visits.

While you are using this medicine, your doctor may want you to drink plenty of fluids and urinate often. This will help prevent kidney problems and keep your kidneys working well. If you have any questions about this, check with your doctor.

Side Effects of This Medicine

Along with its needed effects, a medicine may cause some unwanted effects. Although not all of these side effects appear very often, when they do occur they may require medical attention. Check with your doctor *immediately* if any of the following side effects occur:

More common

Unexplained fever,   Yellowing of eyes
chills, or sore   and skin
throat
Unusual bleeding or
bruising

Less common

Flank or stomach   Unsteadiness when
pain   walking
Joint pain   Swelling of feet or
Loss of appetite   lower legs
Nausea and
vomiting

Rare

Black tarry stools
Sores in the mouth
and on the lips

Other side effects may occur which usually do not require medical attention. These side effects may go away during treatment as your body adjusts to the medicine. However, check with your doctor if any of the following side effects continue or are bothersome:

Less common

Diarrhea
Skin rash or itching

After you stop using this medicine, it may still produce some side effects that need attention. During this period of time check with your doctor if you notice any of the following side effects:

Unexplained fever,   Unusual bleeding or
chills, or sore   bruising
throat

Other side effects not listed above may also occur in some patients. If you notice any other effects, check with your doctor.

THIOTEPA (Systemic)

Thiotepa (thye-oh-TEP-a) belongs to the group of medicines called alkylating agents. It is used by injection to treat some kinds of cancer. Thiotepa is available only on prescription and is to be administered only by or under the immediate supervision of your doctor.

Before Using This Medicine

Thiotepa is a very strong medicine. In addition to its helpful effects in treating your medical problem, it has side effects that could be very serious. Before you receive this medicine, be sure that you have discussed the use of it with your doctor.

In order to decide on the best treatment for your medical problem, your doctor should be told:

—if you have ever had any unusual reaction to thiotepa in the past.

—if you are pregnant or if you intend to have children. This medicine may cause birth defects if either the male or female is using it at the time of conception or if it is used during pregnancy. It may also cause permanent sterility after it has been used for a while. Be sure that you have discussed this with your doctor before using this medicine.

—if you are breast-feeding an infant. Although thiotepa has not been shown to cause problems, the chance always exists.

—if you have any of the following medical problems:

Blood disease
Gout
Infection

Kidney disease
Kidney stones
Liver disease

—if you are taking gout medicine.

—if you have been treated with x-rays or cancer drugs by another doctor.

Proper Use of This Medicine

This medicine sometimes causes nausea, vomiting, and loss of appetite. However, it is very important that you continue to receive the medicine, even if you begin to feel ill. If you have any questions about this, check with your doctor.

Precautions While Using This Medicine

It is very important that your doctor check your progress at regular visits.

While you are using this medicine, your doctor may want you to drink plenty of fluids and urinate often. This will help prevent kidney problems and keep your kidneys working well. If you have any questions about this, check with your doctor.

Before having any kind of surgery, including dental surgery, make sure the doctor or dentist in charge knows that you are taking this medicine.

Side Effects of This Medicine

Along with its needed effects, a medicine may cause some unwanted effects. Although not all of these side effects appear very often, when they do occur they may require medical attention. Check with your doctor if any of the following side effects occur:

More common

Unexplained fever, chills, or sore throat

Unusual bleeding or bruising

Less common

Flank or stomach pain
Joint pain

Swelling of feet and lower legs

Rare

Painful or difficult urination
Skin rash

Tightness of throat
Wheezing

Other side effects may occur which usually do not require medical attention. These side effects may go away during treatment as your body adjusts to the medicine. However, check with your doctor if any of the following side effects continue or are bothersome:

Less common

Dizziness
Hives
Loss of appetite
Loss of hair

Missing menstrual periods
Nausea and vomiting
Pain at place of injection or instillation

This medicine may cause a temporary loss of hair in some people. After treatment with thiotepa has ended, normal hair growth should return.

After you stop using this medicine, it may still produce some side effects that need attention. During this period of time check with your doctor if you notice any of the following:

Unexplained fever, chills, or sore throat

Unusual bleeding or bruising

Other side effects not listed above may also occur in some patients. If you notice any other effects, check with your doctor.

THIOXANTHENES (Systemic)

This information applies to the following medicines:

Chlorprothixene (klor-proe-THIX-een)
Thiothixene (thye-oh-THIX-een)

Some commonly used brand names are:	Generic names:
Taractan
Tarasan*	Chlorprothixene
Navane	Thiothixene

*Not available in the United States.

This medicine belongs to the general family of medicines known as thioxanthenes. It is used in the treatment of nervous, mental, and emotional conditions. This medicine is available only with your doctor's prescription.

Before Using This Medicine

In order to decide on the best treatment for your medical problem, your doctor should be told:

—if you have ever had any unusual reaction to other thioxanthene or phenothiazine medicines. This medicine should not be taken if you are allergic to it.

—if you are pregnant, if you intend to become pregnant, or if you are breast-feeding an infant. Although thioxanthenes have not been shown to cause problems, the chance always exists.

—if you have any of the following medical problems:

Alcoholism	Lung disease
Blood disease	Parkinson's disease
Glaucoma	Prostate enlarge-
Heart or circulation	ment
disease	Stomach ulcers
Liver disease	Urination problems

—if you are now taking any of the following medicines or types of medicine:

Amphetamines	Epinephrine
Antacids	Guanethidine (high
Anticonvulsants	blood pressure
(seizure medicine)	medicine)
Antidiarrhea	Levodopa
medicine	Stomach ulcer
Asthma medicine	medicine

—if you are now taking central nervous system (CNS) depressants such as:

Antihistamines or	Sedatives, tran-
medicine for hay	quilizers,
fever, other aller-	or sleeping
gies, or colds	medicine
Barbiturates	Tricyclic an-
Narcotics	tidepressants
Prescription pain	(medicine for
medicine	depression)

—if you are now taking or have taken within the past 2 weeks monoamine oxidase (MAO) inhibitors such as:

Isocarboxazid	Phenelzine
Pargyline	Tranylcypromine

Proper Use of This Medicine

Do not take more of this medicine or take it more often than your doctor ordered. This is particularly important when it is given to children, since they may react very strongly to the effects of the medicine.

This medicine may be taken with food or a full glass (8 ounces) of water or milk to reduce stomach irritation. Liquid forms of this medicine may be taken undiluted or mixed with milk, water, fruit juice, or carbonated beverages.

Sometimes this medicine must be taken for several weeks before its full effect is reached in the treatment of certain mental and emotional conditions.

If you miss a dose of this medicine, take it as soon as possible. If it is 2 hours or less until your next dose, do not take the missed dose at all and do not double the next one. Instead, go back to your regular dosing schedule. If you have any questions about this, check with your doctor.

Precautions While Using This Medicine

Your doctor should check your progress at regular visits, especially for the first few months you take this medicine.

Do not stop taking this medicine without first checking with your doctor. Your doctor may want you to reduce gradually the amount you are taking before stopping completely.

This medicine will add to the effects of alcohol and other medicines (CNS depressants) that slow down the nervous system. Some examples of CNS depressants are antihistamines or medicine for hay fever, other allergies, or colds; sedatives, tranquilizers, or sleeping medicine; prescription pain medicine or narcotics; barbiturates; medicine for seizures; tricyclic antidepressants (medicine for depression); or anesthetics, including some dental anesthetics. *Check with your doctor before taking any of the above while you are using this medicine.*

This medicine may cause some people to become drowsy or less alert than they are normally, especially during the first few weeks the medicine is being taken. Even if you take this medicine only at bedtime, you may feel drowsy or less alert on arising. *Make sure you know how you react to this medicine before you drive, use machines, or do other jobs that require you to be alert.*

Dizziness, lightheadedness, or fainting may occur, especially when you get up from a lying or sitting position. Getting up slowly may help. If the problem continues or gets worse, check with your doctor.

Sometimes, patients may show signs of restlessness and excitement after taking this medicine. If this occurs, stop taking the medicine and check with your doctor.

This medicine will often make you sweat less, causing your body temperature to increase. Use extra care not to become overheated during exercise or hot weather while you are taking this medicine, since overheating could possibly result in heat stroke. Also, hot baths or saunas may make you feel dizzy or faint while you are taking this medicine.

A few people who take this medicine may become more sensitive to sunlight than they are normally. When you first begin taking this medicine, avoid too much sun or too much use of a sunlamp until you see how you react. If you have a severe reaction, check with your doctor.

Do not take this medicine within an hour of taking antacids or medicine for diarrhea. Taking them too close together may make this medicine less effective.

Try to avoid getting liquid forms of this medicine on the skin or clothing since skin rash and signs of other irritation have been caused by similar medicines.

Side Effects of This Medicine

Along with its needed effects, a medicine may cause some unwanted effects. Although not all of these side effects appear very often, when they do occur they may require medical attention. Check with your doctor if any of the following side effects occur:

More common for chlorprothixene; less common for thiothixene

Fainting	Tic-like (jerky)
Muscle spasms,	movements of
especially of neck	head, face,
and back	mouth, and neck
Restlessness	Trembling and
Shuffling walk	shaking of hands
	and fingers

Less common

Fine, worm-like	Skin rashes
movements of	
tongue	

Rare

Eye problems	Yellowing of eyes
Unexplained sore	and skin
throat and fever	

Other side effects may occur which usually do not require medical attention. These side effects may go away during treatment as your body adjusts to the medicine. However, check with your doctor if any of the following side effects continue or are bothersome:

More common

Blurred vision	Dry mouth
Constipation	Increased sensitivity
Decreased sweating	to sun
Dizziness	Nasal congestion
Drowsiness	Unusually fast
	heartbeat

Less common

Changes in	Difficult urination
menstrual	Swelling of breasts
period	
Decreased sexual	
ability	

Although not all of the side effects listed above have been reported for both of these medicines, they have been reported for at least one of them. However, since chlorprothixene and thiothixene are very similar, any of the above side effects may occur with either of these medicines.

Other side effects not listed above may also occur in some patients. If you notice any other effects, check with your doctor.

THYROID HORMONES (Systemic)

This information applies to the following medicines:

Levothyroxine (lee-voe-thye-ROX-een)
Liothyronine (lye-oh-THYE-roe-neen)
Liotrix (LYE-oh-trix)
Thyroglobulin (thye-roe-GLOB-yoo-lin)
Thyroid (THYE-roid)

This information does not apply to Thyrotropin.

Some commonly used brand names are:	Generic names:
Levothroid	
L-T-S	
Ro-Thyroxine	Levothyroxine
Synthroid	

Cytomel Ro-Thyronine Tertroxin	Liothyronine
Euthroid	Liotrix
Proloid	Thyroglobulin
S-P-T Thyrar Thyrocrine	Thyroid

Thyroid medicines belong to the general group of medicines called hormones. They are used when the thyroid gland does not produce enough hormone. These medicines are available only with your doctor's prescription.

Before Using This Medicine

In order to decide on the best treatment for your medical problem, your doctor should be told:

—if you have ever had any unusual reaction to thyroid medicine in the past.

—if you are pregnant, if you intend to become pregnant, or if you are breast-feeding an infant. Although thyroid hormones have not been shown to cause problems, the chance always exists.

—if you have any of the following medical problems:

Diabetes	Kidney disease
Hardening of the arteries	Underactive adrenal gland
Heart disease	Underactive pituitary gland
High blood pressure	
History of overactive thyroid	

—if you are now taking or have recently taken any of the following medicines or types of medicine:

Anticoagulants (blood thinners)	Diabetes medicine you take by mouth or injection
Cholestyramine	Phenytoin
Cough syrup or cold medicine	Tricyclic antidepressants (medicine for depression)

Proper Use of This Medicine

Use this medicine only as directed by your doctor. Do not use more or less of it, and do not use it more often than your doctor ordered. Your doctor has prescribed the exact amount your body needs and if you take different amounts, you may experience symptoms of an overactive or underactive thyroid. Take it at the same time each day, to make sure it has the best effect.

If you miss a dose of this medicine, take it as soon as possible. If it is almost time for your next dose, do not take the missed dose at all and do not double the next one. Instead, go back to your regular dosing schedule. If you miss more than one dose or if you have any questions about this, check with your doctor.

If your condition is due to a lack of thyroid hormone, you may have to take this medicine for the rest of your life. It is very important that you *do not stop taking this medicine without first checking with your doctor.*

For patients taking the enteric-coated tablet form of thyroid:

• The enteric-coated tablets are to be swallowed whole and must not be chewed or crushed.

Precautions While Using This Medicine

It is very important that your doctor check your progress at regular visits.

If you have some kinds of heart disease, this medicine may cause chest pain or shortness of breath when you exert yourself. *Do not overdo exercise or physical work.* If you have any questions about this, check with your doctor.

Before having any kind of surgery (including dental surgery) or emergency treatment, *tell the doctor or dentist in charge that you are taking this medicine.*

Do not take any other medicine unless prescribed by your doctor. This especially includes over-the-counter (OTC) or nonprescription medicine such as that for colds, cough, asthma, hay fever, or appetite control. Some medicines may increase or decrease the effects of thyroid on your body and cause problems in controlling your condition. Also, thyroid may change the effects of other medicines.

Side Effects of This Medicine

Along with its needed effects, a medicine may cause some unwanted effects. Although not all of these side effects appear very often, when they do occur they may require medical attention. Check with your doctor *immediately* if any of the following side effects occur since they may indicate an overdose or an allergic reaction:

Chest pain	Shortness of breath
Hives	Skin rash
Rapid or irregular heartbeat	

This medicine may take a few days or weeks to have a noticeable effect on your condition. Until it begins to work, you may experience some symptoms. Check with your doctor if the following symptoms continue or are bothersome:

Coldness	Sleepiness
Constipation	Tiredness
Dry, puffy skin	Unusual weight gain
Listlessness	Weakness
Muscle aches	

Other effects may occur if the dose of the medicine is not exactly right. These side effects will go away when the dose is corrected. Check with your doctor if any of the following symptoms occur:

Changes in appetite	Irritability
Changes in	Leg cramps
menstrual	Nervousness
periods	Sensitivity to heat
Diarrhea	Sleeplessness
Fever	Unusual sweating
Hand tremors	Vomiting
Headache	Weight loss

Other side effects not listed above may also occur in some patients. If you notice any other effects, check with your doctor.

THYROTROPIN (Systemic)
Some commonly used brand names are Thyrotron and Thytropar.

Thyrotropin (thye-roe-TROE-pin) belongs to the general group of medicines called hormones. It is used by injection as a test to determine how well your thyroid is working. It is also sometimes used with other treatment for cancer of the thyroid. Thyrotropin is available only on prescription and is to be administered only by or under the immediate supervision of your doctor.

Before Using This Medicine

In order to decide on the best treatment for your medical problem, your doctor should be told:

—if you have ever had any unusual reaction to thyrotropin in the past.

—if you are pregnant, if you intend to become pregnant, or if you are breast-feeding an infant. Although thyrotropin has not been shown to cause problems, the chance always exists.

—if you have any of the following medical problems:

Hardening of the	Underactive adrenal
arteries	gland
Heart disease	Underactive pi-
High blood pressure	tuitary gland

Proper Use of This Medicine

In order for your doctor to properly treat your medical condition, *you must receive every dose of this medicine.* After the last dose, the doctor may want to perform certain tests which are very important.

Side Effects of This Medicine

Along with its needed effects, a medicine may cause some unwanted effects. Although not all of these side effects appear very often, when they do occur they may require medical attention. Check with your doctor *immediately* if any of the following side effects occur:

Rare

Faintness	Skin rash
Itching	Tightness of throat
Redness or swelling	Wheezing
at place of	
injection	

Other effects may occur if the dose of the medicine is not exactly right. Check with your doctor if any of the following symptoms occur:

Chest pain	Rapid or irregular
Irritability	heartbeat
Nervousness	Shortness of breath
	Unusual sweating

Other side effects may occur which usually do not require medical attention. These side effects may go away during treatment as your body adjusts to the medicine. However, check with your doctor if any of the following side effects continue or are bothersome:

More common

Flushing of face	Stomach discomfort
Headache	Unusually frequent
Nausea and	urge to urinate
vomiting	

Other side effects not listed above may also occur in some patients. If you notice any other effects, check with your doctor.

TIMOLOL (Ophthalmic)
A commonly used brand name is Timoptic.

Timolol (TYE-moe-lole) is used in the eye to treat certain types of glaucoma. This medicine is available only with your doctor's prescription.

Before Using This Medicine

In order to decide on the best treatment for your medical problem, your doctor should be told:

—if you have ever had any unusual reaction to timolol in the past. This medicine should not be used if you are allergic to it.

—if you are pregnant, if you intend to become pregnant, or if you are breast-feeding an infant. Although timolol has not been shown to cause problems, the chance always exists.

—if you have any of the following medical problems:

Asthma   Myasthenia gravis
Heart disease

Proper Use of This Medicine

Use this medicine only as directed. Do not use more of it and do not use it more often than your doctor ordered. To do so may increase the chance of too much medicine being absorbed into the body and the chance of side effects.

How to apply this medicine: First, wash hands. Tilt head back and pull lower eyelid away from eye to form a pouch. Drop the medicine into the pouch and gently close eyes. Do not blink. Keep eyes closed for 1 or 2 minutes to allow the medicine to be absorbed.

To prevent contamination of the eye drops, do not touch the applicator tip to any surface (including the eye) and keep the container tightly closed.

If you miss a dose of this medicine and your dosing schedule is one dose to be applied:

Once a day—
Apply the missed dose as soon as possible. Then go back to your regular dosing schedule. But if you do not remember the missed dose until the next day, do not apply it at all. Instead, apply your regularly scheduled dose.

More than once a day—
Apply the missed dose as soon as possible. Then go back to your regular dosing schedule. But if it is almost time for your next dose, do not apply the missed dose at all. Instead, apply your next dose at the regularly scheduled time. Then continue with your regular dosing schedule.

If you have any questions about this, check with your doctor.

Precautions While Using This Medicine

Your doctor should check your eye pressure at regular visits.

Side Effects of This Medicine

Along with its needed effects, a medicine may cause some unwanted effects. Although not all of these side effects appear very often, when they do occur they may require medical attention. Check with your doctor if any of the following side effects occur:

Irritation of eye

Signs of too much medicine being absorbed into the body

Mental confusion or   Unusually slow
depression   heartbeat or
Unusual tiredness or   pulse
weakness   Wheezing or troubled breathing

Other side effects not listed above may also occur in some patients. If you notice any other effects, check with your doctor.

TOLMETIN (Systemic)
A commonly used brand name is Tolectin.

Tolmetin (TOLE-met-in) is used to treat the symptoms of arthritis. It helps relieve inflammation, swelling, stiffness, and joint pain. This medicine is available only with your doctor's prescription.

Before Using This Medicine

In order to decide on the best treatment for your medical problem, your doctor should be told:

—if you have ever had any unusual reaction to aspirin or other salicylates, fenoprofen, ibuprofen, meclofenamate, naproxen, or sulindac.

—if you are pregnant, if you intend to become pregnant, or if you are breast-feeding an infant. Although tolmetin has not been shown to cause problems in humans, the chance always exists.

—if you have any of the following medical problems:

Bleeding problems   Stomach ulcer or
Heart disease   other stomach
High blood pressure   problems
Kidney disease

—if you are now taking any of the following medicines or types of medicine:

Anticoagulants   Inflammation
  (blood thinners)   medicine (for
                           example, aspirin
                           or other arthritis
                           medicine)

Proper Use of This Medicine

In order for this medicine to help you, *it must be taken regularly as ordered by your doctor.* A few days to 1 week may pass before you begin to feel better and up to 2 weeks may pass before you feel the full effects of this medicine.

It is best to take this medicine 30 minutes before meals or 2 hours after meals so that it will get into the blood more quickly. However, to lessen stomach upset, your doctor may want you to take the medicine with food, milk, or antacids. If stomach upset (indigestion, nausea, vomiting, stomach pain, or diarrhea) continues or if you have any questions about how you should be taking this medicine, check with your doctor.

If you miss a dose of this medicine, take it as soon as possible. Then go back to your regular dosing schedule. However, if it is almost time for your next dose, do not take the missed dose at all and do not double the next one. Instead, go back to your regular dosing schedule. If you have any questions about this, check with your doctor.

Precautions While Using This Medicine

Your doctor should check your progress at regular visits in order to make sure that this medicine does not cause unwanted effects.

Stomach problems may be more likely to occur if you take aspirin regularly (for example, every day) or drink alcoholic beverages while being treated with this medicine. Therefore, *do not take aspirin regularly or drink alcoholic beverages while taking this medicine,* unless otherwise directed by your doctor.

Before having any kind of surgery (including dental surgery), tell the doctor or dentist in charge that you are taking this medicine.

This medicine may cause some people to become dizzy, lightheaded, drowsy, or less alert than they are normally. *Make sure you know how you react to this medicine before you drive, use machines, or do other jobs that require you to be alert.*

Side Effects of This Medicine

Along with its needed effects, a medicine may cause some unwanted effects. Although not all of these side effects appear very often, when they do occur they may require medical attention. Check with your doctor if any of the following side effects occur:

Less common

Ringing or buzzing   Swelling of feet or
  in ears   lower legs
Skin rash, hives, or   Unusual weight gain
  itching

Rare

Bloody or black   Shortness of breath,
  tarry stools   troubled
                            breathing,
                            wheezing, or
                            tightness in
                            chest
                          Unexplained sore
                            throat and fever

Other side effects may occur which usually do not require medical attention. These side effects may go away during treatment as your body adjusts to the medicine. However, check with your doctor if any of the following side effects continue or are bothersome:

More common

Headache   Stomach pain or
Nausea   discomfort

Less common

Bloated feeling or   Drowsiness
  gas   Nervousness
Constipation   Vomiting
Diarrhea
Dizziness or
  lightheadedness

Other side effects not listed above may also occur in some patients. If you notice any other effects, check with your doctor.

TOLNAFTATE (Topical)
Some commonly used brand names are Aftate and Tinactin.

Tolnaftate (tole-NAF-tate) belongs to the group of medicines called antifungals. It is applied to the skin to treat some types of fungal infections. This medicine is available without a prescription; however, your doctor may have special instructions on the proper use of tolnaftate for your medical problem.

Before Using This Medicine
In order to decide on the best treatment for your medical problem, your doctor should be told:

—if you have ever had any unusual reaction to tolnaftate in the past. This medicine should not be used if you are allergic to it.

Proper Use of This Medicine
To help clear up your infection completely, *keep using this medicine for 2 weeks after burning, itching, or other symptoms have disappeared,* unless otherwise directed by your doctor.

Keep this medicine away from the eyes.

If you miss a dose of this medicine, apply it as soon as possible. Then go back to your regular dosing schedule. But if it is almost time for your next dose, do not apply the missed dose at all. Instead, go back to your regular dosing schedule. If you have any questions about this, check with your doctor or pharmacist.

Before applying tolnaftate, wash the area to be treated and dry thoroughly. Then apply enough medicine to cover the affected area.

If you are using the powder form of this medicine:

• If the powder is used on the feet, sprinkle it between toes, on feet, and in socks and shoes.

If you are using the aerosol powder form of this medicine:

• Shake well before using.

• From a distance of 6 to 10 inches, spray the powder on the affected areas. If it is used on the feet, spray it between toes, on feet, and in socks and shoes.

• Do not inhale the powder.

• Do not use near heat, near open flame, or while smoking.

• Store away from heat and direct sunlight. Do not puncture, break, or burn container.

If you are using the solution form of this medicine:

• If tolnaftate solution becomes a solid, it may be dissolved by warming the closed container of medicine in warm water.

If you are using the aerosol solution form of this medicine:

• Shake well before using.

• From a distance of 6 inches, spray the solution on the affected areas. If it is used on the feet, spray between toes and on feet.

• Do not inhale the vapors from the spray.

• Do not use near heat, near open flame, or while smoking.

• Store away from heat and direct sunlight. Do not puncture, break, or burn container.

If you are using the spray solution form of this medicine:

• From a distance of 4 to 6 inches, spray the solution on the affected areas. If it is used on the feet, spray between toes and on feet.

• Do not use near heat, near open flame, or while smoking.

Precautions While Using This Medicine
If your skin problem has not improved after using tolnaftate for 4 weeks, check with your doctor.

To help cure the infection and to help prevent reinfection, good health habits are required. These include the following:

• Wash all towels and bedding after each use.

• Use only freshly laundered clothes each time clothing is changed.

If you have any questions about this, check with your doctor, nurse, or pharmacist.

Also, to help prevent reinfection after the period of treatment with this medicine, the powder or spray powder form of this medicine may be used each day after bathing and careful drying.

Side Effects of This Medicine
Along with its needed effects, a medicine may cause some unwanted effects. Although not all of these side effects appear very often, when they do occur they may require medical attention. Check with your doctor or pharmacist if the following side effect occurs:

Irritation of skin not present
before using this medicine

When you apply the spray solution form of this medicine, a mild temporary stinging may be expected.

Other side effects not listed above may also occur in some patients. If you notice any other effects, check with your doctor or pharmacist.

TRETINOIN (Topical)
A commonly used brand name is Retin-A.

Tretinoin (TRET-i-noyn) is applied to the skin to treat acne. This medicine is available only with your doctor's prescription.

Before Using This Medicine

In order to decide on the best treatment for your medical problem, your doctor should be told:

—if you have ever had any unusual reaction to tretinoin in the past. This medicine should not be used if you are allergic to it.

—if you are pregnant, if you intend to become pregnant, or if you are breast-feeding an infant, although tretinoin has not been shown to cause problems.

—if you have either of the following medical problems:

  Eczema
  Sunburn

—if you are now using any topical acne preparation or preparation containing a peeling agent such as benzoyl peroxide, resorcinol, salicylic acid, or sulfur.

—if you are now using any topical alcohol-containing preparation such as after-shave lotion, astringent, cologne, perfume, or shaving cream or lotion.

—if you are now using any of the following preparations:

Abrasive soaps or cleansers	Medicated cosmetics or "cover-ups"
Cosmetics or soaps that dry the skin	Other topical medicine for the skin

Proper Use of This Medicine

It is very important that you use this medicine only as directed. Do not use more of it, do not use it more often, and do not use it for a longer period of time than your doctor ordered. To do so may cause irritation of the skin.

Do not apply this medicine to windburned or sunburned skin or on open wounds.

Do not use this medicine in or around the eyes or mouth, or inside of the nose. Spread the medicine away from these areas when applying.

If you miss a dose of this medicine, apply it as soon as possible. Then go back to your regular dosing schedule. But if you do not remember the missed dose until the next day, do not apply it at all. Instead, go back to your regular dosing schedule. If you have any questions about this, check with your doctor.

This medicine usually comes with patient directions. Read them carefully before using this medicine.

Before applying tretinoin, wash the skin with a mild or nonallergic type of soap and warm water, then gently pat dry. Wait 20 to 30 minutes before applying this medicine to make sure the skin is completely dry.

If you are using the cream or gel form of this medicine:

• Apply enough medicine to cover the affected areas, and rub in gently.

If you are using the solution form of this medicine:

• Using your fingertips, a gauze pad, or a cotton swab, apply enough tretinoin solution to cover the affected areas. If you use a gauze pad or a cotton swab for applying the medicine, avoid getting it too wet, in order to prevent the medicine from running into areas not intended for treatment.

If you are using the swab form of this medicine:

• Using the tretinoin swab, wipe gently over the affected areas.

• Do not use a swab more than once. One swab supplies enough medicine to cover an area the size of the face. If other areas are to be treated, such as the back, use another swab.

Precautions While Using This Medicine

During the first 2 or 3 weeks you are using tretinoin, your skin condition may seem to get worse before it gets better, but this is the way the medicine works. If you have any questions about this, check with your doctor.

You should avoid washing your face too often. Washing it with a mild bland soap 2 or 3 times a day should be enough, unless otherwise directed by your doctor.

You may use cosmetics (nonmedicated) while being treated with tretinoin, unless otherwise directed by your doctor. However, the areas to be treated must be washed thoroughly before the medicine is applied.

During treatment with this medicine, *avoid exposing the treated areas to too much sunlight or to a sunlamp* since exposure may increase the possibility of skin tumors and make the skin more prone to sunburn.

If exposure to too much sunlight cannot be avoided while you are using this medicine, sunscreen preparations may be applied or protective clothing worn over the treated areas.

Some people who use this medicine may become more sensitive to wind and cold temperatures than they are normally. *When you first begin using this medicine, use protection against wind or cold until you see how you react.* If you notice severe skin irritation, check with your doctor.

Side Effects of This Medicine

Along with its needed effects, a medicine may cause some unwanted effects. Although not all of these side effects appear very often, when they do occur they may require medical attention. Check with your doctor if any of the following side effects occur:

> Blistering, crusting, severe burning or redness, or swelling of skin
> Darkening or lightening of the treated skin

After you apply this medicine, a feeling of warmth, mild stinging, or redness may be expected.

After you use this medicine for a few days, some peeling of the skin may be expected.

Other side effects not listed above may also occur in some patients. If you notice any other effects, check with your doctor.

TRIAMTERENE (Systemic)
A commonly used brand name is Dyrenium.

Triamterene (trye-AM-ter-een) is a diuretic. It is commonly used to help reduce the amount of water in the body by increasing the flow of urine. This medicine is available only with your doctor's prescription.

Before Using This Medicine

In order to decide on the best treatment for your medical problem, your doctor should be told:

—if you have ever had any unusual reaction to triamterene in the past. This medicine should not be taken if you are allergic to it.

—if you are pregnant, if you intend to become pregnant, or if you are breast-feeding an infant. Although triamterene has not been shown to cause problems, the chance always exists.

—if you have any of the following medical problems:

Diabetes	Kidney disease
Gout	Liver disease
Heart disease	Pancreas disease

—if you are now taking any of the following medicines or types of medicine:

Diabetes medicine	Other diuretics
Gout medicine	(water pills) or
Laxatives	antihypertensives
Lithium	(high blood
	pressure
	medicine)
	Potassium sup-
	plements

Proper Use of This Medicine

Triamterene may cause you to have an unusual feeling of tiredness when you begin to take it. You may also notice an increase in the amount of urine or in your frequency of urination. After you have taken triamterene for a while, these effects should lessen. In general, in order to keep the increase in urine from affecting your sleep:

• If you are to take a single dose a day, take it in the morning after breakfast.

• If you are to take more than one dose a day, take the last dose no later than 6 p.m., unless otherwise directed by your doctor.

• However, it is best to plan your dose or doses according to a schedule that will least affect your personal activities and sleep. Ask your doctor, nurse, or pharmacist to help you plan the best time to take this medicine.

In order to help remember to take your medicine, try to get into the habit of taking it at the same time each day.

If triamterene upsets your stomach, it may be taken with meals or milk. If stomach upset (nausea, vomiting, stomach pain or cramps) continues, check with your doctor.

If you miss a dose of this medicine, take it as soon as possible. If it is almost time for your next dose, do not take the missed dose at all and do not double the next one. Instead, go back to your regular dosing schedule. If you have any questions about this, check with your doctor.

For patients taking triamterene for high blood pressure:

• Importance of Diet—When prescribing medicine for your condition, your doctor may also prescribe a personal diet for you. Such a diet may be low in sodium (salt). Medicine is usually more effective when this diet is properly followed.

Also, it may be very important for you to go on a reducing diet. However, check with your doctor before going on any diet.

• Many patients who have high blood pressure will not notice any signs of the problem. In fact, many may feel normal. It is very important that you take your medicine exactly as directed and that you keep your doctor's appointments even if you feel well.

• Remember that triamterene will not cure your high blood pressure but it does control it. Therefore, you must continue to take it as directed if you expect to keep your blood pressure down. *You may have to take medicine for the rest of your life.* If high blood pressure is not treated, it can cause serious problems such as heart failure, blood vessel disease, stroke, or kidney disease.

Precautions While Using This Medicine

It is important that your doctor check your progress at regular visits.

Triamterene does not cause a loss of potassium from your body as other diuretics (water pills) do. Therefore, it is not necessary for you to get extra potassium in your diet and too much potassium could even be harmful. Since salt substitutes and low-salt milk may contain potassium, do not use them unless told to do so by your doctor.

Check with your doctor if you become sick and have severe or continuing vomiting or diarrhea. These problems may cause you to lose additional water, which could be harmful, or to lose potassium, which could lessen the medicine's helpful effects.

Caution: Diabetics—This medicine may raise blood sugar levels. While you are using triamterene, be especially careful in testing for sugar in your urine. If you have any questions about this, check with your doctor.

A few people who take this medicine may become more sensitive to sunlight than they are normally. When you begin to take triamterene, avoid too much sun or use of a sunlamp until you see how you react, especially if you tend to burn easily. If you have a severe reaction, check with your doctor.

For patients taking this medicine for high blood pressure:

• *Do not take other medicines unless they have been discussed with your doctor.* This especially includes over-the-counter (nonprescription) medicines for appetite control, asthma, colds, cough, hay fever, or sinus, since they may tend to increase your blood pressure.

Side Effects of This Medicine

Along with its needed effects, a medicine may cause some unwanted effects. Although not all of these side effects appear very often, when they do occur they may require medical attention. *Check with your doctor if any of the following side effects occur, especially since some of them may mean that your body has too much potassium:*

Signs of too much potassium

Irregular heartbeat	Unexplained anxiety
Mental confusion	Unusual tiredness or
Numbness or tin-	weakness
gling in hands,	Weakness or
feet, or lips	heaviness
Shortness of breath	of legs
or difficult	
breathing	

Rare

Bright red tongue	Skin rash or itching
Burning, inflamed	Unexplained sore
feeling in tongue	throat and fever
Cracked corners of	Unusual bleeding or
mouth	bruising
	Weakness

Other side effects may occur which usually do not require medical attention. These side effects may go away during treatment as your body adjusts to the medicine. However, *check with your doctor if any of the following side effects continue or are bothersome, especially since some of them may mean that your body has too little sodium:*

Signs of too little sodium

Drowsiness	Increased thirst
Dryness of mouth	Lack of energy

Less common

Diarrhea
Dizziness

Rare

Headache   Increased sensitivity
                            of skin to sun-
                            light

Triamterene may cause your urine to turn slightly
blue in color. This is not harmful and is to be
expected.

Other side effects not listed above may also occur
in some patients. If you notice any other effects, check with your doctor.

TRIAMTERENE AND HYDROCHLOROTHIAZIDE
(Systemic)

A commonly used brand name is Dyazide.

Triamterene   (trye-AM-ter-een)   and
hydrochlorothiazide (hye-droe-klor-oh-THYE-a-
zide) is a combination of two diuretics. It is commonly used to treat high blood pressure. It is used
also to help reduce the amount of water in the
body by increasing the flow of urine. This
medicine is available only with your doctor's
prescription.

Before Using This Medicine

In order to decide on the best treatment for your
medical problem, your doctor should be told:

—if you are allergic to sulfonamides (sulfa
drugs), thiazide diuretics (water pills), or
triamterene.

—if you are pregnant or if you intend to
become pregnant while using this medicine.
When this medicine is used during pregnancy,
it may cause side effects in the newborn infant.
In addition, although this medicine has not
been shown to cause birth defects, the chance
always exists.

—if you are breast-feeding an infant. Although
triamterene and hydrochlorothiazide have not
been shown to cause problems, the chance
always exists.

—if you have any of the following medical
problems:

Diabetes   Kidney disease
Gout   Liver disease
Heart disease   Pancreas disease
History of lupus
 erythematosus

—if you are now taking any of the following
medicines or types of medicine:

Colestipol   Methenamine
Corticosteroids   Oral anticoagulants
 (cortisone-like   (blood thinners
 medicines)   you take by
Corticotropin   mouth)
 (ACTH)   Other diuretics
Diabetes medicine   (water pills) or
Digitalis glycosides   antihypertensives
 (heart medicine)   (high blood
Gout medicine   pressure
Laxatives   medicine)
Lithium   Potassium sup-
                        plements

Proper Use of This Medicine

This medicine may cause you to have an unusual
feeling of tiredness when you begin to take it.
You may also notice an increase in the amount
of urine or in your frequency of urination.
After you have taken the medicine for a while,
these effects should lessen. In general, in order
to keep the increase in urine from affecting
your sleep:

• If you are to take a single dose a day, take it
in the morning after breakfast.

• If you are to take more than one dose a day,
take the last dose no later than 6 p.m., unless
otherwise directed by your doctor.

• However, it is best to plan your dose or doses
according to a schedule that will least affect
your personal activities and sleep. Ask your
doctor, nurse, or pharmacist to help you plan
the best time to take this medicine.

In order to help remember to take your medicine,
try to get into the habit of taking it at the same
time each day.

If this medicine upsets your stomach, it may be
taken with meals or milk. If stomach upset
(nausea, vomiting, stomach pain or cramps)
continues, check with your doctor.

If you miss a dose of this medicine, take it as soon
as possible. If it is almost time for your next
dose, do not take the missed dose at all and do
not double the next one. Instead, go back to
your regular dosing schedule. If you have any
questions about this, check with your doctor.

For patients taking this medicine for high blood
pressure:

• Importance of Diet—When prescribing
medicine for your condition, your doctor may
also prescribe a personal diet for you. Such a
diet may be low in sodium (salt). Medicine is
usually more effective when a schedule of diet
and exercise is properly followed.

Also, it may be very important for you to go on a reducing diet. However, check with your doctor before going on any diet.

• Many patients who have high blood pressure will not notice any signs of the problem. In fact, many may feel normal. It is very important that you take your medicine exactly as directed and that you keep your doctor's appointments even if you feel well.

• Remember that this medicine will not cure your high blood pressure but it does control it. Therefore, you must continue to take it as directed if you expect to keep your blood pressure down. *You may have to take medicine for the rest of your life.* If high blood pressure is not treated, it can cause serious problems such as heart failure, blood vessel disease, stroke, or kidney disease.

Precautions While Using This Medicine

It is important that your doctor check your progress at regular visits.

This medicine may cause a loss or increase of potassium in your body. Your doctor may have special instructions about eating or drinking foods or beverages that have a high potassium content (for example, orange or other citrus fruit juices), taking a potassium supplement, or using salt substitutes. It is important not to change your diet on your own. Tell your doctor if you are already on a special diet (as for diabetes), or if you are taking a potassium supplement or using salt substitutes. Check with your doctor, nurse, or pharmacist if you need a list of foods which are high in potassium or if you have any questions.

Check with your doctor if you become sick and have severe or continuing vomiting or diarrhea. These problems may cause you to lose additional water and potassium.

Caution: Diabetics—This medicine may raise blood sugar levels. While you are using this medicine, be especially careful in testing for sugar in your urine. If you have any questions about this, check with your doctor.

A few people who take this medicine may become more sensitive to sunlight than they are normally. When you begin to take this medicine, avoid too much sun or use of a sunlamp until you see how you react, especially if you tend to burn easily. If you have a severe reaction, check with your doctor.

Before having any kind of surgery (including dental surgery) or emergency treatment, tell the doctor or dentist in charge that you are taking this medicine.

For patients taking this medicine for high blood pressure:

• *Do not take other medicines unless they have been discussed with your doctor.* This especially includes over-the-counter (nonprescription) medicines for appetite control, asthma, colds, cough, hay fever, or sinus.

Side Effects of This Medicine

Along with its needed effects, a medicine may cause some unwanted effects. Although not all of these side effects appear very often, when they do occur they may require medical attention. *Check with your doctor if any of the following side effects occur, especially since some of them may mean that your body has too much or is losing too much potassium:*

Signs of changes in potassium

Dryness of mouth	Numbness or tin-
Increased thirst	gling in hands,
Irregular heartbeats	feet, or lips
Mood or mental	Unusual tiredness or
changes	weakness
Muscle cramps or	Weak pulse
pain	
Nausea or vomiting	

Rare

Bright red tongue,	Skin rash or hives
burning, inflamed	Unexplained sore
feeling in tongue,	throat and fever
cracked corners	Unusual bleeding or
of mouth	bruising
Severe stomach pain	Weakness
with nausea and	Yellowing of eyes or
vomiting	skin

Other side effects may occur which usually do not require medical attention. These side effects may go away during treatment as your body adjusts to the medicine. However, check with your doctor if any of the following side effects continue or are bothersome:

Less common

Constipation	Increased sensitivity
Diarrhea	of skin to sun-
Dizziness or	light
lightheadedness	Loss of appetite
when getting up	Upset stomach
from a lying or	
sitting position	

This medicine may cause your urine to turn slightly blue in color. This is not harmful and is to be expected.

Other side effects not listed above may also occur in some patients. If you notice any other effects, check with your doctor.

TRICYCLIC ANTIDEPRESSANTS (Systemic)
This information applies to the following medicines:

Amitriptyline (a-mee-TRIP-ti-leen)
Desipramine (dess-IP-ra-meen)
Doxepin (DOX-e-pin)
Imipramine (im-IP-ra-meen)
Nortriptyline (nor-TRIP-ti-leen)
Protriptyline (proe-TRIP-ti-leen)
Trimipramine (trye-MI-pra-meen)

Some commonly used brand names are:	Generic names:
Amitid Amitil Elavil Endep	Amitriptyline
Norpramin Pertofrane	Desipramine
Adapin Sinequan	Doxepin
Imavate Janimine SK-Pramine Tofranil	Imipramine
Aventyl Pamelor	Nortriptyline
Vivactil	Protriptyline
Surmontil	Trimipramine

This medicine belongs to the group of medicines known as tricyclic antidepressants or "mood elevators." It is used to relieve mental depression and depression that sometimes occurs with anxiety. One form of this medicine (imipramine) may be used to treat enuresis (bedwetting). Tricyclic antidepressants are available only with your doctor's prescription.

Before Using This Medicine

In order to decide on the best treatment for your medical problem, your doctor should be told:

—if you have ever had an unusual reaction to any of the tricyclic antidepressants in the past. This medicine should not be taken if you are allergic to it.

—if you are pregnant, if you intend to become pregnant, or if you are breast-feeding an infant. Although tricyclic antidepressants have not been shown to cause problems, the chance always exists.

—if you have any of the following medical problems:

Alcoholism	High blood pressure
Asthma (history of)	Liver disease
Difficult urination	Manic depression
Enlarged prostate	Overactive thyroid
Epilepsy	Schizophrenia
Glaucoma	Stomach or intes-
Heart disease	tinal problems

—if you are now taking *any* other medicines, including over-the-counter (OTC) or nonprescription medicine, especially the following:

Allergy medicine	Other medicine for
Antihistamines	depression
Barbiturates	Pain medicine
Blood pressure medicine	Sedatives
Cold remedies	Seizure medicine
Hay fever medicine	Sleeping medicine
Narcotics	Thyroid medicine
Oral contraceptives	Tranquilizers

—if you are now taking or have taken within the past 2 weeks monoamine oxidase (MAO) inhibitors such as:

Isocarboxazid	Phenelzine
Pargyline	Tranylcypromine

Proper Use of This Medicine

Take this medicine only as directed by your doctor, to benefit your condition as much as possible.

To lessen stomach upset, take this medicine with food, even for a daily bedtime dose, unless your doctor has told you to take it on an empty stomach.

Sometimes this medicine must be taken for several weeks before you begin to feel better.

Keep this medicine out of the reach of children since overdose is especially dangerous in young children.

If you miss a dose of this medicine, take it as soon as possible and then go back to your regular dosing schedule. However, if a once-a-day bedtime dose is missed, do not take that dose in the morning since it may cause disturbing side effects during waking hours. Instead, check with your doctor.

For patients taking the oral liquid form of this medicine:

• This medicine is to be taken by mouth even though it may come in a dropper bottle. The amount you should take is to be measured with the specially marked dropper, and diluted just before you take each dose. Dilute it with about 1/2 glass (4 ounces) of water, milk, citrus fruit juice, or prune juice. Do not mix this medicine with grape juice or carbonated beverages since these may decrease the medicine's activity.

• If your prescription is a liquid form but not in a dropper bottle and the directions on the bottle say to take by teaspoonful, it is not necessary to dilute it before using.

Precautions While Using This Medicine

It is very important that your doctor check your progress at regular visits, in order to allow dosage adjustments and help reduce side effects.

Do not stop taking this medicine without first checking with your doctor. Your doctor may want you to reduce gradually the amount you are using before stopping completely, in order to prevent a possible relapse of your condition, and to reduce the possibility of withdrawal symptoms such as headache, nausea, and/or an overall feeling of uneasy discomfort.

Before having any kind of surgery (including dental surgery) or emergency treatment, tell the doctor or dentist in charge that you are using this medicine.

This medicine will add to the effects of alcohol and other medicines (CNS depressants) that slow down the nervous system. Some examples of CNS depressants are antihistamines or medicine for hay fever, other allergies, or colds; sedatives, tranquilizers, or sleeping medicine; prescription pain medicine or narcotics; barbiturates; medicine for seizures; tricyclic antidepressants (medicine for depression); or anesthetics, including some dental anesthetics. In addition, stomach problems may be more likely to occur if you drink alcoholic beverages while being treated with this medicine. *Check with your doctor before taking any of the above while you are taking this medicine.*

This medicine may cause some people to become drowsy or less alert than they are normally. *Make sure you know how you react to this medicine before you drive, use machines, or do other jobs that require you to be alert.*

Dizziness, lightheadedness, or fainting may occur, especially when you get up from a lying or sitting position. Getting up slowly may help. If this problem continues or gets worse, check with your doctor.

Side Effects of This Medicine

For patients taking this medicine for enuresis (bedwetting):

• Side effects in children taking this medicine for bedwetting usually disappear upon continued drug use. The most common of these are nervousness, sleeping problems, tiredness, and mild upset of the stomach. However, if these side effects continue or are bothersome, check with your doctor.

Along with its needed effects, a medicine may cause some unwanted effects. Although not all of these side effects appear very often, when they do occur they may require medical attention. Check with your doctor if any of the following side effects occur:

Less common

Blurred vision	Irregular heartbeat
Eye pain	(pounding, rac-
Fainting	ing, skipping)
Hallucinations (see-	Problems in
ing, hearing, or	urinating
feeling things that	Shakiness
are not there)	Unusually slow
	pulse

Rare

Seizures	Unexplained sore
Skin rash and	throat and fever
itching	Yellowing of eyes
	and skin

Other side effects may occur which usually do not require medical attention. These side effects may go away during treatment as your body adjusts to the medicine. However, check with your doctor if any of the following side effects continue or are bothersome:

More common

Constipation (if	Nausea
severe check with	Tiredness or
doctor)	weakness (less
Dizziness	common with
Drowsiness (rare	protriptyline)
with protriptyline)	Unpleasant taste
Dry mouth	Unusually fast
Headache	heartbeat
Increased appetite	Weight gain
for sweets	

Less common

Diarrhea	Sleeping difficulty
Excessive sweating	(more common
Heartburn	with protriptyline
Increased sensitivity	especially when
to sunlight	taken late in the
	day)
	Vomiting

Other side effects not listed above may also occur in some patients. If you notice any other effects, check with your doctor.

The effects of this medicine may last for 3 to 7 days after you have stopped taking it. Therefore, stated precautions must be observed during this time.

TRIFLURIDINE (Ophthalmic)
A commonly used brand name is Viroptic.

Trifluridine (trye-FLURE-i-deen) belongs to the general family of medicines called antivirals. Trifluridine ophthalmic preparations are used to help the body overcome virus infections of the eye. They are available only with your doctor's prescription.

Before Using This Medicine

In order to decide on the best treatment for your medical problem, your doctor should be told:

—if you have ever had any unusual reaction to trifluridine. This medicine should not be used if you are allergic to it.

—if you are pregnant, if you intend to become pregnant, or if you are breast-feeding an infant, although trifluridine has not been shown to cause problems.

Proper Use of This Medicine

Bottle is not full; this is to provide proper drop control.

To prevent contamination of the eye drops, do not touch the applicator tip to any surface (including the eye), and keep the container tightly closed.

How to apply this medicine: First, wash hands. Then tilt head back and pull lower eyelid away from eye to form a pouch. Drop medicine into the pouch and gently close eyes. Do not blink.

Keep eyes closed for 1 or 2 minutes to allow medicine to come into contact with the infection.

If you think you did not get the drop of medicine into your eye properly, use another drop.

Do not use this medicine more often or for a longer time than your doctor ordered. To do so may cause problems in the eyes. If you have any questions about this, check with your doctor.

To help clear up your infection completely, *keep using this medicine for the full time of treatment,* even though your symptoms may have disappeared; *do not miss any doses.*

If you do miss a dose of this medicine, apply it as soon as possible. However, if it is almost time for your next application, skip the missed dose and go back to your regular dosing schedule.

Precautions While Using This Medicine

After application of this medicine to the eye, occasional stinging or burning may be expected.

It is very important that you keep your appointment with your doctor. If your symptoms become worse, check with your doctor sooner.

Side Effects of This Medicine

Along with its needed effects, a medicine may cause some unwanted effects. Although not all of these side effects appear very often, when they do occur they may require medical attention. Check with your doctor if any of the following side effects occur:

Rare

Itching, redness, swelling, or other sign of irritation not present before you started using this medicine

Other side effects may occur which usually do not require medical attention. These side effects may go away during treatment as your body adjusts to the medicine. However, check with your doctor if either of the following side effects continues or is bothersome:

More common

Burning or stinging

Other side effects not listed above may also occur in some patients. If you notice any other effects, check with your doctor.

TRIMETHOBENZAMIDE (Systemic)
A commonly used brand name is Tigan.

Trimethobenzamide (trye-meth-oh-BEN-za-mide) is a medicine used to treat nausea and vomiting. It is available only with your doctor's prescription.

Before Using This Medicine
In order to decide on the best treatment for your medical problem, your doctor should be told:

—if you have ever had any unusual reaction to trimethobenzamide in the past. This medicine should not be taken if you are allergic to it.

—if you are allergic or sensitive to benzocaine or other local anesthetics (the suppository form of this medicine contains benzocaine).

—if you are pregnant, if you intend to become pregnant, or if you are breast-feeding an infant. Although trimethobenzamide has not been shown to cause problems in humans, the chance always exists.

—if you have either of the following medical problems:

High fever
Intestinal infection

—if you are now taking any central nervous system (CNS) depressants such as:

Antihistamines or medicine for hay fever, other allergies, or colds	Prescription pain medicine
	Sedatives, tranquilizers,
Barbiturates	or sleeping
Narcotics	medicine
Phenothiazines	Seizure medicine

Proper Use of This Medicine
Trimethobenzamide is used only to relieve or prevent nausea and vomiting. Take it only as directed. Do not take more of it and do not take it more often than your doctor ordered.

Do not use this medicine to treat nausea and vomiting in children unless otherwise directed by your doctor. If you are giving this medicine to a child, be especially careful not to give more than is prescribed since side effects may be more serious in children.

If you are using the rectal suppository dosage form of this medicine:

• How to insert suppository: First remove foil wrapper and moisten the suppository with water. Lie down on side and push the suppository well up into the rectum with finger. If the suppository is too soft to insert because of storage in a warm place, before removing the foil wrapper chill the suppository in the refrigerator for 30 minutes or run cold water over it.

If you must take this medicine regularly and you miss a dose, take the missed dose as soon as possible. However, if it is almost time for your next dose, do not take the missed dose at all and do not double the next one. Instead, go back to your regular dosing schedule. If you have any questions about this, check with your doctor or pharmacist.

Precautions While Using This Medicine
Trimethobenzamide will add to the effects of alcohol and other medicines (CNS depressants) that slow down the nervous system. Some examples of CNS depressants are antihistamines or medicine for hay fever, other allergies, or colds; sedatives, tranquilizers, or sleeping medicine; prescription pain medicine or narcotics; barbiturates; medicine for seizures; tricyclic antidepressants (medicine for depression); or anesthetics, including some dental anesthetics. *Check with your doctor before taking any of the above while you are using this medicine.*

This medicine may cause some people to become dizzy, lightheaded, drowsy, or less alert than they are normally. *Make sure you know how you react to this medicine before you drive, use machines, or do other jobs that require you to be alert.*

When taking trimethobenzamide on a regular basis, make sure your doctor knows if you are taking large amounts of aspirin at the same time (as in arthritis). Effects of too much aspirin, such as ringing in the ears, may be covered by this medicine.

Side Effects of This Medicine
Along with its needed effects, a medicine may cause some unwanted effects. Although not all of these side effects appear very often, when they do occur they may require medical attention. Check with your doctor if any of the following side effects occur:

Back pain	Unexplained sore
Mental depression	throat and fever
Seizures	Unusual feeling of
Severe or continuing vomiting	tiredness
	Yellowing of eyes
Shakiness or tremors	and skin

Other side effects may occur which usually do not require medical attention. These side effects may go away during treatment as your body adjusts to the medicine. However, check with your doctor if any of the following side effects continue or are bothersome:

Blurred vision	Drowsiness
Diarrhea	Headache
Dizziness	Muscle cramps

Other side effects not listed above may also occur in some patients. If you notice any other effects, check with your doctor.

TRIPROLIDINE and PSEUDOEPHEDRINE
(Systemic)

Some commonly used brand names are Actifed, Allerphed, and Tagafed.

Triprolidine (trye-PROE-li-deen) and pseudoephedrine (soo-doe-e-FED-rin) is a combination antihistamine and decongestant. It is used to treat nasal congestion (stuffy nose) and other symptoms of hay fever and other types of allergy. This medicine is available only with your doctor's prescription.

Before Using This Medicine

In order to decide on the best treatment for your medical problem, your doctor should be told:

—if you have ever had any unusual reaction to triprolidine, pseudoephedrine, or similar medicines in the past. This medicine should not be taken if you are allergic to it.

—if you are pregnant or if you intend to become pregnant while using this medicine. Although this medicine has not been shown to cause birth defects or other problems, the chance always exists.

—if you are breast-feeding an infant. Both triprolidine and pseudoephedrine pass into the breast milk and may cause unwanted effects in the infant.

—if you have any of the following medical problems:

Diabetes	High blood pressure
Enlarged prostate	Intestinal blockage
Glaucoma	Overactive thyroid
Heart or blood	Stomach ulcer
vessel disease	Urinary tract
	blockage

—if you are now taking any central nervous system (CNS) depressants such as:

Antihistamines or medicine for hay fever, other allergies, or colds	Narcotics Prescription pain medicine
Barbiturates Medicine for seizures	Sedatives, tranquilizers, or sleeping medicine

—if you are now taking any of the following medicines or types of medicine:

Alkavervir	Nadolol
Amphetamines	Propranolol
Digitalis glycosides (heart medicine)	Protoveratrine A
Guanethidine	Reserpine
Mecamylamine	Tricyclic antidepressants
Medicine for asthma or breathing problems	(medicine for depression)
Methyldopa	Veratrum viride alkaloids
Metoprolol	

—if you are now taking or have taken within the past 2 weeks monoamine oxidase (MAO) inhibitors such as:

Isocarboxazid	Phenelzine
Pargyline	Tranylcypromine

Proper Use of This Medicine

Take triprolidine and pseudoephedrine combination only as directed. Do not take more of it or take it more often than your doctor ordered. To do so may increase the chance of side effects.

Take this medicine with food or a glass of water or milk to lessen stomach irritation, if necessary.

Do not give this medicine to premature or newborn infants, unless otherwise directed by your doctor.

If you must take this medicine regularly and you miss a dose, take the missed dose as soon as possible. However, if it is almost time for your next dose, do not take the missed dose at all and do not double the next one. Instead, go back to your regular dosing schedule. If you have any questions about this, check with your doctor or pharmacist.

Precautions While Using This Medicine

Triprolidine and pseudoephedrine will add to the effects of alcohol and other medicines (CNS depressants) that slow down the nervous system. Some examples of CNS depressants are antihistamines or medicine for hay fever, other allergies, or colds; sedatives, tranquilizers, or sleeping medicine; prescription pain medicine or narcotics; barbiturates; medicine for seizures; tricyclic antidepressants (medicine for depression); or anesthetics, including some dental anesthetics. *Check with your doctor before taking any of the above while you are using this medicine.*

Triprolidine may cause some people to become drowsy, dizzy, or less alert than they are normally. *Make sure you know how you react to this medicine before you drive, use machines, or do other jobs that require you to be alert.*

Other people may become nervous or restless or may have trouble in sleeping due to the pseudoephedrine in this medicine. This may be more likely to occur in children. If you do have trouble in sleeping, take the last dose of this medicine for each day a few hours before bedtime. If you have any questions about this, check with your doctor.

Side Effects of This Medicine

Along with its needed effects, a medicine may cause some unwanted effects. Although not all of these side effects appear very often, when they do occur they may require medical attention. Check with your doctor if any of the following side effects occur:

Rare

Unexplained sore throat and fever	Unusual bleeding or bruising
	Unusual weakness

With high doses

Hallucinations (seeing, hearing, or feeling things that are not there)	Unusually slow heartbeat, shortness of breath, or troubled breathing
Irregular heartbeat	

Other side effects may occur which usually do not require medical attention. These side effects may go away during treatment as your body adjusts to the medicine. However, check with your doctor if any of the following side effects continue or are bothersome:

More common

Drowsiness	Thickening of the bronchial secretions

Less common

Difficult or painful urination	Nervousness, restlessness, or trouble in sleeping (especially in children)
Dizziness	
Dryness of mouth, nose, and throat	
Headache	Skin rash
Loss of appetite	Unusual increase in sweating
Nausea or vomiting	Unusual paleness
	Unusually fast or pounding heartbeat
	Upset stomach or stomach pain

Other side effects not listed above may also occur in some patients. If you notice any other effects, check with your doctor.

TROPICAMIDE (Ophthalmic)
A commonly used brand name is Mydriacyl.

Tropicamide (troe-PIK-a-mide) is used in the eye to dilate (enlarge) the pupil. It is used before eye examinations. This medicine is available only with your doctor's prescription.

Before Using This Medicine

In order to decide on the best treatment for your medical problem, your doctor should be told:

—if you have ever had any unusual reaction to tropicamide in the past. This medicine should not be used if you are allergic to it.

—if you are pregnant, if you intend to become pregnant, or if you are breast-feeding an infant, although tropicamide has not been shown to cause problems.

—if you have any of the following medical problems:

Brain damage (in children)	Spastic paralysis (in children)
Down's syndrome (mongolism)	

Side Effects of This Medicine

When this medicine is applied, some stinging of the eye may be expected.

After this medicine is applied to your eyes, your pupils will become unusually large. This will cause blurring of vision. It will also cause your eyes to become more sensitive to light than they are normally. Wearing sunglasses may help relieve the discomfort from bright light. If these effects continue for longer than 24 hours after the medicine is used, check with your doctor.

Other side effects not listed above may also occur in some patients. If you notice any other effects, check with your doctor.

UNDECYLENIC ACID, COMPOUND
(Topical)
Some commonly used brand names are:

Decylenes	Medaped
Desenex	Quinsana Plus

Compound undecylenic acid (un-de-sill-ENN-ik AS-id) belongs to the group of medicines called antifungals. It is applied to the skin to treat some types of fungal infections. This medicine is available without a prescription; however, your doctor may have special instructions on the proper use of this medicine for your medical condition.

Before Using This Medicine

In order to decide on the best treatment for your medical problem, your doctor should be told:

—if you have ever had any unusual reaction to compound undecylenic acid in the past. This medicine should not be used if you are allergic to it.

—if you are pregnant, if you intend to become pregnant, or if you are breast-feeding an infant, although compound undecylenic acid has not been shown to cause problems.

Proper Use of This Medicine

To help clear up your infection completely, *keep using this medicine for 2 weeks after burning, itching, or other symptoms have disappeared,* unless otherwise directed by your doctor.

Keep this medicine away from the eyes.

If you miss a dose of this medicine, apply it as soon as possible. Then go back to your regular dosing schedule. If you have any questions about this, check with your doctor or pharmacist.

Before applying compound undecylenic acid, wash the area to be treated and surrounding areas,

and dry thoroughly. Then apply enough medicine to cover the affected area.

If you are using the powder form of this medicine:

• If the powder is used on the feet, sprinkle it between toes, on feet, and in socks and shoes.

If you are using the aerosol powder form of this medicine:

• Shake well before using.

• From a distance of 4 to 6 inches, spray the powder on the affected areas. If it is used on the feet, spray it between toes, on feet, and in socks and shoes.

• Do not use this medicine around the eyes, nose, or mouth.

• Do not inhale the powder.

• Do not use near heat, near open flame, or while smoking.

• Store away from heat and direct sunlight. Do not puncture, break, or burn container.

Precautions While Using This Medicine

If your skin problem has not improved after using this medicine for 4 weeks, check with your doctor.

To help cure the infection and to help prevent reinfection, good health habits are required. These include the following:

• Wash all towels and bedding after each use.

• Use only freshly laundered clothes each time clothing is changed.

If you have any questions about this, check with your doctor, nurse, or pharmacist.

Also, to help prevent reinfection after the period of treatment with this medicine, the powder or spray powder form of this medicine may be used each day after bathing and careful drying.

Side Effects of This Medicine

Along with its needed effects, a medicine may cause some unwanted effects. Although not all of these side effects appear very often, when they do occur they may require medical attention. Check with your doctor or pharmacist if the following side effect occurs:

Irritation of skin not present before using this medicine

Other side effects not listed above may also occur in some patients. If you notice any other effects, check with your doctor or pharmacist.

URACIL MUSTARD (Systemic)

Uracil mustard (YOOR-a-sill) belongs to the group of medicines known as alkylating agents. It is used to treat some kinds of cancer as well as some noncancerous conditions. Uracil mustard is available only with your doctor's prescription.

ore Using This Medicine

il mustard is a very strong medicine. In addi-
on to its helpful effects in treating your
medical problem, it has side effects that could
be very serious. Before you take this medicine,
be sure that you have discussed the use of it
with your doctor.

In order to decide on the best treatment for your medical problem, your doctor should be told:

—if you have ever had any unusual reaction to uracil mustard in the past.

—if you are pregnant or if you intend to have children. This medicine may cause birth defects if either the male or female is taking it at the time of conception or if it is taken during pregnancy. It may also cause permanent sterility after it has been taken for a while. Be sure that you have discussed this with your doctor before taking this medicine.

—if you are breast-feeding an infant. Although uracil mustard has not been shown to cause problems, the chance always exists.

—if you have any of the following medical problems:

Blood disease	Kidney disease
Gout	Kidney stones
Infection	Liver disease

—if you are taking gout medicine.

—if you have been treated with x-rays or cancer drugs by another doctor.

Proper Use of This Medicine

Use this medicine only as directed by your doctor. Do not use more or less of it, and do not use it more often than your doctor ordered.

This medicine often causes nausea and vomiting. Even if you begin to feel ill, *do not stop using this medicine without first checking with your doctor.*

If you miss a dose of this medicine, do not take the missed dose at all and do not double the next one. Instead, go back to your regular dosing schedule. If you have any questions about this, check with your doctor.

Precautions While Using This Medicine

It is very important that your doctor check your progress at regular visits.

While you are using this medicine, your doctor may want you to drink plenty of fluids and urinate often. This will help prevent kidney problems and keep your kidneys working well. If you have any questions about this, check with your doctor.

Side Effects of This Medicine

Along with its needed effects, a medicine may cause some unwanted effects. Although not all of these side effects appear very often, when they do occur they may require medical attention. Check with your doctor if any of the following side effects occur:

More common

Unexplained fever, chills, or sore throat	Unusual bleeding or bruising

Less common

Flank and stomach pain	Swelling of feet or lower legs
Joint pain	

Rare

Sores in the mouth and on the lips	Yellowing of eyes and skin

Other side effects may occur which usually do not require medical attention. These side effects may go away during treatment as your body adjusts to the medicine. However, check with your doctor if any of the following side effects continue or are bothersome:

More common

Diarrhea
Nausea and
  vomiting

Less common

Darkening of the skin	Mental depression
	Nervousness
Irritability	Skin rash and
Loss of hair	itching

Rare

Missing menstrual
  periods

This medicine may cause a temporary loss of hair in some people. After treatment with uracil mustard has ended, normal hair growth should return.

After you stop using this medicine, it may still produce some side effects that need attention. During this period of time check with your doctor if you notice any of the following:

| Unexplained fever, chills, or sore throat | Unusual bleeding or bruising |

Other side effects not listed above may also occur in some patients. If you notice any other effects, check with your doctor.

Other side effects may occur which usually do not require medical attention. However, check with your doctor if any of the following side effects continue or are bothersome:

Less common or rare

Headache
Nausea or vomiting

Other side effects not listed above may also occur in some patients. If you notice any other effects, check with your doctor.

UREA (Intra-amniotic)

Intra-amniotic urea (yoor-EE-a) is given by injection to cause abortion. It is available only with your doctor's prescription and is to be administered only by or under the immediate care of your doctor.

Before Using This Medicine

In order to decide on the best treatment for your medical problem, your doctor should be told:

—if you have ever had any unusual reaction to urea in the past. This medicine should not be used if you are allergic to it.

—if you have any of the following medical problems:

| Diabetes | Liver disease |
| Kidney disease | Uterus surgery (history of) |

Proper Use of This Medicine

During the abortion procedure, you should drink fluids to help prevent your body from losing too much water and becoming dehydrated.

Side Effects of This Medicine

Along with its needed effects, a medicine may cause some unwanted effects. Although not all of these side effects appear very often, when they do occur they may require medical attention. Check with your doctor if any of the following side effects occur:

Rare

Irregular heartbeat	Unusual tiredness or
Mental confusion	weakness
Muscle cramps or pain	Weakness and heaviness
Numbness, tingling, pain, or weakness in hands or feet	of legs

UREA (Systemic)

A commonly used brand name is Ureaphil.

Urea (yoor-EE-a) is given by injection, and sometimes by mouth, to treat certain conditions in which there is an increased pressure in the eye, such as glaucoma, or increased pressure on the brain. It may be used before eye surgery to reduce pressure in the eye. It may also be used to help reduce the amount of water in the body by increasing the flow of urine. This medicine is available only with your doctor's prescription.

Before Using This Medicine

In order to decide on the best treatment for your medical problem, your doctor should be told:

—if you have ever had any unusual reaction to urea in the past. This medicine should not be taken if you are allergic to it.

—if you are pregnant, if you intend to become pregnant, or if you are breast-feeding an infant. Although urea has not been shown to cause birth defects or other problems, the chance always exists.

—if you have either of the following medical problems:

| Kidney disease | Liver disease |

Proper Use of This Medicine

For patients taking this medicine by mouth:

• *It is very important that you take this medicine only as directed.* Do not take more of it and do not take it more often than your doctor ordered. To do so may increase the chance of side effects.

• To improve the taste of this medicine, mix with unsweetened grapefruit juice or lemon, lime, or orange juice, pour over cracked ice, and sip through a straw.

• If you miss a dose of this medicine, take it as soon as possible. Then go back to your regular dosing schedule. But if it is almost time for your next dose, do not take the missed dose at all. Instead, take your next dose at the regularly scheduled time. Then continue with your regular dosing schedule. If you have any questions about this, check with your doctor.

Precautions While Using This Medicine

For patients taking this medicine by mouth:

• In some patients, headaches may occur while this medicine is being used. To help prevent or relieve the headache, lie down for about 60 minutes after taking this medicine. If headaches become severe or continue, check with your doctor.

Side Effects of This Medicine

Along with its needed effects, a medicine may cause some unwanted effects. Although not all of these side effects appear very often, when they do occur they may require medical attention. Check with your doctor if any of the following side effects occur:

For patients taking this medicine by injection:
Less common or rare

Fever	Unusual ner-
Redness, swelling,	vousness
or pain at the	Unusually fast
place of injection	heartbeat

For patients taking this medicine by injection or by mouth:
Less common or rare

Irregular heartbeat	Seizures
Mental confusion	Trembling
Muscle cramps or	Unusual tiredness
pain	or weakness
Numbness, tingling,	Weakness and
pain, or weakness	heaviness of legs
in hands or feet	

Other side effects may occur which usually do not require medical attention. These side effects may go away during treatment as your body adjusts to the medicine. However, check with your doctor if any of the following side effects continue or are bothersome:

For patients taking this medicine by injection or by mouth:
More common

Headache	Unusual dryness of
Nausea or vomiting	mouth or in-
	creased thirst

Other side effects not listed above may also occur in some patients. If you notice any other effects, check with your doctor.

VALPROIC ACID (Systemic)
A commonly used brand name is Depakene.

Valproic (val-PROE-ik) acid belongs to the group of medicines called anticonvulsants. It is used to control certain seizures in the treatment of epilepsy. This medicine is available only with your doctor's prescription.

Before Using This Medicine

In order to decide on the best treatment for your medical problem, your doctor should be told:

—if you have ever had any unusual reaction to valproic acid in the past. This medicine should not be taken if you are allergic to it.

—if you are pregnant or if you intend to become pregnant while using this medicine. While valproic acid has not been shown to cause birth defects or other problems in humans, the chance always exists.

—if you are breast-feeding an infant. Although valproic acid has not been shown to cause problems, the chance always exists, since it passes into the breast milk.

—if you have any of the following medical problems:

Blood disease	Liver disease
Kidney disease	

—if you are now taking any of the following medicines or types of medicine:

Anticoagulants	Other anticon-
(blood thinners)	vulsants (sei-
Aspirin	zure medicine,
Dipyridamole	especially
	clonazepam,
	phenobarbital,
	phenytoin, or
	primidone)
	Sulfinpyrazone

—if you are now taking central nervous system (CNS) depressants such as:

Antihistamines or	Prescription pain
medicine for hay	medicine
fever, other aller-	Sedatives, tran-
gies, or colds	quilizers,
Barbiturates	or sleeping
Narcotics	medicine
	Tricyclic antidepres-
	sants (medicine
	for depression)

—if you are now taking or have taken within the past 2 weeks monoamine oxidase (MAO) inhibitors such as:

Isocarboxazid   Phenelzine
Pargyline   Tranylcypromine

Proper Use of This Medicine

This medicine must be taken exactly as directed by your doctor in order to prevent seizures and reduce the possibility of side effects.

To lessen stomach upset take this medicine immediately after meals or with food.

If you are taking the capsule form of valproic acid, it should be swallowed whole without chewing or breaking to prevent irritation of the mouth and throat.

If you miss a dose of this medicine and remember within 6 hours, take it as soon as possible. Then go back to your regular dosing schedule. Do not double doses. If you have any questions about this, check with your doctor.

Precautions While Using This Medicine

Your doctor should check your progress at regular visits, especially for the first few months you take this medicine.

Do not stop taking this medicine without first checking with your doctor. Your doctor may want you to gradually reduce the amount you are taking before stopping completely. Stopping the medicine suddenly may result in seizures.

Before having any kind of surgery (including dental surgery) or emergency treatment, tell the doctor or dentist in charge that you are taking this medicine.

This medicine will add to the effects of alcohol and other medicines (CNS depressants) that slow down the nervous system. Some examples of CNS depressants are antihistamines or medicine for hay fever, other allergies, or colds; sedatives, tranquilizers, or sleeping medicine; prescription pain medicine or narcotics; barbiturates; medicine for seizures; tricyclic antidepressants (medicine for depression); or anesthetics, including some dental anesthetics. *Check with your doctor before taking any of the above while you are using this medicine.*

This medicine may cause some people to become drowsy or less alert than they are normally. *Make sure you know how you react to this medicine before you drive, use machines, or do other jobs that require you to be alert.*

Your doctor may want you to carry a medical identification card or bracelet stating that you are taking this medicine.

Side Effects of This Medicine

Along with its needed effects, a medicine may cause some unwanted effects. Although not all of these side effects appear very often, when they do occur they may require medical attention. Check with your doctor if any of the following side effects occur:

Rare

Skin rash   Yellowing of eyes
Unusual bleeding or   and skin
  bruising

Other side effects may occur which usually do not require medical attention. These side effects may go away during treatment as your body adjusts to the medicine. However, check with your doctor if any of the following side effects continue or are bothersome:

More common

Diarrhea   Stomach or in-
Indigestion   testinal cramps
Nausea or vomiting

Less common

Constipation   Hair loss (slight
Drowsiness   and temporary)

Rare

Dizziness   Headache
Fatigue   Lack of coordina-
                         tion

Other side effects not listed above may also occur in some patients. If you notice any other effects, check with your doctor.

VIDARABINE (Ophthalmic)
A commonly used brand name is Vira-A.

Vidarabine (vye-DARE-a-been) belongs to the general family of medicines called antivirals. Vidarabine ophthalmic preparations are used to help the body overcome virus infections of the eye. They are available only with your doctor's prescription.

Before Using This Medicine

In order to decide on the best treatment for your medical problem, your doctor should be told:

—if you have ever had any unusual reaction to vidarabine. This medicine should not be used if you are allergic to it.

—if you are pregnant, if you intend to become pregnant, or if you are breast-feeding an infant, although vidarabine has not been shown to cause problems in humans.

Proper Use of This Medicine

To prevent contamination of the eye ointment, do not touch the applicator tip to any surface (including the eye). After using, wipe the tip of the ointment tube with a clean tissue and keep the tube tightly closed.

How to apply this medicine: First, wash hands. Then pull the lower eyelid away from eye to form a pouch. Squeeze a thin strip of ointment into the pouch. A 1.25-cm (approximately 1/2-inch) strip of ointment is usually enough unless otherwise directed by your doctor. Gently close eyes and keep them closed for 1 or 2 minutes to allow medicine to come into contact with the infection.

Do not use this medicine more often or for a longer time than your doctor ordered. To do so may cause problems in the eyes. If you have any questions about this, check with your doctor.

To help clear up your infection completely, *keep using this medicine for the full time of treatment,* even though your symptoms may have disappeared; *do not miss any doses.*

If you do miss a dose of this medicine, apply it as soon as possible. However, if it is almost time for your next application, skip the missed dose and go back to your regular dosing schedule.

Precautions While Using This Medicine

After application, eye ointments usually cause your vision to blur for a few minutes.

It is very important that you keep your appointment with your doctor. If your symptoms become worse, check with your doctor sooner.

Side Effects of This Medicine

Along with its needed effects, a medicine may cause some unwanted effects. Although not all of these side effects appear very often, when they do occur they may require medical attention. Check with your doctor if any of the following side effects occur:

Increased sensitivity of eyes to light
Itching, redness, swelling, pain, burning, or other sign of irritation not present before you started using this medicine

Other side effects may occur which usually do not require medical attention. These side effects may go away during treatment as your body adjusts to the medicine. However, check with your doctor if any of the following side effects continue or are bothersome:

Excess flow of tears
Feeling of something in the eye

Other side effects not listed above may also occur in some patients. If you notice any other effects, check with your doctor.

VINBLASTINE (Systemic)
Some commonly used brand names are Velban and Velbe*.

---

*Not available in the United States.

Vinblastine (vin-BLAS-teen) belongs to the group of medicines known as antineoplastic agents. It is used by injection to treat some kinds of cancer as well as some noncancerous conditions. Vinblastine is available only on prescription and is to be administered only by or under the immediate supervision of your doctor.

Before Using This Medicine

Vinblastine is a very strong medicine. In addition to its helpful effects in treating your medical problem, it has side effects that could be very serious. Before you receive this medicine, be sure that you have discussed the use of it with your doctor.

In order to decide on the best treatment for your medical problem, your doctor should be told:

—if you have ever had any unusual reaction to vinblastine in the past.

—if you are pregnant or if you intend to have children. This medicine may cause birth defects if either the male or female is taking it at the time of conception or if it is taken during pregnancy. It may also cause permanent sterility after it has been taken for a while. Be sure that you have discussed this with your doctor before taking this medicine.

—if you are breast-feeding an infant. Although vinblastine has not been shown to cause problems, the chance always exists.

—if you have any of the following medical problems:

Blood disease   Kidney stones
Gout   Liver disease
Infection

—if you are taking gout medicine.

—if you have been treated with x-rays or cancer drugs by another doctor.

Proper Use of This Medicine

This medicine is sometimes given together with certain other medicines. If you are using a combination of drugs, it is important that you receive each medicine at the proper time. If you are taking some of these medicines by mouth, ask your doctor, nurse, or pharmacist to help you plan a way to take them at the right time.

This medicine often causes nausea and vomiting. However, it is very important that you continue to receive the medicine, even if you begin to feel ill. Your doctor may prescribe another medicine to help relieve stomach upset. If you have any questions about this, check with your doctor.

Precautions While Using This Medicine

It is very important that your doctor check your progress at regular visits.

While you are using this medicine, your doctor may want you to drink plenty of fluids and urinate often. This will help prevent kidney problems and keep your kidneys working well. If you have any questions about this, check with your doctor.

Side Effects of This Medicine

Along with its needed effects, a medicine may cause some unwanted effects. Although not all of these side effects appear very often, when they do occur they may require medical attention. Check with your doctor if any of the following side effects occur:

More common

Unexplained fever, chills, or sore throat

Less common

Flank or stomach pain	Swelling of feet and lower legs
Joint pain	Unusual bleeding or bruising

Rare

Black tarry stools	Numbness or tingling in fingers and toes
Difficulty in walking	
Dizziness	
Double vision	Pain in fingers and toes
Drooping eyelids	
Headache	Pain in testicles
Jaw pain	Sores in the mouth and on the lips
Mental depression	
	Weakness

Other side effects may occur which usually do not require medical attention. These side effects may go away during treatment as your body adjusts to the medicine. However, check with your doctor if any of the following side effects continue or are bothersome:

More common

Loss of hair
Nausea and vomiting

Less common

Muscle pain

Rare

Blisters on the skin	Loss of appetite
Constipation	Skin rash and itching
Diarrhea	
Increased sensitivity of skin to sunlight	Stomach pain
	Swollen, sore tongue

This medicine often causes a temporary loss of hair. After treatment with vinblastine has ended, normal hair growth should return.

If vinblastine accidentally seeps out of the vein into which it is injected, it may damage the skin and cause some scarring. Tell the doctor right away if you notice redness, pain, or swelling at the place of injection.

Other side effects not listed above may also occur in some patients. If you notice any other effects, check with your doctor.

VINCRISTINE (Systemic)
A commonly used brand name is Oncovin.

Vincristine (vin-KRIS-teen) belongs to the group of medicines known as antineoplastic agents. It is used by injection to treat some kinds of cancer as well as some noncancerous conditions. Vincristine is available only on prescription and is to be administered only by or under the immediate supervision of your doctor.

Before Using This Medicine

Vincristine is a very strong medicine. In addition to its helpful effects in treating your medical problem, it has side effects that could be very serious. Before you receive this medicine, be sure that you have discussed the use of it with your doctor.

In order to decide on the best treatment for your medical problem, your doctor should be told:

—if you have ever had any unusual reaction to vincristine in the past.

—if you are pregnant or if you intend to have children. This medicine may cause birth defects if either the male or female is taking it at the time of conception or if it is taken during pregnancy. It may also cause permanent sterility after it has been taken for a while. Be sure that you have discussed this with your doctor before taking this medicine.

—if you are breast-feeding an infant. Although vincristine has not been shown to cause problems, the chance always exists.

—if you have any of the following medical problems:

Blood disease	Kidney stones
Gout	Liver disease
Infection	Nerve or muscle disease

—if you are now taking isoniazid or gout medicine.

—if you have been treated with x-rays or cancer drugs by another doctor.

Proper Use of This Medicine

This medicine is often given together with certain other medicines. If you are using a combination of drugs, it is important that you receive each medicine at the proper time. If you are taking some of these medicines by mouth, ask your doctor, nurse, or pharmacist to help you plan a way to take them at the right time.

This medicine sometimes causes nausea and vomiting. However, it is very important that you continue to receive the medicine, even if you begin to feel ill. If you have any questions about this, check with your doctor.

This medicine frequently causes constipation and stomach cramps. Your doctor may want you to take a laxative or stool softener; however, do not decide to take these medicines on your own without first checking with your doctor.

Precautions While Using This Medicine

It is very important that your doctor check your progress at regular visits.

While you are using this medicine, it may be necessary to drink plenty of fluids and urinate often to help prevent kidney problems and keep your kidneys working well. Ask your doctor if this is necessary for you.

Side Effects of This Medicine

Along with its needed effects, a medicine may cause some unwanted effects. Although not all of these side effects appear very often, when they do occur they may require medical attention. Check with your doctor if any of the following side effects occur:

More common

Constipation	Numbness or tingling in fingers and toes
Difficulty in walking	
Double vision	Pain in fingers and toes
Drooping eyelids	
Flank or stomach pain	Pain in testicles
	Stomach cramps
Headache	Swelling of feet or lower legs
Jaw pain	
Joint pain	Weakness

Less common

Agitation	Inability to sleep
Bed-wetting	Lack of sweating
Confusion	Loss of appetite
Dizziness or lightheadedness when getting up from a lying or sitting position	Mental depression
	Painful or difficult urination
	Seizures
Hallucinations (seeing, hearing, or feeling things that are not there)	Unusual decrease or increase in urination

Rare

Cough	Unexplained fever, chills, or sore throat
Shortness of breath	
Sores in the mouth and on the lips	Unusual bleeding or bruising

Other side effects may occur which usually do not require medical attention. These side effects may go away during treatment as your body adjusts to the medicine. However, check with your doctor if any of the following side effects continue or are bothersome:

More common

Loss of hair

Less common

Bloating	Nausea and
Diarrhea	vomiting
Loss of weight	Skin rash

This medicine often causes a temporary loss of hair. After treatment with vincristine has ended, normal hair growth should return.

If vincristine accidentally seeps out of the vein into which it is injected, it may damage some tissues and cause scarring. Tell the doctor right away if you notice redness, pain, or swelling at the place of injection.

After you stop using this medicine, it may still produce some side effects that need attention. During this period of time check with your doctor if you notice any of the following:

Blurred or double vision	Hearing problems
	Mental problems
Difficulty in walking	Squinting of eyes
	Tiredness
Extreme thirst and increase in urination	Vomiting
Headache	

Other side effects not listed above may also occur in some patients. If you notice any other effects, check with your doctor.

VITAMINS AND FLUORIDE (Systemic)

This information applies to the following medicines:

Multiple Vitamins and Fluoride
Vitamins A, D, and C, and Fluoride

Some commonly used brand names are*:	Generic name:
Vita-Flor	
Adeflor	
Mulvidren-F	
Novacebrin with Fluoride	Multiple Vitamins
Vi-Penta F	and Fluoride
Poly-Vi-Flor	
V-Daylin with Fluoride	

Cari-Tab	Vitamins A, D, and
Tri-Vi-Flor	C, and Fluoride

---

*Specific vitamin content varies among products.

This medicine is a combination of vitamins and fluoride. Vitamins are used when the daily diet does not include enough of the vitamins needed for good health.

Fluoride has found to be helpful in reducing the number of cavities in the teeth. It is usually present naturally in drinking water. However, some areas of the country do not have a high enough level of fluoride in the water. To make up for this, extra fluorides may be added to the diet. Some children may require both dietary fluorides and fluoride treatments by the dentist. Use of a fluoride toothpaste or rinse may be helpful, as well.

Taking fluorides does not replace good dental habits. These include eating a good diet, brushing teeth frequently, and having regular dental checkups.

This medicine is available only with your physician's or dentist's prescription.

Before Using This Medicine

In order to decide on the best treatment for your medical problem, your physician or dentist should be told:

—if you have ever had any unusual reaction to medicines containing fluorides.

—if you have any of the following medical problems:

Heart disease	Osteosclerosis (bone
Kidney disease	disease)
	Underactive thyroid
	gland

Proper Use of This Medicine

Take this medicine only as directed by your physician or dentist. Do not take more of it and do not take it more often than ordered. Taking even slightly too much fluoride over a period of time may cause unwanted effects.

If you miss a dose of this medicine, take it as soon as you remember. However, if it is almost time for the next dose, do not take the missed dose at all and do not double the next one. Instead, go back to your regular dosing schedule. If you have any questions about this, check with your physician or dentist.

For patients taking the chewable tablet form of this medicine:

• Tablets should be chewed or crushed before they are swallowed.

• This medicine works best if it is taken at bedtime, after the teeth have been thoroughly brushed.

For patients taking the oral liquid form of this medicine:

• This medicine is to be taken by mouth even though it comes in a dropper bottle. The amount to be taken is to be measured with the specially marked dropper.

• *Always store this medicine in the original plastic container.* It has been designed to give you the correct dose. Also, fluoride will interact with glass and should not be stored in glass containers.

• This medicine may be dropped directly into the mouth or mixed with cereal, fruit juice, or other food.

Precautions While Using This Medicine

The level of fluoride present in the water is different in different parts of the country. If you move to another area, check with a physician or dentist in the new area as soon as possible to see if this medicine is still needed or if the dose needs to be changed.

Inform your physician or dentist as soon as possible if you notice white, brown, or black spots on the teeth. These are signs of too much fluoride.

Keep this medicine out of reach of children, since overdose is especially dangerous in children.

Side Effects of This Medicine

Along with its needed effects, a medicine may cause some unwanted effects. Although not all of these side effects appear very often, when they do occur they may require medical attention. When the correct amount of this medicine is used, side effects usually are rare. However, *stop taking this medicine and check with your physician immediately* if any of the following side effects occur as they may be symptoms of overdose:

Black tarry stools	Stomach cramps or
Bloody vomit	pain
Diarrhea	Tremors
Drowsiness	Unusual excitement
Faintness	Unusual increase in
Nausea and	saliva
vomiting	Watery eyes
Shallow breathing	Weakness

Check with your physician or dentist also if the following side effects occur:

Constipation	Sores in the mouth
Loss of appetite	and on the lips
Pain and aching of	Stiffness
bones	Weight loss
Skin rash	White, brown, or
	black discoloration of teeth

Other side effects not listed above may also occur in some patients. If you notice any other effects, check with your physician or dentist.

XANTHINES (Systemic)

This information applies to the following medicines:

Aminophylline (am-in-OFF-i-lin)
Dyphylline (DYE-fi-lin)
Oxtriphylline (ox-TRYE-fi-lin)
Theophylline (the-OFF-i-lin)

Some commonly used brand names are:	Generic names:
Aminodur	
Aminophyl*	
Amphylline*	
Corophyllin*	Aminophylline
Lixaminol	
Mini-Lix	
Somophyllin	
Aerophylline*	
Airet	
Dilin	
Dilor	Dyphylline
Lufyllin	
Neothylline	
Protophylline*	
Choledyl	Oxtriphylline
Accurbron	
Aerolate	
Asthmophylline*	
Bronkodyl	
Elixicon	
Elixophyllin	
Physpan	
Slophyllin	Theophylline
Somophyllin-T	
Theobid	
Theoclear	
Theodur	
Theolair	
Theolixir	
Theophyl	
Theospan	

* Not available in the United States.

Xanthines belong to the group of medicines called bronchodilators. They are given by mouth, by injection, or rectally to treat bronchial asthma, chronic bronchitis, emphysema, and other lung diseases. They relieve wheezing, shortness of breath, and troubled breathing. Also, aminophylline may be given by injection to stimulate the heart in certain conditions and to relieve pain in certain gallbladder conditions. These medicines are available only with your doctor's prescription.

Before Using This Medicine

In order to decide on the best treatment for your medical problem, your doctor should be told:

—if you have ever had any unusual reaction to aminophylline, caffeine, dyphylline, oxtriphylline, theobromine, or theophylline.

—if you are pregnant or if you intend to become pregnant while using this medicine. Use of aminophylline, oxtriphylline, or theophylline during pregnancy may cause unwanted effects in the newborn infant. In addition, although the xanthines have not been shown to cause birth defects or other problems, the chance always exists.

—if you are breast-feeding an infant. Theophylline passes into the breast milk and may cause irritability or other side effects in infants of mothers taking either aminophylline, oxtriphylline, or theophylline. This does not apply to dyphylline.

—if you have any of the following medical problems:

Heart disease	Overactive thyroid
High blood pressure	Stomach ulcer (or
Kidney disease	history of)
Liver disease	

—if you are now taking any of the xanthines and are also taking any of the following medicines or types of medicine:

Lithium	Propranolol
Other medicine for	
asthma or	
breathing	
problems	

—if you are now taking aminophylline, oxtriphylline, or theophylline and are also taking any of the following medicines:

Clindamycin	Lincomycin
Erythromycin	Troleandomycin

Proper Use of This Medicine

Use this medicine only as directed by your doctor. Do not use more of it, do not use it more often, and do not use it for a longer period of time than your doctor ordered. To do so may increase the possibility of side effects.

If you miss a dose of this medicine and remember within an hour or so of the missed dose, take it right away. Then go back to your regular dosing schedule. But if you do not remember until later, do not take the missed dose at all and do not double the next one. Instead, go back to your regular dosing schedule. If you have any questions about this, check with your doctor.

If you are taking this medicine by mouth:

• *This medicine works best when taken with a glass of water on an empty stomach* (either 30 minutes to 1 hour before meals or 2 hours after meals) since that way it will get into the blood sooner. However, in some cases your doctor may want you to take this medicine with meals or right after meals to lessen stomach upset. If you have any questions about how you should be taking this medicine, check with your doctor.

• There are several different forms of xanthines capsules and tablets. If you are taking:

—chewable tablets, chew the tablets before swallowing.

—enteric-coated tablets, swallow the tablets whole.

—extended-release capsules, swallow the capsule whole. Do not crush, break, or chew before swallowing. If the capsule is too large to swallow, you may mix the contents of the capsule with jam, jelly, or applesauce and swallow without chewing.

—extended-release tablets, swallow the tablets whole. Do not break, crush, or chew before swallowing.

If you are using aminophylline enema or theophylline enema:

• This medicine usually comes with patient directions. Read them carefully before using this medicine.

• If crystals form in the solution (for aminophylline enema only), dissolve them by placing the closed container of solution in warm water.

• If burning or other irritation of the rectal area occurs after you use this medicine and it continues or becomes worse, check with your doctor.

If you are using aminophylline suppositories or theophylline suppositories:

• Some suppositories must be kept in the refrigerator, while others do not. If the suppositories ordered by your doctor must be refrigerated, let them warm at room temperature for a few minutes before using. If the suppositories do not have to be refrigerated and are kept in an unusually warm place, chill them in the refrigerator for about 30 minutes before using; or place them in cold water in their foil wrapping for a few minutes just before using.

• How to insert suppository: First remove the foil wrapper and moisten the suppository with water. Lie down on side and push the suppository well up into rectum with finger.

• If burning or other irritation of the rectal area occurs after you use this medicine and it continues or becomes worse, check with your doctor.

Precautions While Using This Medicine

Your doctor should check your progress at regular visits, especially for the first few weeks after you begin using this medicine.

This medicine may add to the central nervous system stimulant effects of caffeine-containing beverages such as tea, coffee, cocoa, and cola drinks. *Avoid drinking large amounts of these beverages while using this medicine.* If you have any questions about this, check with your doctor.

Side Effects of This Medicine

Along with its needed effects, a medicine may cause some unwanted effects. Although not all of these side effects appear very often, when they do occur they may require medical attention. Check with your doctor if any of the following side effects occur:

Less common or rare
   Skin rash or hives

Possible signs of overdose

Bloody or black	Unusually fast,
tarry stools	pounding, or ir-
Cloudy urine	regular heartbeat
Increased urination	Vomiting up blood
Mental confusion	or material that
Muscle twitching	looks like coffee
Unusual thirst	grounds
Unusual tiredness or	
weakness	

Other side effects may occur which usually do not require medical attention. These side effects may go away during treatment as your body adjusts to the medicine. However, check with your doctor if any of the following side effects continue or are bothersome:

More common (less common with dyphylline)

Headache	Stomach pain
Irritability	Trouble in sleeping
Nausea	Vomiting
Nervousness or rest-	
lessness	

Less common

Diarrhea	Loss of appetite
Dizziness or light-	Unusually fast
headedness	breathing
Flushing or redness	
of face	

Other side effects not listed above may also occur in some patients. If you notice any other effects, check with your doctor.

XYLOMETAZOLINE (Nasal)

Some commonly used brand names are:

4-Way Long Acting	Sine-Off Once-A-
Neo-Synephrine II	Day
Otrivin	Sinex Long-Acting
Rhinall Long Acting	Sinutab Long Act-
	ing Sinus Spray

Xylometazoline (zye-loe-met-AZ-oh-leen) is used for the temporary relief of congestion or stuffiness in the nose caused by hay fever or other allergies, colds, or sinus trouble. This medicine is available without a prescription; however, your doctor may have special instructions on the proper use or dose for your medical condition.

Before Using This Medicine

In order to decide on the best treatment for your medical problem, your doctor should be told:

—if you have ever had any unusual reaction to xylometazoline or to other nasal decongestants in the past. This medicine should not be used if you are allergic to it.

—if you are pregnant, if you intend to become pregnant while using this medicine, or if you are breast-feeding an infant. Although xylometazoline has not been shown to cause problems, the chance always exists.

—if you have any of the following medical problems:

Blood vessel disease	Heart disease
Diabetes	High blood pressure
Glaucoma	Overactive thyroid

—if you are now taking tricyclic antidepressants (medicine for depression).

—if you are now taking or have taken within the past 2 weeks monoamine oxidase (MAO) inhibitors such as:

Isocarboxazid	Phenelzine
Pargyline	Tranylcypromine

Proper Use of This Medicine

Use this medicine only as directed. Do not use more of it, do not use it more often, and do not use it for longer than 3 days, unless otherwise directed by your doctor. To do so may make your runny or stuffy nose worse and may also increase the chance of side effects.

For patients using the nose drops:

• How to use the nose drops: Blow nose gently. Tilt head back while standing or sitting up, or lie down on a bed and hang head over the side. Place the drops into each nostril and keep head tilted back for a few minutes to allow medicine to spread throughout the nose.

Rinse the dropper with hot water and dry with a clean tissue. Replace the cap right after use.

For patients using the nose spray:

• How to use the nose spray: Blow nose gently. With head upright, spray the medication into each nostril. Sniff briskly while squeezing bottle quickly and firmly. For best results, spray once into each nostril, wait 3 to 5 minutes to allow medicine to work, then blow nose gently and thoroughly. Repeat until complete dose is used.

Rinse the tip of the spray bottle with hot water taking care not to suck water into the bottle, and dry with a clean tissue. Replace the cap right after use.

To avoid the spread of infection, do not use the container for more than one person.

If you miss a dose of this medicine and you remember within an hour or so of the missed dose, use it right away. Then go back to your regular dosing schedule. But if you do not remember until later, do not use the missed dose at all and do not double the next one. Instead, go back to your regular dosing schedule. If you have any questions about this, check with your doctor or pharmacist.

Side Effects of This Medicine

Along with its needed effects, a medicine may cause some unwanted effects. Although not all of these side effects appear very often, when they do occur they may require medical attention. When this medicine is used for short periods of time at low doses, side effects usually are rare. However, check with your doctor or pharmacist if any of the following occur:

Increase in runny or
 stuffy nose

Possible signs of too much medicine being absorbed into the body

Blurred vision	Pounding or
Headache or light-	unusually fast
headedness	heartbeat
Irregular heartbeat	Trouble in sleeping
	Unusual nervousness

Other side effects may occur which usually do not require medical attention. These side effects may go away during treatment as your body adjusts to the medicine. However, check with your doctor or pharmacist if any of the following side effects continue or are bothersome:

Burning, dryness, or stinging of inside of nose	Sneezing

Other side effects not listed above may also occur in some patients. If you notice any other effects, check with your doctor or pharmacist.

Index

Brand names are in *italics*. There are many brands and different manufacturers of drugs on the market. The listing of selected United States and Canadian brand names is intended only for ease of reference. There are additional brand names that have not been included. The inclusion of a brand name does not mean the USPC has any particular knowledge that the brand listed has properties different from other brands of the same drug, nor should it be interpreted as an endorsement by the USPC. Similarly, the fact that a particular brand has not been included does not indicate that the product has been judged to be unsatisfactory or unacceptable.

E

M

Q

R

T

Y

Z

KEEPING CURRENT

You can stay informed about the medicines described in this book and the drug-use issues in the news through a subscription to the ABOUT YOUR MEDICINES NEWSLETTER.

Published every other month, each issue will bring you timely articles and updated drug information from the same experts who produced this book and the authoritative United States Pharmacopeia (USP)—National Formulary (NF) and the USP Dispensing Information used by physicians, dentists, pharmacists, and nurses in their professional work.

Even if you only take an occasional aspirin or vitamin, you owe it to yourself to know more about these and all the medicines available to you over-the-counter or on prescription by staying informed ABOUT YOUR MEDICINES.

About Your Medicines Newsletter:
$3.00/yr* (6 issues).

Subscription orders must be prepaid and should be sent to:

USP DI, Publications Department
12601 Twinbrook Parkway
Rockville, MD 20852
(301)881-0666

*Maryland residents add 5% sales tax.

Clip and return to: USP DI, Publications Dept., 12601 Twinbrook Pkwy., Rockville, MD 20852

Enclosed is my check or money order for $3.00* made payable to USPC. Please enter my subscription to the ABOUT YOUR MEDICINES NEWSLETTER for one year.

NAME_____

ADDRESS_____

CITY_____

STATE_____ ZIP CODE_____

*Maryland residents add 5% sales tax.

Please check the appropriate boxes below. Then tell us what kind of information you would like to see included in the ABOUT YOUR MEDICINES NEWSLETTER.

AGE: ☐ Under 35 ☐ 35 to 54 ☐ 55 or over
I have special training in the health-care area. ☐ Yes ☐ No
If yes, please indicate area_____

I would like to see the following kind of information in your newsletter:

Your comments regarding the information in this book—*The Physicians' and Pharmacists' Guide to Your Medicines*—are welcome.